Histopathology Specimens

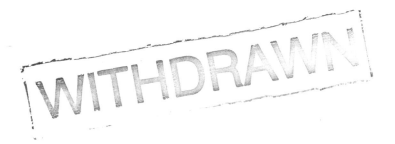

Derek C. Allen and R. Iain Cameron (Eds)

Histopathology Specimens

Clinical, Pathological and Laboratory Aspects

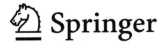 Springer

Derek C. Allen, MD, FRCPath
Consultant Pathologist, Histopathology Laboratory,
Belfast City Hospital Trust, Belfast UK

R. Iain Cameron, MB, BCh FRCS
Specialist Registrar in Histopathology, Histopathology Laboratory,
Belfast City Hospital Trust, Belfast UK

British Library Cataloguing in Publication Data
Histopathology specimens : clinical, pathological and laboratory aspects
   1. Histology, Pathological – laboratory manuals
   I. Allen, Derek C. (Derek Creswell) II. Cameron, R. Iain
   616'. 07583
ISBN 1852335971

Library of Congress Cataloging-in-Publication Data
A catalog record for this book is available from the Library of Congress

ISBN 978-1-85233-597-7 Springer-Verlag London Berlin Heidelberg
a member of BertelsmannSpringer Science+Business Media GmbH

Typeset by Florence Production Ltd., Stoodleigh, Devon
Printed and bound in the United States of America
28/3830–543210 Printed on acid-free paper

In memory of Dr Heather Elliott

Preface

The reorganisation of cancer services has emphasised the importance of histopathology specimens in patient management and highlighted the pivotal role the histopathologist has as part of the multidisciplinarian team. The specimens require careful, detailed and consistent handling to ascertain multiple prognostic factors relevant to appropriate management of individual patients. This must stem from a background knowledge of the relevant anatomy, clinical presentation and investigation of disease, the common pathological processes and how they affect both tissues and patient outlook. Specimen handling ought to reflect investigative techniques, e.g., CT/MRI scanning and the operative surgical procedures used. Histopathology reports must be prompt and accurate using classifications and documenting locoregional spread that match therapeutic options and prognostic groups.

The multidisciplinarian team extends to the histopathology laboratory to include medical pathologists, biomedical scientists and secretarial staff. The purpose of this book is to educate and better equip all those involved in the histopathology specimen process for their task. An emphasis is placed on a standardised approach to specimen handling and reporting to achieve consistently high quality. Practical outworking of this process involves informed clinicopathological correlation, active communication, supervision and feedback within and between the clinical and laboratory teams.

Hopefully the reader will find the content pragmatic and practicable representing our current practice. No one method is exclusively right – other options exist and are of equal merit given due care and consistency. What is certain is that techniques will inevitably change in the light of new developments and will be incorporated into the histopathology specimen process.

The authors gratefully acknowledge the use of illustrations from P. Hermanek, R.V.P. Hutter, L.H. Sobin, G. Wagner, Ch. Wittenkind (eds). TNM Atlas: Illustrated Guide to the TNM/pTNM Classification of Malignant Tumours. 4th edn. Berlin Heidelberg New York. Springer 1997, and, Allen D C. Histopathology Reporting – Guidelines for Surgical Cancer. London. Springer 2000.

Grateful appreciation is expressed to Melissa Morton (medical editor), Eva Senior and the staff at Springer, and all our colleagues in the Belfast City Hospital and Royal Victoria Hospital Histopathology Laboratories. Mrs Debbie Greene provided particular secretarial expertise.

Acknowledgement is made of Mr Brian Duggan (urological specialist registrar) for his clinical comments on the urology specimens section.

Derek Allen, Iain Cameron
Belfast

Contents

Gastrointestinal Specimens

Derek C Allen, R Iain Cameron

Breast Specimens

TF Lioe

Head and Neck Specimens

Séamus S Napier with clinical comments by David S Brooker, Derek J Gordon, Richard W Kendrick, William J Primrose and Colin FJ Russell

Eye, Muscle and Nerve Specimens
Roy W Lyness

Gynaecological Specimens
W Glenn McCluggage

Urological Specimens
Declan M O'Rourke, Maurice B Loughrey

Pelvic and Retroperitoneal Specimens
Maurice B Loughrey, Damian T McManus

Skin Specimens
Maureen Y Walsh

Cardiothoracic Specimens and Vessels
Kathleen M Mulholland

Osteoarticular and Soft Tissue Specimens

Richard I Davis

Haemopoietic Specimens

Lakshmi Venkatraman, W Glenn McCluggage, Peter A Hall

Miscellaneous Specimens

Damian T McManus

Contributors

Dr Derek C Allen
Consultant Pathologist
Histopathology Laboratory
Belfast City Hospital Trust
Belfast
UK

Mr David S Brooker
Consultant ENT Surgeon
Royal Victoria Hospital
Belfast
UK

Dr R Iain Cameron
Specialist Registrar in Histopathology
Histopathology Laboratory
Belfast City Hospital Trust
Belfast
UK

Dr Richard I Davis
Consultant Pathologist
Institute of Pathology
Royal Victoria Hospital
Belfast
UK

Mr Derek J Gordon
Consultant Plastic Surgeon
Ulster Hospital
Belfast
UK

Prof. Peter A Hall
Consultant Pathologist
Department of Pathology
Royal Victoria Hospital
Belfast
UK

Mr Richard W Kendrick
Consultant Oral and Maxillofacial Surgeon
Ulster Hospital
Belfast
UK

Dr T F Lioe
Consultant Histo/cytopathologist
Belfast City Hospital Trust
Belfast
UK

Dr Maurice B Loughrey
Specialist Registrar in Pathology
Belfast City Hospital
Belfast
UK

Dr Roy W Lyness
Consultant Pathologist
Histopathology Laboratory
Belfast City Hospital Trust
Belfast
UK

Dr W Glenn McCluggage
Consultant Pathologist
Department of Pathology
Royal Group of Hospitals Trust
Belfast
UK

Dr Damian T McManus
Consultant Pathologist
Histopathology Laboratory
Belfast City Hospital Trust
Belfast
UK

Dr Kathleen M Mulholland
Specialist Registrar in Histopathology
Histopathology Laboratory
Belfast City Hospital Trust
Belfast
UK

Dr Séamus S Napier
Consultant in Oral Histopathology
Royal Group of Hospitals Trust
Belfast
UK

Dr Declan M O'Rourke
Consultant Pathologist
Histopathology Laboratory
Belfast City Hospital Trust
Belfast
UK

Mr William J Primrose
Consultant ENT Surgeon
Royal Victoria Hospital
Belfast
UK

Mr Colin F J Russell
Consultant Surgeon
Royal Victoria Hospital
Belfast
UK

Dr Lakshmi Venkatraman
Specialist Registrar in Histopathology
Department of Histopathology
Institute of Pathology
Royal Victoria Hospital
Belfast
UK

Dr Maureen Y Walsh
Consultant Dermatopathologist
Institute of Pathology
Royal Victoria Hospital
Belfast
UK

Introduction

Derek C Allen, R Iain Cameron

1. The Role of Histopathology Specimens

Histopathology specimens are a vital cornerstone in patient care. They not only establish a tissue diagnosis but are crucial in clinical management decisions and provide important prognostic data. They are nodal events in a patient's illness, shaping the choice of relevant medical and surgical therapies and determining follow-up routines. The data they provide are used to assess the efficiency of current and new treatment regimes and to monitor the impact of population screening programmes. Clinical governance has recognised their key role in auditing not only individual clinicians but the patterns and quality of overall health care provision. Biomedical research with advances in investigations and therapy would flounder without them. They are therefore a precious resource to be handled with great care by sufficient numbers of appropriately trained and experienced personnel. The data generated are of a confidential nature privy to the patient, consultant clinician or general practitioner and the reporting pathologist. This information may be shared as appropriate with other directly involved health care professionals, e.g., in the context of multidisciplinary team meetings, but laboratory practice (e.g., telephoned results, report authorisation) must be geared to protect patient confidentiality at all times. The patient not only has a right to see and have explained the information in his/her specimen but must undergo a process of informed consent prior to the clinical procedure. Thus the nature, purpose, extent and side effects of the procedure are explained in understandable terms. This process extends to the laboratory as contemporary surgical consent forms require to seek from the patient permission for disposal and use of the tissue not only for diagnosis but also educative, audit and research purposes. Additionally, research projects should be verified by an appropriate research ethics committee. Patient denial of any of these uses must then be communicated to the laboratory and incorporated into the handling and disposal procedures. The histopathology specimen report forms a permanent part of the patient's medical record and as such may be used as medico-legal evidence in negligence and compensation cases. These various factors serve to emphasise the importance of the care that should be taken with these specimens by histopathology laboratory personnel.

2. The Handling of Histopathology Specimens

Specimen transportation, accession, dissection, audit and reporting are considered.

Specimen transportation: There must be close liaison between pathology and clinical staff to ensure appropriate transportation of specimens between the operating theatre and the laboratory, e.g., prompt transport of fresh specimens, or the provision of special fixatives. This must be reflected in shared protocols, a user information manual and education of the portering staff.

Specimen accession: Allocation of a unique laboratory number and accurate computer registration of patient details are fundamental to maintenance of a meaningful and practicable histopathology database. This is important not only to individual patient care (e.g., a sequence of biopsies) but also for provision of statistics, e.g., download to cancer registries.

Specimen dissection: Traditionally, the role of medical pathologists in specimen dissection is now also being done by an increasing number of biomedical scientists (BMSs) as has been the situation for several decades in some laboratories in America (Pathologist Assistants) and Northern Ireland. BMSs, trainee and consultant pathologists are all appropriate to the task provided that several principles are adhered to:

● The histopathology specimen and its report remain the overall responsibility of the reporting consultant pathologist.
● There is close proximity and ready availability of active consultant pathologist supervision before, during and after handling of the specimen.
● There is workforce stability and staff are prepared to work together as a team. The working unit comprises a variable combination of two people (junior/senior, medic/BMS) fulfilling the roles of dissector/writer/supervisor with active consultant pathologist supervision.
● Staff recognise that acquisition of dissection skills is an at-the-bench apprenticeship based on sufficient knowledge, time, experience and supervision. This knowledge-base requires insight into normal anatomy, clinical presentation and investigations relevant to request form information, common pathological conditions and their effect on specimens, surgical considerations in production of the specimen, and core report data tailored to patient management and prognostic information. Consequently, the chapters in this book are structured accordingly under these headings. The cut-up supervisor plays a vital role in passing on verbal knowledge but this is supplemented by various means, e.g., publications (in-house protocols, ACP broadsheets, textbooks) or training courses. A structured training programme facilitates learning and progression.

Staff must also be familiar with the laboratory process of checking patient details, specimen labelling and past history (cytology, biopsy, treatment), the importance of specimen opening for adequate fixation, demonstration of resection margins and use of orthodox or digital photography. Knife etiquette and sampling blocks of appropriate thickness and fixation are crucial. The supervising pathologist must provide active feedback as to the significance and adequacy of these blocks. Line diagrams are an invaluable communication tool between dissector and reporters. Specimens not infrequently need to be revisited prior to report authorisation or following new information gained from the multidisciplinary team meeting. Retention of "wet" specimens must be sufficiently long (minimum four weeks) to allow this process to happen.

● Dissectors should only work to their individual level of experience and competence – this is determined by the structured training programme, audit process (see below) and categorisation of specimens according to their complexity.
● Dissectors should actively seek supervisor input if a specimen is usually complex, novel, shows an unusual variation on a usual theme, or if they have any doubt.

Specimen dissection audit: The quality of specimen dissection must be meaningfully monitored and the majority of this is done actively at the laboratory bench by the consultant pathologist/BMS supervisor team as part of the specimen dissection pre-/peri-/post-view and reporting feedback procedures. In addition, this team should carry out formal periodic audit and assessment of dissectors' skills. This combination of approaches forms the basis for an individual dissector's continued practice and progression between specimen categories (see appendix). It also identifies areas of subspecialist expertise or if there is need of further training. It must be recognised that category progression cannot be proscribed by rigid time frames but rather related to the aptitude of the individual dissector and spectrum of workload that is encountered.

Specimen reporting: Histopathology specimen reports remain the responsibility of an appropriately trained and experienced medical pathologist.

Sample protocols for general specimen handling, categorisation and laboratory abbreviations are included in the appendices to this section.

3. The Core Data in Histopathology Specimens

Specimen dissection must be geared to provide information relevant to the clinician who is managing the patient. Reports must be timely, i.e., prompt, but in the context of an adequate period of fixation so that acquisition of accurate data is not compromised. The report content must not only come to an interpretationally accurate diagnosis but also be qualified by assessment of various prognostic indicators. In the field of surgical cancer pathology this is reflected by the trend towards set-format reports or minimum datasets for the common cancers. Thus, the core content should include gross specimen description, tumour histological type and grade, extent of local tumour spread, lymphovascular invasion, lymph node involvement, relationship to primary excision margins and any associated pathology.

Gross description: Clear distinction should be made between biopsy and resection specimens as they are handled differently and represent different nodal points in a patient's illness. This should be reflected in the use of appropriate SNOMED T (topography) and P (procedure) codes – this also facilitates audit of biopsy and resection – proven cancer numbers and correlation with other techniques such as cytology, radiology and serum markers. The site, distribution, size, edge and appearance of a tumour within an organ greatly influences the specimen handling and creation of a diagnostic short list for microscopy. For example, a gastrointestinal malignant lymphoma may be multifocal, pale and fleshy with prominent mesenteric lymphadenopathy whereas a carcinoma is more usually ulcerated and annular, firm and irregular with more localised lymph node disease and vascular involvement.

Histological tumour type: There are marked prognostic and therapeutic differences between the diagnoses of carcinoma, sarcoma, germ cell tumour and malignant lymphoma. This is further highlighted within a given anatomical site, e.g., lung, where a diagnosis of carcinoma can be of various subtypes requiring either primary surgical (squamous cell carcinoma) or chemo-/radio-therapeutic (small cell carcinoma) approaches and with very different biological outcomes.

Histological tumour differentiation or grade: Tumour differentiation or grade reflects the similarity to the ancestral tissue of origin and degree of cellular pleomorphism, mitoses and necrosis. It, too, greatly influences choice of therapy and prognosis, e.g., low-grade versus high-grade gastric lymphoma (antibiotics versus chemotherapy/surgery) or grade I (surgery alone) versus grade III (surgery and chemotherapy) breast cancer.

An accurate histological tumour type and grade cannot be ascertained unless there is appropriate specimen handling with adequate fixation.

Extent of local tumour spread: Prognosis of a given cancer may be influenced by the character of its invasive margin (circumscribed/infiltrative) but is largely determined by its pathological stage, i.e., the depth or extent of spread in the organ and degree of lymph node involvement. This is then updated by other information, e.g., evidence of distant metastases, to formulate a clinical stage upon which management is based. The TNM (Tumour Nodes Metastases) classification is the international gold standard for the assessment of spread of cancer and translates into hard data some of the descriptive language used in histopathology reports, facilitating communication within the multidisciplinary team. The post-surgical histopathological classification is designated pTNM and is based on pre-treatment, surgical and pathological information.

pT: requires resection of the primary tumour or biopsy adequate for evaluation of the highest pT category or extent of local tumour spread. Due to tumour heterogeneity this is contingent upon adequate numbers of well-orientated blocks. Where possible, multiple tumours are individually staged and the highest pT category used for management decisions.

pT0: no histological evidence of primary tumour.

PTis: carcinoma in-situ.

pT1–4: increasing size and/or local extent of the primary tumour histologically.

pN: requires removal of nodes sufficient to evaluate the absence of regional node metastasis and also the highest pN category. Where possible all regional nodes in a resection specimen should be sought and harvested for histology.

pN0: no regional lymph node mestastasis histologically.

pN1–3: increasing involvement of regional lymph nodes histologically.

pM: requires microscopic examination of positive body cavity fluid cytology or distant metastases – the latter may not be available to the pathologist and is therefore designated on clinical or radiological grounds.

Other descriptors include unifocality (pT1a) versus multifocality (pT1b), lymphatic invasion (L), venous invasion (V), classification during or after multimodality therapy (ypT), recurrent tumour (rpT) and multiple primary tumours (pTm). Qualifying tumours in the TNM system are carcinoma, malignant mesothelioma, malignant melanoma, gestational trophoblastic tumours, germ cell tumours and retinoblastoma.

Lymphovascular invasion: Usually defined histologically in blocks from the tumour edge or slightly away from it and more likely to be associated with cancers that show local recurrence, lymph node involvement, submucosal spread and satellite lesions. This has implications for blocking of resection specimens and their margins. Some cancers (hepatocellular carcinoma, renal cell carcinoma) have a propensity for vascular involvement and care should be taken to identify this on gross specimen dissection and microscopy as it alters the tumour stage and is a marker for distant haematogenous spread.

Lymph nodes: The pN category relates to the total node yield and the number that are involved. Nodal yields are used to audit the care of dissection by the pathologist, adequacy of resection by the surgeon and the choice of operation, e.g., axillary node sampling versus clearance in breast cancer. All regional nodes should be sampled and although ancillary techniques exist (xylene clearance, revealing solutions) there is no substitute for time spent on careful dissection. Care should be taken not to double count the same node, and those small nodes ($\geq$ 1 mm with an identifiable subcapsular sinus) in the histological slides immediately adjacent to the tumour should not be ignored. TNM rules state that direct extension of primary tumour into a regional node is counted as a nodal metastasis as is a tumour nodule with the form and smooth contour of a lymph node in the connective tissue of a lymph drainage area (e.g., mesorectum) even if there is no histological evidence of residual lymphoid tissue. A tumour nodule with an irregular contour is classified in the pT category, i.e., as discontinuous extension. Dissection and submission of separate deposits is therefore important. When size is a criterion for pN classification, e.g., breast carcinoma, measurement is of the metastasis, not the entire node and will usually be made from the histological slides. Micrometastases ($\leq$ 2 mm) are designated pN1 (mi) and isolated tumour cells (< 0.2 mm) pN0 as they are not regarded as having metastatic potential. Most busy general laboratories submit small nodes (< 5 mm) intact or bisected and a mid-slice of larger ones. Additional slices are processed pending microscopy. The limit node is the nearest node to the longitudinal and/or apical resection limits and suture ties. Some specimens, e.g., transverse colectomy, will have more than one and they should be identified as such. Extra-capsular spread is an adverse indicator more usually recognised histologically but should be noted on gross inspection if near to or impinging upon a resection margin, e.g., axillary clearance in breast carcinoma.

Excision margins: The clearance of excision margins has important implications for patient follow-up, adjuvant therapy and local recurrence of tumour. Measurements should be made on the gross specimen and checked against the histological slide. Painting of the margins by ink supplemented by labelling of the blocks is important. Paint adheres well to fresh specimens but also works on formalin-fixed tissue. India ink or alcian blue are commonly used. Commercially available multi-coloured inks are helpful particularly if there are multiple margins as in breast carcinoma. If the intensity of the colour on the slide is low it can be easily checked against the paraffin block. Paint is usually applied to margins prior to dissection but can be re-applied for further emphasis after obtaining the block along its edge. The relevance of particular margins (longitudinal, quadrant, transverse, circumferential and anatomical) varies according to specimen and cancer type and is further discussed in their respective organ systems. In general terms, involvement of longitudinal margins can be by direct, discontinuous or multifocal spread, e.g., oesophageal carcinoma. Positive circumferential radial margins are an indicator of potential local recurrence and a gauge of cancer spread, local anatomy and the extent of surgical excision. Peritoneal or pleural serosal disease allow potential trans-coelomic spread to other abdominopelvic organs, or transpleural spread to the chest wall.

TNM classifies local resection as:

R0: No residual tumour.
R1: Microscopic residual tumour (proven by tumour bed biopsy or cytology) and in effect if tumour involves (to within $\leq$ 1 mm) the resection margin.
R2: Macroscopic residual tumour.

Other pathology: Predisposing, concurrent and associated conditions should be noted, blocked and documented, e.g., colorectal carcinoma and adenomatous polyps, gastric carcinoma and gastric atrophy or synchronous malignant lymphoma (MALToma).

4. Ancillary Techniques in Histopathology Specimens

The vast majority of histopathology specimens can be adequately reported by close attention to careful gross description, dissection and block selection and microscopy of good quality formalin-fixed paraffin sections stained with haematoxylin and eosin. However, key ancillary techniques are also used in a proportion of cases (see Chapter 45). Some examples follow.

Frozen sections: Confirmation of parathyroidectomy, assessment of operative resection margins in cancer surgery, cancer versus inflammatory lesions at laparotomy.

Histochemical stains: Demonstration of mucin in adenocarcinoma, congophilia in amyloid and organisms (pyogenic bacteria, tubercle, fungus) in infection.

Immunofluorescence: Glomerular deposits in renal biopsies, deposition of immunoglobulin and complement in blistering skin disorders.

Immunohistochemistry: The surgical pathologist's "second H and E" is invaluable in assessing tumour type, prognosis and treatment, e.g., carcinoma (cytokeratins) versus malignant lymphoma (CD45) and malignant melanoma (S100), or better prognostic and hormone respon-sive breast cancer (oestrogen receptor positive). Tumour antigenic profile is also of use in specifying the site of origin for a metastasis, e.g., prostate carcinoma (PSA positive).

Electron microscopy: Valuable in renal biopsy diagnosis, and tumours where morphology and immunohistochemistry are inconclusive, e.g., malignant melanoma (pre-/melanosomes) and neuroendocrine carcinoma (neurosecretory granules).

Molecular and chromosomal studies: Immunoglobulin heavy chain and T cell receptor gene rearrangements in the confirmation of malignant lymphoma and the characterisation of various cancers (malignant lymphoma, sarcoma and some carcinomas, e.g., renal) by specific chromosomal changes.

Quantitative methods: Prognostic indicators include the Breslow depth of invasion in malignant melanoma, muscle fibre typing and diameter in myopathies and the mitotic activity index in breast carcinoma.

5. Diagnostic Cytology

Fine needle aspiration, exfoliative and body cavity fluid cytology all provide valuable complementary information in diagnosis and staging (see Chapter 45). The direct smear and cytospin preparations are supplemented by formalin-fixed, paraffin-processed cell blocks of cell sediments and needle core fragments (mini-biopsies) which can combine good morphology and robust immunohistochemistry. Correlation between the cytology and histopathological findings is pivotal to accurate diagnosis (e.g., lung cancer) and staging (e.g., pelvic washings in gynaecological cancer). Cytology may also provide a diagnosis where biopsy fails due to sampling error, inaccessibility of the lesion or biopsy crush artefact.

Appendix 1

Specimen Dissection – A Working Practice

1. Log the specimen into the day book and allocate a laboratory number.
2. Point out any urgent, fresh or inadequately fixed specimens to a supervisory BMS so that appropriate action can be taken. Record on the request form.
3. With a supervisory BMS, categorise the specimens (see Appendix 2) and make a provisional allocation of work.
4. Send the request form of specimen categories C, D and E to the secretarial office for registration and attachment of any computer back history. Return the forms to the laboratory staff so that specimen dissection can proceed. Categories A and B are usually loaded into the processing cassettes before registration.
5. Preview – consult with the supervisory medical pathologist about the more complex specimens (mainly categories C, D and E) to confirm categorisation, reassign categorisation or to discuss the special needs/work allocation of particular specimens. The medical pathologist authorises request forms at this stage.
6. Cut-up
    - work in pairs, one to dissect and describe, the other to write, prepare cassettes, cross-check data, observe and confirm findings. The second person can also have a supervisory, training role as appropriate.
    - check and sign off request form and specimen container label details, i.e.,
        - Patient name.
        - Patient date of birth.
        - Patient unit number.

     – Specimen type, parts and numbering.
     – Laboratory reference number and cassette labels.
- dissect to your level of experience and competence to obtain an accurate description and relevant blocks and also to allow a subsequent meaningful review process.
- float out the cassettes with their blocks in formalin.
- set the specimens (mainly categories C, D and E) aside on and covered by appropriately numbered wet paper towels with the corresponding request form beside them.

7. Review – consult with the supervisory medical pathologist about the more complex specimens (mainly categories C, D and E). He/she will carry out a review with direct feedback to the dissector regarding the quality of macroscopic descriptions, diagrams and appropriateness of blocks. At this stage the cut-up of individual specimens will either be confirmed and the request form authorised, or further description, diagnostic possibilities or supplementary blocks indicated. The supervisory pathologist will mark certain cases for subsequent reporting because of either a special interest or unusual/complex features to the case.

8. Enclose the specimens in moist numbered paper towels in correspondingly numbered plastic bags and store in that day's plastic tray. Small specimens (mainly categories A and B) are individually wrapped in their numbered paper towels along with any spare cassette labels and enclosed in a plastic bag marked with the dissector's initials and those of his/her working partner. Some individual specimens will be retained in formalin-filled containers, e.g., lymph nodes and some complex cases, as indicated at the review discussion. Specimens are disposed of after four weeks once it has been ensured that the surgical histopathology report has been satisfactorily completed, authorised and dispatched.

9. For specific specimens of interest that they have cut, dissectors are to note the laboratory reference number and to obtain subsequent feedback on the diagnosis, descriptions and appropriateness of blocks. Trainee pathologists are encouraged to report and sign out cases that they have cut.

10. Knife etiquette – wipe instruments in between block selection and different specimens to avoid tissue carry-in. Use a sharp knife on well-fixed specimens.

11. Remember – if in doubt, ASK. Problems can be resolved by discussion and staff should always be prepared to point out potential errors. Work as a team.

Appendix 2

Specimen Dissection – Guidelines for Categorisation of Specimens According to Complexity (RCPath., Recommendations).

These are intended to be broad guideline definitions to act as a baseline that departments and individual consultants may see fit to modify. The review system will permit the recognition of situations in which clinical or anatomical circumstances indicate the category as per protocol is inappropriate.

Basic Definitions

A. Specimens only requiring transfer from container to tissue cassette.
B. Specimens requiring transfer, but with standard sampling, counting, weighing or slicing.
C. Simple dissection required with sampling needing a low level of diagnostic assessment and/or preparation.
D. Dissection and sampling required needing a moderate level of assessment.
E. Specimens requiring complex dissection and sampling methods.

Category A

- All small biopsies (endoscopic, synovial, etc.).
- Uterine curettings.
- Simple products of conception.
- Bone marrow trephines.
- Testicular biopsies.
- Cervical punch biopsies.
- Needle biopsies (excluding those requiring special procedures, e.g., renal, muscle).
- Skin curettings and skin biopsies not requiring dissection.

Category B

- Vasa deferentia.
- Fallopian tubes.
- Sebaceous cysts.
- Small lipomas.
- Unremarkable tonsils.
- Unremarkable nasal polyps.
- Temporal arteries.
- Thyroglossal cysts.
- Molar pregnancy.
- Transcervical endometrial resection.
- Prostatic chippings.
- Lymph nodes.

Category C

- Appendix.
- Gall bladder.
- Large gastrointestinal polyps.
- Meckel's diverticulum.
- Diverticular disease.
- Ischaemic bowel.
- Thyroid – non-tumour.
- Salivary gland – non-tumour.
- Placenta.
- Uterus – routine hysterectomy.
- Cervical cone biopsy.
- Muscle and cardiac biopsy.
- Small soft tissue tumours.
- Femoral head.
- Renal biopsy.
- Skin biopsies – benign – requiring dissection.
- Simple small benign breast biopsies.

Category D

- Orchidectomy – non-neoplastic.
- Simple small ovarian cysts and tumours.
- Salivary gland – tumours.
- Thyroid – tumours.

- Pigmented skin lesions.
- Gastrectomy – benign ulcer.
- Complex (non-neoplastic) gastrointestinal resections.

Category E

- Ovarian tumours.
- Uterine carcinoma (including cervical carcinoma).
- Vulvectomy.
- Gastrointestinal carcinoma.
- Oesophagectomy.
- Renal resections.
- Bladder resections.
- Prostatectomy.
- Penile carcinoma.
- Orchidectomy – neoplastic.
- Localised wide lump breast excisions.
- Mastectomy.
- Bone tumours.
- Neck dissection.
- Mandibulectomy.

Appendix 3: Laboratory Abbreviations

g(s)	gram(s)
kg	kilogram
mm	millimetre
ml	millilitre
cm	centimetre
F.W.L	fragments with levels
all processed	all tissue processed
processed intact	tissue processed intact
fix	undergoing further formalin fixation
retained	tissue retained in formalin
mes	mesentery
ser	serosa

bisected

mid section

block in three

multiple serial sections

quadrants

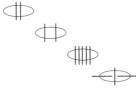

Appendix 4: Levels and Label Coding

A. Specimens to be cut through three levels with 100 μm between each level are:

ENDOSCOPIC BIOPSIES

- Vocal Cord.
- Bronchial.
- Oesophageal.
- Gastric.
- Duodenal.
- Jejunal (also require examination under the dissecting microscope).
- Colonic.
- Rectal.
- Bladder.

NEEDLE BIOPSIES

- Liver.
- Pancreas.
- Breast.
- Prostate.
- Renal.

MISCELLANEOUS

- Cervical punch biopsies.
- Small skin biopsies.
- Temporal artery (embed transversely).
- Cell blocks.

B. Cassettes are identified either by a microwriter or the use of perforated paper labels placed perpendicular to and protruding from the end of the cassette. They may also be colour coded to designate an urgent specimen or specimen type, e.g., gastric biopsy.

Gastrointestinal Specimens

Derek C Allen and R Iain Cameron

General Comments

1. Oesophagus

2. Stomach

3. Pancreas, Duodenum, Ampulla of Vater and Extrahepatic Bile Ducts

4. Small Intestine

5. Colorectum

6. Appendix

7. Anus

8. Gall Bladder

9. Liver

10. Abdominal Wall, Umbilicus, Hernias, Omentum and Peritoneum

General Comments

1. Anatomy

The type of histopathology resection specimen received is dictated by the nature of any previous operations and the current disease process, its distribution and degree of local spread within the organ and to adjacent structures. Resection surgery must provide adequate clearance of longitudinal and deep circumferential radial margins. It must also take into account the lymphovascular supply to achieve satisfactory anastomoses and the regional lymph node drainage for an adequate radical cancer operation. Site location within any given organ may influence the nature of the pathological abnormality and surgical procedure undertaken, e.g., anterior resection for high rectal cancer versus abdominoperineal resection for low rectal cancer, or mid-oesophagus (squamous carcinoma) versus distal oesophagus (adenocarcinoma). Multifocal distribution may be seen in both inflammatory (Crohn's disease) and neoplastic (malignant lymphoma) disorders. Inflammatory disease can be mucosa confined (ulcerative colitis), transmural (Crohn's disease) or mixed (ischaemic colitis). Tumour growth may be predominantly polypoid and intraluminal with only a minor mural component and variable presentation depending on the organ involved, e.g., symptomatic dysphagia due to oesophageal polypoid carcinoma, or asymptomatic iron deficiency anaemia with a caecal carcinoma. Often, cancer ulcerates and deeply invades the wall, stenosing and obstructing the proximal bowel with early access to mesenteric nodes, lymphovascular channels and peritoneum, and potential perforation. Alternatively, the tumour may be characterised by an intact mucosa and incipient thickening of the wall with a tendency for longitudinal spread and skip lesions (diffuse gastric carcinoma – linitis plastica). Thus, normal anatomy is variably distorted by differing disease processes and this must be considered in handling the specimen to obtain appropriate management and prognostic data, e.g., depth of local tumour spread, peritoneal and regional lymph node involvement and excision margin clearance. Allowance must also be made for variation in normal anatomy between and within individuals. For example, harvest of lymph nodes from the mesorectum is scant compared to the sigmoid mesocolon, and in some patients few mesorectal nodes will be found. This is also made more difficult by preoperative radiotherapy, emphasising the importance of taking into account the previous treatment history and request form information. The surgical histopathology specimen also acts as an audit tool for surgical practice and expertise, e.g., rates of anterior resection versus abdominoperineal resection, or completeness of mesorectal excision in rectal cancers. Thus, preoperative and operative techniques alter the specimen anatomy, resulting in differing management and prognostic implications for an equivalent degree of tumour spread in similar specimens from different patients.

2. Clinical Presentation and Investigations

Site-specific symptomatology and investigations are alluded to in the relevant chapters but some general features can be noted. Clinical presentation can be non-specific such as weight loss or anaemia, or focussed on either the upper (nausea, vomiting, haematemesis) or lower (abdominal pain, bleeding per rectum, change in bowel habit) gastrointestinal tract. An iron-deficiency anaemia as measured by the haemoglobin level; red blood cell indices and serum iron/ferritin levels often means occult blood loss from ingestion of NSAIDs or from the surface of an ulcer or polypoid lesion. Serum albumin levels are decreased due to the reduced food intake, protein-losing enteropathy or liver disease. The erythrocyte sedimentation rate (ESR) and C-reactive protein (CRP) are increased in neoplasia, vasculitis and acute flare-up of chronic inflammatory bowel disease. Peripheral white blood cell counts and body temperature are often elevated in acute infection or neoplasia, e.g., leukaemia. Features of malabsorption can be due to either small intestinal or pancreatic disease. Liver function and coagulation tests are altered in hepatic and biliary disease.

Various general radiological investigations are also helpful in diagnosing gastrointestinal disorders.

- CXR (chest X-ray) – to detect metastatic deposits in the lung fields or any enlargement of the lung hilum, heart or aorta that might compress the oesophagus. Also to show air under the diaphragm following perforated duodenal ulcer.
- Straight erect abdominal X-ray (AXR) – to demonstrate calcification in pancreatitis or bowel loops distended by fluid levels due to intestinal obstruction.
- ELUS (endoluminal ultrasound) and MRI (magnetic resonance imaging) scans – to gauge the depth of spread of a tumour through the gastrointestinal wall into adjacent structures and assess locoregional lymph node enlargement.
- CT (computerised coaxial tomography) scan chest/abdomen/pelvis – to gauge the extent of local and metastatic tumour spread.
- PET (positron emission tomography) scan – to help distinguish local tumour recurrence from inflammation and radiotherapy fibrosis.
- USS (ultrasound scan) abdomen/pelvis – to detect gall stones; biliary tract dilatation; cysts in the liver, pancreas, appendix or retrorectal space; and mixed solid/cystic abdominopelvic tumours.

Serological markers of use in diagnosing and also detecting recurrence of gastrointestinal cancer are CA19–9 (pancreatic carcinoma), alpha-fetoprotein (AFP – hepatocellular carcinoma) and carcinoembryonic antigen (CEA – colorectal carcinoma).

Diagnostic laparoscopy allows inspection and biopsy of the peritoneal cavity in various disorders, e.g., tuberculous peritonitis, or staging of tumour spread from a gastric carcinoma – a finding that would contraindicate primary surgical resection of the stomach. The mainstay of investigation is gastrointestinal endoscopy and biopsy.

3. Biopsy Specimens

Flexible Endoscopy

Gastrointestinal mucosal biopsy specimens are obtained by flexible endoscopy due to its ease of operation and relative lack of complications. Flexible endoscopes are complex pieces of equipment consisting of a flexible shaft with a manoeuvrable tip and a control head which the operator holds. The control head is connected to a light source. Other channels such as air, water, suction, etc. pass through the light source. A channel for the passage of therapeutic or diagnostic instruments is located in the control head. The picture from the tip is transmitted to a television screen.

Upper endoscopy involves informed consent, fasting for six hours, intravenous sedation and passage of the endoscope via a mouthguard with direct inspection of the oesophagus, stomach and duodenum, which can be biopsied in relevant areas. Measurements are printed on the shaft of the endoscope so that the operator knows the position of the tip relative to the incisor teeth. Lower endoscopy requires adequate bowel preparation to remove faecal debris and careful insufflation of air via the endoscope to dilate the bowel and allow navigation of the various contours. Due to the fragility of the tissues in some conditions, e.g., toxic megacolon or ischaemic colitis, endoscopy may be contraindicated to avoid perforation.

Specimen Collection

In diagnostic endoscopy tissue biopsies will usually be taken, sometimes supplemented by cytology specimens, and there are various accessories designed for this function.

- Forceps: these consist of a pair of sharpened cups attached by a metal cable to a control handle. The forceps are passed down the channel within the endoscope. The cups are opened and closed by an assistant pulling and pushing the plastic handle. The site for biopsy is approached perpendicularly and firm pressure is applied while the cups are closed. In the oesophagus the approach is tangential and so forceps with a central spike can be used to prevent them from "sliding" off the tissue to be biopsied. At least six tissue samples should be taken from a lesion. Biopsies of ulcers should include samples from the four quadrants and the base, although basal specimens often only yield necrotic slough. If malignancy is suspected it is prudent to take several specimens from the same place as this allows the outer necrotic layer to be penetrated. With polypoid lesions the crown and base of the polyp as well as the adjacent flat mucosa should be adequately sampled. In some conditions, such as Barrett's metaplasia or chronic ulcerative colitis, segments of mucosa are sequentially sampled and mapped by multiple serial biopsies to detect precancerous epithelial dysplasia. Site distribution of lesions is also helpful in differential diagnosis, e.g., ulcerative colitis versus Crohn's disease. The biopsy forceps are withdrawn through the endoscope each time and the tissue sample removed from them by an assistant. A final larger biopsy can be taken if the tissue sample is held in the cups of the forceps while the endoscope is removed.

  The tissue sample is then either put directly into fixative, or after placement onto an orientation millipore (cellulose) filter or polycarbonate strip, preferably mucosal surface upwards to avoid flattening the glandular or villous architecture.
- Cytology brushings: small-spiralled brushes on a metal cable can be used for surface cytology of a lesion. The brush is retracted into a covering plastic sleeve, which protects the specimen during withdrawal. It is then either promptly made into direct smears or cut off and placed in a suitable transport medium for laboratory processing.
- Fine needle aspiration cytology (FNAC): FNAC can sample submucosal, mural and extrinsic lesions not accessible to mucosal biopsy. The syringe needle contents are gently expelled into suitable transport medium, promptly transported to the laboratory and cytocentrifuged onto glass slides for staining and interpretation.

Mucosal biopsies are generally 2–4 mm diameter and 1 mm deep but this varies with patient anatomy, the success of the endoscopy procedure and the nature and configuration of the lesion. Biopsy site and technique also influence specimen size. For example, pinch biopsies obtained via the colonoscope are smaller than rectosigmoidoscopy samples using grasp or jumbo forceps or a strip technique where glucose solution or saline is injected submucosally. A wider-diameter biopsy channel can accommodate jumbo forceps or a suction capsule, the latter being of use where mucosal orientation (reflux oesophagitis) or deeper tissues (submucosa for the assessment of Hirschsprung's disease) are required.

Mucosal polyps vary in size and appearance. For example, in the colorectum metaplastic polyps are often 1–2 mm diameter while adenomas can be similar but are not infrequently larger (1–2 cm) with a distinct head and stalk or even sessile. Small polyps may be removed in-toto by usual biopsy forceps, or monopolar hot biopsy forceps which results in variable diathermy distortion of the mucosal detail. Stalked adenomas are suitable for total excision by an electrosurgical snare. This is facilitated by elevation of the mucosa after submucosal injection of adrenaline, glucose or saline – a technique that is also used for local endoscopic mucosal resection of sessile lesions.

Needle biopsy cores of liver and pancreas are obtained endoscopically, percutaneously or at operation transabdominally by a variety of needles of differing lengths and calibre. They can be spring-loaded or manually operated with the cutting edge of the needle delivering a core of tissue into its lumen. The needle is then retracted and withdrawn with careful removal of its contents and placement into formalin fixative. The procedure may be done blind, under X-ray control or at operation direct vision, depending on the individual case. The patient should have an adequate coagulation status and during the procedure vascular structures avoided to minimise any risk of bleeding. Endoscopic, percutaneous or transabdominal FNAC can traverse abdominal viscera with no detrimental effect to sample abdominal and retroperitoneal masses not accessible to usual endoscopic procedures.

Specimen Handling

Fragments, non-orientated:

- usually multiple fragments, free floating in fixative, non-orientated.
- count.
- place in cassette between foam insert pads or loosely wrap in moist filter paper.
- insert levels label.
- align in the block at the embedding stage as this facilitates microscopic assessment and fragments are not missed.
- separate specimens: use separate cassettes and site identification labels appropriate to the request form information.
- cut through multiple levels.

Fragments, orientated:

- this allows better assessment of mucosal architecture and site distribution of lesions, e.g., colonic strip biopsy in chronic inflammatory bowel disease.
- filter paper: count the fragments and note any that have detached. Process intact between foam insert pads or covered by moist filter paper to preserve orientation for embedding and cutting through multiple levels.
- polycarbonate strip (Figure 1): the endoscopist allows a 2–4 minute period of air drying prior to formalin fixation, ensuring adherence of the mucosal fragments to the strip which is designated according to a pre-agreed protocol, e.g., the cut pointed end is distal or anorectal. Strict alignment of the fragments on the strip by the clinician is essential as it is embedded intact

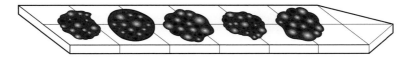

Figure 1. Colonoscopic biopsies mounted on a polycarbonate or Millipore strip.

and on its edge for cutting to allow representation of all the fragments at the same level in the block. Count the fragments and cut through multiple levels.

Polyps (Figure 2):

- non-orientated fragments: these are handled as indicated above.
- snare specimens:
  - ≤ 1 cm diameter – bisect vertically down through the stalk/base and embed both cut surfaces face down. Cut through multiple levels.
  - > 1 cm diameter – obtain a central, vertical mid-slice (3 mm thick) down through and to include an intact stalk/base. Embed face down in the block and the lateral trimmings in a separate block. Cut both through multiple levels. If there is a long stalk an initial transverse section of its resection margin may be taken.
- local mucosal resection: endoscopic or transabdominal is used for stalked polyps (see above) or sessile lesions. Ideally, the latter should be submitted by the surgeon to the laboratory already carefully pinned out onto a cork board or piece of card. Remove and paint the deep and lateral mucosal resection margins. Obtain multiple vertical transverse serial slices (3 mm thick) to include the lesion and underlying base. Where the lesion edge is to within 3 mm of the mucosal margin, sample at right angles to it from a 10 mm slice. Embed the slices face down in the block and cut through multiple levels.

Wedge biopsy:

- usually derived from the edge of a perforated ulcer detected at surgical laparotomy for an acute abdomen. Its base is oversewn and a biopsy taken if the edges show any unusual features, e.g., rolled margins.
- with the mucosal surface upwards bisect or cut into multiple vertical serial slices. Embed the slices face down and cut through multiple levels.

Needle core biopsy:

- up to 1.5 cm long and 1–2 mm diameter, core size is influenced by the patient's anatomy, the nature of the lesion being biopsied, the needle that is used and operator expertise. Some scirrhous carcinomas can be difficult to sample whereas other disease processes lead to fragmentation of the core, e.g., cirrhosis of the liver. Skinny needle cores can be particularly fine requiring careful handling and even painting or immersion in dye (e.g., alcian blue) prior to embedding so that the tissue can be seen when the block is faced at cutting.
- count and measure the maximum core length (mm).
- place intact in cassette between foam insert pads or loosely wrap in moist filter paper.
- cut through multiple levels.

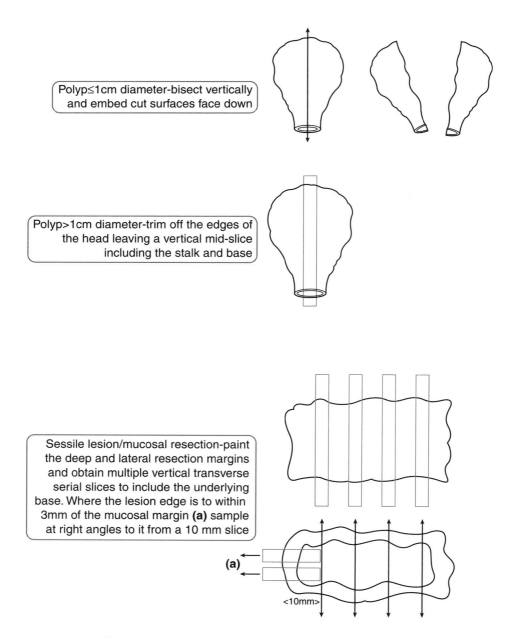

Polyp≤1cm diameter-bisect vertically and embed cut surfaces face down

Polyp>1cm diameter-trim off the edges of the head leaving a vertical mid-slice including the stalk and base

Sessile lesion/mucosal resection-paint the deep and lateral resection margins and obtain multiple vertical transverse serial slices to include the underlying base. Where the lesion edge is to within 3mm of the mucosal margin **(a)** sample at right angles to it from a 10 mm slice

(a)

<10mm>

Figure 2. Gastrointestinal mucosal polyps and local mucosal resections.

Fresh tissue:

- the vast majority of specimens are submitted in formalin fixative but some cases require fresh tissue for frozen sections, e.g., acetylcholinesterase staining in Hirschsprung's disease, or an inflammatory versus malignant lesion at diagnostic laparotomy.

4. Resection Specimens

Fixation

Ideally, specimens are submitted fresh to the laboratory to facilitate sampling for research and measurements as fixation results in considerable shrinkage (15–30% on average) and discrepancy between clinical and pathological dimensions, e.g., margins of tumour clearance. It also allows cleaning out of the specimen and either partial or total opening for pinning out and fixation. This avoids specimen distortion and ultimately allows dissection appropriate to the specimen and tumour type, e.g., the assessment of circumferential resection margins. Adequate fixation of a cleaned, opened specimen requires 36–48 hours immersion in formalin. Where it is normal practice to submit resection specimens to the laboratory already in fixative, the theatre staff should be instructed on how to partially open and clean out the specimen but to avoid transecting the tumour segment and compromising margin assessment.

Margins

Longitudinal, circumferential and anatomical margins are considered.

- Longitudinal margins: circumferential, transverse sections are taken in non-neoplastic disorders such as ischaemia or chronic inflammatory bowel disease to assess involvement. In cancer resections, separate anastomotic rings are often submitted and these constitute the longitudinal margins rather than those of the main specimen. In the absence of an anastomotic ring the longitudinal margin should be circumferentially sampled although if the tumour is close ($\leq$ 0.5–1 cm) to it a longitudinal block may be more practicable. The significance of longitudinal margin clearance varies, e.g., a macrosopic tumour clearance of 2–3 cm in an anterior resection for rectal cancer is considered satisfactory whereas it is not for diffuse gastric or oesophageal cancers where multifocal epithelial and discontinuous submucosal or mural skip lesions can occur. Longitudinal margins should be blocked first prior to dissection of the tumour to avoid knife carry-in of tumour fragments.
- Circumferential radial margin (CRM): this gives an assessment of the extent of lateral or radial spread of a tumour and its adequacy of excision, features that are strongly related to subsequent local recurrence and morbidity. Prior to dissection the CRM should be painted and both macroscopic and microscopic measurements of tumour clearance are then made. In the mesorectum direct tumour spread or tumour within a lymph node or lymphatic to within $\leq$ 1 mm of the CRM is considered involved. CRM involvement may indicate the need for postoperative radio- or chemotherapy. The amount and completeness of excision of circumferential tissues depends on the anatomical site and expertise of the surgeon. For example, adventitial tissues in an oesophagectomy specimen may be scant whereas the posterior and lateral mesorectum is usually 2–3 cm deep. The success of total mesorectal excision relates to surgical training and the available time resources to carry out an adequate

procedure but is an important part of auditing surgical practice. The significance of tumour at the mesocolic edge or that of the gastric lesser omentum is less established but should be reported by the pathologist.

- Anatomical margins: the serosa or peritoneum is a visceral margin and breech of it allows the tumour to access the abdominal and pelvic cavities with potential for transcoelomic spread, e.g., diffuse gastric cancer with bilateral ovarian metastases (Krukenberg tumours). Thus, gastrointestinal cancers may present clinically with deposits at another abdominopelvic site and this should be borne in mind on assessment of tumour macroscopic and microscopic appearances. Tumour at and ulcerating the serosa represents either pT3 (stomach) or pT4 (small and large intestines) disease and is a decision factor in selection for postoperative chemotherapy. It should be distinguished from the commoner finding of carcinoma in a subserosal inflammatory fibrous reaction but not at its free surface. The serosa overlying the tumour should be painted prior to dissection to help determine the presence of involvement.

Once appropriate blocks are obtained their circumferential edge can be repainted to ensure adequate margin demonstration.

Dissection

Cancer resections: for optimal demonstration of the deepest point of tumour spread, its relationship to the CRM and correlation with ELUS/CT cross sectional imaging multiple, serial, 3–4 mm thick slices of the cancer in the transverse axis are recommended. The slices can then be laid out in sequence and a photographic or digital record provided. Generally, four or five blocks of the tumour and wall are selected to adequately define the pT stage. Some pathologists leave the tumour segment unopened during fixation and transverse slicing to keep the CRM intact – others open it carefully avoiding suspect areas of the CRM to ensure adequate tumour fixation and ascertain tumour measurements. Either approach is justifiable as long as it is done with care and consistency. Sometimes the local anatomy or proximity of the tumour to a longitudinal margin necessitate dissection in the longitudinal plane. Such a block can be useful in a poorly differentiated carcinoma when the adjacent mucosa may show a point of origin or clue as to its histological type. Mucosal blocks away from the tumour may also demonstrate its histogenesis, e.g., metaplasia/dysplasia/cancer sequence in the stomach, or multifocality. Multiple colonic cancers are blocked and reported individually.

All regional lymph nodes should be sampled as size alone is not a reliable indicator of metastatic involvement and pN staging relates to total and involved numbers of nodes. Small nodes seen histologically in the tumour blocks are also counted and may only measure ≥ 1 mm diameter but are recognisable by their subcapsular sinus. A limit node is identified adjacent to a mesenteric pedicle suture tie – some specimens, e.g., transverse colon, may have more than one. Dukes staging for colorectal cancer varies according to whether the limit node is involved (C2) or not (C1). Techniques such as xylene clearance have been advocated to increase nodal yields but in general there is no substitute for experienced, careful dissection. A target number can be useful, e.g., a harvest of eight nodes will identify the vast majority of Dukes C colorectal carcinomas. Preoperative radio-/chemotherapy can lead to marked tumour degeneration and fibrotic reaction compromising nodal yields and identification of residual primary tumour or nodal deposits. Most general laboratories submit small nodes (< 5 mm) intact or bisected, and a mid-slice of larger ones. It is important that the same node is not counted twice.

Non-neoplastic resections: an important descriptive feature in differential diagnosis is disease distribution, e.g., diffuse, segmental, mucosal or transmural. Overt lesions may show only end-stage non-specific florid ulceration and reactive changes – the disease distribution and changes in the intervening mucosa give important diagnostic clues. For example, ulcerative colitis is mucosal and diffuse, Crohn's disease segmental and transmural with intervening aphthous ulcers, chronic ischaemic stricture is preferentially located at the splenic flexure and clostridium difficle infection shows mucosal pseudomembranes. Non-neoplastic colonic specimens therefore require sequential labelled blocks of abnormal and normal (e.g., every 10 cm) areas. As the mucosa is arranged in transverse folds, long-axis blocks are taken. Longitudinal limits are transverse sectioned to look for disease involvement and although mesenteric nodes are usually reactive only, they may show helpful diagnostic pointers such as granulomas in Crohn's disease. In ischaemic conditions, mesenteric vessels are also sampled for signs of vasculitis or embolic thrombi. Some vascular anomalies, e.g., angiodysplasia of the colon, may require close liaison with the surgical and radiological teams necessitating perioperative injection of radio-opaque contrast medium. In some cases, e.g., gastric resections, it is not possible to tell macroscopically if the ulcer, adjacent mucosa or regional nodes are benign or malignant or to gauge the extent of mural spread – dissection and block selection must be sufficiently comprehensive to allow for this.

1 Oesophagus

1. Anatomy

The oesophagus is a tubular structure, approximately 25 cm long, extending from the laryngeal part of the pharynx at the level of the 6th cervical vertebra, passing through the diaphragm at the level of the 10th thoracic vertebra to join the stomach at the oesophagogastric (OG) junction (Figure 1.1). For purposes of practicality during endoscopic procedures, the site of a lesion in the oesophagus is given as the distance from the upper incisor teeth. As it is approximately 16 cm from the upper incisor teeth to the proximal oesophageal limit, the OG junction is at approximately 40–41 cm. The oesophagus traverses the neck, thorax and enters the abdominal cavity and so can be anatomically divided into three sub-sites:

1. Cervical oesophagus: 2–3 cm long and extends from the proximal oesophageal limit (C6) to the thoracic inlet, which is marked by the surface landmark of the suprasternal notch of the sternum (breast bone).
2. Intrathoracic oesophagus: approximately 21 cm long and extends from the thoracic inlet to the oesophageal hiatus in the diaphragm. At 25 cm from the upper incisor teeth the oesophagus is constricted by the aortic arch and the left main bronchus crossing its anterior surface.
3. Abdominal oesophagus: 1–1.5 cm long and extends from the oesophageal hiatus in the diaphragm to the right side of the stomach. It is covered anterolaterally by peritoneum and comes into close relationship with the left lobe of liver.

An internal landmark of relevance to determining the site of origin of an oesophagogastric tumour is the OG junction where the pale oesophageal squamous mucosa meets the glandular mucosa of the gastric cardia. The OG junction can be somewhat irregular in outline (the Z line) and does not necessarily correspond to the lower physiological valve or sphincter. External landmarks are distal oesophagus orientated to adventitial fat while the junctional area and proximal stomach relate to a covering of serosa or peritoneum. Thus, a tumour of the distal oesophagus or OG junction can spread through the wall either to adventitial fat of the mediastinum or the abdominal peritoneum. Adventitial fat is disposed laterally, but absent anteriorly and posteriorly where the oesophagus is adjacent to the heart and vertebral column respectively. Note that the adventitia of the mid-oesophagus may also relate to a serosal surface – that of resected mediastinal pleura.

As well as determining the position of the lesion within the oesophagus by its anatomical site, it can also be defined by its relative position in the upper, middle or lower third of the oesophagus. This is of relevance clinically as the lymphovascular drainage is considered in these terms and is therefore important in cancer surgery.

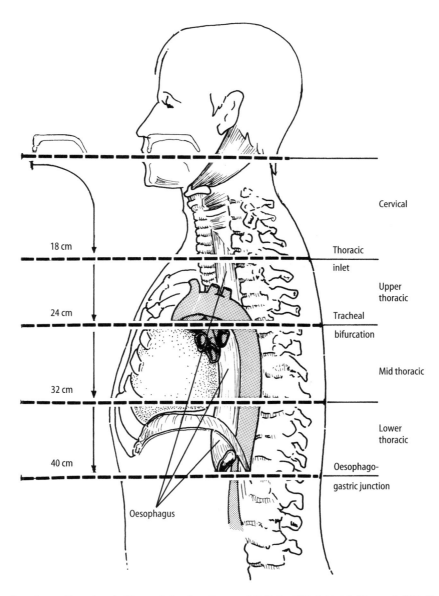

18 cm

24 cm

32 cm

40 cm

Oesophagus

Cervical

Thoracic
inlet

Upper
thoracic

Tracheal
bifurcation

Mid thoracic

Lower
thoracic

Oesophago-
gastric junction

Figure 1.1. Oesophagus. Reproduced with permission from Hermanek P, Hutter RVP, Sobin LH, Wagner G, Wittekind Ch (eds.). TNM Atlas: illustrated guide to the TNM/pTNM classification of malignant tumours, 4th edition. Springer-Verlag: Berlin and Heidelberg, 1997.

The regional lymph nodes are, for the cervical oesophagus, the cervical nodes including
supraclavicular nodes and, for the intrathoracic oesophagus, the perioesophageal,
subcarinal, mediastinal and perigastric nodes, excluding those at the origin of the coeliac artery

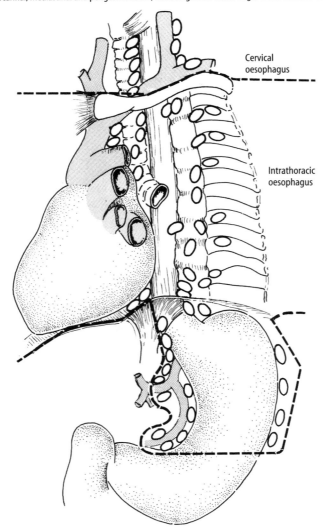

Figure 1.2. Oesophagus: regional lymph nodes. Reproduced with permission from Hermanek P, Hutter RVP, Sobin LH, Wagner
G, Wittekind Ch (eds.). TNM Atlas: illustrated guide to the TNM/pTNM classification of malignant tumours, 4th edition. Springer-
Verlag: Berlin and Heidelberg, 1997.

Lymphovascular drainage (Figure 1.2)

- Upper third – deep cervical nodes.
- Middle third – superior and posterior mediastinal nodes.
- Lower third – nodes along the left gastric blood vessels and the coeliac nodes.

Venous drainage from the middle third (azygos vein) into the lower third (gastric vein) leads to the formation of a porto-systemic anastomosis and, with raised portal venous pressure (e.g., as in liver cirrhosis), the possibility of the formation of oesophageal varices (dilatation of oesophageal veins).

2. Clinical Presentation

Patients with oesophageal disease may be asymptomatic, but usually experience one or more of the following: chest pain, heartburn (a retrosternal burning sensation), reflux of food and dysphagia (difficulty swallowing). Dysphagia can be painful (odynophagia) or progressive due to benign or malignant strictures, i.e., initially for solid foods, e.g., meat, then soft foods and ultimately liquids. Patient localisation of the site of obstruction can be poor. Occult bleeding can lead to iron-deficiency anaemia while haemorrhage (haematemesis) can be potentially life threatening (varices) or self-limiting due to linear tears of the OG junction mucous membrane after prolonged vomiting (Mallory–Weiss syndrome).

3. Clinical Investigations

Endoscopy and biopsy.
CXR to detect any enlargement of the heart, mediastinal lymph nodes or pulmonary hilum that might extrinsically press on the oesophagus. Barium swallow to outline the contour of the oesophageal lumen and wall and assess motility/swallowing.
For biopsy proven cancer – ELUS and CT scan chest and abdomen to determine the pretreatment tumour stage.
24 hour pH monitoring – has a high diagnostic sensitivity for reflux oesophagitis. Oesophageal manometry can assess the effectiveness of motility, e.g., achalasia, scleroderma.

4. Pathological Conditions

Non-neoplastic Conditions

Reflux oesophagitis: usually due to hiatus hernia (slippage of the OG junction into the thorax) resulting in gastro-oesophageal reflux (GOR) of acid and bile; there is poor correlation with symptoms, endoscopy and biopsy being normal in 20–30% of cases. Otherwise well-orientated biopsies show basal zone hyperplasia and prominent vascularised connective tissue papillae. This is superseded by inflammatory infiltrates of neutrophils and eosinophils, surface erosion, full-thickness ulceration and ultimately fibrous stricture formation (10% of cases). It may require operative dilatation (often repeatedly) to relieve dysphagia and although it usually has a smooth outline it may be difficult to distinguish endoscopically from a malignant growth. Prior to this, treatment of GOR is either medical (weight loss, antacids), or occasionally surgical. This is usually done laparoscopically by wrapping the fundus of the stomach around the distal oesophagus (Nissen fundoplication) to maintain lower oesophageal tone and retain it in the abdominal cavity.

Infective oesophagitis: may be seen in otherwise healthy individuals but is more commonly encountered where there is alteration of either local or systemic immunity (e.g., AIDS). Underlying ulceration, broad-spectrum antibiotics, diabetes, corticosteroid therapy and immunosuppressive drugs can all alter the local gut flora resulting in superimposed infection. Causative agents are: candidal fungus, herpes simplex virus (HSV 1 and 2), cytomegalovirus (CMV), and atypical mycobacteria.

Miscellaneous: other causes of oesophagitis, ulceration and/or stricture are: drugs (e.g., NSAIDs, aspirin), mediastinal radiotherapy, motility disorders (e.g., achalasia), Crohn's disease and direct injury (foreign body, prolonged nasogastric intubation, corrosive ingestion).

Incidental endoscopic findings are inflammatory or fibrovascular polyps of the OG junction.

Neoplastic Conditions

Benign tumours: these are rare in surgical material, e.g., squamous papilloma, leiomyoma or granular cell tumour.

Oesophageal carcinoma: predisposing conditions to oesophageal cancer include diverticula, achalasia and Plummer–Vinson syndrome (elderly females, iron-deficiency anaemia, upper oesophageal web). Predisposing lesions to oesophageal cancer are squamous cell dysplasia and Barrett's metaplasia/dysplasia.

Squamous cell dysplasia/carcinoma in-situ: macroscopically inapparent but seen histologically adjacent to, overlying, or distant from squamous cell carcinoma.

Barrett's metaplasia or <u>columnar</u> epithelium <u>lined</u> lower <u>oesophagus</u> (CLO): seen in about 10% of patients with hiatus hernia and/or GOR. It arises from erosion with differentiation of multipotential stem cells to metaplastic small intestinal or gastric glandular epithelia. The Barrett's segment appears as a velvety area proximal to the OG junction surrounded by pale squamous mucosa. It can be multifocal or continuous. The segment is either classical/long ($\geq$ 3 cm), short (< 3 cm), or ultra-short (junctional). About 10% of Barrett's cases develop mucosal dysplasia and/or adenocarcinoma, representing an increased risk of 30–40 times that of the general population. Barrett's metaplasia positive for mucosal dysplasia is classified as either low-grade or high-grade. The latter has a strong (40–60%) association with concurrent or subsequent adenocarcinoma, indicating the need for immediate clinicopathological reassessment and consideration of surgery. The appearances of Barrett's metaplasia can also be altered by its treatment with antacid medication, laser ablation or photodynamic therapy.

Squamous cell carcinoma: forms 30–40% of oesophageal cancers and is typically seen in the mid-oesophagus of elderly patients. It is usually moderately differentiated and keratinising, ulcerates or strictures with rolled, irregular margins, involves a long segment of oesophagus and has spread through the full thickness of the wall at presentation. Palliation can be achieved by radiotherapy, ablative laser therapy or the insertion of an expanding metal stent or tube to relieve obstruction. Primary surgical resection is the treatment of choice in a medically fit patient with a locally confined lesion < 5 cm in length. If more extensive than this, resection can be facilitated by preoperative radio-/chemotherapy which produces signs of tumour regression (degeneration, necrosis, fibrosis, keratin granulomas) in some 50–60% of cases, but often makes identification of tumour on gross inspection of the specimen difficult. Perforation with potentially fatal mediastinitis is a possible complication of preoperative therapy and endoscopy of malignant strictures. Bronchoscopy is also done to exclude the possibility of a primary lung cancer invading the oesophagus which would preclude primary resection as do haematogenous and distant nodal metastases or invasion of mediastinal vessels and main structures.

Variants of squamous carcinoma are: verrucous carcinoma (warty, slow growth), basaloid carcinoma (aggressive) and spindle cell/polypoid carcinoma (carcinosarcoma – intermediate prognosis).

Adenocarcinoma: forms 50–60% of oesophageal cancers and arises in the distal oesophagus/OG junction often secondary to intestinal-type Barrett's metaplasia and dysplasia. The incidence of this tumour has greatly increased in the last twenty years due in part to antibiotic eradication of helicobacter pylorii with loss of its gastric acid suppressor effect resulting in more GOR disease. As well as extensive radial spread through the wall out to the CRM it can spread upwards undermining the oesophageal squamous mucosa and downwards to the proximal stomach where clear distinction from a primary gastric carcinoma can be difficult. Clues as to site of origin are both anatomical (oesophageal if > 50% of the tumour is above the OG junction) and histological in the adjacent mucosa (oesophagus – Barrett's metaplasia/dysplasia; stomach – gastric mucosal dysplasia). Adenocarcinoma is usually ulcerated with irregular rolled margins or polypoid, and histologically tubular or papillary with an intestinal glandular pattern, but sometimes of diffuse signet ring cell type. Treatment of choice for locally confined disease is primary surgical resection supplemented by chemotherapy if indicated by subsequent pathological staging of the resection specimen. Current clinical trials are examining whether preoperative chemotherapy has any role to play.

Other features: oesophageal cancer tends to show multifocality (15–20%). Examination of specimen proximal and distal surgical margins is therefore important. "Early" or superficial squamous carcinoma is confined to the mucosa or submucosa with or without regional lymph node involvement and is of better prognosis than "advanced" or deep muscle invasive carcinoma. Involvement of the perioesophageal CRM is partly dependent on individual patient anatomy but is also an indicator of extent of tumour spread, adequacy of surgical resection and potential local recurrence due to residual mediastinal disease.

Other cancers: rare but can include small cell carcinoma, malignant melanoma, leukaemia/malignant lymphoma, metastatic cancer (e.g., lung or breast), leiomyosarcoma, and Kaposi's sarcoma (AIDS).

Prognosis: prognosis of oesophageal cancer is poor (five-year survival 5–15%) relating mainly to depth of spread and lymph node involvement, i.e., tumour stage, and involvement of longitudinal and circumferential excision margins. Early or superficial carcinoma does significantly better – 55% → 88% five-year survival depending on the depth of mucous membrane invasion.

5. Surgical Pathology Specimens – Clinical Aspects

Biopsy Specimens

Two main types of oesophageal endoscopy exist, namely rigid and flexible. Rigid oesophagoscopy is only occasionally used to provide larger biopsies when previous flexible endoscopy samples have proven non-diagnostic. Specific lesions such as polyps or ulcers necessitate multiple targeted biopsies which may be supplemented by brush cytology of the mucosal surface. Mapping and annual/biennial surveillance of flat mucosa for Barrett's metaplasia and dysplasia is achieved by multiple segmental (every 2 cm) and quadrantic biopsies. The basis of an oesophageal stricture may be easier to demonstrate if malignant in nature because of carcinoma ulcerating the squamous epithelium, whereas a benign peptic stricture due to submucosal or mural fibrosis is often not accessible to mucosal biopsy. Endoscopic biopsy of achalasia or oesophageal webs is often unrewarding as it provides intact surface mucosa only.

Resection Specimens

The surgical techniques for resecting oesophageal tumours fall into two broad categories: those which employ a chest incision (thoracotomy) and those which do not (transdiaphragmatic hiatal procedures). The type of procedure used depends on the general level of health of the patient, any previous operations, the preference of the operating surgeon, the position of the tumour in the oesophagus (see Table 1.1) and the choice of oesophageal substitute, i.e., stomach, jejunum or colonic interposition. Ideally the surgeon should strive for a 5 cm longitudinal margin of clearance with adenocarcinoma and 10 cm for squamous carcinoma.

a) *Ivor Lewis technique* – in this operation upper abdominal and right thoracotomy incisions are made. The proximal stomach is divided and the oesophagus is transected proximal to the tumour. The distal stomach is then raised into the chest and an oesophagogastric anastomosis is fashioned.

b) *Thoracoabdominal oesophagectomy* – a continuous incision extending from the midline of the upper abdomen running obliquely across the rib margin and posterolateral aspect of the chest wall is made. The left diaphragm is divided and this gives access for potential en bloc resection of the oesophagus, stomach, gastric nodes and, if required, the spleen and distal pancreas. An oesophagojejunal or oesophagogastric anastomosis is fashioned in the neck.

c) *Transhiatal oesophagectomy* – depending on whether a total or distal oesophagectomy is to be performed, two variations of this procedure are used:
   - 'Two-field approach' – the entire oesophagus and stomach is mobilised via upper abdominal and oblique neck incisions. The cervical oesophagus is divided and anastomosed to stomach, which had been mobilised and raised high into the posterior mediastinum.
   - Distal oesophagectomy with proximal gastrectomy – (for distal oesophageal/junctional tumours). Only an upper abdominal incision is used, with the distal oesophagus being mobilised and an oesophagogastric anastomosis fashioned in the chest.

Although transhiatal resection for diseases of the thoracic oesophagus used to be uncommon, it is now more commonly used, reducing the physiological insult experienced with a thoracotomy.

Whenever possible the stomach should be used in the anastomosis and with appropriate mobilisation the stomach will reach the neck in virtually all patients. If the tumour is limited to the OG junction, the entire greater curvature of the gastric fundus (shaded area in Figure 1.3), including the point which usually reaches most cephalad to the neck (* in Figure 1.3), may be preserved while still obtaining a 4–6 cm gastric margin distal to the malignancy.

Table 1.1.   Choice of surgical procedure in oesophageal neoplasia

Proximal 1/3 tumours	Pharyngo-oesophagectomy.
Middle 1/3 tumours	Ivor Lewis technique Thoracoabdominal oesophagectomy Two field transhiatal oesophagectomy
Lower 1/3 tumours	Ivor Lewis technique Thoracoabdominal oesophagectomy Transhiatal oesophagectomy
Barrett's	Transhiatal oesophagectomy

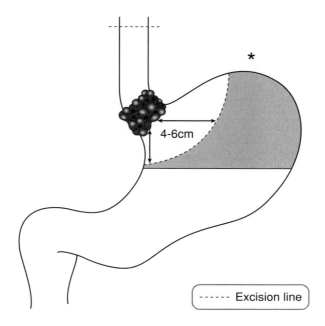

Figure 1.3.   Transhiatal oesophagectomy with limited proximal gastrectomy.

There are several benefits in performing a total thoracic oesophagectomy with cervical anastomosis: maximum clearance of surgical margins is obtained while the risk of mediastinitis, sepsis and GOR that can be seen with an intrathoracic anastomosis is diminished.

6. Surgical Pathology Specimens – Laboratory Protocols

Biopsy Specimens

See Gastrointestinal Specimens – General Comments (page 6)

Resection Specimens

Specimen

most oesophageal resections are for neoplastic conditions: partial oesophagectomy, total thoracic oesophagectomy (TTO), oesophagectomy with limited gastrectomy, oesophagogastrectomy.

Initial procedure

- by palpation and with the index finger locate the lumenal position of the tumour.
- paint the overlying external CRM comprising adventitial fatty connective tissue and any related serosa.
- open longitudinally with blunt ended scissors cutting on the opposite side of the tumour. Open proximal stomach along the greater curvature continuous with the oesophageal cut.

Alternatively, some pathologists prefer to leave the tumour segment unopened for fixation and subsequent transverse slicing.

- measurements:
  - oesophagus – length (cm), width (cm).
  - proximal stomach – lengths (cm) along lesser and greater curvatures.
  - tumour – length × width × depth (cm) or maximum dimension (cm).
  - distances (cm) to the proximal and distal limits of resection.
  - distance (cm) to the OG junction if the tumour is mid-oesophageal in location.
  - distance (cm) above/below the OG junction if the tumour is distal oesophageal or junctional in location.
  - > 50% tumour bulk above OG junction = oesophageal in origin (Siewert I).
  - > 50% tumour bulk below OG junction = proximal gastric in origin (Siewert III).
  - tumour bulk equally straddles OG junction = junctional in origin (Siewert II).
  - note that the junction may be obscured by tumour and external landmarks (oesophagus – adventitia; stomach – serosa) should also be used in determining the location.
  - Barrett's mucosa – location/length (cm).
- photograph.
- fixation by immersion in 10% formalin for 48 hours preferably pinned out on a cork board in the opened position but not placed under tension (to avoid splitting).

Description

- tumour – polypoid: spindle cell carcinoma/carcinosarcoma.
  - warty/verrucous: verrucous carcinoma.
  - nodular/plaque: superficial carcinoma.
  - fungating/strictured/ulcerated/infiltrative edge: usual carcinoma.
  - multifocal.
  - regression and scarring.
- mucosa – Barrett's mucosa (velvety appearance).
- wall – tumour confined to mucous membrane, in the wall or through the wall.
- other – achalasia, diverticulum, mucosal web, perforation.

Blocks for histology (Figure 1.4)

- sample the proximal and distal limits of surgical resection – complete circumferential transverse section (oesophagus) or multiple circumferential blocks (proximal stomach).
- alternatively, if separate anastomotic doughnuts are submitted, take one complete circumferential transverse section of each.
- serially section the bulk of the tumour transversely at 3–4 mm intervals.
- lay the slices out in sequence and photograph.
- sample a minimum of four blocks of tumour and wall to show the deepest point of circumferential invasion.
- sample two longitudinal blocks of tumour and adjacent mucosa, proximal and distal to the gross lesion respectively.
- sample one block of oesophagus proximal to the tumour, and one block of oesophagus (or proximal stomach) distal to the tumour.
- sample any abnormal background mucosa, e.g., multiple sequential blocks may be required to map the extent of Barrett's metaplasia.
- if tumour is not seen grossly, sequentially sample and correspondingly label unremarkable and abnormal areas of mucosa.

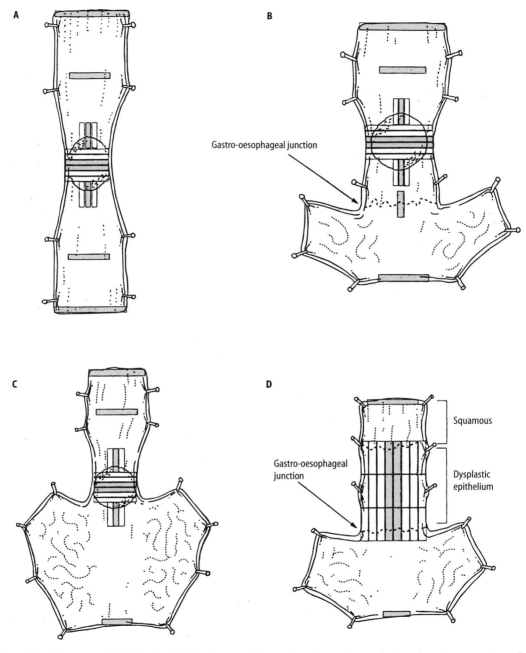

Figure 1.4. Recommended blocks for histology in resected oesophageal neoplasms. **A.** Oesophagectomy specimen. **B.** Oesophago-gastrectomy specimen containing tumour above the gastro-oesophageal junction. **C.** Oesophago-gastrectomy specimen containing tumour at the gastro-oesophageal junction. **D.** Resected specimen for high-grade dysplasia/in situ carcinoma. Shaded blocks represent the recommended minimum number to be sampled. Reproduced with permission from Ibrahim, NBN. Guidelines for handling oesophageal biopsies and resection specimens and their reporting. J Clin Pathol 2000;53:89–94.

- count and sample all lymph nodes.
- sample the mid-point and proximal surgical limit (as marked by the surgeon) of any separate proximal segment of normal oesophagus excised to facilitate pull-through of the oesophagogastric anastomosis to the neck.

Histopathology report

- tumour type: adenocarcinoma/squamous carcinoma/other

- tumour differentiation:

	adenocarcinoma	squamous carcinoma
well	> 95% glands	keratinisation/intercellular bridges
moderate	50–95% glands	
poor	< 50% glands	no keratinisation/inter-cellular bridges

- tumour edge: pushing/infiltrative/lymphoid response

- extent of local tumour spread

pTis carcinoma in situ
pT1   tumour invades lamina propria or submucosa
pT2   tumour invades muscularis propria
pT3   tumour invades adventitia
pT4   tumour invades adjacent structures eg trachea, bronchus, lung.

Note also any invasion of the proximal gastric serosa or mediastinal pleura.
   Siewert I tumours are staged as oesophageal under TNM and Siewert II and III cancers as gastric in origin.

- lymphovascular invasion – present/not present. Note perineural invasion.
- regional lymph nodes

Thoracic oesophagus: perioesophageal, subcarinal and mediastinal/perigastric nodes excluding those at the origin of the coeliac artery, which are classified as a distant metastasis (pM1)

pN0 no regional lymph node metastasis
pN1 metastasis in regional lymph node(s).

- excision margins

proximal and distal limits of tumour clearance (cm)
   separate proximal oesophageal and distal gastric anastomotic doughnuts – involved/not involved
   deep circumferential radial margin of clearance (mm).

- other pathology

squamous dysplasia, Barrett's metaplasia/dysplasia, radio-/chemotherapy necrosis and tumour regression, perforation, achalasia, oesophageal web, diverticulum.

2 Stomach

1. Anatomy

The stomach is a dilated portion of the gastrointestinal tract which has three main functions; storage of food, mixing food with gastric secretions and control of the rate of release of food to the small intestine for further digestion and absorption. It is a J-shaped organ and much of it lies under the cover of the lower ribs. It has an anterior and posterior surface, two openings (the proximal cardiac and the distal pyloric orifices) and two curvatures (greater and lesser) (Figure 2.1). Although relatively fixed at both ends, the intervening part is mobile and can undergo considerable variation in shape. The stomach is usually divided into the following parts:

Fundus – dome shaped and projects upwards and to the left of the cardiac orifice.
Body – extends from the level of the cardiac orifice to the incisura angularis (a constant notch at the junction of the lesser curve and antrum). The incisura is an important endoscopic landmark.
Antrum – extends from the incisura to the proximal part of the pylorus.
Pylorus – the most tubular part of the stomach and its thick muscular wall forms the physiological and anatomical pyloric sphincter, marked by a slight constriction on the surface of the stomach. The pylorus, which is approximately 2.5 cm long, joins the first part of the duodenum.

The cardiac orifice is where the abdominal part of the oesophagus enters the stomach. Although no anatomical sphincter is present, a physiological mechanism exists which prevents gastro-oesophageal regurgitation.

The lesser curvature forms the right border of the stomach, extending from the cardiac orifice to the pylorus. The greater curvature extends from the left of the cardiac orifice, over the fundus to the inferior part of the pylorus. Peritoneum completely surrounds the stomach and leaves its curvatures as double layers called omenta which contain fat, lymph nodes and vessels. The lesser omentum extends from the lesser curve to the liver. The gastrosplenic omentum extends from the upper part of the greater curve to the spleen, while the greater omentum runs to the transverse colon from the lower part.

The mucous membrane of the gastric body is thrown into numerous longitudinal folds or rugae. This facilitates flattening of the mucosa when the stomach is distended by food. The mucosal surface contains millions of gastric pits or foveolae that lead to mucosal glands. The mucosal surface is composed of columnar, mucin-secreting epithelium (surface mucus – foveolar cells), while deeper in the gastric pits are mucus neck cells. The gastric glands vary depending on their anatomic region (Figure 2.1):

Cardia: mucin-secreting cells.
Fundus/body: parietal cells (acid), chief cells (pepsin) and scattered endocrine cells.
Antrum/pylorus: endocrine (mostly gastrin G cells) and mucin-secreting cells.

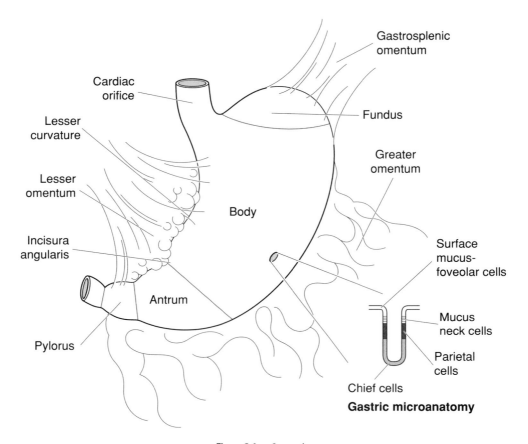

Figure 2.1.   Stomach.

Lymphovascular supply

The entire arterial supply of the stomach is derived from the coeliac artery which arises from the aorta. Veins drain into the portal system. The lymphatics drain to the coeliac lymph nodes. The so-called N1 and N2 node groups (12 in total) are situated along the arterial supply (Figure 2.2). N1 nodes are within 3 cm of the primary malignancy and N2 nodes more than 3 cm from the tumour.

The main nerve supply to the stomach is from the anterior and posterior vagal trunks, with the innervation of the pylorus being mainly derived from the anterior vagus.

2. Clinical Presentation

Patients with gastroduodenal disease may be asymptomatic or experience one or more of the following: upper abdominal (epigastric) pain, dyspepsia ("indigestion"), vomiting which may be projectile if there is pyloric outflow obstruction, haematemesis (vomiting blood), melaena (altered blood per rectum) or dysphagia if there is a proximal gastric lesion.

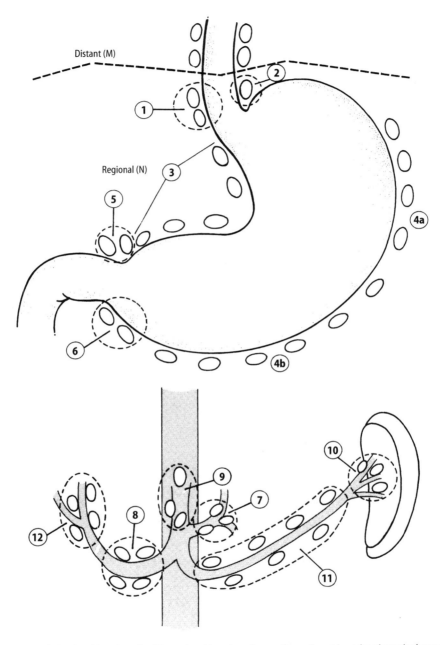

Figure 2.2. Stomach: Regional lymph nodes. The regional lymph nodes are the perigrastric nodes along the lesser (*1, 3, 5*) and greater (*2, 4a, 4b, 6*) curvatures, the nodes located along the left gastric (*7*), common hepatic (*8*), splenic (*10, 11*) and coeliac arteries (*9*) and the hepatoduodenal nodes (*12*). Involvement of other intra-abdominal lymph nodes such as the retropancreatic, mesenteric and para-aortic is classified as distant metastasis. Reproduced from Hermanek P, Hutter RVP, Sobin LH, Wagner G, Wittekind Ch (eds.). TNM atlas: illustrated guide to the TNM/pTNM classification of malignant tumours, 4th edition. Springer-Verlag: Berlin and Heidelberg, 1997.

3. Clinical Investigations

- Endoscopy and biopsy.
- Erect CXR to detect "air under the diaphragm" in a perforation and also metastatic tumour deposits in the lungs.
- Barium swallow will outline the mucosal surface and detect delayed emptying caused by pyloric outflow obstruction.
- For biopsy-proven cancer – ELUS and CT scan chest, abdomen and pelvis to determine the pretreatment tumour stage.
- Peritoneal aspiration of ascitic fluid for malignant cells and staging laparoscopy with peritoneal biopsy.
- Gastric function tests – peak acid output is measured by the pentagastrin test and will differentiate "hypersecretors" from "non-hypersecretors" – important if surgery is to be considered for duodenal peptic ulcer disease.

4. Pathological Conditions

Non-neoplastic Conditions

Acute gastritis: acute haemorrhagic/erosive gastritis is usually antral and drug related (aspirin, NSAIDs, alcohol), or, less commonly in the body secondary to shock and hypoperfusion, e.g., post trauma, sepsis or burns, and therefore not biopsied. Acute neutrophilic gastritis is seen in food poisoning, sepsis and *Helicobacter pylorii* (HP) infection.

Chronic gastritis: with poor correlation between symptoms, endoscopic appearances and histology it is very common in biopsy material and is autoimmune, bacterial or chemical in nature (types A, B and C). The latter is usually antral, related to drug ingestion or bile reflux and comprises a reactive mucosa with a lack of inflammatory cells. Autoimmune gastritis affects the corpus resulting in a spectrum of atrophic gastritis and gastric atrophy with hypochlorhydria, pernicious anaemia and a predisposition to gastric cancer. It is associated with other autoimmune diseases, e.g., diabetes and mucosal damage is mediated by circulating antibodies to gastrin receptors on the parietal cells. The anaemia is due to lack of gastric intrinsic factor with decreased vitamin B12 absorption in the terminal ileum. HP infection is the commonest form of chronic gastritis and increases in incidence with age. The Gram negative, curved bacillus is readily identified (H and E, Cresyl Violet, Giemsa) lying under the surface mucous layer damaging the epithelium and producing a chronic inflammatory reaction in the lamina propria with focal neutrophil polymorph cryptitis. Treatment is by antibiotic eradication.

The *Sydney System* classifies and grades chronic gastritis based on an assessment of histological (neutrophils, chronic inflammation, atrophy, intestinal metaplasia), topographical (antral/corpus predominant or pangastritis) and aetiological (HP, drugs) factors.

Chronic gastritis predisposes to peptic ulceration, gastric carcinoma and malignant lymphoma. Unusual variants such as lymphocytic, granulomatous or eosinophilic gastritis are occasionally seen – infective gastritis occurs in immunosuppressed patients (e.g., CMV) or opportunistically overlying ulceration (e.g., candida fungus).

Peptic ulceration: there are two patient groups:

1. HP antral gastritis → loss of acid regulatory feedback → hyperchlorhydria → duodenitis → duodenal gastric metaplasia with HP colonisation → further duodenitis and duodenal ulcer (DU), or

2. HP pangastritis → hypoacidity → weakening of the mucosal mucous barrier → further gastritis → erosion and gastric ulceration (GU).

Further risk factors include smoking, alcohol and drugs (NSAIDs, aspirin, steroids). DU outnumbers GU (4:1). Benign gastric ulcers are usually on the lesser curve in the vicinity of the incisura.

Complications include acute or chronic bleeding from the ulcer base, perforation with peritonitis, penetration and fistula to an adjacent organ (e.g., colon or pancreas), fibrotic repair resulting in mechanical obstruction such as pyloric stenosis, and rarely, cancer. Surgery for peptic ulceration has decreased dramatically in the last two decades with the evolution of effective anti-ulcer treatments based largely on antibiotic eradication of HP infection and acid suppression (H$_2$ receptor antagonists, proton pump inhibitors (PPIs)). It is now reserved for those peptic ulcers refractory to medical treatment, in which complications have arisen or there is a suspicion of malignancy. Acute haemorrhage is managed conservatively by laser, electrocoagulation or injection of sclerosant.

Hyperplastic polyps: commonest in the antrum and up to 1.5 cm in size, they form 60% of gastric mucosal polyps and are characterised by dilated, hyperplastic glands in oedematous, inflamed lamina propria. Single or multiple, they probably represent healing of the mucosa after erosion – malignant change is extremely rare although there can be cancer elsewhere in the stomach.

Other non-neoplastic polyps: rare, e.g., hamartomatous polyps (Peutz Jegher's/Cronkhite – Canada syndromes), inflammatory fibroid polyp, or common, such as fundic gland cyst polyps – small, multiple, gastric body, cystic dilatation of specialised glands, incidental or associated with PPI therapy/familial adenomatous polyposis coli (FAPC).

Note that various diseases can present as polypoidal gastric folds or hypertrophic gastropathy, e.g., Ménétrier's disease (hypochlordydria, protein loss from elongated gastric pits), Zollinger–Ellison syndrome (pancreatic/duodenal gastrinomas, hyperchlorhydria, multiple peptic ulcers), Crohn's disease, carcinoma or malignant lymphoma.

Neoplastic Conditions

Predisposing conditions: predisposition to gastric neoplasia occurs with HP gastritis, gastric atrophy and previous partial gastrectomy with gastroenterostomy. Antecedent lesions include incomplete intestinal metaplasia (type IIb/III large intestinal variant) and epithelial dysplasia. Dysplasia occurs in flat (commonest), sessile or polypoid mucosa and is categorised as low- or high-grade corresponding to categories 3 and 4 of the Vienna Consensus Classification of Gastrointestinal Epithelial Neoplasia (Table 2.1).

Low-grade dysplasia requires endoscopic follow-up while high-grade dysplasia should be considered for surgical resection due to the strong association (30–80%) with concurrent or subsequent cancer. Polypoid adenomatous dysplasia comprises 8% of gastric polyps but has a 30–40%

Table 2.1. Vienna classification of gastrointestinal epithelial neoplasia

Category	Neoplasia/Dysplasia
1	negative
2	indefinite
3	non-invasive low grade
4	non-invasive high grade
5	invasive – either intramucosal, submucosal or beyond

risk of malignancy related to size, villous architecture and grade of dysplasia. Local resection (endoscopic or surgical) is necessary for full histological assessment.

Adenocarcinoma: forms the majority of gastric malignancy and classically antral (50%) or lesser curve (15%) in site but with an increasing incidence in the proximal stomach and cardia, in part due to HP eradication and loss of its acid suppression effect. Histological patterns are intestinal (50%), diffuse (20%) or mixed/solid (25%) showing correlation with macroscopic appearances and behaviour. Intestinal carcinomas arise from intestinal metaplasia/dysplasia, form ulcerated or polypoid lesions with expansile margins and show lymphovascular spread to regional nodes, liver, lung, adrenal gland and bone. Diffuse carcinomas (signet ring cells) form diffusely infiltrating linitis plastica (leather bottle stomach) undermining the mucosa with transmural spread to the peritoneum where seedlings and classical Krükenberg tumours (bilateral ovarian secondaries) occur. Gastric cancer may be multifocal – resection margins are routinely checked. Distal cancers can involve proximal duodenum, and proximal cancers the distal oesophagus. Tubule-rich, mucin-poor tumours with a circumscribed edge have a better prognosis than tubule-poor, mucin-rich tumours with an infiltrative edge. Depth of spread is defined as early gastric cancer (EGC) confined to the mucous membrane ± regional node involvement, or advanced muscle coat invasive disease which has a much worse prognosis. EGC (10% of cases) can be multifocal in distribution and raised, flat or ulcerated in morphology.

Other carcinomas are rare (e.g., parietal cell, medullary) or metastatic in nature (e.g., breast, lung, kidney, malignant melanoma).

Carcinoid tumour: of gastric endocrine or enterochromaffin-like (ECL) cell origin.
- Multiple (benign): atrophic gastritis/gastric atrophy → hypochlorhydria → hypergastrinaemia → ECL hyperplasia → microcarcinoidosis (multiple, mucosal, 1–3 mm). If < 1 cm, endoscopic removal is sufficient: if 1–2 cm in size, treatment is by polypectomy or local resection as they have uncertain malignant potential.
- Single or sporadic (aggressive): surgical resection if > 2 cm in size, invasion beyond submucosa, angioinvasion or cellular atypia (including necrosis or mitoses). Functionally secreting tumours are also potentially malignant.

Gastrointestinal mesenchymal or stromal tumours (GISTs): spindle or epithelioid cell in type, a minority are leiomyomatous or neural and a majority stromal (CD34, CD117 (c-kit) positive) in character with absent or incomplete myogenic/neural features. Malignancy cannot be accurately predicted but indicators are: size (> 5 cm), cellularity and atypia, tumour necrosis and haemorrhage, infiltrative margins and mitotic activity (> 5/50 high power fields). Malignant spread is to peritoneum and liver. Biopsy proof can be problematic as GISTs are submucosal/mural lesions covered by intact mucosa except for a classical central area of "apple-core" ulceration.

Malignant lymphoma: primary with disease bulk in the stomach and regional nodes, or secondary to systemic nodal disease. Single, multiple, plaque-like, ulcerated or as thickened folds, it has a rubbery, fleshy appearance. The majority are of B cell MALT (mucosa associated lymphoid tissue) type and strongly associated with HP chronic gastritis. Low- or high-grade, the former can be difficult to diagnose, requiring an accumulation of histological, immunohistochemical and molecular evidence over a number of biopsy episodes. Cardinal features are the density and uniformity of the lymphoid infiltrate, loss and destruction of mucosal glands, demonstration of immunoglobulin light chain restriction and heavy chain gene rearrangements. High-grade lymphoma transforms from a low-grade lesion or presents de novo and must be distinguished immunohistochemically from poorly differentiated carcinoma. Rarely, there can be an association between MALToma and concurrent or subsequent adenocarcinoma.

Prognosis: the majority of patients with gastric cancer present with advanced disease and prognosis is poor (20–35% five-year survival) relating to histological type, differentiation, excision margin involvement and, crucially, stage of disease. Following a positive endoscopic biopsy the tumour is staged radiologically and laparoscopically to determine suitability for radical surgery. Current trials are examining the role of preoperative chemotherapy, which traditionally has been limited to palliative treatment of advanced disease. EGC has a better prognosis (80–95% five-year survival) and may be amenable to local mucosal resection but is converted to completion gastrectomy if the cancer shows unfavourable features such as > 50% surface ulceration, poor differentiation, lymphovascular invasion or involvement of the submucosa or specimen base.

Carcinoid tumours are of low-to intermediate-grade malignancy – 70–80% five-year survival. Low-grade MALTomas are indolent (65–95% five-year survival) whereas high-grade lesions are more aggressive (40–55% five-year survival). Treatment options for gastric lymphoma after appropriate typing, grading and staging (CT scan, bone marrow trephine) include HP eradication, chemotherapy and surgery, the latter particularly if there are anatomical alterations, e.g., gastric outlet obstruction.

GISTs are primarily resected and recurrent abdominal or metastatic liver deposits treated by specific chemotherapy (STI 571 agent).

5. Surgical Pathology Specimens – Clinical Aspects

Biopsy Specimens

Flexible endoscopy is the cornerstone for investigation and diagnosis of gastric-related symptoms. Biopsies for gastritis should be taken according to the Sydney protocol from antrum, body and incisura and any abnormal areas. Specific lesions such as ulcers need multiple biopsies from the base and margin quadrants. A peptic ulcer has a classic endoscopic appearance in that it is round/oval and sharply "punched out" with straight walls. Heaping up of mucosal margins is rare in benign ulcers and should raise the suspicion of malignancy. Size does not reliably differentiate between benign and malignant ulcers as 10% of benign ulcers are greater than 4 cm in diameter. Tumours covered by intact mucosa such as diffuse gastric carcinoma or GISTs are often difficult to demonstrate by mucosal biopsy and endoscopic FNA may be employed.

Resection Specimens

Benign Conditions

As alluded to above, surgery for chronic peptic ulceration is now unusual. It aims to remove the gastric ulcer and the gastrin-producing G cells that drive acid secretion. This is accomplished by a Bilroth I distal gastrectomy with a gastroduodenal anastomosis (Figure 2.3). Alternatively, blockage of gastric innervation is achieved by transecting the vagus nerve trunks as they emerge through the diaphragmatic hiatus (truncal vagotomy) resulting in reduced gastric secretions and motility. Because of the latter, a drainage procedure, either pyloroplasty or gastrojejunostomy must also be done. This approach is used in elderly frail patients or for refractory DU. Highly selective vagotomy preserves pyloric innervation, negating the need for a drainage procedure. The now-rare Bilroth II gastrectomy for DU comprises a distal gastrectomy with oversewing of the duodenal stump and fashioning of a gastrojejunal anastomosis of either Polya or Roux-en-Y type. The latter prevents bile reflux as the distal duodenum is joined to the jejunum some 50 cm distal to the gastrojejunal anastomosis.

Bilroth I gastrectomy with gastroduodenal anastomosis

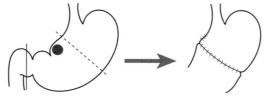

Vagotomy with drainage

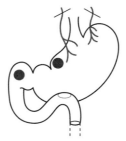

Bilroth II gastrectomy with gastrojejunal anastomosis

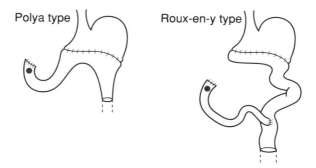

Figure 2.3.   Gastric surgery for gastroduodenal peptic ulceration.

Malignant Conditions

Curative gastric surgery should involve removal of the tumour with a 5 cm rim of "normal" tissue and the related lymph nodes. The surgeon may prefer to perform a partial or total gastrectomy depending on the site and type of tumour (e.g., diffuse carcinoma) and medical fitness of the patient.

Total gastrectomy: this can be done with or without radical lymph node dissection. Both procedures employ an upper midline abdominal incision. In a total gastrectomy without radical lymph node dissection (D1 resection) the stomach is removed with the lesser and greater omenta (which contain local lymph nodes). In this resection nodes may also be found along the greater curvature and the gastrosplenic omentum. A radical gastrectomy (D2 resection) involves removal of the stomach, lesser omentum – with careful dissection of nodes along the hepatic artery and coeliac plexus, greater omentum and gastrosplenic omentum. Nodes should also be removed from along the portal vein, splenic artery and the retropancreatic area. In Japan an even more radical procedure is popular which involves en-bloc resection of the stomach, spleen, distal pancreas and associated lymph node groups.

Good margin clearance is crucial and so the oesophagus is divided as far proximally as is needed and occasionally this may involve entering the chest. The distal margin of resection is formed by division of the first part of the duodenum. Continuity is restored by an oesophagojejunostomy with a Roux-en-Y diverting limb for the duodenal stump.

Partial gastrectomy: the type of procedure employed will depend on the site of the tumour:

● proximal tumours – tumours in the vicinity of the OG junction may arise in the distal oesophagus and infiltrate distally, or in the cardia/fundus and infiltrate proximally. Various procedures may be employed (see Oesophagus, page 18):
  – transhiatal distal oesophagectomy with proximal gastrectomy for tumours of the distal oesophagus/OG junction/cardia.
  – transhiatal distal oesophagectomy with total gastrectomy for tumours of the cardia with extensive distal spread.
  – a more extensive oesophagectomy (via either a two-field approach or thoracotomy) with proximal/total gastrectomy for junctional tumours with extensive proximal spread.
● distal tumours – either a Bilroth I or Bilroth II procedure with the latter being favoured as the anastomosis is wider (important if there is local recurrence) and further away from the likely site of recurrence.

6. Surgical Pathology Specimens – Laboratory Protocols

Biopsy and Local Mucosal Resection Specimens

See Gastrointestinal Specimens – General Comments (page 6)

Resection Specimens

Specimen

● the majority of gastric resections are for neoplastic conditions. However because of the difficulty in reliably distinguishing between benign and malignant gastric ulcers on gross inspection it is practical to use the same handling procedures. Irregular elevated mucosal margins and absence of radial mucosal folds are possible pointers to malignancy. Benign ulcers usually do not occur on the greater curvature.
● partial gastrectomy (proximal or distal), total/radical gastrectomy, variable amounts of lesser and greater omental fat including unspecified or separately named regional lymph node groups, with or without spleen removed because of either direct involvement by gastric cancer or for technical reasons eg operative access or capsular tear at surgery.

Initial procedure

● by palpation and with the index finger locate the lumenal position of the tumour/ulcer.
● open the specimen along the curvature opposite to and avoiding the tumour/ulcer.
● measurements:
  – distal oesophagus, greater curvature, duodenal cuff – lengths (cm).

- tumour/ulcer:
    - length × width × depth (cm) or maximum dimension (cm).
    - distances (cm) to the proximal and distal limits of excision.
    - distances (cm) to the OG junction. If > 50% of the tumour/ulcer bulk is below the junction designate as gastric in origin (Siewert III), if straddling it consider as a junctional lesion (Siewert II). External landmarks may be helpful: oesophagus is orientated to adventitia, stomach to serosa.
- photograph.
- paint any relevant area of serosa and omental margin suspicious of tumour involvement or close to its edge.
- fixation by immersion in 10% formalin for 48 hours either gently packed with formalin-soaked lint, or if suitable, pinned out on a cork board in the opened position.

Description

- tumour/ulcer site
    - distal oesophagus/cardia/fundus/corpus/antrum/pylorus/lesser curve/greater curve/ anterior/posterior/multifocal/extension to duodenum or oesophagus.
- tumour
    - polypoid/ulcerated/scirrhous/mucoid/irregular margins: usual carcinoma.
    - thickened, non-expansile wall/intact granular mucosa: diffuse gastric carcinoma.
    - plaque/granular mucosa/depressed/multifocal: EGC.
    - plaque/thickened folds/ulcerated/fleshy/multifocal: malignant lymphoma.
    - nodular/ulcerated/yellow: carcinoid tumour.
    - polypoid/mural/dumb-bell shaped/apple-core ulceration:GIST.
- ulcer
    - mucosal edges: flat/punched out/elevated.
    - base: blood vessels/perforation/penetration (e.g., pancreas or fistula present).
- mucosa: oedematous/atrophic/granular/thickened.
- wall
    - tumour: confined to mucous membrane, in the wall or through the wall.
    - ulcer: perforation/penetration.
- serosa: involved by tumour/coated in exudate.
- omenta: involved by tumour: circumscribed/irregular margin.
    - maximum deposit size (cm).
    - distance of tumour from the omental edge (mm).

Blocks for histology (Figure 2.4)

- sample the proximal and distal limits of resection – complete circumferential transverse sections (duodenum, oesophagus) or multiple circumferential blocks (mid-stomach).
- alternatively, if separate anastomotic doughnuts are submitted – one complete circumferential transverse section of each.
- count and sample all lymph nodes (lesser/greater omenta, splenic hilum) and process separately any named lymph nodes.
- sample a minimum of four blocks of tumour and wall to show any serosal involvement and the deepest point of omental invasion. Serial transverse slices (3–4 mm thick) or quadrant sections may be used according to the anatomy of the lesion and adjacent structures.

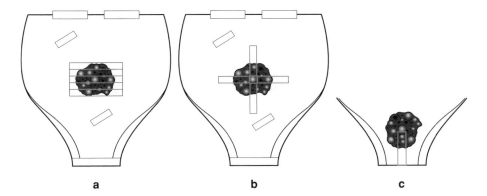

Figure 2.4. Distal gastrectomy – serial, transverse slices (**a**) or quadrant sections (**b**) may be used according to the anatomy of the lesion and adjacent structures. A longitudinal limit block (**c**) may be taken if the tumour is close (< 0.5 cm to it).

- – tumour ulcer: four sections to include the ulcer base, edge, adjacent mucosa and wall.
- – tumour polyp: two sections from the body of the polyp and a minimum of two from the underlying base and wall.
- – linitis plastica: six transmural blocks as a gross lesion is often not evident and the extent of local spread may vary.
- – GISTs: roughly one block per centimetre diameter to include mucosal, mural and extramural components of the tumour.
- – omental tumour: representative blocks in relation to the nearest omental edge/serosa.
- ● sample any other satellite lesions or abnormal areas of mucosa.
- ● sample non-neoplastic gastric mucosa away from the tumour/ulcer (two blocks).
- ● serially slice, at 1 cm intervals, spleen and pancreas (if present) and sample two blocks.

Histopathology report

- ● tumour type
  - – adenocarcinoma: intestinal/diffuse/mixed/mucin-rich/mucin-poor.
  - – malignant lymphoma.
  - – GIST.
- ● tumour differentiation
  - – adenocarcinoma – well/moderate/poor defined as tubule-rich or tubule-poor.
  - – malignant lymphoma – MALToma/centrocytic/follicle centre cell/other.
  - – low-grade/high-grade.
  - – GIST – spindle cell/epithelioid.
    - – cellularity/atypia/mitoses/necrosis/margins/size.
    - – leiomyomatous/neural/stromal (CD34, CD117).
- ● tumour edge – pushing/infiltrative/lymphoid response.
- ● extent of local tumour spread (for carcinoma).
  - – pTis	carcinoma in situ: intraepithelial tumour without invasion of the lamina propria.
  - – pT1	tumour invades lamina propria or submucosa.
  - – pT2	tumour invades muscularis propria (pT2a) or subserosa or lesser/greater omenta (pT2b).
  - – pT3	tumour penetrates serosa (visceral peritoneum) without invasion of adjacent structures.

- pT4   tumour invades adjacent structures (spleen, transverse colon, liver, diaphragm, pancreas, abdominal wall, adrenal gland, kidney, small intestine, retroperitoneum).
  - EGC = pT1 ± lymph node involvement.
  - advanced carcinoma = pT2/pT3/pT4 ± lymph node involvement.
- lymphovascular invasion – present/not present.
- regional lymph nodes
  - perigastric, hepatoduodenal, nodes along the left gastric, common hepatic, splenic and coeliac arteries. Also for the gastrooesophageal junction – paracardial, diaphragmatic, lower mediastinal paraoesophageal. Other intra-abdominal lymph nodes are distant metastases (pM1).
  - pN0   no regional lymph node metastasis.
  - pN1   1 to 6 involved regional node(s).
  - pN2   7 to 15 involved regional nodes.
  - pN3   more than 15 involved regional nodes.
- excision margins
  - proximal and distal limits of tumour clearance (cm).
  - separate proximal oesophageal/gastric and distal gastric/duodenal anastomotic doughnuts – involved/not involved/presence of mucosal dysplasia.
  - deep circumferential omental margin of clearance (mm).
  - deep margin of clearance (mm) in polypectomy and endoscopic mucosal resection specimens.
- other pathology
  - satellite foci, polyps, intestinal metaplasia, dysplasia, gastric atrophy, *Helicobacter* gastritis, MALToma, hypertrophic gastropathy (e.g., Ménétrier's disease, Zollinger–Ellison Syndrome), ECL cell hyperplasia/microcarcinoidosis.

3 Pancreas, Duodenum, Ampulla of Vater and Extrahepatic Bile Ducts

1. Anatomy

Duodenum

The small intestine is divided into three parts: duodenum, jejunum and ileum. The duodenum is C-shaped and joins the gastric pylorus to the proximal jejunum by curving around the head of the pancreas. It is 25 cm long and receives the openings of the common bile and pancreatic ducts. The proximal 2.5 cm is covered on its anterior and posterior surfaces by peritoneum, the remainder being retroperitoneal. The duodenum, for purposes of description, is divided into four parts (D1–4). At the duodenojejunal junction the intestine turns forward – this being called the duodenojejunal flexure.

The mucosa of the duodenum is thick and thrown into numerous circular folds called *plicae circulares*. The common bile duct and the major pancreatic duct pierce the medial wall of D2, approximately half way along its length. At this point there is a small elevation called the major duodenal papilla (see below).

Lymphovascular Supply

The arterial supply originates from the coeliac artery and the superior mesenteric artery. Venous drainage is to the portal system. The lymphatics follow the course of the arteries, i.e., those from the proximal half drain to the coeliac nodes and those from the distal duodenum drain to the superior mesenteric nodes via the periduodenal nodes.

Pancreas, Ampulla of Vater and Extrahepatic Bile Ducts

The pancreas is a soft, lobulated retroperitoneal organ which is both an endocrine and exocrine gland. The exocrine portion produces enzymes (lipases, proteases) which are conveyed to the duodenum by the pancreatic duct and are concerned with digestion. The endocrine portion (including the islets of Langerhans) produces hormones such as insulin and glucagon. The pancreas is subdivided as follows (Figure 3.1):

- *Head* – that part to the right of the left border of the superior mesenteric vein. It lies within the concavity of the duodenum. The *uncinate process*, a part of the head, extends from the left posterior to the superior mesenteric vessels.
- *Body* – lies between the left border of the superior mesenteric vein and the left border of the aorta.
- *Tail* – lies to the left of the aorta and comes into contact with the hilum of the spleen. Anteriorly the pancreas has a thin covering capsule.

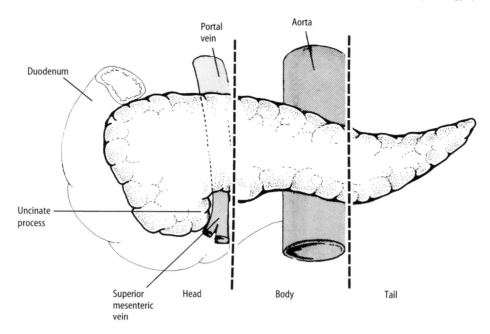

Figure 3.1. Pancreas. Reproduced with permission from Hermanek P, Hutter RVP, Sobin LH, Wagner G, Wittekind Ch (eds.). TNM Atlas: illustrated guide to the TNM/pTNM classification of malignant tumours, 4th edition. Springer-Verlag: Berlin and Heidelberg, 1997.

The extrahepatic bile ducts consist of the right and left hepatic ducts, common hepatic duct and common bile duct (Figure 3.2). The hepatic ducts emerge from the porta hepatis of the liver and converge to form the common hepatic duct. This descends for 4 cm until it is joined from the right side by the cystic duct when it becomes the common bile duct. This is 8 cm long and descends in the free edge of the lesser omentum while in the distal part of its course it lies in a groove on the posterior surface of the pancreatic head. The main pancreatic duct runs the length of the gland and just before the ducts enter the duodenum they converge. Together they open into the ampulla of Vater, a small flask-shaped dilated channel situated in the duodenal wall. The ampulla then opens into the duodenal lumen by the major duodenal papilla (Figure 3.2). The distal part of both ducts and the ampulla are surrounded by muscle fibres, this being termed the sphincter of Oddi. The extrahepatic bile duct system may be subject to a number of variations in its anatomy between individuals.

Lymphovascular Supply

The arterial supply of the pancreas is from the same vessels that supply the duodenum, and venous drainage is to the portal system. The lymphatics follow the arteries to the peripancreatic, pancreaticoduodenal and pyloric nodes, and ultimately to the coeliac and superior mesenteric nodes (Figure 3.3).

The arterial supply to the bile ducts is complex, originating from both the coeliac and superior mesenteric arteries. The lymphatics flow to the infrahepatic, peripancreatic, periduodenal, coeliac and superior mesenteric nodes.

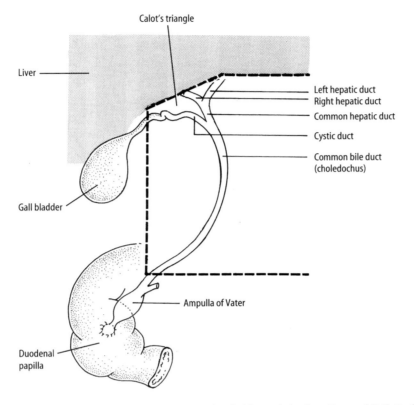

Figure 3.2. Ampulla of Vater and extrahepatic bile ducts. Reproduced with permission from Hermanek P, Hutter RVP, Sobin LH, Wagner G, Wittekind Ch (eds.). TNM Atlas: illustrated guide to the TNM/pTNM classification of malignant tumours, 4th edition. Springer-Verlag: Berlin and Heidelberg, 1997.

2. Clinical Presentation

The symptomatology of duodenal peptic ulceration has been discussed in the previous chapter. Duodenal neoplasms, although rare, may lead to epigastric pain and obstructive jaundice if present in the region of the ampulla.

Classically acute pancreatitis presents with severe epigastric pain which radiates to the back. Chronic pancreatitis produces less acute, but often intractable, epigastric pain. Complications of acute pancreatitis such as shock, infection of necrotic tissue, bowel ileus, metabolic disturbance and multiorgan failure produce characteristic clinical features.

Bacterial infection in the bile ducts is usually due to secondary infection of obstructed ducts and leads to cholangitis with pain, fever, rigors and jaundice. If severe, the cholangitis may become "ascending" and cause liver abscesses.

Neoplasms of the head of pancreas (excluding the uncinate process), ampulla of Vater and extrahepatic bile ducts lead to obstructive jaundice. Tumours elsewhere in the pancreas do not and so will present later. Obstructive jaundice, because of a lack of absorption of fat and increased excretion of bilirubin in the urine, leads to light-coloured faeces and dark urine. In general, pancreatic and bile duct neoplasms result in vague, poorly localised epigastric pain, anorexia and weight loss.

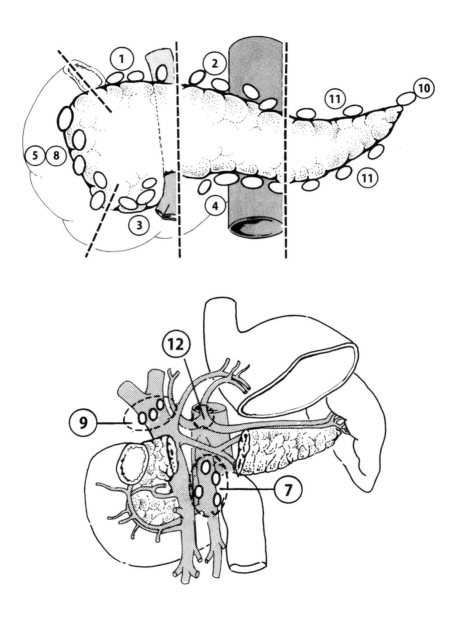

Figure 3.3.   Pancreas and ampulla of Vater: regional lymph nodes are peripancreatic (1–4, 11), pancreaticoduodenal (5, 8), splenic hilar (10), proximal mesenteric (7), common bile duct (9) and coeliac (12). Reproduced with permission from Hermanek P, Hutter RVP, Sobin, LH, Wagner, G, Wittekind, Ch. (Eds). TNM Atlas: Illustrated guide to the TNM/pTNM classification of malignant tumours, 4th edition. Springer-Verlag: Berlin and Heidelberg, 1997.

Tumours of the endocrine pancreas may produce characteristic clinical features because of the hormones they produce:

- insulinoma – psychiatric/neurological symptoms
- gastrinoma – Zollinger–Ellison syndrome
- glucagonoma – diabetes mellitus and skin rash
- VIPoma – watery diarrhoea, hypokalaemia and achlorhydria (WHDA) syndrome.

3. Clinical Investigations

The investigation of duodenal peptic ulcer disease was discussed in the previous chapter.

- Urea and Electrolytes (U and E) – electrolyte imbalance may occur in acute pancreatitis and certain endocrine tumours.
- Serum amylase – elevated in acute pancreatitis.
- Clotting screen – may be deranged in obstructive jaundice because of lack of absorption of fat-soluble vitamins which are required in the synthesis of certain clotting factors.
- Liver function tests – obstructive jaundice picture (elevated alk phos and α GT – see page 109).
- CA19–9 – serum marker of pancreatic malignancy.
- CXR – to detect pulmonary metastases.
- AXR – 10% of gallstones are radio-opaque. Air in the biliary tree may also be seen if there has been previous surgery or a biliary–intestinal fistula.
- USS – to diagnose acute pancreatitis and may detect gall stones in the bile ducts. Tumours less than 1 cm will not be detected. It will also confirm the presence of obstructive jaundice by demonstrating dilated intrahepatic ducts.
- CT (chest, abdomen and pelvis) and MRI scan – will detect primary tumour and any metastatic spread.
- Intravenous cholangiogram – certain contrast agents are excreted by the liver and so will opacify the bile ducts – these can then be visualised radiologically.
- Percutaneous transhepatic cholangiogram (PTC) – another method of visualising the bile ducts is by injecting contrast into the right lobe of the liver.
- Radionucleotide scanning – good for showing obstruction and inflammation in the bile ducts.
- OGD/ERCP – may be used for both diagnostic and therapeutic purposes (see below).
- Peritoneal aspiration – for malignant cells in ascitic fluid.
- Percutaneous FNAC or needle core biopsy – may provide a preoperative diagnosis.
- Staging laparoscopy with biopsy.
- Doppler studies of the portal vein and angiography may be used to ensure that the vessels are not involved by tumour.
- Serum gut hormone levels and octreotide isotope uptake scan – pancreatic and duodenal endocrine tumours.

4. Pathological Conditions

Non-neoplastic Conditions

Duodenum: duodenitis and DU have been previously discussed – gastric metaplasia, or nodular gastric heterotopia in D1 and Brunner's gland hyperplasia are also encountered in biopsies of the proximal duodenum. Biopsy for coeliac disease is considered under small intestine (page 53).

Ampulla of Vater: inflammatory polyps of the duodenal papilla are small, pedunculated and often ulcerated. Partly traumatic in origin due to passage of calculi from the biliary tree, distinction from neoplasia at OGD/ERCP can be difficult and biopsy is required.

Pancreas: the distal pancreatic duct forms a common channel with the terminal common bile duct in 50–60% of patients resulting in a strong association between pancreatitis and biliary tract disease.

Acute pancreatitis: with an overall mortality of 10–15% it is rarely biopsied or resected. The commonest causes are gall stones, sphincter spasm or incompetence with reflux of duodenal fluid and bile, alcohol, trauma and hypothermia. It is due to release of pancreatic enzymes comprising pancreatic haemorrhage, necrosis and inflammation with saponification and chalky calcification of abdominal fat. It is usually a self-limiting process but critical complications include sepsis, shock, bowel paralysis or perforation. Treatment is resuscitative and supportive – operative intervention can include removal of obstructing gall stones (by ERCP) or infected necrotic tissue (necrosectomy).

Chronic pancreatitis: commonly due to excess alcohol intake, there is correlation between radiological calcification, pancreatic endocrine and exocrine dysfunction and the severity of histological changes. Complications include abscess, systemic fat necrosis and pancreatic pseudocyst. Caused by distruption of the duct system due to obstruction by calculus or tumour, a pseudocyst has a thick fibrous wall lined by granulation tissue but no epithelium. It can rupture into the peritoneal cavity or splenic artery. Treatment is by endoscopic or transabdominal drainage either internally to stomach or duodenum, or externally to skin. Surgical excision is used if small and localised to the body or tail, or if the pseudocyst is thick-walled and not appropriately sited for drainage.

The commonest biopsy expression of chronic pancreatitis is that seen adjacent to a pancreatic tumour or secondary to an ampullary tumour due to duct obstruction. The acinar and stromal changes can mimic pancreatic carcinoma, making interpretation difficult especially on frozen section. Chronic pancreatitis tends to retain its lobular architecture, lacks malignant cytological changes and shows no invasion of nerve sheaths or peripancreatic fat.

Extrahepatic bile ducts: stricture of the common bile duct may be caused by passage of a calculus with or without ascending cholangitis and secondary infection, but is more usually after surgical trauma due to inadvertent injury to or ligation of the duct. Treatment aims to re-establish free drainage of bile to the bowel either by a bypass or stenting procedure (see below).

Neoplastic Conditions

Ampullary adenocarcinoma: arising from adenomatous dysplasia of either the periampullary duodenal or intra-ampullary duct mucosae, it is one of the commonest causes of death in FAPC. Adenoma may be amenable to local excision but radical surgical resection is often required for large lesions and because a surface biopsy showing epithelial dysplasia may harbour underlying invasive adenocarcinoma. Most cases have a well-defined intestinal pattern but in a minority it can be difficult to separate adenocarcinoma of the duodenal papilla, ampulla, distal pancreatic duct and distal common bile duct as they can share similar well-to-moderately differentiated tubular and ductular patterns. Detailed examination of the exact anatomical location in the resection specimen is required and sometimes the only conclusion possible is adenocarcinoma of the ampullary–pancreatico–biliary region. Secondary involvement of the ampulla by pancreatic cancer can occasionally be specified based on the histological features and pattern of mucosal spread.

Benign pancreatic exocrine tumours: congenital cysts (Von Hippel Lindau Syndrome), acquired retention cyst, serous cystadenoma (elderly, macro-/microcystic, fluid filled, central scar, clear cuboidal epithelium).

Pancreatic exocrine tumours of malignant potential: intraductal papillary/mucinous and mucinous cystic tumours with a benign, borderline and malignant spectrum of behaviour related to the degree of epithelial dysplasia and extent of invasion into pancreatic parenchyma and peripancreatic fat. Often, in middle-aged women and uni- or multicystic, they show indolent growth with local spread to the abdomen but prior to this are potentially resectable. Solid pseudopapillary tumour – young females, pseudopapillae of uniform cells, cystic with necrosis, of low malignant potential, often benign.

Pancreatic exocrine carcinoma: arising from dysplastic pancreatic duct epithelium and forming the vast majority of pancreatic tumours, 80–90% are adenocarcinomas which are graded according to the degree of gland formation. Most (70–80%) arise in the pancreatic head with a minority in the body or tail and occasionally multifocal. Perineural invasion is characteristic and diagnostically helpful in biopsies. There is limited suitability for resection (5–10% of cases only). Node negative tumours of the pancreatic head < 3 cm in size may be resected by a Whipple's procedure with an average increase in survival of 1 year but a majority present with locally advanced disease into regional nodes and retroperitoneal tissues. Treatment is mainly palliative – pain control, nutritional support and relief of jaundice by open or laparoscopic bypass, or endoscopic stent insertion to combat biliary obstruction.

Other cancers: unusual but include pleomorphic carcinoma, acinar cell carcinoma, small cell carcinoma, malignant lymphoma (usually from an adjacent nodal lymphoma) and sarcoma, which often represents spread from a primary sarcoma of gut or retroperitoneum.

Pancreatic endocrine tumours: single or multiple and forming a minority of pancreatic tumours they can be small (< 1–2 cm), well circumscribed and pale or yellow in colour. They are positive for general neuroendocrine markers (chromogranin, synaptophysin) and specific peptides, e.g., insulin, glucagon, gastrin. Many (60–85%) are associated with a functional hormonal syndrome, e.g., Zollinger–Ellison syndrome due to pancreaticoduodenal gastrinomas. The pancreas is also involved in 80–100% of type I multiple endocrine neoplasia (MEN) syndrome comprising hyperplasia or tumours of parathyroid, pituitary, adrenal glands and pancreas (usually gastrinoma). Histology does not reliably predict behaviour and better indicators of potential malignancy are functionality and established metastases – insulinoma (85% benign), gastrinoma (60–85% malignant), size > 3 cm, site (e.g., duodenal), invasion of vessels, nodes, adjacent organs and liver.

Extrahepatic bile duct carcinoma: there is an increased incidence in various disorders including ulcerative colitis, sclerosing cholangitis, gall stones and congenital bile duct anomalies. The majority (50–75%) arise in the upper third (including the hilum) with lesser numbers in the middle and distal thirds (10–25% each) or even diffuse and multifocal. Sometimes polypoid but often nodular, ulcerated, sclerotic or strictured, prognosis relates to the stage of disease, location and histological grade. There is characteristic perineural invasion often with involvement of regional lymph nodes, peritoneum or the liver (upper third tumours) at presentation. Other rare cancers are carcinoid tumour, malignant melanoma, lymphoma/leukaemia and in childhood, embryonal rhabdomyosarcoma.

Prognosis: prognosis of pancreatic ductal adenocarcinoma is poor with the majority of patients dead within a number of months. Chemotherapy may have a limited palliative role in some patients. Cystadenocarcinomas are relatively rare but potentially resectable. Pancreatic endocrine tumours have an indolent time course with a 50% 10-year survival and potential chemoresponsiveness even in the presence of metastases. Ampullary carcinoma has a five-year survival of 25–50%, improving to 80–85% if early stage (pT1) disease confined to the sphincter of Oddi. Distal bile duct cancers may be potentially resected with 25% five-year survival. Sclerosing bile duct carcinoma at the hilum (Klatskin tumour) can have an indolent course but the majority of bile duct cancers present late with very limited survival and only palliative biliary drainage (open bypass or laparoscopic/endoscopic stent insertion) is justified.

5. Surgical Pathology Specimens – Clinical Aspects

Biopsy Specimens

The endoscopic technique for the diagnosis of benign lesions of the duodenum has been discussed previously. Endoscopic biopsy of duodenal and ampullary tumours is by OGD or ERCP. Demarcation of ampullary tumours is important as they have a better prognosis and are more amenable to resection than those in the pancreas proper.

ERCP (*endoscopic retrograde cholangiopancreatography*) has many applications in both the investigation and, in certain cases, treatment of biliary and pancreatic disease. However, the ERCP scope differs in that the camera views from the side (lateral view) and not from the end (forward view) as in the gastroscope. This allows the major duodenal papilla to be viewed relatively easily when the tip of the scope is 60–70 cm from the incisor teeth.

Diagnostic techniques – the papilla is cannulated by a catheter passed through the scope. Contrast is then injected at intervals to outline the duct system and radiographs, which appear on a monitor, are taken to check the position of the catheter. The bile duct (cholangiography) and the pancreatic duct (pancreatography) are cannulated in turn and radiographs taken which will provide clues to the aetiology of the condition, e.g., stones, stricture, etc. The following specimens can be taken by ERCP:

- bile and pancreatic juice for cytology.
- brushings from the ducts for cytology.
- FNAC specimens from the duct systems (or duodenum) are useful in submucosal lesions.
- biopsies can be taken from the ampulla or relevant duct system.

ERCP can also be used for *therapeutic procedures:*

- sphincterotomy (division of the sphincter of Oddi) can be performed in patients with a history of common bile duct stones to allow free drainage.
- stone extraction can be performed using a balloon catheter or basket.
- dilatation of stricture using a balloon catheter.
- both benign and malignant biliary strictures may be stented (a palliative procedure in the latter) to reduce jaundice.

ERCP is not without its complications, two of the most common being acute pancreatitis (1–3% of cases) and cholangitis.

Resection Specimens

Neoplastic Lesions – Duodenum, Ampulla, Distal Common Bile Duct and Exocrine Pancreas

At the time of presentation, pancreatic carcinoma is beyond resection in more than 80% of patients. Also, given the advanced age of presentation in the vast majority of patients, over 95% of cases are treated palliatively. However, if the patient is fit, the tumour is less than 3 cm, does not involve major vessels and has not metastasised then a curative procedure may be considered.

Although the type of operation will depend on the site and size of tumour, the curative procedure of choice for duodenal, ampullary, distal common bile duct and pancreatic tumours is a standard *Kausch–Whipple pancreaticoduodenectomy (PD)* – *"Whipple's procedure"*.

This procedure involves a transverse subcostal incision and initial exploration to assess operability. It then involves the en bloc resection of the pancreatic head (with a variable amount of body depending on the location and size of the tumour), distal two thirds of the stomach, duodenum (and proximal 10 cm of jejunum), gall bladder and common bile duct (Figure 3.4a), which may be extended proximally for distal common bile duct tumours. There are many methods (up to 70!) of reconstruction after PD. One of the most popular is the formation of the following (Figure 3.4b):

I.   Pancreaticojejunostomy (end to end).
II.   Hepaticojejunostomy (end to side) – anastomosis of the hepatic duct to the jejunum.
III. Gastrojejunostomy (end to side).
IV.   Jejunojejunostomy (side to side) – this decompresses the proximal jejunal loop and reduces jejuno-gastric reflux.

If there is involvement by tumour of the body and tail, the procedure can be modified to a *total* PD, which includes resection of the body and tail of the pancreas plus or minus the spleen.

For some small ampullary and periampullary (i.e., head of pancreas, distal common bile duct and duodenum) tumours, a *pylorus-preserving PD* is performed. This is essentially identical to a standard PD except that the distal stomach and proximal 3 cm of duodenum are left in situ thus retaining the food storage and release functions of the stomach.

A *distal pancreatectomy* consists of resection of the body and tail of the pancreas, usually including the spleen. This procedure may be used for tumours which are thought to be benign (e.g., cystadenoma) in the distal pancreas.

In all the above procedures, the pancreatic resection margin should be sent for frozen section examination to ensure adequate excision.

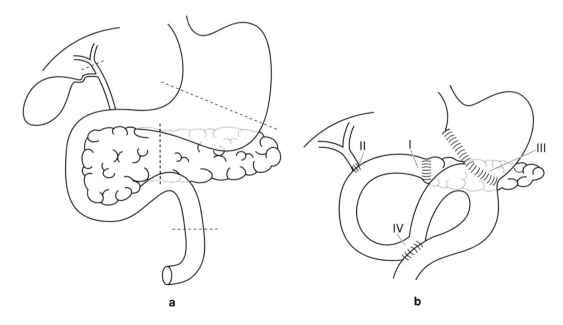

Figure 3.4.   Whipple's procedure – (**a**) limits of resection and (**b**) reconstruction anastomoses.

Neoplastic Lesions of the Endocrine Pancreas

The goals of surgery for tumours of the endocrine pancreas are twofold:

- To locate and excise all abnormal tissue.
- To differentiate between benign and malignant tumours by conducting a search for metastatic deposits.

Localisation of tumours may be carried out by a combination of preoperative imaging (MRI, octreotide scanning) and intraoperative palpation and USS. Once the tumour has been localised, there are two main methods of excision:

- Enucleation – excision of the tumour and a surrounding segment of normal pancreas can be carried out if the tumour is small (< 1.5 cm) and superficial.
- Resection – for larger tumours which are deep-seated, a formal pancreatic resection is required, i.e., a distal pancreatectomy for distal tumours or a proximal pancreatectomy (duodenum-preserving resection of the pancreatic head) for proximal tumours. A PD procedure is only rarely required for large tumours in the head of pancreas or duodenum.

Neoplastic Lesions of the Extrahepatic Bile Ducts

Cancer of the bile ducts (cholangiocarcinoma) is treated palliatively in 80–90% of cases and resection should only be considered in localised tumours without metastatic spread. When surgical resection is considered the type of procedure will depend on the site of tumour:

- Tumours in the distal common bile duct (i.e., lying behind the duodenum and pancreas) – Whipple's procedure.
- Tumours proximal to this and distal to the confluence of the right and left hepatic ducts – wide excision of the supraduodenal biliary tree, gall bladder and related nodes. A length of jejunum is isolated in a Roux-en-Y loop and an end-to-side hepaticojejunal anastomosis allows biliary drainage.
- Tumours proximal to the hepatic confluence require the above plus a relevant liver resection (see Chapter 9).

Palliation for distal common bile duct tumours is most commonly done by ERCP stenting. Other methods of operative palliation (i.e., "bypass" techniques) are:

- Choledochoduodenostomy – proximal common bile duct is anastomosed to D1.
- Hepaticojejunostomy – can be used in more proximal biliary tumours (i.e., common hepatic duct/proximal common bile duct).

For proximal biliary (hilar) tumours, a segment III hepaticojejunostomy can be used. In this the liver is divided to the left of the falciform ligament until the segment III duct is visualised. An anastomosis is then fashioned between this and a Roux-en-Y loop of jejunum.

Non-neoplastic Lesions

Two of the most common complications of *acute pancreatitis* requiring surgical intervention are:

- Necrotising pancreatitis – surgical intervention has a mortality rate of 60% and involves removal of necrotic tissue from the pancreas and retroperitoneal spaces, and drainage of fluid collections.

- Pancreatic pseudocyst – cystogastrostomy – a pseudocyst in the lesser sac is drained into the stomach via an opening in the posterior wall of the stomach.

In *chronic pancreatitis* the following procedures may be employed:

- The pain associated with chronic pancreatitis is caused by obstruction of the pancreatic duct leading to duct hypertension. The *Frey operation* (localised resection of the pancreatic head and side-to-side pancreaticojejunostomy) is designed to decompress the duct.
- When there is disruption of the duct distal to the head, a distal pancreatectomy is indicated.
- Occasionally, when the disease is maximal in the head, a Whipple's procedure may be employed. Another option would be a duodenum-preserving resection of the pancreatic head or total pancreatectomy.

Bile duct stones may be removed laparoscopically or by an open procedure if they cannot be removed by ERCP. Strictures may be stented or bypassed using one of the techniques described above.

6. Surgical Laboratory Specimens – Laboratory Protocols

Biopsy and Local Mucosal Resection Specimens

See Gastrointestinal Specimens – General Comments (pages 6 and 7).

Resection Specimens

Specimen
- Most pancreatic resections are for neoplastic conditions although operative intervention may be indicated for debridement of necrotic tissue in acute pancreatitis, trauma to a major duct or removal of the pancreatic head or pseudocyst in chronic pancreatitis. Resections are either local for pseudocyst or cystic neoplasms, or radical for ampullary, pancreatic head or bile duct cancers. Carcinoma of the body and tail usually presents late and is irresectable.
- To demonstrate the lesion and its relationship to the surgical margins the pancreas is cut into multiple parallel slices in either vertical coronal or horizontal planes, the latter allowing correlation with CT scan cross-sectional images.
- Specimens may be opened and partially incised to aid fixation prior to complete dissection.
- The presence of any surgically labelled structures, e.g., portal vein, or stents should be noted.

Local Resection of Cystic Lesions
- weight (g) and maximum dimension (cm).
- capsule: intact/deficient/smooth/nodular/adhesions/circumscribed/lobulated.
- cut surface: uni-/multilocular/septate/solid areas (cm)/contents – fibrin, mucoid, serous fluid.
- photograph.
- paint the external surface.
- fixation by immersion in 10% formalin for 48 hours.
- sample one block per centimetre diameter of the tumour/cyst to include thin, nodular and solid areas of its wall and internal aspect.
- sample adjacent tissues to include the resection margins and any other structures.

Local Resection of Pancreatic Head in Chronic Pancreatitis

- weight (g) and dimensions (cm): then fix in 10% formalin for 48 hours.
- serially slice perpendicular to the pancreatic duct.
- inspect and describe, e.g., haemorrhage, abscess, necrosis, calculi, calcification.
- select five representative blocks.

Necrosectomy Specimen

- number of pieces, total weight (g) and maximum dimension (cm).
- fix in 10% formalin for 48 hours.
- serially slice, inspect and describe, e.g., haemorrhage, abscess, necrosis, calculi, calcification, tissues present.
- select five representative blocks.

Distal Pancreatectomy (Figure 3.5)

- orientate – cut end is proximal, distal end is uncut ± spleen.
- weight (g) and measurements – length × width × depth (cm).

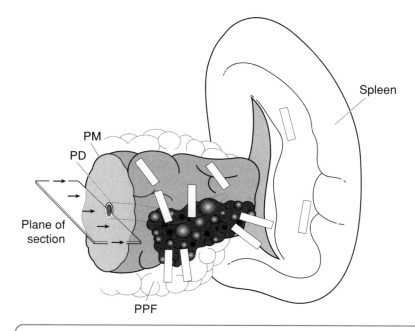

1. Sample resection margins: PD   pancreatic duct
                               PM   proximal pancreatic margin
2. Sample tumour in relation to pancreas, pancreatic duct, peripancreatic fat (PPF) and its margins and spleen.
3. Sample all regional lymph nodes , non-tumourous pancreas and spleen.

Figure 3.5.   Distal pancreatectomy.

- paint the proximal cut margin and the external surfaces using different colours of ink for the various anatomical and surgical aspects – superior, inferior, anterior capsule, posterior retroperitoneal.
- fixation by immersion in 10% formalin for 48 hours.
- transverse section the proximal margin to include the duct.
- serially section the pancreas at 3–4 mm intervals in a horizontal plane parallel to its long axis.
- lay the slices out in sequence and photograph.
- tumour: size (cm), edge (circumscribed/irregular), appearances, consistency, relationship to the pancreatic duct, distances (mm) to the specimen edges.

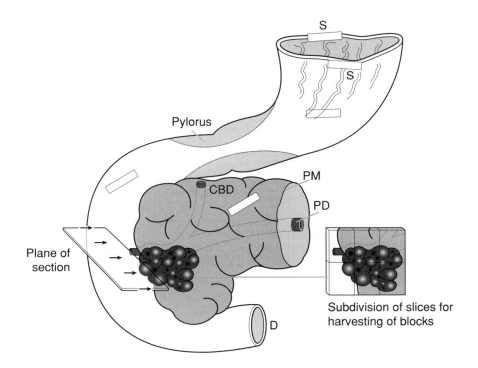

1. Sample resection margins: S   stomach
                              D   distal duodenum
                              CBD common bile duct
                              PD pancreatic duct
                              PM pancreatic margin
2. Sample tumour in relation to the ampulla, pancreas, duct structures, duodenum and peripancreatic tissues including the painted anatomical and surgical margins.
3. Sample duodenum and stomach.
4. Sample all regional lymph nodes and non-tumourous pancreas.

Figure 3.6.   Whipple's procedure for carcinoma of ampulla of Vater, head of pancreas or distal common bile duct

- sample a minimum of five blocks of tumour in relation to pancreas, pancreatic duct, peripancreatic fat and its margins, and spleen.
- sample all regional lymph nodes, pancreas and spleen.

Whipple's Procedure (Figure 3.6)

Initial Procedure

- open with scissors by cutting along the lesser curvature of the stomach and the free border of the duodenum.
- measurements:
  - lengths (cm) of distal sleeve of stomach and duodenum, and parts present (D1–4).
  - dimensions (cm) of pancreas, and parts present (head, body).
  - lengths of gall bladder and bile duct (cm).
- fixation by immersion in 10% formalin for 24–36 hours.
- sample the following surgical margins: proximal gastric, distal duodenal, distal pancreatic face to include the pancreatic duct, and proximal common bile duct.
- paint the external anatomical and surgical margins using different colours of ink and label appropriately – superior, inferior, anterior capsule, posterior retroperitoneal, medial (superior mesenteric vein).
- carefully insert a fine probe into the distal end of the pancreatic duct and gently advance, if possible, to the ampulla.
- place the specimen flat on the bench and with a long, sharp knife use the probe as a guide to horizontally hemisect it, cutting through the peripancreatic duodenum and pancreas. Alternatively, a vertical coronal slice may be used.
- further 24 hours fixation may be required.
- photograph.

Description

- tumour
  - site: duodenal mucosa or papilla/ampulla/pancreas (duct/parenchyma)/bile duct.
  - size: length × width × depth (cm) or maximum dimension (cm).
  - appearance: polypoid/diffuse/ulcerated – ampullary/bile duct tumours.
    - cystic/papillary/mucoid/scirrhous/thickening – pancreatic exocrine tumours.
    - circumscribed/pale/homogeneous – pancreatic endocrine tumours.
  - edge: circumscribed/irregular.
- pancreatic and bile ducts: dilatation/stenosis/extrinsic or intraduct tumour/stent.
- pancreas: indurated/oedematous/fat necrosis.
- peripancreatic lymph nodes: location/number/size.
- other organs: involvement of duodenum or stomach, etc.

Blocks for Histology (Figure 3.6)

- resection margins (see above).
- serial 3–4 mm cuts parallel to the plane of hemisection provide suitable slices for subdividing and harvesting of blocks.
- sample the tumour (a minimum of six blocks) in relation to the ampulla, pancreas, duct structures, duodenum, and peripancreatic tissues including the painted and labelled anatomical/surgical margins.

- sample uninvolved pancreas, stomach and duodenum.
- count and sample all lymph nodes.
- if other organs are present (total or regional pancreatectomy – pancreaticoduodenectomy, gastrectomy, splenectomy, portal vein, transverse colectomy, mesocolon, omentum and regional nodes): describe, weigh, measure, paint and block according to the macroscopic degree of tumour spread. Label the blocks as to their site of origin.

Proximal Extrahepatic Bile Duct Cancer Resection

- bile duct segment – site: common bile duct/common hepatic duct/right or left hepatic duct/ cystic duct.
    - length × diameter (cm).
    - dilated/ulcerated/strictured/cyst and maximum dimension (cm) of lesion.
    - calculi.
- tumour – maximum dimension (cm).
    - site: common bile duct/common hepatic duct/right or left hepatic duct/cystic duct/ intraduct/mural/extramural/involvement of liver.
    - appearance: strictured/ulcerated/nodular/polypoid.
- hepatic resection – segment(s).
    - dimensions (cm) and maximum dimension (cm) of tumour present.
- biliary stent – not present/present/placement (within or outside the lumen).
- gall bladder – present/not present/involved by tumour.
- sample the distal bile duct limit (circumferential transverse section) and the proximal bile duct limit or the hepatic resection margin (two or three blocks).
- paint the external adventitial CRM.
- serially section the specimen transversely at 3–4 mm intervals.
- sample five or six blocks to demonstrate the worst point of tumour invasion in relation to the CRM, liver, gall bladder, proximal and distal surgical limits.
- sample all lymph nodes.

Histopathology Report

- tumour type – ampulla/bile duct: adenocarcinoma
    - pancreas: benign/of low malignant potential/adenocarcinoma/endocrine tumour/other.
- tumour differentiation/grade:
    - ampullary/bile duct adenocarcinoma: well/moderate/poor.
    - pancreatic carcinoma

well/grade 1	> 95% glands
moderate/grade 2	50–95% glands
poor/grade 3	5–49% glands
undifferentiated/grade 4	< 5% glands

- tumour edge – pushing/infiltrative/lymphoid response.
- extent of local tumour spread

Ampulla.

pTis carcinoma in situ.
pT1   tumour limited to the ampulla or sphincter of Oddi.
pT2   tumour invades duodenal wall.
pT3   tumour invades pancreas.

pT4   tumour invades peripancreatic soft tissues, or other adjacent organs or structures.

Pancreas.

pTis carcinoma in situ.
pT1   tumour limited to the pancreas, < 2 cm maximum dimension.
pT2   tumour limited to the pancreas, > 2 cm dimension.
pT3   tumour extends beyond pancreas, but without involvement of coeliac axis or superior
      mesenteric artery.
pT4   tumour involves coeliac axis or superior mesenteric artery.

Extrahepatic bile ducts.

pT1   tumour confined to the bile duct.
pT2   tumour invades beyond the wall of the bile duct.
pT3   tumour invades the liver, gall bladder, pancreas, and/or unilateral tributaries of the portal
      vein (right or left) or hepatic artery (right or left).
pT4   tumour invades any of the following: main portal vein or its tributaries bilaterally, common
      hepatic artery, or other adjacent structures, e.g., colon, stomach, duodenum, abdominal wall.

● lymphovascular invasion – present/not present. Perineural space or lymphovascular invasion is present in up to 50% of pancreaticobiliary carcinomas with spread to regional nodes
  at diagnosis. Involvement of large named vessels, e.g., portal vein, is a major determinant of
  postoperative survival.
● regional lymph nodes: peripancreatic, pancreaticoduodenal, pyloric and proximal mesenteric. Also coeliac (for head of pancreas tumour), and tail of pancreas/splenic hilum nodes
  (for body/tail of pancreas tumours). Also cystic duct, pericholedochal and periportal (for
  extrahepatic bile duct tumours).

pN0   no regional lymph node metastasis.
pN1   metastasis in regional lymph node(s).

● excision margins.
  – proximal gastric and distal duodenal limits of tumour clearance (cm).
  – distal pancreatic surgical margin/common bile duct margin of tumour clearance (mm) –
    also, is mucosal dysplasia present?
  – peripancreatic edge tumour clearance (mm) – superior/inferior/anterior capsule/poste-
    rior retroperitoneal/medial (superior mesenteric vein). The peripancreatic circumferen-
    tial margin is the most commonly involved.
  – for extrahepatic bile duct cancer – tumour clearance (mm) of the distal and proximal
    bile duct, hepatic and radial resection margins.
● other pathology.
  – duodenal adenoma(s), secondary pancreatitis, fat necrosis, calculi, ulcerative colitis,
    sclerosing cholangitis, choledochal cysts.

4 Small Intestine

1. Anatomy

The small intestine is the longest part of the gastrointestinal tract and is divided into the duodenum (discussed previously), jejunum and ileum (Figure 4.1). It is primarily concerned with digestion and absorption of food. Together, the jejunum and ileum measure approximately 6 metres (jejunum 2.5 m/ileum 3.5 m) in the adult. The jejunum commences at the duodenojejunal junction (flexure) and the ileum ends at the ileocaecal valve (two horizontal folds of mucosa that project around the orifice of the ileum as it joins the caecum). A fan-shaped fold of peritoneum (the small intestinal mesentery) attaches the small intestine to the posterior abdominal wall. The long edge of the mesentery completely encloses the intestine, allowing it to be mobile, while the short "root", which is attached to the posterior abdominal wall, admits blood vessels, lymphatics and nerves which supply the intestine by traversing the mesentery.

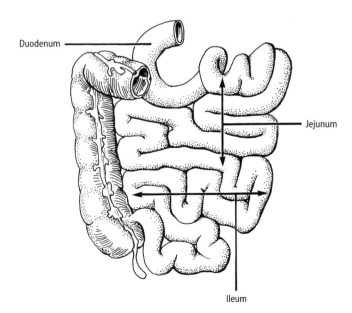

Figure 4.1. Small intestine. Reproduced with permission from Hermanek P, Hutter RVP, Sobin, LH, Wagner, G, Wittekind, Ch. (Eds). TNM Atlas: Illustrated guide to the TNM/pTNM classification of malignant tumours, 4th edition. Springer-Verlag: Berlin and Heidelberg, 1997.

Although there is a gradual change from jejunum to ileum, in general the jejunum tends to be located in the upper part of the abdominal cavity, is thicker-walled with more prominent *plicae circulares* (permanent mucosal folds) and has more numerous *Peyer's patches* (aggregations of lymphoid tissue).

Histologically, the mucosa of the small intestine projects into the lumen in the form of finger-like structures covered by ciliated epithelium. These projections are called *villi* and increase the surface area for absorption. The circular and longitudinal muscle layers are continuous.

Lymphovascular Supply

The arterial supply of the jejunum and ileum is from the superior mesenteric artery. Numerous intestinal branches run in the mesentery and anastomose with one another to form "arterial arcades", which in turn supply the intestine. Venous drainage is via the superior mesenteric vein to the portal system. Lymphatics traverse through a series of mesenteric nodes and ultimately drain to the superior mesenteric nodes situated at the origin of the superior mesenteric artery.

2. Clinical Presentation

Patients with small-intestinal disease may present with vague symptoms and signs such as poorly localised dull central (periumbilical) abdominal pain. If there is full-thickness inflammation the peritoneal somatic pain receptors are stimulated and the pain becomes more severe and localised. A patient with an obstructing lesion will classically present with vomiting, colicky abdominal pain (cramps), absolute constipation (i.e., neither flatulence or faeces passed per rectum) and abdominal distension.

Bleeding into the lumen of the small intestine may lead to hypovolaemic shock and altered blood (melaena) per rectum. Intussusception produces a mixture of blood and mucus – "redcurrant jelly stool" particularly in infants. Perforation, although rare (e.g., trauma, Meckel's diverticulum) will lead to a generalised peritonitis. A heart murmur or irregular pulse may provide a diagnostic clue in embolic small intestinal infarction.

The presentation of Crohn's disease may be insidious or acute, with symptoms including diarrhoea, anorexia and weight loss. Various forms of fistulae (abnormal connection between two epithelial lined structures) may occur including an enterovesical fistula (between small intestine and urinary bladder) which leads to gas in the urine (pneumaturia) and repeated urinary tract infections. Enterocolic and enteroenteric (between adjacent small bowel loops) fistulae may also occur. Enterocutaneous fistulae usually only happen after previous surgery. One of the differential diagnoses of a right iliac fossa mass is Crohn's disease with a peri-intestinal abscess around the distal ileum.

Several conditions, including Crohn's disease, may lead to a protein-losing enteropathy, resulting in generalised oedema. Melanin spots may be seen in the buccal mucosa and lips of those with Peutz–Jegher's syndrome.

3. Clinical Investigations

- U&E – electrolyte imbalance due to malabsorption.
- LFT's/albumin – liver enzymes may be deranged in Crohn's disease and hypoalbuminaemia will occur in protein-losing enteropathy.
- Folate, B12 and iron studies – pernicious anaemia in Crohn's disease.

- Erect CXR – air under the diaphragm in a perforation.
- Erect and supine AXR – will detect gas shadows and fluid levels in distended loops of small intestine in obstruction.
- Small bowel series – radiological contrast is drunk and abdominal images are taken at regular intervals to outline the mucosal surface of the small intestine and to measure the transit time. This is particularly useful for obstructing lesions and Crohn's disease, and may also detect a Meckel's diverticulum.
- Barium enema – will demonstrate an ileocolic intussusception and may be used as a therapeutic procedure (see below).
- Sinogram/fistulogram – useful to delineate the extent of the complications of Crohn's disease.
- CT scan – useful in delineating an abdominal (e.g., right iliac fossa) mass.
- Radioisotope scanning – can be used in cases of repeated gastrointestinal haemorrhage of unknown aetiology and will localise heterotopic gastric mucosa in a Meckel's diverticulum. Radiolabelled red blood cells may show a site of active bleeding.
- Selective arteriography (superior mesenteric) – will aid identification of a site of small intestinal bleeding. This may detect angiodysplasia of the small intestine providing the bleeding rate is greater than 2 ml/minute.
- Enteroscopy – allows direct visualisation of small intestinal mucosa.
- Distal duodenal biopsy and serology (anti-gliadin/endomysial and transglutaminase antibodies) in coeliac disease.

4. Pathological Conditions

Non-neoplastic Conditions

Duodenitis and duodenal ulcer (DU): HP distal gastritis leads to hyperchlorhydria, duodenitis with surface gastric metaplasia, colonisation by HP, further duodenitis and ulceration. Occurring mainly in the cap and first part of the duodenum, DU is invariably benign and only rarely biopsied at laparotomy for perforation if its mucosal edges are irregular. DU is successfully treated by HP eradication – occasionally it is due to other causes, e.g., NSAIDs, Crohn's disease or Zollinger–Ellison syndrome.

Coeliac disease: traditionally investigated by Crosby capsule biopsy of the proximal jejunum, it is now assessed by a combination of coeliac serology and distal duodenal biopsies taken at flexible OGD. Cardinal features are an excess of surface intra-epithelial lymphocytes, villous atrophy and crypt hyperplasia. Proof is by clinical improvement on a gluten-free diet and deterioration on subsequent rechallenge. It is present thoughout the small intestine and can be complicated by malignant lymphoma or adenocarcinoma. Other conditions can produce similar mucosal changes, e.g., *Giardia lamblia* infestation, lactose intolerance or post-infective enteritis, but are usually not gluten responsive. *Giardia* is a kite-shaped flagellate protozoon present in the intervillous mucus causing diarrhoea with or without mucosal inflammation – it typically affects children or the elderly.

Crohn's disease (regional enteritis): a pan-gastrointestinal inflammatory condition of uncertain aetiology, lesions can occur anywhere from the mouth to the anus. It is characterised by segmental, transmural chronic inflammation associated with linear and fissuring ulceration, and, in 40% of cases non-caseating epithelioid and giant cell granulomas present either in the mucous membrane, bowel wall or regional lymph nodes. The terminal ileum, ileum and colon, or colon alone are affected in decreasing order of frequency. Macroscopically there are skip lesions comprising stenotic ring strictures and hosepipe segments, serosal fat encroachment (fat wrapping), fissure ulcers with fistulae to other organs and abscess formation, and ulceration which can be pin-point (aphthous), linear or contiguous. Perianal fissures or fistulae are also often present. Due to its segmental distribution subsequent recurrence elsewhere in the gut is not infrequent. Complications can be gastrointestinal, e.g., adenocarcinoma or malignant lymphoma, or extraintestinal such as liver disease, amyloid or arthritis.

Other causes of ileitis include backwash ileitis in ulcerative colitis, ileo-caecal tuberculosis or yersinial infection. Viral adenitis of the mesenteric lymph nodes can also mimic ileitis or appendicitis. Relatively common viral or bacterial gastroenteritis rarely provide histopathology material. Immunodeficency, e.g., AIDS, predisposes to various opportunistic infections (giardia lamblia, mycobacterium avium intracellulare, CMV, etc.) and malignancies (malignant lymphoma, Kaposi's sarcoma) that need to be considered on duodenal or terminal ileal biopsy.

Meckel's diverticulum: in 2% of people, 2 inches long, 2 feet from the ileo-caecal valve and "too" important to forget, this is a remnant of the foetal vitellointestinal duct comprising an outpouching of the ileal wall on its antemesenteric border with or without a fibrous cord attaching it to the umbilicus. Its wall is continuous with the ileal muscle coat and the small intestinal lining not infrequently shows heterotopic gastric or pancreatic tissue. Complications (4% of cases) include peptic diverticulitis with ulceration, haemorrhage or perforation, intussusception, or rarely malignancy.

Obstruction: broadly, small intestinal obstruction is either due to loss of peristaltic bowel movement (paralytic ileus), or is mechanical in nature. Ileus is commonly seen in the postoperative period of abdominal surgery and is self-limiting although it is also encountered in various metabolic disturbances and can be difficult to manage – histopathology specimens are rarely provided. Mechanical obstruction is due to blockage of the bowel lumen or distortion of its wall. Common causes are primary or secondary malignancy, ulceration with ring stricture/diaphragm formation (Crohn's disease, NSAIDs), incarceration within a hernia, or extrinsic compression by postoperative adhesions or fibrous bands. The proximal bowel dilates, fills with fluid and ultimately becomes atonic – sepsis or ischaemia are possible complications. Particular forms of enteric obstruction are volvulus where a loop of bowel twists around its mesenteric pedicle, and intussusception where a lumenal or mural abnormality (e.g., tumour) acts as a nidus for peristalsis to propel a proximal segment (the intussusception) forwards and inside a receiving distal segment (the intussuscipiens). The intussusception can be benign or malignant in nature and variable in site, e.g., ileal–ileal or ileal–caecal. Handling of all these specimens is targeted at determining the nature of the obstructing abnormality, its distribution and completeness of excision and the presence and extent of secondary changes such as inflammation or ischaemia.

Inflammatory fibroid polyp: an inflammatory mucosal pseudotumour of unknown aetiology that can form the apex of an intussusception, it comprises oedematous and inflamed fibrovascular granulation tissue with an infiltrate of eosinophils.

Diaphragm disease: due to chronic ingestion of NSAIDs it comprises multiple diaphragm-like mucosal ring strictures with variable lumen stenosis and intervening compartmentalisation and sacculation. The strictures have a triangular cross sectional profile of fibrovascular connective tissue and are probably partly ischaemic in nature. Presentation is with subacute obstruction.

Ischaemia: acute, subacute or chronic depending on the nature, severity and rapidity of onset of the cause. Acute ischaemia is characterised by haemorrhagic necrosis of bowel wall that becomes paper thin and gangrenous with subsequent electrolyte imbalance, sepsis and shock. Chronic ischaemia comprises ulcerated segments or strictures with replacement of bowel wall by fibrovascular connective tissue, evidence of secondary vascular thickening and haemosiderin deposition. Examination of these specimens must include assessment of resection limit viability and any abnormality of the mesenteric vessels. Common causes are arterial, such as mesenteric artery embolism or thrombosis (particularly if superimposed on a low flow state due to mesenteric atheroma or cardiogenic hypotension), or venous thrombosis. The latter is usually due to obstruction of venous flow by bowel entrapment within a hernia, or kinking of its mesentery by a fibrous band or adhesion resulting from previous surgery. Less usual causes of ischaemia are systemic vasculitis (e.g., polyarteritis) or amyloid deposition which thickens and occludes mesenteric and mural vessels. Drugs must always be considered as a cause of isolated ulcers or chronic ischaemic segments, especially NSAIDs.

Hernia: herniation of the bowel can be either internal or external. Internal hernias are into anatomical spaces, e.g., the lesser omental sac or across fibrous bands, which can be acquired (postoperative) or congenital (e.g., persistent vitellointestinal duct). External hernias involve protrusion of the peritoneum ± bowel into the layers of the abdominal wall (particularly at the site of a previous surgical incision), groin or femoral canal. They can be intermittent and reducible or irreducible with the risk of secondary ischaemic changes. The surgical specimens are dealt with elsewhere (see Chapter 10).

Non-neoplastic polyps: in the duodenum these include gastric heterotopia, Brunner's gland hyperplasia/adenoma and pancreatic heterotopia. Small intestine is the commonest site for Peutz–Jegher's syndrome, which is autosomal dominant comprising oral pigmentation and pangastrointestinal polyposis – the polyps have a branching smooth muscle core and twisting of the polyp can produce glandular herniation into the submucosa and mimicry of adenocarcinoma. The terminal ileum can show mucosal nodular lymphoid hyperplasia which is usually of unknown aetiology but is occasionally linked to immunodeficiency. A protruberant ileo-caecal valve or fatty hyperplasia of its submucosa can simulate a tumour on radiological investigation.

Neoplastic Conditions

Forming less than 10% of all bowel tumours, duodenal/jejunal lesions tend to be adenomas or adenocarcinoma whereas carcinoid tumour and malignant lymphoma have a predilection for the ileum.

Adenoma: relatively unusual in the small bowel but commoner in D2 particularly in FAPC where there is a strong association with periampullary adenocarcinoma. Surgical removal is either by endoscopy or duodenotomy with thorough assessment of the ampullary region to exclude underlying tumour that would necessitate radical resection. Adenomas can also occur sporadically in the jejunum or ileum giving rise to adenocarcinoma.

Adenocarcinoma: duodenal cancers (70% of cases) are often polypoid while distal lesions are ulcerated and napkin ring-like. Presentation is late with regional lymph node metastases and serosal involvement due to the fluid content of the small bowel and consequent lack of symptoms. Prognosis is poor and incidence is increased in Crohn's disease and coeliac disease.

Carcinoid tumour: single or multiple, carcinoid tumour is of intermediate-grade malignancy, metastatic potential relating to size (> 1–2 cm), angioinvasion, invasion beyond the submucosa and functionality. It produces vasoactive peptides, e.g., serotonin that cause vascular thickening and elastotic stromal fibrosis which distorts the bowel wall leading to subacute obstruction or intussusception. Metastatic deposits in the liver result in the peptides accessing the systemic venous circulation and carcinoid syndrome – facial flushing, asthma and thickening of cardiac valves. Carcinoid tumours can be ulcerated or nodular, and are usually yellow. Other neuroendocrine lesions occur in the duodenum and include gastrinoma as part of Zollinger–Ellison syndrome, somatostatinoma and gangliocytic paraganglioma, both of which may be associated with von Recklinghausen's syndrome (neurofibromatosis).

Malignant lymphoma: solitary or multifocal, primary or secondary to systemic nodal disease, the vast majority are non-Hodgkin's in type. Established disease is ulcerated, segmental and rubbery or fleshy in appearance. Many are MALT derived of B cell character and variably low- or high-grade, prognosis relating to the grade and stage of disease. Unusual variants of malignant lymphoma include multiple lymphomatous polyposis (ileo-colonic nodular polyps of mantle cell lymphoma), ileo-caecal Burkitt's lymphoma in children and immunosuppressed patients, and enteropathy-associated T cell lymphoma (EATCL). EATCL is strongly associated with coeliac disease, either occult or clinically established of short or long duration. Presentation can be with perforated ulcerative jejunitis, a change in response to the gluten free diet or with abdominal pain/mass.

Gastrointestinal mesenchymal or stromal tumours (GISTs): spindle or epithelioid cell in type, a minority are leiomyomatous or neural and a majority stromal (CD34, CD117 (ckit) positive) in character with absent or incomplete myogenic/neural features. Malignancy cannot be accurately predicted but indicators are: size (> 2–5 cm), cellularity and atypia, tumour necrosis and haemorrhage, infiltrative margins and mitotic activity (> 5/30–50 high power fields). Small-intestinal GISTs tend to behave more aggressively than their equivalent gastric counterparts with spread to the abdominal peritoneum and liver. There is differing opinion as to whether the neural variant GANT (gastrointestinal autonomic nerve tumour) is of worse prognosis. The tumour can be polypoid, mural or dumb-bell shaped with an extramural component. Occasionally they arise primarily in the small bowel mesentery or retroperitoneum with no attachment to gastrointestinal wall.

Metastases: the small intestine is particularly prone to involvement by metastatic adenocarcinoma either from other abdominopelvic sites, e.g., stomach, pancreas, colorectum and ovary, or due to distant spread, e.g., lung, breast, malignant melanoma. Deposits can be nodular, ulcerate or stricture the bowel wall mimicking a primary lesion – designation as a primary small intestinal adenocarcinoma therefore necessitates exclusion of spread from a more common site or evidence of a point of origin, e.g., an adjacent mucosal adenoma. Alternatively, the deposits may be as diffuse peritoneal seedlings. Malignant melanoma can be pigmented.

Prognosis: small bowel adenocarcinoma is unusual being fifty times less common than colorectal cancers. Presentation is late with poor prognosis (10–30% five-year survival). Carcinoid tumour has an overall five-year survival rate of 50–65% with smaller (< 1–2 cm), early lesions confined to the bowel wall being more favourable. Prognosis is better for low-grade B cell lymphomas (44–75% five-year survival) than high-grade B or T cell lymphomas (25–35% five-year survival) and is strongly grade- and stage-dependent. GISTs are of intermediate behaviour and recurrent lesions may respond to specific chemotherapy.

5. Surgical Pathology Specimens – Clinical Aspects

Biopsy Specimens

Biopsy specimens can be obtained from the ileocaecal valve and terminal ileum by colonoscopy. They can also be obtained during laparotomy by either enteroscopy or wedge resection of a serosal lesion. In enteroscopy an incision is made in the wall of the small intestine and an endoscope is passed along the small intestinal lumen to view the region of interest. The endoscope can also be introduced orally and the surgeon can guide it through the stomach and small intestine during a laparotomy.

Resection Specimens

Although small intestine may be resected as part of another procedure, e.g., right hemicolectomy, in primary small bowel resection the goals of surgery are removal of the lesion and restoration of intestinal continuity. However, the exact procedure will depend on the type of lesion to be dealt with.

Neoplastic Conditions

Tumours: the type of resection will depend on the site of the tumour, e.g., a distal tumour will require a right hemicolectomy. For more proximal lesions the operation of choice is a local resection with en bloc resection of a wedge of mesentery (Figure 4.2).

At least 5 cm of intestine on either side of the tumour should be removed with an end-to-end anastomosis to re-establish continuity. Occasionally, a hamartomatous polyp may be removed by making a longitudinal elliptical incision in the intestinal wall to include the base of the polyp. Closure should be done transversely to avoid luminal narrowing.

Non-neoplastic Conditions

Small intestinal resection in non-neoplastic conditions is essentially similar to that for neoplastic disease in that the affected length of intestine is resected, with continuity being restored by a hand-sewn end-to-end anastomosis. Some specific conditions are discussed below:

Crohn's disease: small bowel resection is usually reserved for those individuals for whom medical treatment has failed or who are suffering complications, e.g., obstruction (due to strictures), peri-intestinal abscess, fistula formation or perforation. Essentially, the extent of resection is limited to the macroscopically involved intestine as extensive resection does not reduce the risk of recurrent lesions and may lead to short bowel syndrome if subsequent resections are necessary.

If there are multiple areas of stricturing these need not be resected in order to preserve intestinal length. Instead, a "widening procedure" called a stricturoplasty may be employed. In this procedure the strictured region is incised longitudinally, the walls retracted and the incision then sutured transversely (Figure 4.3).

Infarction: at laparotomy the infarcted intestine will appear dusky and should be resected until there is active bleeding from the ends that are going to form the anastomosis. A primary anastomosis may be fashioned or in cases of extensive intraperitoneal leakage or uncertain intestinal viability, an ileostomy (or jejunostomy) and distal mucus fistula can be fashioned. Essentially, an ileostomy (or jejunostomy) is produced by bringing the cut opened end of the intestine out

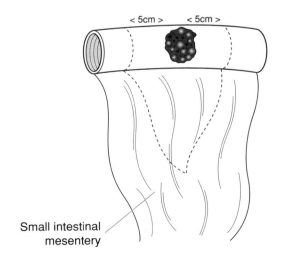

Figure 4.2. Resection of tumour in small intestine.

through an opening in the abdominal wall where it is sutured in place. A special ileostomy bag is then fitted to collect the effluent.

Meckel's diverticulum: they are usually only resected if symptomatic or found incidentally during another procedure. Essentially, the diverticulum is excised with the opening in the intestinal wall closed in a transverse fashion to avoid luminal narrowing. If the diverticulum is large or broad based a limited ileal resection may be required.

Intussusception: barium enema can be used both as a diagnostic procedure, and if the reservoir of barium is elevated 1 metre above the abdomen, hydrostatic reduction under radiological screening can be attempted. Reduction is signified when barium flows freely to the proximal loops of ileum. If hydrostatic reduction fails, or there is evidence of perforation/peritonitis, operative management is indicated. In this, reduction may be facilitated by squeezing the distal colon and pushing the intussuscepted intestine proximally. If this is unsuccessful then resection of the affected segment should be carried out.

6. Surgical Pathology Specimens – Laboratory Protocols

Biopsy Specimens

See Gastrointestinal Specimens – General Comments (page 6). Formal Crosby capsule jejunal biopsies are larger than flexible OGD distal duodenal samples. They are usually submitted on filter paper to allow orientation and inspection of the mucosal surface under a dissecting microscope and correlation with histology. Finger-like, cerebriform and mosaic patterns correspond to normal, partially atrophic and flat mucosae. respectively.

Resection Specimens

Specimen

- resection of small intestine can be for specific conditions such as Meckel's
- diverticulum or ischaemia, or for obstruction due to various inflammatory, mechanical and neoplastic disorders.

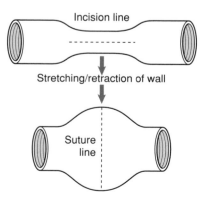

Figure 4.3.   Small intestinal stricturoplasty.

Meckel's Diverticulum

● measurements:
   – ileal base or segment – length × diameter (cm).
   – diverticulum – length × diameter (cm).
● open the ileum longitudinally with blunt-ended scissors along its mesenteric border opposite the diverticulum, and then cut at right angles to this along the diverticulum towards its tip (Figure 4.4). Photograph before and after dissection.
● paint the external aspect of the diverticulum and fix by immersion in 10% formalin for 36–48 hours.
● inspect and describe the diverticulum (especially its tip), e.g., heterotopic mucosa, ulceration, perforation, abscess, fibrous bands or tumour.
● inspect and describe the ileal segment, e.g., inflammation, ischaemia or signs of intussusception.
● transverse section the proximal and distal ileal limits of resection or ileal/diverticulum base.
● sample normal-appearing ileum, diverticulum and its tip.
● sample additional blocks as indicated by any macroscopic abnormalities present.

Ischaemia

● measurements:
   – small bowel segment – length and maximum diameter (cm).
   – mesentery – length × depth (cm).
● inspect and describe: hyperaemia/duskiness of the serosa, perforation, constriction bands across the bowel or mesentery.
● open longitudinally with blunt-ended scissors along the mesenteric border – inspect for mucosal thinning, ulceration, haemorrhage, necrosis, perforation, stricture formation, or any underlying tumour that might have precipitated volvulus or intussusception.
● fix by immersion in 10% formalin for 36–48 hours.
● transverse section the proximal and distal limits of resection.
● sample (five blocks minimum) representative macroscopically normal and abnormal areas as indicated (Figure 4.5).
● sample mesentery with constituent vessels (a minimum of two blocks).
● sample mesenteric lymph nodes.

Obstructive Enteropathy

● the resection specimen is dictated by the site and nature of the abnormality and extent of any complications that are present. For example, jejunal ring diaphragm disease results in resection of the radiologically and macroscopically involved segment whereas Crohn's terminal ileitis produces a limited right hemicolectomy. Intussusception complicated by ischaemia needs a more extensive resection than would be otherwise necessary. A cancer operation will necessitate more radical dissection of mesentery and regional lymph nodes. In some instances it is not possible clinically or macroscopically to distinguish between inflammatory and neoplastic ulcers or strictures – handling of the specimen must therefore cover these various options pending histopathological assessment.

Initial Procedure

● open longitudinally with blunt ended scissors along the mesenteric border avoiding any obvious areas of tumour or perforation.

Tip perforation or heterotopic tissue

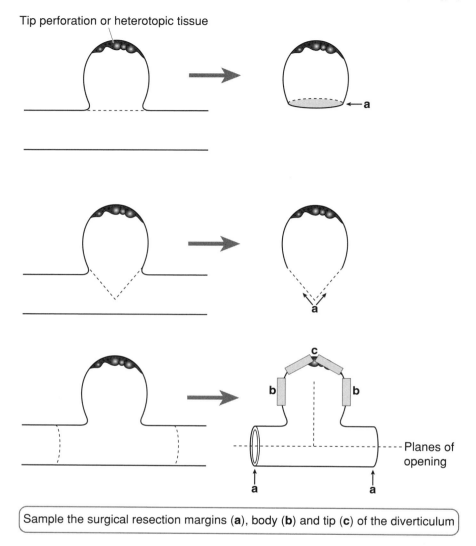

Sample the surgical resection margins (**a**), body (**b**) and tip (**c**) of the diverticulum

Figure 4.4.   Meckel's diverticulum – specimens.

- measurements:
  - lengths and maximum diameter (cm) of the parts present – duodenum, jejunum, ileum, caecum, ascending colon, appendix.
  - lengths (cm) of ischaemic, strictured or hose-pipe segments, intussusception.
  - maximum dimensions (cm) of any perforation(s), ulcer(s), polyp(s) and tumour(s).
  - distances (cm) of the abnormality from the proximal and distal resection limits.
- photograph.
- gently pack the bowel lumen with formalin-soaked lint and fix by immersion in 10% formalin for 48 hours.

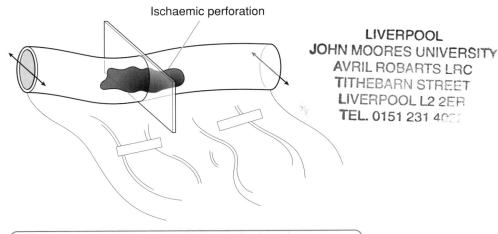

Ischaemic perforation

Transverse section the surgical limits and the bowel to represent normality and any lesion that is present. Sample the mesenteric vessels

Figure 4.5.   Small bowel ischaemia.

Description

- tumour   – site: duodenal/jejunal/ileal/ileo-caecal valve.
                           lumenal/mural/extramural/mesenteric.
  – size: length × width × depth (cm) or maximum dimension (cm).

  – appearance: polypoid/nodular – inflammatory fibroid polyp, carcinoid, malignant melanoma, adenoma, carcinoma, multiple lymphomatous polyposis, GIST.

  ulcerated/stricture – carcinoma, carcinoid, malignant lymphoma, metastatic carcinoma.

  fleshy/rubbery – GIST, malignant lymphoma.

  multifocal – metastases (carcinoma, melanoma), carcinoid, malignant lymphoma.

  adjacent atrophic mucosa – EATCL
  – edge: circumscribed/irregular

- Crohn's Disease
  – cobblestone mucosa/ulceration (aphthous, linear, confluent)/ring strictures/hose-pipe segments/fat wrapping/fistula/polyps or tumour/lymphadenopathy/sharp demarcation at the ileo-caecal valve/caecal or colonic disease/adhesions/abscess formation.

- diaphragm disease
  - ring strictures – number, width, lumen aperture, intervening sacculation, mucosal ulceration.

- extrinsic compression
  - constriction band/extrinsic tumour/lumen stenosis/mucosal ulceration/proximal dilatation.

- intussusception
  - apex (inflammatory fibroid polyp, tumour, Meckel's, mesenteric lymphadenopathy)/ischaemia/perforation/ileo-ileal/ileo-caecal.

Blocks for Histology (Figure 4.6)

Non-neoplastic Conditions

- sample by circumferential transverse sections the proximal and distal limits of resection.
- sample macroscopically normal bowel.
- sample representative blocks (a minimum of five) of any abnormality that is present to include its edge and junction with the adjacent mucosa, e.g., ulceration, stricture, fistula, perforation, serosal adhesions or constriction band, intussusception apex. These can be taken transversely or longitudinally depending on the anatomy and the abnormality present.
- sample mesenteric lymph nodes and any adjacent structures, e.g., caecum, appendix or ileo-caecal valve.

Neoplastic Conditions

- sample the nearest longitudinal resection margin if tumour is present to within < 2 cm of it.
- sample macroscopically normal bowel – usually one section but several if a multifocal condition, e.g., FAPC or EATCL is suspected.
- serially section the bulk of the tumour transversely at 3–4 mm intervals.
- lay the slices out in sequence and photograph.
- sample (four blocks minimum) tumour and wall to show the deepest point of circumferential invasion. With tumours < 1 cm diameter fewer blocks will be possible. Include adjacent mucosa where feasible.
- count and sample all lymph nodes – identify a suture tie limit node.
- sample multifocal serosal tumour seedlings as indicated by inspection and palpation.

Histopathology Report

Ischaemia

- necrosis – mucosal/transmural/gangrenous.
- resection limits – ischaemic/viable.
- mesenteric vessels – thrombosis/embolism/vasculitis.
- miscellaneous – constriction band/volvulus/intussusception/stricture.

Crohn's Disease

- chronic transmural inflammation/granulomas/fissures/fistulae/abscess formation/ileal confined/ileo-caecal/appendiceal or resection limit disease/malignancy.

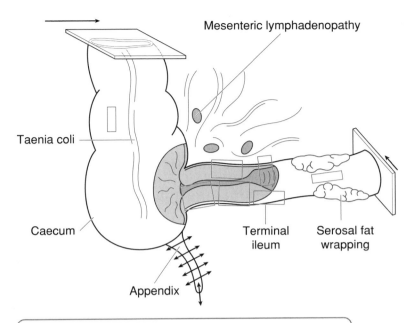

1. Transverse section the surgical limits
2. Process the appendix as usual
3. Sample normal ileum and colon
4. Sample representative blocks of the
   hose pipe segment, any ulceration and adjacent mucosa.
5. Sample mesenteric lymph nodes

Figure 4.6. Right hemicolectomy for Crohn's disease.

Intussusception

● apex/secondary ulceration, stricture, ischaemia or perforation/site (ileo-ileal/ileo-caecal).

Neoplastic Conditions

● tumour type
  – adenocarcinoma/malignant lymphoma/GIST.
● tumour differentiation
  – adenocarcinoma   well/moderate/poor.
  – malignant lymphoma   MALToma/centrocytic/follicle centre cell/Burkitt's/other.
                          low-grade/high-grade.
  – GIST   spindle cell/epithelioid.
             cellularity/atypia/necrosis/mitoses/margins/size.
             leiomyomatous/neural/stromal (CD34, CD117).
● tumour edge
  – pushing/infiltrative/lymphoid response.

- extent of local tumour spread (for carcinoma).
  - pTis   carcinoma in situ
  - pT1   tumour invades lamina propria or submucosa
  - pT2   tumour invades muscularis propria
  - pT3   tumour invades through the wall into subserosa or perimuscular connective tissues (mesentery or retroperitoneum) with extension $\leq$ 2 cm.
  - pT4   tumour perforates the serosa or invades other organs/structures, e.g., mesentery > 2 cm, small bowel loops, abdominal wall.
- lymphovascular invasion – present/not present
- regional lymph nodes
  - duodenum: pancreatioduodenal, pyloric, hepatic, superior mesenteric nodes.
  - ileum/jejunum: mesenteric.
  - terminal ileum: ileocolic, posterior caecal.
  - pN0   no regional lymph node metastasis.
  - pN1   metastasis in regional lymph node(s).
- excision margins
  - proximal, distal and mesenteric limits of tumour clearance (cm).
- other pathology
  - FAPC, Peutz–Jegher's syndrome, Crohn's disease, coeliac disease, EATCL.

5 Colorectum

1. Anatomy

The colon and rectum together measure between 125 and 140 cm in the adult. The colon is divided into the caecum (10 cm), ascending (15 cm), transverse (40 cm), descending (25 cm) and sigmoid (25–40 cm) colons. The rectum measures approximately 13–15cm (Figure 5.1). The main function of the colon is absorption of water and electrolytes and the storage of faecal material until it can be excreted. The caecum is that part that lies below the ileocaecal valve and receives the opening of the appendix. It is completely surrounded by peritoneum allowing it to be mobile in the right iliac fossa. The base of the appendix is attached to the posteromedial surface of the caecum. The ascending colon extends upwards from the caecum to the inferior surface of the right lobe of liver. Here it becomes continuous with the transverse colon by turning sharply

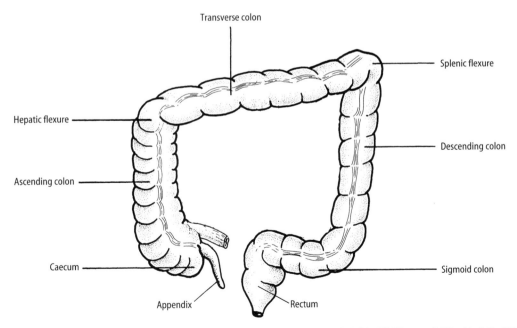

Transverse colon

Splenic flexure

Hepatic flexure

Descending colon

Ascending colon

Caecum

Sigmoid colon

Appendix

Rectum

Figure 5.1.   Colorectum. Reproduced with permission from Hermanek P, Hutter RVP, Sobin, LH, Wagner, G, Wittekind, Ch. (Eds). TNM Atlas: Illustrated guide to the TNM/pTNM classification of malignant tumours, 4th edition. Springer-Verlag: Berlin and Heidelberg, 1997.

to the left, forming the right colic or hepatic flexure. The ascending colon is bound to the posterior abdominal wall by peritoneum covering its front and sides. The transverse colon extends from the hepatic flexure to the left, hanging downwards and then ascending to the inferior surface of the spleen where it turns sharply downwards to form the left colic or splenic flexure. The transverse colon is completely surrounded by peritoneum with the transverse mesocolon being attached to its superior border (the length of the transverse mesocolon accounts for the variability in the position of the transverse colon) and the greater omentum to its lower border. The descending colon extends downwards from the splenic flexure to the left side of the pelvic brim. It is bound to the posterior abdominal wall by peritoneum covering its sides and front. The sigmoid colon is continuous with the descending colon and hangs as a loop into the pelvic cavity. It is completely surrounded by peritoneum and a fan-shaped piece of mesentery attaches it to the posterior abdominal wall, thus allowing mobility. The rectum begins as a continuation of the sigmoid colon in front of the third sacral vertebra and follows the curvature of the sacrum and coccyx to where it pierces the pelvic floor to become continuous with the anal canal. Peritoneum covers the anterior and lateral surfaces of the upper third and the anterior surface of the middle third, the lower third being devoid of a peritoneal covering. At the junction of the middle and lower third the peritoneum is reflected onto the posterior surface of the upper vagina in the female to form the rectovaginal pouch (pouch of Douglas) (Figure 5.2) and onto the upper part of the posterior bladder in the male forming the rectovesical pouch. The extent of serosal covering in the colorectum in illustrated in Figure 5.3. The rectum is surrounded by a bi-lobed encapsulated fatty structure which is bulkier posterolaterally than anteriorly – the mesorectum.

The small and large intestines differ in their appearance in a number of ways:

- The longitudinal muscle in the small intestine forms a continuous layer whereas in the colon it comprises three bands called *taeniae coli*. However, in the rectum the taeniae coli come together to form a broad band on the anterior and posterior surfaces.
- The wall of the colon is sacculated whereas the small intestine is smooth.
- The colon has "fatty tags" called *appendices epiploicae*.
- The permanent mucous membrane folds (*plicae circulares*) in the small intestine are not present in the colon.

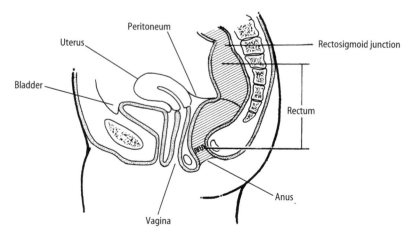

Figure 5.2.   Rectosigmoid and peritoneal reflection (lateral view). Reproduced with permission from Hermanek P, Hutter RVP, Sobin, LH, Wagner, G, Wittekind, Ch. (Eds). TNM Atlas: Illustrated guide to the TNM/pTNM classification of malignant tumours, 4th edition. Springer-Verlag: Berlin and Heidelberg, 1997.

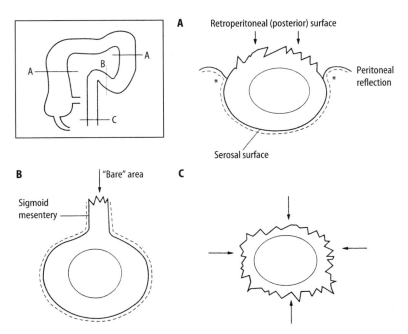

Figure 5.3. Extent of serosal covering of the large intestine. Arrows indicate the "bare" non-peritonealised areas of different levels. A. The ascending and descending colon are devoid of peritoneum on their posterior surface. B. The sigmoid colon is completely covered with peritoneum, which extends over the mesentery. C. The lower rectum lies beneath the pelvic peritoneal reflection. The asterisks in A indicate the sites where serosal involvement by tumour is likely to occur. Reproduced with permission from Burroughs SH, Williams GT. ACP best practice no. 159. Examination of large-intestine resection specimens. J Clin Pathol 2000;53:344–349.

Microscopically, the colonic mucosa is made up of tubular crypts lined by columnar epithelium with mucin-secreting goblet cells and endocrine cells also being present.

Lymphovascular Supply

Embryologically the gastrointestinal tract is divided into three segments (fore, mid and hindgut) with each region being supplied by its own artery:

- Coeliac artery supplies the foregut (distal oesophagus to the mid-portion of the second part of the duodenum).
- Superior mesenteric artery supplies the midgut (mid-portion of the second part of the duodenum to the junction of the proximal two thirds and distal third of the transverse colon).
- Inferior mesenteric artery supplies the hindgut (distal third of the transverse colon to the junction of the superior and inferior half of the anal canal).

The rectum is also supplied by branches of the internal iliac artery. The anastomosis of the colic arteries around the concavity of the colon forms the marginal artery. The venous drainage of the colon is to the portal venous system and the rectum to the inferior mesenteric and internal iliac veins.

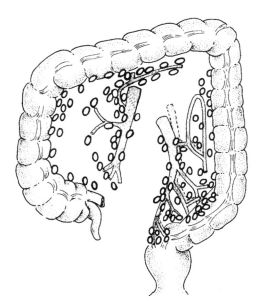

Figure 5.4.   Colorectum: regional lymph nodes. The regional lymph nodes are the pericolic and perirectal and those located along the ileocolic, right colic, middle colic, left colic, inferior mesenteric, superior rectal (haemorrhoidal) and internal iliac arteries. Reproduced with permission from Hermanek P, Hutter RVP, Sobin, LH, Wagner, G, Wittekind, Ch. (Eds). TNM Atlas: Illustrated guide to the TNM/pTNM classification of malignant tumours, 4th edition. Springer-Verlag: Berlin and Heidelberg, 1997.

The lymphatics accompany the colic vessels draining to the superior and inferior mesenteric nodes. Those from the rectum drain into nodes (pararectal nodes) situated in the perirectal connective tissue (mesorectum) and thence to the superior mesenteric and internal iliac nodes (Figure 5.4).

2. Clinical Presentation

There is considerable variability in the clinical presentation of colorectal disease.

Angiodysplasia usually presents with persistent occult bleeding or repeated small bleeds. In colonic ischaemia/infarction there may be a history of arrhythmia or cardiac failure, and it may present acutely with abdominal pain and bloody diarrhoea or less acutely with stricturing and symptoms of obstruction. Infective conditions usually lead to diarrhoea, crampy abdominal pain and fever. A careful drug history should be obtained if pseudomembranous colitis is suspected. Inflammatory bowel disease may have an indolent presentation with lethargy, anorexia and weight loss. However, more characteristic symptoms of ulcerative colitis include bloody diarrhoea (> 10 stools/day), urgency and abdominal pain. Peritonitis and systemic sepsis may occur with toxic megacolon and perforation. Colorectal Crohn's disease characteristically presents with diarrhoea. Obstruction due to stricturing may occur and fistulae leading to specific symptoms (e.g., colovesical – pneumaturia and recurrent urinary infection; rectovaginal – faecal discharge per vagina). Perianal fissures/fistulae and anorectal sepsis are relatively common in Crohn's disease. Extra-gastrointestinal manifestations of inflammatory bowel disease include finger-clubbing and erythema nodosum. Diverticular disease may present insidiously with lower abdominal pain or fistula formation (e.g., colovesical), or acutely as acute diverticulitis (abdominal pain, diarrhoea and localised peritonitis), pericolic abscess, obstruction (due to stricturing), perforation (gener-alised peritonitis) or haemorrhage (relatively rare).

Adenomatous polyps are usually asymptomatic, but large villous adenomas in the rectum may illicit an alteration in bowel habit, mucus per rectum (may cause pruritis ani), tenesmus (a sensa-tion of incomplete evacuation) and electrolyte loss (particularly potassium). Colorectal carcinoma is usually asymptomatic early in its existence and later may present with non-specific sympto-matology such as an alteration in bowel habit, mucus PR, abdominal mass or discomfort and PR bleeding (may be occult and can lead to iron deficiency anaemia). As a rule the more proximal the tumour the darker the blood. Tumours in the right colon are more likely to be ulcerated and so tend to present with PR bleeding, whereas tumours of the left colon are often constrictive and present with obstruction – this is compounded by the fact that the faecal material is more solid in the distal colon. Perforation may occur either through the tumour itself or distant and prox-imal to it due to obstruction and back pressure, e.g., in the caecal pouch. Rectal tumours can lead to tenesmus, and local invasion may produce back pain and sciatica (involvement of the sacral plexus), rectovaginal fistula, etc. Liver metastases may cause clinical jaundice.

3. Clinical Investigations

FBP – iron deficiency anaemia as a result of PR bleeding.

U & E – electrolyte disturbance in diarrhoea/mucus PR.

LFTs – deranged in liver metastases or in the hepatobiliary manifestations of Crohn's disease.

C-reactive protein/ESR – allows the activity of inflammatory bowel disease to be monitored.

Stool culture – rule out infective colitis.

Faecal occult blood – will detect occult bleeding.

CXR – will detect pulmonary metastases.

AXR – will show signs of colonic obstruction. Any dilatation of the colon > 6 cm in diameter heralds the onset of toxic megacolon. In ischaemic colitis there will be dilated colon with char-acteristic "thumbprinting". In colovesical fistula gas is present in the bladder. Free intraperitoneal gas will be seen in colonic perforation. In patients being investigated for chronic constipation radio-opaque markers are ingested and an AXR is taken five days later with passage of < 80% of the markers considered abnormal.

Barium enema – widely used investigation in colorectal disease. There will be characteristic "thumbprint" filling defects caused by oedematous mucosa in ischaemia/infarction. The extent of ulcerative colitis can be assessed and in Crohn's disease it will show skip lesions, areas of stric-turing and any fistulae. It will reveal the presence of diverticula. Barium enema is useful in the detection of large polyps and carcinomas with constricting tumours producing a characteristic "apple-core" lesion. However, it will not reliably define rectal lesions.

CT scan – will detect a pericolic abscess (can be drained under CT guidance) and is useful in showing the site of a tumour and any metastatic spread.

MRI scan and ELUS – allow assessment of local tumour spread for staging purposes.

PET scan – helps to distinguish recurrent carcinoma from post-radiotherapy fibrosis in the pelvis.

Angiography – will demonstrate a bleeding point. e.g., in angiodysplasia if there is active bleeding > 2 ml/min.

Cytology – examination of ascitic fluid or peritoneal washings.

Endoscopy and biopsy – inspection and biopsy of the mucosa, determination of disease distri-bution, solitary or multiple lesions.

Laparoscopy – staging laparoscopy may be undertaken and any peritoneal deposits biopsied.

CEA serum levels – elevated in colorectal neoplasia particularly in metastatic or recurrent disease.

4. Pathological Conditions

Non-neoplastic Conditions

These comprise inflammatory (acute or chronic), mechanical, ischaemic and iatrogenic disorders.

Inflammatory Disorders

Acute proctocolitis: infective or drug induced, e.g., antibiotics, there is preservation of the mucosal architecture and acute inflammation with biopsies only being submitted if symptoms persist beyond several weeks. Infective cases (*Campylobacter, Shigella, Salmonella*) are usually self-limited and culture-positive in only 40% of cases. Drug-induced inflammation often responds to its withdrawal.

Chronic proctocolitis: characterised by disturbance of the mucosal architecture and a chronic inflammatory cell infiltrate ± foci of active inflammation. Commonly due to idiopathic chronic inflammatory bowel disease (CIBD) but also seen overlying diverticulosis and pneumatosis coli, in infection (*Shigella*, amoebiasis, schistosomiasis), obstructive enterocolitis and with drugs. Microbiological culture, travel and drug history should always be ascertained in patients with chronic diarrhoea.

CIBD – ulcerative colitis and Crohn's disease: the latter has been discussed previously but can present either as isolated colonic disease or associated with ileitis. It is a segmental, transmural chronic inflammatory condition and there is often rectal sparing but anal disease (fissure, fistula, abscess) present. The segmental distribution, focality of inflammation, presence of granulomas and ileal component are all useful diagnostic pointers in colonoscopic biopsy or resection specimens. Recurrence elsewhere in the gut is not uncommon despite surgical resection and because of this Crohn's disease is a contraindication to pouch formation in restorative proctocolectomy. Occasionally it presents isolated to the appendix or sigmoid colon coexisting with diverticulitis.

In contrast to this, ulcerative colitis is a diffuse, chronic, active mucosal inflammatory condition involving the rectum and a contiguous length of large intestine, e.g., left-sided proctocolitis or pancolitis. It is of variable severity with episodic exacerbations and remissions – acute fulminant colitis may be complicated by severe haemorrhage, toxic dilatation or megacolon, perforation and peritonitis. Other complications include mucosal dysplasia and malignancy (usually adenocarcinoma) in extensive disease of long standing duration (pancolitis > 10 years). Villiform or polypoid DALMs (dysplasia-associated lesions or masses) can be difficult to distinguish from the much more common inflammatory mucosal polyps and may harbour underlying adenocarcinoma. Alternatively, dysplasia may occur in flat mucosa, and colonoscopic surveillance of chronic colitis involves sequential mucosal sampling as well as target biopsy of any macroscopic abnormality. Biopsy orientation onto a polycarbonate strip aids subsequent localisation of any histological abnormalities. Macroscopically ulcerative colitis shows mucosal granularity, linear or confluent ulceration and polyps of varying size. The terminal ileum is only involved in severe pancolitis over a length of 1–2 cm (backwash ileitis) and although there is usually proctitis the rectum may be spared due to treatment effects, e.g., predsol enemas. Extraintestinal effects include arthritis, iritis and, in the liver, sclerosing cholangitis which can lead to cirrhosis and cholangiocarcinoma.

In a minority of cases clear distinction cannot be made between ulcerative colitis and Crohn's disease on macroscopic and microscopic examination – so-called indeterminate colitis.

Diversion proctocolitis: follows faecal stream diversion, e.g., after ileostomy or colostomy for tumour, trauma or CIBD. The defunctioned segment develops florid reactive lymphoid hyperplasia which can be mucosal or transmural, mimicking or superimposed on an underlying inflammatory disorder such as CIBD. Persistent severe symptoms may neccessitate surgical excision of the segment, e.g., the rectal stump following colectomy for ulcerative colitis.

Microscopic colitis: minimal inflammation may be apparent grossly or histologically for various reasons, e.g., treated CIBD, post infection, drug ingestion, uraemia, stercoral trauma, etc. However, microscopic colitis which causes chronic, voluminous watery diarrhoea is radiologically and colonoscopically normal. It occurs in middle-aged to elderly women and has variable associations with HLA type, autoimmune diseases and NSAID ingestion. Diagnosis is by histology with a normal architecture and transmucosal infiltrate of chronic inflammatory cells. Its main variants, collagenous and lymphocytic colitis, show a thickened subepithelial collagen band and excess surface intraepithelial lymphocytes, respectively. Not infrequently there is spontaneous resolution or response to anti-inflammatory therapy.

Infective proctocolitis: investigation includes microbiological culture with microscopy for cysts (amoebiasis) and ova (schistosomiasis). Infection should be considered particularly where there is a history of travel or immunosuppression, e.g., AIDS, chemotherapy or post transplant. In immunosuppression, infection with unusual opportunistic organisms can occur, e.g., cryptosporidiosis, atypical mycobacteria.

Mechanical Disorders

Melanosis coli: characterised by pigmented macrophages in the lamina propria that impart a dusky mucosal appearance mimicking ischaemia. The pigment is lipofuscin and degenerative in nature, and is thought to relate to cellular apoptosis. There is an association with use of laxatives and bowel dysmotility.

Volvulus: usually comprises a markedly dilated atonic sigmoid colon in either Africans (due to a high-fibre diet with bulky stools), or constipation-related acquired megacolon in the elderly. The sigmoid loop twists on its mesentery, obstructs and may become secondarily ischaemic. Resection specimens are often dilated, thinned and featureless. Melanosis coli may be present. Congenital megacolon and Hirschsprung's disease are discussed elsewhere (see page 232).

Pneumatosis coli: submucosal gas cysts lined by macrophages and giant cells with overlying mucosal chronic inflammation or pseudolipomatosis. There is an association with volvulus, constipation, diverticulosis and chronic obstructive airways disease. Pathogenesis relates to retroperitoneal tracking of air into the bowel mesentery, abnormal luminal gas production linked to the increased intraluminal pressure seen in the above disorders, and introduction of gas during endoscopy. About 50% of cases resolve but recurrent or severe lesions may require colectomy of the involved segment.

Obstructive enterocolitis: continuous or segmental areas of inflammation or ulceration adjacent to or distant from an obstructing distal lesion, e.g., annular carcinoma or diverticulosis. Small bowel may also be involved with mimicry of Crohn's disease. A dilated, thinned caecal pouch can become ischaemic and perforate.

Diverticulosis: very common in Western society due to a low-fibre diet, high intraluminal pressure and subsequent transmural mucosal herniation in the sigmoid colon through points of vessel entry from the mesentery. Presentation is with altered bowel habit, per rectum bleeding, left iliac fossa pain or a mass. The latter implies diverticulitis with possible perforation and pericolonic reaction/abscess formation. Portal pyaemia, liver abscesses and peritonitis can ensue. The diverticular segment is thickened and contracted with muscle coat hypertrophy and visible diverticular pouches in the muscularis and mesenteric fat. They may be filled and obstructed with faecal or vegetable debris, and ulcerated with a coating of pericolonic exudate and abscess. The concertina-like redundant mucosal folds can show crescentic colitis due to abrasion of their tips by the passing faecal stream. Occasionally, the chronic inflammation may be transmural and granulomatous mimicking or co-existing with Crohn's disease. Treatment is often conservative, e.g., by diet alteration, but severe or complicated cases require colectomy. Co-presentation with an occult carcinoma within the strictured segment must be excluded by careful pathological examination.

Mucosal prolapse: a mechanism producing reactive mucosal changes of crypt hyperplasia, smooth-muscle thickening of the lamina propria and variable surface erosion. It is common to a number of situations including: solitary rectal ulcer syndrome (SRUS), inflammatory cloacogenic polyp, diverticular-related crescentic colitis, mucosa adjacent to a polyp, stricture or tumour, stercoral trauma and the mucocutaneous junction of stomas. In SRUS there is a history of abnormal anterior rectal wall descent due to straining at defaecation. This results in induration of the wall that can mimic a plaque of tumour on palpation and rectoscopy. Biopsy is diagnostic and treatment is usually conservative, related to better stool habit – occasional cases require resection of the involved sleeve of mucous membrane with apposition and plication of the intervening muscle (Delorme's procedure).

Ischaemic Disorders

The pathogenesis of intestinal ischaemia has been previously discussed and in the large intestine is often due to mesenteric vascular insufficiency because of systemic hypotension (myocardial infarction, cardiac arrhythmia, blood loss) or mesenteric atheroma/thrombosis/embolism. Acute lesions may resolve if mucosa-confined but are potentially fatal if transmural. Late or chronic ischaemia has a predilection for the splenic flexure and rectosigmoid watershed areas of vascular supply. This can result in non-specific ulceroinflammatory and stricturing lesions – end-stage changes that can be produced by various other conditions, e.g., CIBD, infection (*E. coli* 0157:H7 bacterium), pseudomembranous colitis due to *Clostridium difficle* overgrowth, obstructive enterocolitis and stercoral trauma. Occasional cases are due to vasculitis or amyloid infiltration. Assessment of resection limit viability and mural/mesenteric vessels is necessary in ischaemia.

A vascular abnormality that can present with an iron deficiency anaemia in elderly patients is colonic angiodysplasia. Thought to be degenerative in nature due to increased intraluminal pressure compressing mural vessels, the commonest site is the caecum. Operative injection of radio-opaque contrast may be needed to demonstrate areas of vascular ectasia so that targeted blocks can be sampled. The ectatic vessels involve the submucosa and lamina propria.

Iatrogenic Disorders

This includes drugs, radiation therapy and graft versus host disease.

Drugs: NSAIDs should always be considered in the presence of any unusual colitis, localised ulceration, stricture, perforation or mucosal diaphragm formation. Antibiotics can commonly cause dysfunctional diarrhoea, an acute proctocolitis, or, particularly in the elderly, pseudomembranous colitis. The latter is due to the production of C. difficile toxin leading to ischaemic-type lesions with yellow surface plaques of acute inflammatory and fibrinous pseudomembrane. Severe cases result in end-stage ulceration and colectomy may be indicated although initial treatment is with appropriate antibiotics.

Radiation therapy: acute and chronic phases with the potential for mucosal healing and usually produced by radiotherapy for pelvic (uterine cervix, rectum, prostate) or retroperitoneal cancer. Acute radiation proctocolitis is normally self-limited and seldom biopsied. Chronic changes result in mucosal atrophy, hyaline fibrosis, vascular thickening and strictures.

Graft versus host disease: immunosuppressed bone marrow transplant patients risk developing a range of acute and chronic changes similar to those seen in radiation damage.

Neoplastic Conditions

Simple hyperplastic or metaplastic polyps are benign and more prevalent in the left colon with increasing age. They are sometimes associated with malignancy if sessile, right sided and incorporating a degree of epithelial dysplasia (serrated adenoma). Adenomatous polyp is the commonest precancerous lesion.

Adenoma: designated as tubular, tubulovillous or villous depending on the relative proportions of glands and fronds present and composed of low- or high-grade dysplastic epithelium. Increasing in frequency with age and in the left colon the risk of malignancy relates to the size (> 2 cm = 40–50% risk), degree of villous morphology and grade of dysplasia. Tubular adenomas are nodular and tend to develop a distinct stalk whereas villous lesions are sessile. Stalked adenomas can twist and prolapse resulting in glandular herniation into the submucosa that mimics invasive carcinoma – the presence of haemosiderin and lack of stromal fibrous desmoplasia are useful histological clues. Invasive carcinoma is defined by the presence of neoplastic epithelium infiltrating submucosa and in stalked adenomas polypectomy may be considered therapeutic if the tumour is well-to-moderately differentiated, does not show lympho-vascular invasion or involvement of the diathermied base. Otherwise, colonic resection is required, and, therefore, good orientation of the adenoma to its stalk and assessment of the base are crucial. In contrast, invasion in a sessile adenoma accesses true mural submucosa and colonic resection is usually considered more appropriate unless the patient is very elderly or medically unfit. Local mucosal resection is an option but further radical surgery is required if the cancer involves muscle coat, the base of the specimen, lymphovascular channels or is poorly differentiated.

It is not unusual for patients to have several adenomas but in FAPC there are hundreds or thousands with progression to colorectal cancer 20–30 years earlier than average. There is also a strong association with duodenal adenomas and periampullary carcinoma.

Flat adenomas are less common and difficult to identify macroscopically without the use of a hand lens or dye spray technique. They have proportionately higher grades of dysplasia and frequency of carcinoma and may account for a proportion of the 30% of carcinomas without an identifiable adenoma at their edge.

Adenocarcinoma: comprising the vast majority of colorectal malignancies, 80–85% are moder-ately differentiated adenocarcinoma of no special type. A minority are mucinous, signet ring cell or poorly differentiated. Distribution is throughout the colorectum although rectosigmoid is the commonest site (50% of cases) – 10–15% of sporadic cases are multiple occurring either synchronously or subsequently. Predisposing conditions are chronic ulcerative colitis, FAPC and hereditary non-polyposis colorectal cancer (HNPCC). In HNPCC there is a tendency for right-sided cancers – which may be multiple, mucinous or poorly differentiated – and a family history of cancer at a younger age, also involving other sites, e.g., stomach, uterus, ovary, kidney and breast. Its genetic basis is different from that of sporadic colorectal cancer due to a deficiency in the DNA mismatch repair genes.

As previously noted, the cancer site and its macroscopic growth pattern influence clinical presentation. Important prognostic indicators are the extent of local tumour spread, a circum-scribed or infiltrative margin, involvement of the serosa, longitudinal or mesocolic/mesorectal resection margins and tumour perforation. Tumour present to within ≤ 1 mm defines involve-ment of the mesenteric margin irrespective of whether it is nodal, lymphovascular or direct spread. Generally, a macroscopic clearance of 2–3 cm from a longitudinal margin is satisfactory unless histology shows the cancer to be unusually infiltrative or poorly differentiated. A minimum target of eight but preferably all mesenteric lymph nodes should be counted and sampled and a suture tie limit node identified – in some colectomy specimens this may mean more than one. Involvement of adjacent organs or structures (e.g., abdominal wall) is documented and predis-posing lesions such as adenoma(s) or colitis represented. Multiple tumours are dissected and staged individually with respect to mural and nodal spread.

Other cancers: carcinoid tumours are usually small, incidental, mucosal polyps; GISTs are rare and malignant lymphoma can complicate ulcerative colitis or AIDS.

Prognosis: relates mainly to the depth of tumour spread, lymph node involvement and adequacy of local excision with overall five-year survival 35–40%. Cancers confined to the mucous membrane or wall do much better than those that invade beyond this or show nodal disease. Adverse prognostic indicators also include a mucinous character, poor differentiation, tumour perforation, obstruction and resection margin involvement. It is estimated that about 50% of patients are cured, 10% die from local recurrence and 40% from lymphatic and vascular spread. Treatment is surgical excision with adjuvant chemotherapy for cancers showing poor differentiation; nodal, peritoneal and extramural vascular spread; tumour perforation or resection margin involvement. Rectal cancers often receive five-day, short-course, preoperative radiotherapy in an attempt to downstage the lesion or facilitate resection – this usually does not produce the marked macroscopic and histological features of regression that can be seen with the alternative six-week-long course of adjuvant therapy that is given to clinically fixed tumours.

5. Surgical Pathology Specimens – Clinical Aspects

Biopsy Specimens

A number of procedures can be undertaken to obtain biopsy specimens from the colorectal mucosa:

Proctoscopy is used to inspect the distal rectum and anal canal.

Sigmoidoscopy can be carried out by using either a rigid or flexible sigmoidoscope. Rigid sigmoidoscopy is usually done without bowel preparation at the bedside or in the outpatient clinic. A hollow, rigid plastic tube measuring 25 cm in length with an attached light and air supply is inserted into the rectum up to the distal sigmoid colon. Forceps can be passed through the tube to biopsy any lesion visualised. The scope is also used to assess tumour fixation and its distance from the anus. Flexible sigmoidoscopy (and colonoscopy) involve formal bowel preparation. A flexible fibre optic endoscope is inserted and works in the same way as an upper GI endoscope, with a controllable tip and ports for inserting instruments, e.g., forceps, snare, etc. This should visualise up to the proximal sigmoid colon.

Colonoscopy is carried out using a colonoscope, which is essentially a longer sigmoidoscope, with scopes of different lengths available (range from 140 to 185 cm). An experienced endoscopist should be able to pass the endoscope through the ileocaecal valve to visualise the terminal ileum. Intraoperative endoscopy can be used during a laparotomy to, for instance, locate lesions, e.g., polyps found by barium enema, that require localised resection and which cannot be palpated by the surgeon.

Biopsy specimens can be taken from the colonic mucosa by forceps passed through the endoscope in much the same way as that used in upper GI endoscopy. The colonoscopic management of polyps is important and depends on the size and type of polyp:

- Large pedunculated polyps can be removed by "snaring". A circular wire is passed over the polyp onto its stalk. An electrical current is passed along the wire to coagulate the vessels in the base of the stalk, which is then transected by closing the wire. If the stalk is large, adrenaline can be injected into the base to minimise bleeding. The polyp is retrieved by using the snare, a Dormia basket or suction.
- Smaller polyps (5–7 mm) can also be snared and removed by suction.
- Polyps < 5 mm can be removed by "hot biopsy". Biopsy forceps grasp the polyp and a current is applied to electrocoagulate the base; the head of the polyp is then pulled off by the forceps.
- Broad-based sessile polyps can either be removed piecemeal using the snare or by *injection polypectomy*. This involves injecting adrenaline solution into the submucosa around the

polyp, raising it, and allowing it to be snared completely. This method can be used for polyps up to 5 cm in diameter.

● In patients with multiple small polyps, these can be highlighted by spraying dye onto the mucosa. This will reveal polyps 0.5 mm and larger as pale areas on a blue background.

● If the endoscopist is concerned that a polyp may be malignant the site of polypectomy can be marked by tattooing the bowel mucosa with India ink. This allows the site to be revisited at a later date.

Submucosal lesions can be sampled by endoscopic FNA. Colonoscopy may also be used as a therapeutic tool, e.g., foci of angiodysplasia may be coagulated using hot biopsy forceps.

Resection Specimens

Resection of the colon and rectum is performed for a wide variety of both non-neoplastic and neoplastic conditions (Table 5.1), the type of procedure depending on the site and nature of the lesion, e.g., a malignant tumour will require a more extensive resection than that for a large adenomatous polyp. Likewise, the extent of mesenteric resection will depend on the type of lesion, i.e., wide mesenteric resection for neoplastic lesions and limited resection for non-neoplastic conditions. It also depends on the "intention" of the surgery for a malignant condition, i.e., a wide mesenteric resection with proximal ligation of vessels and hence removal of lymph node groups if the intention is curative, or limited mesenteric resection if the disease is advanced and the intention is palliative. The variety of terms used to describe the different types of colonic resection (colectomy) is depicted in Figure 5.5. Choice is also determined by the distribution or multiplicity of lesions detected at preoperative colonoscopy.

Resection in Neoplastic Conditions

Adenomatous polyps: as discussed above, the majority of adenomatous lesions can be removed by endoscopic techniques. However, large sessile polyps > 5 cm in diameter and occupying more than one third of the colon circumference should be removed by a localised resection. Sessile adenomas in the rectum can be removed by *transanal submucosal resection.* In this procedure adrenaline solution is infiltrated into the submucosa around the lesion and the mucosa is incised

Table 5.1.   Colorectal resections

Specific	diverticular disease volvulus pneumatosis coli colonic angiodysplasia rectal stump (CIBD, diversion proctitis) rectal mucosa (prolapse)
Ulceroinflammatory	ulcerative colitis Crohn's disease pseudomembranous colitis ischaemia
Neoplasia	large or multiple adenomas carcinoma malignant lymphoma

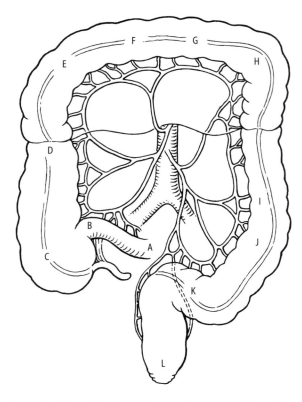

Figure 5.5. Types of colonic resection. From Rob and Smith's operative surgery of the colon, rectum and anus, 5th edition. Fielding LP, Goldberg SM (Eds), 1993. Reprinted with permission of Elsevier Science.

A → C:	Ileocaecectomy
±A + B → D:	Ascending colectomy
±A + B → F:	Right hemicolectomy
±A + B → G:	Extended right hemicolectomy
±E + F → G ± H:	Transverse colectomy
G → I:	Left hemicolectomy
F → I	Extended left hemicolectomy
J + K	Sigmoid colectomy
±A + B → J:	Subtotal colectomy
±A + B → K:	Total colectomy
±A + B → L:	Total proctocolectomy
L:	Proctectomy

by scissors 1 cm from the lesion. This can then be easily lifted off the circular muscle in a single piece and the mucosal defect is closed by sutures. Occasionally, large rectal polyps may require formal proctectomy or anterior resection.

Malignant lesions: the type of resection for colonic tumours will depend on the site of the lesion and the intent of the surgery. As previously stated, the colonic lymphatics accompany the main blood vessels and the extent of resection depends on the lymphatic clearance required. In cancer operations of curative intent the affected colon with its lymphovascular mesenteric pedicle is resected. Continuity is restored by either an ileocolic or colocolic end-to-end anastomosis.

However, on occasion an end ileostomy/colostomy may be required if the surgeon thinks that primary anastomosis would be compromised (e.g., if there is extensive intraperitoneal contamination).

The curative resection of rectal tumours may be carried out by one of two methods:

- *Anterior resection of rectum* – in this procedure the rectum is mobilised by entering the fascial plane around the mesorectum. This allows the rectum to be removed en bloc with the mesorectum which contains the initial draining lymphovascular channels and nodes (low anterior resection and total mesorectal excision – TME) (Figure 5.6a). Continuity is re-established by a stapling device forming an end-to-end colorectal anastomosis. Occasionally, in low anastomoses, a protective loop colostomy/ileostomy may be fashioned to divert the faecal stream. This can be closed at a later date. To obtain an adequate length of colon to form a safe anastomosis the splenic flexure will usually need to be mobilised. On occasions the spleen may be damaged during this mobilisation and a splenectomy would then have to be performed. In cases where the tumour is in the proximal rectum, a high anterior resection and mesorectal division can be employed. This entails division of the rectum and mesorectum 5 cm distal to the tumour and allows a larger rectal stump for anastomosis.
- *Abdominoperineal (AP) resection of rectum* – in this procedure the rectum is mobilised as above and the colon is divided at the apex of the sigmoid. The anal canal and distal rectum are then resected from below via the perineal route (Figure 5.6b). The entire rectum (and mesorectum) and anus are then removed en bloc. The perineal wound is closed and a permanent end colostomy is fashioned in the left iliac fossa using the transected end of the sigmoid colon.

Until the early 1980s anterior resection was used in less than 50% of patients with rectal tumours, i.e., those in the proximal rectum. However, it is now used for approximately 90% of tumours in the rectum. Initially it was feared that, because less tissue is excised and the clearance of the distal margin is not as great during anterior resection, there would be increased local recurrence rates if anterior resection was used for low rectal tumours. However, it appears that the degree of lateral clearance is similar in the two procedures and that a distal clearance of 2 cm is adequate to prevent local recurrence. Given the physical and psychological problems associated with a permanent colostomy, and the higher incidence of bladder and sexual problems in patients undergoing AP resection, it is felt that a sphincter-saving procedure (i.e., anterior resection) should be employed whenever possible. However, tumours extending to less than 2 cm from the anorectal junction (i.e., less than 6 cm from the anal verge) should be treated by AP resection.

Occasionally, in a medically unfit patient, localised resection is used for a well-differentiated, pT1 rectal cancer that is < 3 cm diameter. Accurate preoperative staging is crucial in selection of these patients and some may then need to proceed to salvage resection if adverse pathological features are identified in the pathological specimen, e.g., poor differentiation, lymphovascular involvement or invasion of muscle coat. Sometimes patients with obstructing cancers undergo partial laser ablation or stenting to restore intestinal continuity and avoid the risk of perforation. This may even allow resection to be carried out more safely at a later date.

Resection in Non-neoplastic Conditions

Hartmann's procedure – this is one of the most commonly used emergency operations for colorectal disease. Although this was initially devised for the elective treatment of proximal rectal tumours, it is now usually used in the emergency setting to treat conditions such as perforated diverticular disease (most commonly), perforated tumour, etc. The procedure itself is defined as resection of the sigmoid colon (and a variable length of proximal rectum if required) with the fashioning of a terminal end colostomy and closure of the rectal stump. The colostomy may be reversed at a later date by forming an end-to-end colorectal anastomosis.

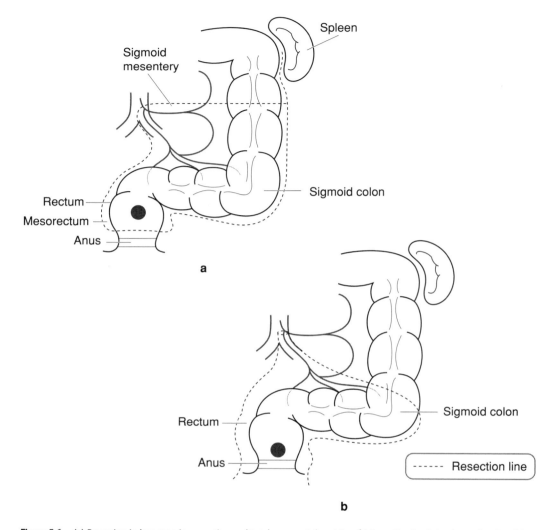

Figure 5.6 (**a**) Resection in low anterior resection and total mesorectal excision (**b**) Resection in abdominoperineal excision.

Non-acute presenting diverticular disease is usually treated surgically by either sigmoid colectomy or left hemicolectomy depending on the extent of the disease.

Surgery in colorectal inflammatory bowel disease – the surgical management of colorectal Crohn's disease is similar to that in the small intestine (see Chapter 4); namely, surgical intervention is reserved for those in whom medical management has failed (i.e., minimal resection of the diseased segment) or who are suffering complications, e.g., obstruction, pericolic abscess, fistula, etc.

As in Crohn's disease, close liaison between surgeons and physicians is required in the management of ulcerative colitis. Emergency surgery is needed in cases of acute severe colitis and/or toxic megacolon. The procedure of choice is a subtotal colectomy and end ileostomy with the

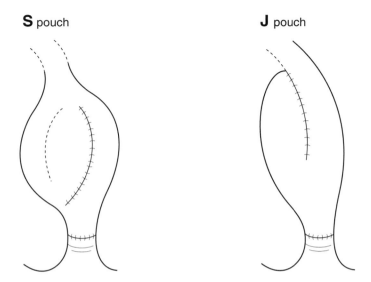

Figure 5.7. Two popular designs of ileal pouch.

proximal end of the rectum brought to the surface in the form of a mucus fistula. This spares an already sick patient the added trauma of pelvic surgery and, if ulcerative colitis is confirmed by histological examination, allows an ileoanal pouch procedure to be considered in the future. Prior to the mid-1970s, patients with refractory ulcerative colitis underwent a panproctocolectomy (removal of the colon, rectum and anus) with a permanent end ileostomy. However, in 1976 the procedure of *restorative proctocolectomy* was introduced and removed the need for a permanent ileostomy in suitable patients. In this procedure the entire colon and rectum are removed and the mucosa may be stripped from the upper anus above the dentate line (some surgeons prefer to leave this mucosa intact as it is thought to improve future continence). An ileal reservoir (pouch) is formed (Figure 5.7) and an ileoanal anastomosis is fashioned. A protective loop ileostomy is formed as close to the ileal pouch as possible and this can be closed at a later date (usually 2–3 months) after healing has been completed. A proportion of these patients (approximately 10%) may develop "pouchitis" – increased frequency of stool and feeling generally unwell. The exact aetiology of this is unknown but some feel it may be due to bacterial overgrowth in the pouch.

Angiodysplasia – if bleeding is severe enough to require surgical intervention, and if conservative treatment such as endoscopic coagulation has been unsuccessful, the procedure of choice will be dictated by the site of the bleeding point(s). However, if the site of bleeding cannot be discovered a total colectomy with ileorectal anastomosis (or end ileostomy, rectal mucus fistula and reversal at a later date) may be required.

6. Surgical Pathology Specimens – Laboratory Protocols

Biopsy Specimens

For biopsy specimens and local mucosal resections, see Gastrointestinal Specimens – General Comments (pages 6–8).

Resection Specimens

Specimen

Colorectal specimens are received for a range of either specific, ulceroinflammatory or neoplastic conditions (Table 5.1). These can be complicated by obstruction with or without associated enterocolitis or perforation, or show evidence of background disease such as CIBD or FAPC. The resection specimen is dictated by the site and nature of the abnormality and extent of any complications or predisposing lesions that are present.

Initial Procedure

In general, specimens are measured, opened with blunt-ended scissors along the antemesenteric border and then blocked longitudinally (but see diverticular disease and tumour) following gentle washing out of faecal debris, pinning out with avoidance of unnecessary traction, and immersion in 10% formalin fixative for 48 hours. Photographs may be taken before and after dissection.

When opening avoid areas of perforation or tumour. Tumour segments may either be left unopened for fixation and subsequent transverse slicing or carefully opened – the latter gives better fixation but the cut should be guided by palpation with the index finger to avoid disturbing the relationship of the tumour to the circumferential margin.

Specific Conditions

Diverticular Disease

- measurements: length × diameter (cm) of the thickened colonic segment.
- inspect and describe: perforation, pericolonic exudate or abscess.
- open and fix.
- serially transverse section at 5 mm intervals.
- sample (five blocks minimum) the diverticula, any associated inflammation or thickened mucosa that might represent crescentic colitis, mucosal prolapse or tumour.
- sample mesenteric lymph nodes.

Volvulus, Pneumatosis Coli, Rectal Stump, Rectal Mucosa in Prolapse

- measurements: length × maximum diameter (cm).
- open and fix.
- inspect and describe.
    - volvulus – dilatation, thinning, melanosis, stercoral ulceration, ischaemia, perforation.
    - pneumatosis – mucosal cobbling, blebs or gas cysts, inflammation, ulceration, perforation.
    - rectal stump – mucosal granularity, ulceration, polyps, fistulae, tumour.
    - rectal mucosal prolapse – mucosal granularity, thickening, induration, ulceration.
- sample (six blocks minimum) macroscopically normal and abnormal areas as indicated.
- sample mesenteric lymph nodes.

Ulceroinflammatory and Neoplastic Conditions

- open and inspect.
- measurements:
    - lengths and maximum diameter (cm) of the parts present – terminal ileum, appendix, colon, rectum, anus.

- lengths (cm) of ischaemic, inflamed or strictured segments.
- maximum dimensions (cm) of any perforation(s), ulcer(s), polyp(s) or tumour(s).
- distances (cm) of the abnormality from the proximal and distal resection limits.
- distances (cm) of the polyp/tumour/ulcer from the anorectal dentate line and relationship to the peritoneal reflection (above/straddling/below) and colorectal circumference (anterior/posterior/right or left lateral).
- distances (cm) of tumour from the serosa and nearest aspect of the mesocolic/mesorectal CRM.

- note the completeness of mesorectal excision, its capsular integrity or any deficiencies present.
- photograph.
- paint any aspect of the serosa or mesocolic/mesorectal margin adjacent to or overlying tumour or perforation.
- gently pin out and fix for 48 hours.

Description

- tumour – site: ileocaecal valve/caecum/colon (which segment, flexure)/rectum (above, straddling or below the peritoneal reflection and upper, mid or lower, anterior, posterior or lateral)/anus.

  lumenal/mural/extramural/mesenteric.

  – size: length × width × depth (cm) or maximum dimension (cm).

  – appearance: polypoid/nodular – adenoma, carcinoma, carcinoid, multiple lymphomatous polyposis, GIST.

  ulcerated/stricture – carcinoma, malignant lymphoma, metastatic carcinoma.

  fleshy/rubbery – malignant lymphoma, GIST.

  multiple – adenomas, carcinoma (primary or metastatic), malignant lymphoma.

  – edge: circumscribed/irregular.

  – perforation.

  – adjuvant therapy changes: necrosis, ulceration, fibrosis.
- CIBD
  - ulcerative colitis: contiguous/diffuse mucosal distribution, granularity, ulceration (linear/confluent), inflammatory polyps, synechiae, nodular or sessile DALMs, tumour, mucosal reversion with healing and atrophy, backwash ileiitis, treatment-related rectal sparing.
  - Crohn's disease: segmental/transmural distribution, cobblestone mucosa, ulceration (aphthous/linear/confluent), stricture, fat wrapping, fistula, polyps or tumour, lymphadenopathy, adhesions, abscess formation, ileal/anal disease.
- ischaemia – serosal hyperaemia/constriction band, mucosal hyperaemia/haemorrhage/ulceration/necrosis, wall thinning/perforation/stricture.

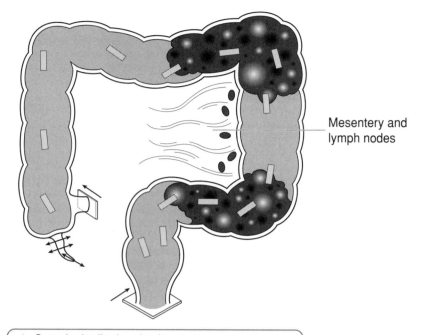

Mesentery and
lymph nodes

1. Sample the ileal and colorectal resection limits
2. Process the appendix as usual
3. Sample representative blocks of any abnormality
   including the junction with adjacent mucosa
4. Sequentially sample normal bowel
5. Sample mesenteric lymph nodes

Figure 5.8. Ulceroinflammatory colorectal conditions.

- pseudomembraneous colitis – pseudomembranes (adherent/yellow), mucosal granularity/ erosion/ulceration, stricture.
- obstructive enterocolitis – ulceration or stricture (contiguous or distant, diffuse or segmental), dilatation, wall thinning, perforation, ileal component.

Blocks for Histology

Ulceroinflammatory conditions (Figure 5.8)

- sample by circumferential transverse sections the proximal and distal limits of resection.
- sample macroscopically normal bowel.
- sample representative longitudinal blocks (a minimum of six) of any focal abnormality that is present to include its edge and junction with the adjacent mucosa, e.g., ulceration, stricture, fistula, perforation, pseudomembranes, inflammatory polyps, serosal adhesions or constriction bands. Also
  – CIBD: sequential labelled samples at 10 cm intervals from caecum to anus and additional blocks from any unusual nodular or sessile abnormality (DALM).

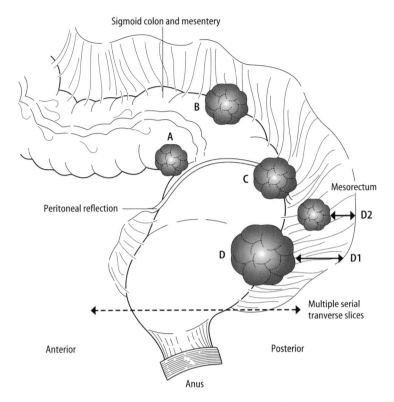

Figure 5.9. Rectal carcinoma. The upper anterior rectum is invested in peritoneum. The anterior mesorectum is thinner (0.75–1 cm) than the posterior mesorectum (1.5–3 cm). Cut the resection specimen into multiple serial transverse slices about 3–4 mm thick. Blocks for histology are:

Above the reflection	A	tumour, rectal wall and serosa
	B	tumour, rectal wall and serosa
		tumour, rectal wall and mesentery
At the reflection	C	tumour, rectal wall and serosa
		tumour, rectal wall and mesorectum
Below the reflection	D	tumour, rectal wall and mesorectum
	D1	distance (mm) of the deepest point of continuous tumour extension to the nearest point of the painted CRM
	D2	distance (mm) of the deepest point of discontinuous tumour extension (or in a lymphatic, node or vessel) to the nearest point of the painted CRM

Reproduced with permission from Allen DC. Histopathology Reporting: Guidelines for Surgical Cancer. Springer-Verlag: London, 2000.

- ischaemia: sample the mesenteric vessels.
- sample mesenteric lymph nodes and any other structures, e.g., appendix or terminal ileum.

Neoplastic conditions (Figure 5.9)

- sample the nearest longitudinal resection margin if tumour is present to within < 3 cm of it.

- sample macroscopically normal bowel and representative blocks of other mucosal lesions that are present, e.g., adenomatous polyps (if multiple, particularly those > 1 cm diameter).
- serially section the bulk of the tumour transversely at 3–4 mm intervals.
- lay the slices out in sequence and photograph.
- note and measure the relationship of the deep aspect of the tumour to the nearest site orientated point of the serosa and the CRM. Note serosal tumour perforation or CRM involvement (≤ 1 mm).
- sample (four blocks minimum) tumour and wall to demonstrate these relationships. With bulky mesentery/mesorectum the block may have to be split and appropriately labelled for loading in the cassettes.
- count and sample all lymph nodes and identify a suture tie limit node. Take care to count the nodes in the tumour slices and also those in the mesentery away from the tumour, e.g., sigmoid mesocolon in a rectal cancer.
- sample multifocal serosal seedlings as indicated by inspection and palpation.

Histopathology Report

- Ulcerative colitis:
    - Site-related disease activity (healed/quiescent/mild/moderate/severe), rectal sparing, appendiceal and caecal skip lesions, backwash ileiitis, toxic dilatation, superimposed infection (e.g., CMV), DALMs, carcinoma or lymphoma.
- Crohn's disease:
    - chronic transmural inflammation, granulomas, fissures/fistulae, abscess formation, segmental distribution/appendiceal/ileal disease, malignancy.
- Ischaemia:
    - necrosis – mucosal/transmural/gangrenous.
    - resection limits – ischaemic/viable.
    - mesenteric vessels – thrombosis/embolism/vasculitis.
    - miscellaneous – constriction band/volvulus/stricture.
- Pseudo membranous colitis:
    - pseudomembranes, ulceration, necrosis, perforation, strictures.
- Obstructive enterocolitis:
    - note ulceration/perforation/stricture/distribution and features specific to the aetiological abnormality.

Neoplastic conditions

- tumour type – adenocarcinoma/malignant lymphoma/other.
- tumour differentiation.
    - adenocarcinoma.
        - well or moderate/poor.
    - malignant lymphoma.
        - MALToma/centrocytic/follicle centre cell/Burkitt's/other.
        - low-grade/high-grade.
- tumour edge – pushing/infiltrative/lymphoid response.
- extent of local tumour spread (for carcinoma).
    - pTis   carcinoma in situ: intraepithelial (within basement membrane) or invasion of lamina propria (intramucosal) with no extension through muscularis mucosae into submucosa.
    - pT1   tumour invades submucosa.

- – pT2   tumour invades muscularis propria.
- – pT3   tumour invades through the wall into subserosa or non-peritonealised peri-colic/perirectal tissues.
- – pT4   tumour invades other organs or structures (e.g., other bowel loops via the serosa) and/or perforates visceral peritoneum.
- lymphovascular invasion – present/not present.
- regional lymph nodes.
  - – pericolic, perirectal, those located along the ileocolic, colic, inferior mesenteric, superior rectal and internal iliac arteries.
  - – pN0   no regional lymph node metastasis.
  - – pN1   1–3 involved regional lymph node(s).
  - – pN2   4 or more involved regional lymph nodes.
  - – Dukes' stage:
  - – A   tumour limited to the wall, node negative.
  - – B   tumour beyond the wall, node negative.
  - – C_1 nodes positive, apical node negative.
  - – C_2 apical node positive.
  - – D   distant metastases.
- excision margins.
  - – proximal and distal longitudinal (cm) and mesocolic/mesorectal circumferential (mm) limits of tumour clearance.
- other pathology.
  - – adenoma(s), FAPC, ulcerative colitis, Crohn's disease, schistosomiasis.

6

Appendix

1. Anatomy

The vermiform ("worm-like") appendix is a vestigial organ in the right iliac fossa. Although there is considerable variability in its length and position, the base of the appendix is always found attached to the posteromedial surface of the caecum, approximately 2 cm below the ileocaecal valve. The base is the only part of the appendix which is fixed, the remainder being free, thus accounting for the great variability in the position of the body and tip (Figure 6.1). It is completely surrounded by peritoneum which is continuous with the mesentery of the small intestine, this connection being termed the mesoappendix. Again, the size of the mesoappendix is variable and the distal appendix may occasionally be devoid of a mesenteric covering. As was stated, the position of the appendiceal base is constant, the surface landmark of this being one third the way along a line drawn from the right anterior superior iliac spine to the umbilicus – *McBurney's point*. Internally, the base can be found by following the taeniae coli of the caecum to the base of the appendix where they converge to form a continuous appendiceal longitudinal muscle coat.

Histologically, the appendiceal lumen is lined by colonic-type columnar epithelium with abundant lymphoid follicles (which decrease with age) in the submucosa. There are continuous circular and longitudinal muscle coats.

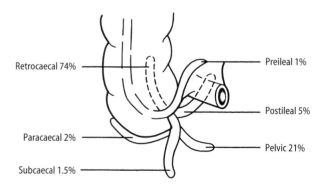

Figure 6.1. The various positions of the appendix. Reproduced from Mann CV, Russell RCG, Williams NS. (eds.) Bailey and Love's short practice of surgery. Chapman & Hall: London, 1995.

Lymphovascular supply

The appendix is supplied by terminal branches of the superior mesenteric artery and vein. Lymphatics drain to nodes in the mesoappendix and subsequently to superior mesenteric nodes.

2. Clinical Presentation

Acute appendicitis (and its complications) is among the most common surgical emergencies encountered. Classically it presents initially with vague, colicky central abdominal (periumbilical) pain which is associated with vomiting and anorexia. When the inflammation becomes transmural a localised peritonitis is illicited and the pain becomes sharp in nature, localised in the right iliac fossa and associated with pyrexia. Palpation reveals signs of localised peritonitis in the vicinity of *McBurney's point.*

As was stated above, the position of the body and tip of the appendix is variable and so the nature of the symptoms and signs will vary accordingly – e.g., flank pain and tenderness in retrocaecal appendicitis. Although perforation of the appendix usually remains localised (due to "walling off" by the greater omentum) occasionally it may lead to a generalised peritonitis.

The list of differential diagnoses for acute appendicitis is myriad and includes ectopic pregnancy, torsion of an ovarian cyst, Meckel's diverticulitis, urinary tract infection, terminal ileitis, endometriosis, etc.

An appendiceal abscess (which usually develops three days after a bout of acute appendicitis) can usually be palpated by a combination of abdominal and rectal examination. Differential diagnoses of an appendiceal mass also include carcinoma of the caecum, Crohn's terminal ileitis and ovarian carcinoma.

3. Clinical Investigations

- FBP – white cell count will be elevated in > 75% of cases of acute appendicitis.
- Pregnancy test – will be positive in an ectopic pregnancy.
- Urinalysis – to test for a urinary tract infection.
- USS – can demonstrate a swollen appendix and will detect a pelvic mass.
- CT scan – can delineate the nature of an "appendiceal mass".
- Laparoscopy – can be used to differentiate acute appendicitis from gynaecological conditions. It will also detect a small mass in the appendix, such as a mucocoele, and may be used to biopsy suspected deposits of pseudomyxoma peritonei.

4. Pathological Conditions

The appendix may be resected incidentally as part of a radical cancer operation, e.g., right hemicolectomy for caecal carcinoma, or, opportunistically at laparotomy, for other reasons, e.g., Meckel's diverticulectomy. However, the vast majority of appendices are removed because of clinically significant primary inflammation and a small minority for neoplasia.

Non-neoplastic Conditions

Appendicitis: caused by epithelial ulceration then infection by bowel bacteria, it may be precipitated by an underlying structural abnormality such as a diverticulum, or more commonly,

Table 6.1.   Obstructive causes of appendicitis

Faecolith	hardened, impacted faecal debris
Foreign body	vegetable matter, fruit pips
Tumour	carcinoid adenocarcinoma appendix or caecal base
Mucosal lymphoid hyperplasia	mesenteric adenitis, infectious mononucleosis, *Yersinia enterocolitica* infection
Endometriosis	

by luminal obstruction for one of various reasons (Table 6.1). It is characterised by transmural acute neutrophilic inflammation with the serosal component eliciting signs of peritonism. There is usually close correlation between the macroscopic and histological findings with acute appendicitis resulting in serosal congestion, inflammatory exudate and adherence of fat. Serious complications can arise from the resultant mural necrosis with wall thinning, gangrene and perforation potentially leading to generalised peritonitis, periappendicular abscess formation, portal vein pyaemia and hepatic abscesses. In general, the high risk of morbidity and mortality serves to emphasise the crucial importance of early diagnosis and therapeutic appendicectomy. Chronic appendicitis is a more controversial entity but in a minority of cases the inflammation may resolve leaving only residual thickening of the tissues.

Other unusual causes of sub-acute appendicitis are: granulomatous appendicitis (Crohn's disease, sarcoidosis, TB, schistosomiasis, but usually isolated and idiopathic), measles, CMV or secondary to ulcerative colitis. Periappendicitis or serosal inflammation without a mucosal or mural component should be noted as this may indicate inflammation emanating from another abdominopelvic organ, e.g., pelvic inflammatory disease (salpingitis) or colonic diverticulitis. In the older patient such an exudate must also be closely scrutinised for evidence of peritoneal spread of carcinoma cells.

Fibroneural obliteration of the appendiceal tip and body is now regarded as an age-related physiological phenomenon rather than representing evidence of previous inflammation.

Neoplastic Conditions

Carcinoid tumour: forming over 80% of appendiceal tumours, carcinoid tumour of classical type is usually small (< 1 cm diameter) and found as an incidental finding at the appendiceal tip with or without associated appendicitis. It can be a histological finding only amidst the inflammation, or macroscopically discernible as a firm, pale-yellow mass replacing the lumen and wall. It has a variable nested and tubular pattern of uniform neuroendocrine cells that are positive with chromogranin antibody. Despite showing transmural, serosal and lymphovascular spread, appendicectomy is usually totally therapeutic and recurrence is only seen in a very small number of cases where the lesion is greater than 2 cm diameter or there is involvement of the appendiceal base, caecal wall, mesoappendix or local lymph nodes. Conversely, the much less common mucin-rich goblet cell carcinoid (adenocarcinoid/crypt cell carcinoma) more frequently involves the appendiceal base with potential for nodal metastases, local invasion of the caecal pouch and transcoelomic peritoneal spread. Because of this, goblet cell carcinoid may require consideration for right hemicolectomy. Due to the difficulties in distinguishing between carcinoid tumour and inflammatory fibrotic reaction the appendiceal tip and base are sampled and separately identified as part of the routine blocking procedure to assess adequacy of tumour excision if present.

Adenoma: tubular, tubulo-villous or villous and more often sessile than polypoid comprising low- or high-grade dysplastic epithelium. It may be associated with synchronous/metachronous polyps or tumours elsewhere in the colorectum, FAPC, mucocoele (see below) or adenocarcinoma of the appendix or adjacent caecal pouch.

Adenocarcinoma: a relatively unusual lesion that may be mucinous and cystic, secondary involvement of the proximal appendix from the caecal pouch is more common than a primary appendiceal lesion. More recently, attention in the literature has focused on the association with ovarian mucinous borderline tumours (see pseudomyxoma peritonei). Very occasionally, mixed adenocarcinoma–carcinoid tumours occur. Other cancers metastatic to the appendix are from ovary, stomach, breast and lung.

Mucocoele: macroscopic distension of the appendiceal lumen by abundant mucus often with marked thinning of the wall. Obstructed or non-obstructed in character, the former represents a retention cyst lined by attenuated and atrophic but normal mucosa. Non-obstructed mucocoele is due to oversecretion of mucus by an abnormal mucosal lining that can be either hyperplastic, adenomatous or adenocarcinomatous in nature. Extrusion of mucus through the wall to the serosa results in pseudomyxoma peritonei which is localised to the periappendiceal tissues or generalised in the peritoneal cavity. The latter is refractory to surgical debridement with reaccumulation over a prolonged time course of months to years resulting in bowel obstruction and death. It is due to spillage of either atypical or frankly malignant appendiceal epithelium into the peritoneal cavity whereas mucocoele due to benign hyperplastic or cystadenomatous epithelium more often results in a self-limited localised reaction.

It is now recognised that there is a strong association between generalised pseudomyxoma peritonei, appendiceal mucinous tumours and bilateral ovarian mucinous borderline tumours, with the latter regarded as metastases from the appendiceal lesion.

Prognosis: carcinoid tumours less than 2 cm diameter are generally adequately treated by local appendicectomy. Those that are larger, involve the base or are of goblet cell type may require right hemicolectomy. Prognosis of mucocoele depends on the nature of the underlying mucosal epithelium and degree of spillage into the peritoneum. Adenocarcinoma treated by appendicectomy alone does worse (20% five-year survival) than when right hemicolectomy is performed (60–65% five-year survival) – outlook is tumour grade and stage dependent.

5. Surgical Pathology Specimens – Clinical Aspects

Biopsy Specimens

Not applicable.

Resection Specimens

Appendicectomy

Although the appendix may be removed laparoscopically or in the course of other procedures for diagnostic and/or staging purposes (e.g., suspected ovarian malignancy), the operation of choice in acute appendicitis is open appendicectomy. In the case of an "uncomplicated appendicitis" a muscle splitting *Gridiron* oblique incision centred over McBurney's point is used. The caecum is delivered into the wound and the taeniae coli are followed to the base of the appendix. The appendicular vessels in the mesoappendix are divided and ligated. The appendiceal base is crushed and ligated, and the appendix is divided distal to the ligation.

If appendiceal perforation with generalised peritonitis is present preoperatively, a midline incision may be employed to facilitate better access to the abdominal cavity. This will allow an adequate laparotomy examination and peritoneal lavage to be carried out and so will lessen the risk of postoperative abscess formation.

In the case of an appendiceal abscess, the patient may be initially treated conservatively with antibiotics and close clinical supervision, followed by an interval appendicectomy at a later date. However, if there is diagnostic doubt or worsening symptomatology (e.g., increasing pyrexia), early operative intervention is indicated. Although a simple appendicectomy may suffice, a right hemicolectomy may be needed if a large mass is present.

Right Hemicolectomy

The technique of right hemicolectomy (removal of the terminal ileum, caecum and proximal ascending colon) is described in detail elsewhere (see Chapter 5).

As well as for a large appendiceal mass, other lesions of the appendix requiring a right hemi-colectomy include primary adenocarcinoma and, as previously discussed, a minority of carcinoid tumours.

6. Surgical Pathology Specimens – Laboratory Protocols

Resection Specimens

Specimen

- handle similarly whether as part of a radical cancer resection specimen or a simple appen-dicectomy. The former will require sampling of adjacent structures and locoregional lymph nodes.
- some appendicectomies are submitted in several pieces due to difficulties in surgical exci-sion. This precludes assessment of the base unless a surgical clamp mark is visible.

Initial Procedure

- orientate the tip (rounded end) and the base (clamp marked).
- measurements:
  - appendix – length (cm) × maximum diameter (cm).
  - mesoappendix – maximum dimension (cm).
  - exudate (serofibrinous/mucin)/perforation/mucocoele/tumour – maximum dimension (cm) and distances (cm) from the tip and base.
- photograph before and after blocking as appropriate.
- fix in 10% formalin for 24–36 hours.

Description

- tumour   nodular/yellow: carcinoid.
                  cystic: cystadenoma/adenocarcinoma.
                  ulcerated/stricture/polypoid: adenocarcinoma/goblet cell carcinoid.
- wall   tumour confined to mucous membrane, in the wall or through the wall.
- mesoappendix   maximum dimension (cm) of abscess/tumour/mucin deposits.
- mucocoele   maximum diameter (cm)/intact or ruptured/mucin coating (location and extent).
- diverticulum   maximum diameter (cm) and location.
- appendicitis   exudate/perforation/gangrene: location and extent.

Blocks for Histology (Figure 6.2)

- trim off any excess mesenteric fat and only process that which appears abnormal.
- process in one cassette a 1–1.5 cm longitudinal slice from the tip along with a transverse section from the base.
- serially section the rest of the appendix transversely at 3 mm intervals with a sharp scalpel.
- sample five to six slices, approximately one slice per 1–1.5 cm length and process in a separate cassette from that of the tip/base.
- sample any area of mural thinning or focal lesion as indicated by gross inspection.
- if part of a formal cancer resection specimen, e.g., right hemicolectomy, dissect and sample as previously described.

Histopathology Report

- appendicitis
  - cause: faecolith, tumour, diverticulum, endometriosis.
  - type: acute (transmural/gangrenous/perforation/abscess).
            granulomatous.
            periappendicular.
- mucocoele
  - obstructed/non-obstructed.
  - intact/ruptured.
  - mucosal hyperplasia/adenoma/adenocarcinoma.
  - pseudomyxoma: localised/generalised/nature of the epithelium present.

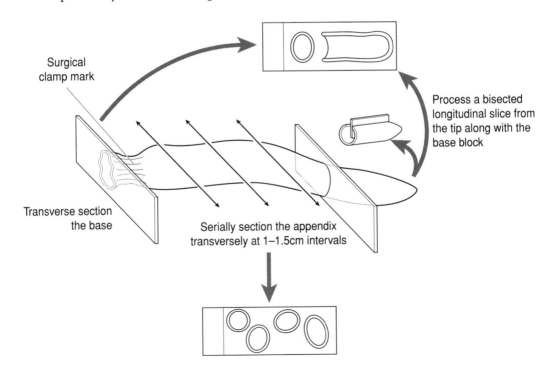

Surgical clamp mark

Process a bisected longitudinal slice from the tip along with the base block

Transverse section the base

Serially section the appendix transversely at 1–1.5cm intervals

Figure 6.2.   Appendicectomy specimen.

- carcinoid tumour
    - type: classical/goblet cell.
    - size: < or > 2 cm.
    - spread: mesoappendix, appendiceal base.
- adenocarcinoma – see Colorectal carcinoma. In the TNM system, appendix is an anatomical subsite of colorectum.

7 Anus

1. Anatomy

The anal canal (anus) is 4 cm long and is continuous with the rectum above the pelvic floor. The mucous membrane of the upper half of the anal canal is lined by columnar epithelium and supplied by autonomic nerves, being sensitive only to stretch. The lower half is lined by stratified squamous epithelium and has a somatic nerve supply, being sensitive to pain, touch, etc. There is a transition zone with a sharp demarcation between the two types of mucosa, termed the *dentate line*. The circular muscle layer is thickened around the upper anal canal to form the internal (involuntary) sphincter. A sheath of striated muscle encloses this – the external (voluntary) sphincter. The longitudinal muscle coat descends between the internal and external sphincters. The ischiorectal fossa is a fat-filled space on either side of the anal canal between it and the bony pelvis (Figure 7.1).

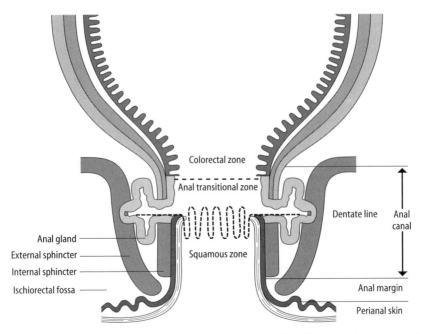

Figure 7.1. The anatomy of the anal canal. Reproduced from Williams GR, Talbot IC. Anal carcinoma: a histological review. Histopathology 1994;25:507–516

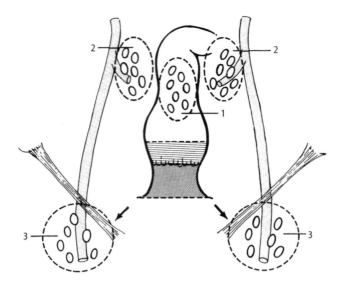

Figure 7.2. Anus: regional lymph nodes. Perirectal (1), internal iliac (2) and inguinal (3). Reproduced from Hermanek P, Hutter RVP, Sobin LH, Wagner G, Wittekind Ch (eds.). TNM Atlas: illustrated guide to the TNM/pTNM classification of malignant tumours, 4th edition. Springer-Verlag: Berlin and Heidelberg, 1997.

Lymphovascular Supply

The upper half is supplied by the superior rectal artery (a branch of the inferior mesenteric artery) and the lower half by the inferior rectal artery (a branch of the internal iliac artery). The veins correspond to the arteries and the lymphatics from the upper and lower halves drain to the inferior mesenteric and superficial inguinal nodes, respectively (Figure 7.2).

2. Clinical Presentation

Anorectal conditions are relatively common in surgical practice and present in a number of ways including pain, itch, bleeding, discharge, pyrexia, a mass or inguinal lymphadenopathy. An accurate diagnosis is crucial to successful treatment of the condition.

3. Clinical Investigations

- FBP – occasionally chronic bleeding can lead to iron deficiency anaemia.
- Serology – if a syphilitic ulcer is suspected.
- Blood glucose – in those with recurrent anorectal sepsis to rule out diabetes mellitus.
- Microbiology – pus from an abscess should be cultured and antibiotic sensitivities obtained.
- Proctoscopy – used to inspect the anus and anorectal ring. Biopsy of lesions above the dentate line can be taken without anaesthesia.
- Sigmoidoscopy/colonoscopy – should be undertaken when an anorectal condition is thought to be secondary to inflammatory bowel disease.

- MRI scan – useful in delineating the course of complicated fistulae and with ELUS the extent of local tumour spread. CT scan (chest, abdomen and pelvis) will demonstrate local and distant metastases.
- Trucut needle biopsy – used when there is suspicion of recurrent or residual tumour in the ischiorectal fossa.

4. Pathological Conditions

Non-neoplastic Conditions

Haemorrhoids (piles): comprising engorgement of submucosal veins, they are common and predisposed to by increased pelvic pressure, e.g., constipation, pregnancy, obesity, pelvic tumour. They bulge into the anal canal and are traumatised by straining at stool and hard faeces. Complications include bleeding, reversible prolapse into the anal canal or persistent prolapse outside the anal margin – these so-called external haemorrhoids which are located below the dentate line and covered by anal skin are particularly prone to painful strangulation and thrombosis which is an indication for surgical excision.

Skin tags: fibrous skin tags at the anal margin can indicate various abnormalities, e.g., a previous thrombosed external haemorrhoid, Crohn's disease, fissure or fistula.

Fissure-in-ano: a tear at the anal margin that often follows the passage of a constipated stool, it is usually posterior and midline in location. It is painful and may be marked by a skin tag at its distal aspect. Multiple fissures can complicate Crohn's disease.

Anorectal abscesses: resulting from infection of anal submucosal glands, they are perianal, ischiorectal, submucous or pelvirectal in location. Underlying Crohn's disease or diabetes must always be excluded in anorectal sepsis.

Fistula-in-ano: an abnormal communication between two epithelial surfaces, commonly the anal canal and perineal skin. The majority arise from infection of anal glands resulting in an anorectal abscess that tracks and opens, discharging onto the perineum externally and the anal canal internally. Associated conditions such as Crohn's disease, ulcerative colitis and mucinous carcinoma must be excluded histologically.

Prolapse: a consequence of mucosal prolapse at this site is inflammatory cloacogenic polyp. It arises at the internal margin comprising a mixture of thickened low rectal and high anal glandular and squamous mucosae associated with hypertrophic muscularis mucosae. These polyps are often excised to exclude the possibility of adenoma or carcinoma which can share similar clinical appearances.

Neoplastic Conditions

Benign tumours: these are rare, e.g., granular cell tumour.

Human papilloma virus (HPV): a common aetiological agent associated with a spectrum of anal viral lesions, preneoplasia (anal intraepithelial neoplasia – AIN) and carcinoma, as well as concurrent lesions of the uterine cervix. HPV subtypes 16/18 are particularly neoplasia-progressive in this viral – AIN – carcinoma sequence.

Anal margin/perianal skin carcinoma: commonly well-differentiated keratinising squamous carcinoma with predisposing conditions being viral warts (condyloma accuminatum), giant condyloma of Buschke–Löwenstein and Bowen's disease (squamous cell carcinoma in-situ) of anal skin. Variants include the exophytic, indolent verrucous carcinoma. Treatment is primarily by local surgical excision as for skin carcinoma.

Anal canal carcinoma: a squamous cell carcinoma with variable degrees of squamous, basaloid (synonym: cloacogenic/non-keratinising small cell squamous carcinoma) and ductular differentiation. Proximal canal cancers are poorly differentiated and basaloid whereas distal anal cancers are well differentiated and more overtly squamous in character. There is an increased incidence in Crohn's disease, smoking, immunosuppression and sexually transmitted diseases. At diagnosis, many have spread through sphincteric muscle into adjacent soft tissues (vagina, urethra etc.) and 5–10% have haematogenous metastases to liver, lung and skin. Primary therapy is concurrent radio-/chemotherapy with good preservation of anal sphincter function and tumour response. Abdominoperineal or exenterative resection is reserved for extensive (e.g., vaginal involvement), recurrent or non-responsive tumours. Inguinal node disease may require block dissection of the groin. Many arise in the vicinity of the dentate line from the transitional/cloacal zone with upwards submucosal spread, presenting as an ulcerated tumour of the lower rectum from which it must be distinguished by biopsy as rectal cancer requires surgical resection.

Other cancers: a not-uncommon differential diagnosis is a low rectal carcinoma with distal spread into the anal canal. Relatively rare cancers are mucinous adenocarcinoma in an anal fistula, anal gland adenocarcinoma, extra-mammary Paget's disease (associated with low rectal adenocarcinoma, anal gland adenocarcinoma, or isolated), malignant melanoma and leiomyosarcoma.

Prognosis: perianal carcinoma 85% five-year survival, anal canal carcinoma 65–80% five-year survival. Adverse indicators are advanced stage or depth of spread, inguinal node involvement and post-treatment pelvic and perineal recurrence. Malignant melanoma is aggressive with poor outlook, the prognosis of leiomyosarcoma is related to tumour grade.

5. Surgical Pathology Specimens – Clinical Aspects

Biopsy Specimens

The anal canal is best inspected by proctoscopy. The proctoscope is a rigid disposable tube with a light source attached, which is inserted with the patient in the left lateral position. Forceps can be passed through the tube to biopsy any visible lesion. Biopsy specimens may also be received from the walls/roof of areas of anorectal sepsis to rule out granulomatous inflammation.

Resection Specimens

Resection of Neoplastic Disease

Anal carcinoma – small lesions (< 2 cm) present at the anal verge are usually treated by local excision with a 2 cm margin of skin around the tumour. The resection should extend down to the perianal fat. For larger tumours, or extensive tumours of the anal canal that are unresponsive to radio-/chemotherapy, abdominoperineal resection is the procedure of choice. A 2 cm margin of perineal skin should be excised around the tumour and there should be a radical ischiorectal resection. If there is metastatic spread to superficial inguinal nodes then a radical groin dissection may be considered.

Resection of Non-neoplastic Lesions

Fissure-in-ano – acute fissures can usually be treated conservatively by introducing stool-softening measures. However, a chronic anal fissure can be treated by either anal dilatation or lateral internal sphincterotomy.

Haemorrhoids – if haemorrhoids are small and asymptomatic then no treatment is necessary except for measures to avoid constipation. Non-prolapsing piles are probably best treated by injection sclerotherapy. Larger prolapsing piles above the dentate line are treated by rubber-band ligation. Both the above procedures can be performed during routine proctoscopy without anaesthesia. Piles too large to band and/or which extend below the dentate line can be treated by formal haemorrhoidectomy. The procedure most commonly used involves excision of the three main piles, with preservation of the intervening anal mucosa. The wounds are left open to heal by secondary intention.

Anorectal abscess/fistula – an abscess is drained under general anaesthetic, after thorough proctoscopic/sigmoidoscopic examination, by incision and laying open the abscess cavity. The surgical treatment of fistula-in-ano depends on the position of the tracts and is often complicated. Essentially, the general principle of anorectal fistula surgery is to lay open the primary tract and drain any secondary tracts while maintaining sphincter function. It is crucial to continence to preserve the function of the upper part of the external sphincter and so laying open "high" fistulae is not advised. Instead, a permanent *seton* suture is passed through the tract and allows drainage while the secondary tract heals. The primary tract should then heal after removal of the suture.

6. Surgical Pathology Specimen – Laboratory Protocols

Biopsy Specimens

Elliptical incisional and excisional biopsies of the perineal skin and anal margin are handled similarly to skin biopsies. Anal canal biopsy fragments are processed as previously described – see Gastrointestinal Specimens – General Comments (page 6). Specific points of note are:

Haemorrhoids: typically nodular and 1–2 cm in diameter with a smooth covering mucosa and ectatic submucosal vessels. Bisect vertically down through the epithelial surface and process both halves. With larger or multiple specimens a mid-slice of each is taken.

Skin tags: count and measure, process intact, vertically bisect or take a representative mid-slice according to size.

Fissure-in-ano: not usually excised although biopsy fragments of granulation tissue from its edge may be submitted.

Anorectal abscess: usually heavily inflamed ellipses of tissue from the covering skin, lateral or deep aspects of the abscess wall. Measure, process intact, vertically bisect or take a representative mid-slice according to size.

Fistula-in-ano (Figure 7.3): rarely resected but typically a small skin ellipse often with a punctate opening on the surface, minimal subcutaneous tissue and a stringy attachment which may be up to several centimetres long – the fistulous tract. It may also be submitted in fragments if excision was difficult. Measure the skin ellipse, its opening and the tract. Take a block vertically through the skin to include the punctum and represent any subcutaneous abscess. Sample multiple transverse sections of the fistulous tract and label a transverse deep resection limit block.

Cloacogenic polyp: measure, vertically bisect or take representative slices. Prior to this paint the deep and lateral margins in case it turns out to be polypoid tumour.

Neoplastic Conditions

Anal margin/perianal skin lesions such as condyloma, Bowen's disease or carcinoma are handled as for skin specimens.

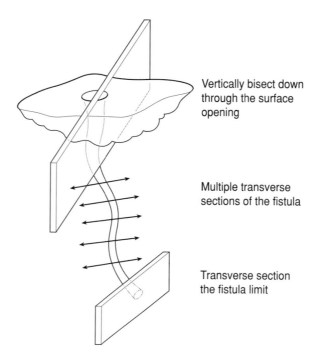

Vertically bisect down
through the surface
opening

Multiple transverse
sections of the fistula

Transverse section
the fistula limit

Figure 7.3.   Fistula-in-ano.

Anal canal carcinoma if resected will either be because of recurrent or extensive disease in the context of abdominoperineal resection or pelvic exenteration specimens where the tumour spread may be partially masked by fibrotic radio-/chemotherapy changes. For general comments see Gastrointestinal Specimens – Colorectum (Chapter 5) and Pelvic Exenterations Specimens (Chapter 34).

Specific points of note in abdominoperineal resection for anal canal carcinoma are:

- open the canal longitudinally with blunt-ended scissors on the opposite side of the tumour having previously painted the external CRM.
- the tumour is frequently submucosal ± overlying mucosal ulceration. Pale and variably fleshy to scirrhous in character, pigmentation and rubbery/fleshy qualities should raise the possibility of malignant melanoma or leiomyosarcoma, respectively. Mucinous carcinoma may occur in a fistula while anal gland carcinoma is also submucosal and sclerotic.
- the relationships and distances (mm) to the anal margin/perianal skin and anorectal dentate line.
- upward or downward spread to the lower rectum and perianal skin, respectively.
- the extent of mucosal/mural/extramural spread and distances (mm) to the nearest longitudinal and radial margins (perianal skin, site-orientated apsect of the CRM). Note that the CRM comprises a tube of perianal levator musculature which also forms a tight neck or constriction at its junction with the lower edge of the mesorectum.
- serially section the tumour transversely at 3–4 mm intervals. Sample a minimum of four blocks of tumour and wall to show the deepest point of invasion in relation to the painted

CRM. Sample a longitudinal block of tumour and proximal/distal limit if close (< 0.5–1 cm) to it.

Histopathology report

- tumour type – anal canal squamous carcinoma/other.
- tumour differentiation – basaloid/keratinising/non-keratinising/ductular component.
- tumour edge – pushing/infiltrative/lymphoid response.
- extent of local tumour spread
  - pTis   carcinoma in situ.
  - pT1   tumour ≤ 2 cm in greatest dimension.
  - pT2   2 cm < tumour ≤ 5 cm in greatest dimension.
  - pT3   tumour > 5 cm in greatest dimension.
  - pT4   tumour of any size invading adjacent organ(s), e.g., vagina, urethra, bladder.
- lymphovascular invasion – present/not present.
  - anal margin/perianal skin lesions: inguinal nodes.
  - anal canal lesions: perirectal, internal iliac, inguinal nodes in that order.
  - pN0   no regional lymph node mestastasis.
  - pN1   metastasis in perirectal lymph node(s).
  - pN2   metastasis in unilateral internal iliac and/or unilateral inguinal lymph node(s).
  - pN3   metastasis in perirectal and inguinal lymph nodes and/or bilateral internal iliac and/or bilateral inguinal lymph nodes.
- excision margins
  - proximal rectal and distal perianal/perineal limits of tumour clearance (cm).
  - deep circumferential radial margin of clearance (mm).
- other pathology
  - Condylomatous warts or giant condyloma, Bowen's disease, anal fistula, Crohn's disease, AIN, radio-/chemotherapy necrosis and tumour regression.

8 Gall Bladder

1. Anatomy

The gall bladder is a sac which lies on the inferoposterior surface of the liver. It is divided into the fundus (rounded portion which projects below the liver), body (lies in contact with the liver) and neck (becomes continous with the cystic duct). Stones may cause a dilatation at the junction of the neck and cystic duct known as Hartmann's pouch. The gall bladder is two-thirds surrounded by peritoneum which binds the non-peritonealised adventitial aspect of the body and neck to the under surface of the liver. The cystic duct is 4 cm long and joins the neck of the gall bladder to the right side of the common hepatic duct to form the common bile duct. The course of the cystic duct shows great variation between individuals. The gall bladder is concerned with the concentration, storage and delivery of bile. To aid the concentration process the mucous membrane is thrown into permanent folds. The bile salts emulsify fats in the duodenum and so facilitate their digestion and absorption. When fatty food enters the duodenum, endocrine cells release hormones which lead to contraction of the gall bladder and relaxation of the sphincter of Oddi, thus allowing bile to be delivered to the duodenum. The mucous membrane of the cystic duct is raised in the form of a spiral fold. This is thought to assist in keeping the lumen patent. An important surgical landmark (where the cystic artery can be found) is *Calot's triangle*, which is formed by the common hepatic duct, the cystic duct and the liver (Figure 3.2).

Lymphovascular Supply

The main arterial supply to the gall bladder is from the right hepatic artery via the cystic artery, which runs through Calot's triangle. The cystic vein drains directly to the portal system. Lymphatics from the gall bladder and bile ducts pass to the cystic node (situated near the gall bladder neck) and then through the infrahepatic nodes. At the distal end of the common bile duct they pass into the peripancreatic and periduodenal nodes, and ultimately drain to the coeliac and superior mesenteric nodes (Figure 8.1).

2. Clinical Presentation

There is considerable overlap in the clinical features of gall bladder and extrahepatic bile duct disease. Gallstones are often asymptomatic. However, if there is gall bladder outlet obstruction by a stone then progressively severe right-upper-quadrant "colicky" pain (biliary colic), associated with nausea and vomiting, may be felt. If the stone remains impacted the gall bladder may become infected and acutely inflamed (acute cholecystitis) – this leads to severe constant right-upper-quadrant pain, pyrexia and signs of localised peritonitis. This can progress to an empyema

The regional lymph nodes are the cystic duct node and the pericholedochal, hilar, peripancreatic (head only), periduodenal, periportal, coeliac and superior mesenteric nodes

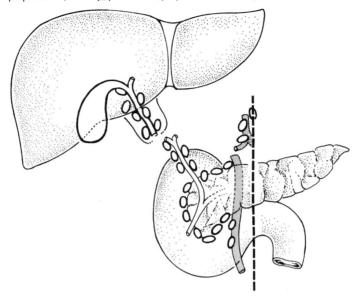

Figure 8.1. Gall bladder: regional lymph nodes. Reproduced from Hermanek P, Hutter RVP, Sobin LH, Wagner G, Wittekind Ch (eds.). TNM Atlas: illustrated guide to the TNM/pTNM classification of malignant tumours, 4th edition. Springer-Verlag: Berlin and Heidelberg, 1997.

(pus-filled gall bladder). Stone impaction may also lead to a mucocoele, i.e., a dilated gall bladder in which the bile has been resorbed but mucus secretion continues. A mucocoele is heralded by a palpable gall bladder and dull right-upper-quadrant pain. Occasionally in the elderly the gall bladder may perforate leading to generalised peritonitis. Gallstones localised to the cystic duct will occasionally cause obstructive jaundice, especially if the duct is short as the inflammation and oedema around the cystic duct impedes the flow of bile through the adjacent common bile duct (Mirizzi syndrome). Gallstone ileus (small-bowel obstruction due to impaction of a stone at the ileocaecal valve after the formation of a fistula between the gall bladder and duodenum) is a rare complication of cholecystitis.

Gall bladder carcinoma may present in a similar manner to gallstone disease, although weight loss and jaundice are additional features, obstructive jaundice being caused by metastatic spread to nodes which compress the bile ducts.

3. Clinical Investigations

There is considerable overlap in the investigation of gall bladder and extrahepatic bile duct disease.

- FBC – elevated WCC in cholecystitis.
- AXR – 10% of stones are radio-opaque; gas in the gall bladder wall (emphysematous chole-cystitis) is a serious complication of cholecystitis seen most commonly in diabetics; in

gallstone ileus it will show the classic triad of small-intestinal obstruction, gallstone in the right iliac fossa and gas in the biliary tree.

- USS – sensitive for stones > 4 mm.
- Oral cholecystogram – oral contrast is taken and this is absorbed from the gut, bound to albumin in the portal vein, and subsequently secreted in bile. Radiological imaging of the gall bladder is then carried out 10 hours after ingestion. Although largely replaced by USS, this investigation is still indicated when the clinical symptoms are strongly suggestive of gall-stones and the USS is negative.
- Radionucleotide scanning – high sensitivity in acute cholecystitis.
- Percutaneous drainage – under radiological guidance can be used to drain the gall bladder in, e.g., empyema.
- CT scan (chest, abdomen and pelvis), cholangiography (percutaneous or at ERCP) – to demonstrate a tumour mass, invasion of the liver and compression of bile ducts.

4. Pathological Conditions

Non-neoplastic Conditions

Cholelithiasis (gall stones): the commonest aetiological agent in gall bladder pathology and clas-sically occurring in fair, fat, fertile, females in their forties. Mixed stones are the most frequent (80%) formed from an amalgam of bile, cholesterol and calcium, and comprising biliary sludge, calculous gravel or multiple, faceted, laminated stones. Occasionally, stones can be pure such as dark bilirubinate pigment stones in a congenital haemolytic disorder, e.g., spherocytosis, or soli-tary, large, yellow and cholesterol rich.

Acute cholecystitis: 95% of cases are due to impaction of a stone in the cystic duct resulting in stasis, a bile-induced chemical reaction and then secondary infection. The acute inflammation often subsides with conservative medical treatment but can persist producing an empyema – perforation and bile peritonitis are unusual. In a mucocoele the wall may calcify and form a "porcelain" gall bladder.

Chronic cholecystitis: invariably associated with calculi, there are varying degrees of mucosal and transmural chronic inflammation, thickening of the muscularis, perimuscular fibrosis and adherence to the liver bed. Indicators of chronicity are mucosal pseudopyloric metaplasia and transmural mucosal herniation to form Rokitansky–Aschoff sinuses. These mucosal pouches can inspissate with bile and mucus becoming inflamed and forming extramural abscesses which may only partly resolve leaving a marked xanthogranulomatous histiocytic inflammatory reaction that encases the gall bladder. Prominent sinus formation at the fundus can similarly mimic a mucosal polyp or tumour; so-called cholecystitis glandularis proliferans. Unusual variants of chronic cholecysitis are follicular (reactive lymphoid aggregates), eosinophilic (often acalculous and chemical in nature) and malakoplakia. Due to the strong association with pancreatitis, fat necrosis and calcification may be seen.

Cholesterolosis: a relatively common finding of yellow mucosal flecks ("strawberry" gall bladder) due to accumulation of cholesterol-laden macrophages in the lamina propria. It is usually incidental and not associated with hypercholesterolaemia.

Oleogranulomas: the cystic duct lymph node is not infrequently enlarged and submitted along with the cholecystectomy specimen. It often contains oleogranulomas comprising fat spaces surrounded by histiocytes presumably representing a gall bladder drainage phenomenon.

Neoplastic Conditions

Adenoma: relatively uncommon in surgical material, adenomas can be polypoid or sessile, tubular, tubulovillous or villous and comprise variably dysplastic epithelium. The dysplasia may be multifocal and the proximal cystic duct margin should be checked for this.

Carcinoma: usually occurs in late-middle-aged females and many (50–75%) present already with regional lymph node metastasis and involvement of the gall bladder bed, liver or other direct spread to duodenum, stomach, colon and peritoneum. Calculi (80–90% of cases), chronic inflammatory bowel disease and sclerosing cholangitis are risk factors. Often clinically inapparent and found incidentally as diffuse thickening of the wall at cholecystectomy for gall stones, 10–20% are initially diagnosed by histology of routine blocks, there having been no macroscopic suspicion of tumour. Fundal in location (60%) and grossly diffuse (70%) or polypoid (30%), the vast majority (95%) are adenocarcinomas of tubular or papillary patterns arising from a sequence of intestinal metaplasia–dysplasia–carcinoma. Assessment of the depth of invasion can be difficult and extension of carcinoma in situ into Rokitansky–Aschoff sinuses must be distinguished from true invasion of the wall. Perineural involvement is characteristic. Gall bladder cancer may therefore be encountered either in the context of an incidental finding in a simple cholecystectomy, or infrequently as an electively planned extended cholecystectomy (with or without segmental resection of liver) with radical lymph node dissection.

Other cancers: rare but can include embryonal rhabdomyosarcoma (children), leiomyosarcoma and malignant lymphoma, or metastatic carcinoma especially transcoelomic – stomach, pancreas, ovary, bile ducts, colon and breast.

Prognosis: better if lesions are of papillary type, low histological grade and confined to the mucous membrane, when resection is potentially curative (90% five-year survival). However, many cases present with disease beyond the gall bladder, involvement of liver (25% five-year survival) and overall 5–10% five-year survival figures.

5. Surgical Pathology Specimens – Clinical Aspects

Resection Specimens

Benign Conditions

In benign disease the gall bladder may be removed either laparoscopically or by an open procedure.

Laparoscopic cholecystectomy is now by far the most popular method. There are no absolute contraindications except for those that apply to other operative procedures, e.g., poor anaesthetic risk. However, previous abdominal surgery with resultant fibrous adhesions and obesity may make a laparoscopic approach difficult. It may have to be abandoned and converted to an open cholecystectomy. In a laparoscopic cholecystectomy an initial small infraumbilical stab wound is made and a spring-loaded Veress needle is passed through the abdominal wall into the peritoneal cavity. A CO_2 supply is then connected to the needle and gas is insufflated into the abdomen to produce a pneumoperitoneum. The needle is then removed and the incision extended and deepened. A sheath is then inserted and the laparoscope is passed through this to make the optic port. The image from the laparoscope is transferred to a monitor and can be viewed by the surgeon. Three other incisions (ports) are made under direct visualisation: for retraction and irrigation; for tools such as an electrosurgical hook, scissors, etc.; and for grasping forceps. An initial examination of all areas of the abdomen is performed, including the pelvis. The fundus of the gall bladder is then grasped, the cystic artery and duct in Calot's triangle both clipped and divided.

If cholangiography with or without exploration of the common bile duct is required, a cannula is passed into the common bile duct via an opening in the cystic duct before clipping. The gall bladder is then dissected from the liver bed and the contents removed by suction. It is then placed in a bag and removed through the optic port.

Open cholecystectomy is used in the few cases deemed inappropriate for laparoscopic chole-cystectomy via a Kocher's incision parallel to the right subcostal margin.

Gall Bladder Cancer

Careful patient selection for surgery of gall bladder cancer is essential and only relatively fit patients with localised tumours and no evidence of metastatic spread should be considered. However, despite this the results of surgery remain poor with 90% of patients dying within 12 months.

A right subcostal incision is used and a complete examination of the abdomen undertaken. If there is no invasion of the bile ducts and no or only superficial liver invasion, an *extended cholecystectomy* is performed. In this, after determination of the depth of liver invasion by intra-operative USS, the gall bladder and the hepatic gall bladder bed are removed in the form of a wedge resection. A regional lymph node dissection is carried out by removing the lymph nodes draining the gall bladder as far as the coeliac nodes.

If the tumour extends more deeply into the liver, then a *segmental liver resection* (usually IV and V or IV, V and VI) will be required. Very occasionally, if the tumour has spread to the extra-hepatic bile ducts, a segmental liver resection and extrahepatic duct resection is required. Rarely, a liver resection and an extended Whipple's procedure may be used. Palliation can involve bypass surgery or stenting to relieve gastric outlet obstruction or jaundice.

6. Surgical Pathology Specimens – Laboratory Protocols

Biopsy Specimens

Not applicable.

Resection Specimens

Specimen

Most cholecystectomy specimens are now done laparoscopically rather than by open surgery and submitted opened or unopened containing 5–10 ml of bile fluid. Occasionally, specimens are received in several pieces if operative access has been technically difficult. The proximal end comprises a variable length of cystic duct adjacent to which an enlarged lymph node may be present.

Initial Procedure

- measurements:
    gall bladder – length × maximum diameter (cm).
    cystic duct – length × maximum diameter (cm).
    lymph node – number and maximum diameter (cm).
- open longitudinally from the fundus towards the cystic duct with blunt-ended scissors, draining off the bile and noting any contents.
- photograph if appropriate.

- paint the external serosal and adventitial aspects if there is any suspicion of tumour.
- fixation by immersion in 10% formalin for 36–48 hours.

Description

- received – opened/unopened/intact/deficient/perforated/fragments.
- adventitia – adhesions/rim of liver/tumour.
- serosa – adhesions/exudate/perforation/tumour.
- wall – thickness (cm)/fibrosis/tumour/thinning/necrosis/perforation/sinuses/abscess/calcification.
- mucosa – tumour: polypoid/nodular/ulcerated/diffuse/mucinous.
    - length × width × depth (cm) or maximum dimension (cm).
    - location (fundus/body/neck/cystic duct) and distance (mm) to the cystic duct limit.
    - confined to mucous membrane, in the wall or through the wall.
- cholesterolosis/ulceration/haemorrhage/polyps/glandularis proliferans.
- contents – bile/mucus/stones (size, number, shape, mixed, pigment, cholesterol)/fibrin/pus.
- cystic duct – stone impaction/dilatation/lymph node.

Blocks for Histology: (Figure 8.2)

- sample by circumferential transverse section the proximal cystic duct limit.
- sample the cystic duct lymph node and any other separately submitted named nodes.
- serially transverse section the gall bladder at 3–4 mm intervals with either a sharp knife or scissors.
- usually one broken transverse ring will suffice for histology in the absence of any macroscopic abnormality.
- sample gross lesions with multiple transverse blocks as indicated, e.g., ulceration, perforation, tumour, abscess, polyps, wall thickening. Demonstrate tumour in relation to the serosa and adventitia including its resection margin.

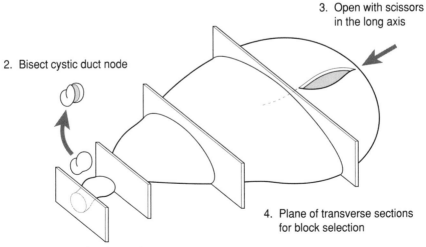

3. Open with scissors in the long axis

2. Bisect cystic duct node

4. Plane of transverse sections for block selection

1. Transverse section the cystic duct proximal limit

Figure 8.2.   Opening and transverse sectioning the gall bladder.

- if part of a radical cancer resection – describe and measure the attached segments of liver and bile ducts, and the relationship of any tumour to them and their resection limits. Sample multiple blocks to demonstrate these relationships. Sample all regional lymph nodes.

Histopathology Report

- non-neoplastic
  - inflammation: acute/chronic/xanthogranulomatous.
  - necrosis/perforation/abscess/empyema/fistula.
  - mucocoele.
- tumour type – adenocarcinoma/other.
- tumour differentiation – well/moderate/poor.
- tumour edge – pushing/infiltrative/lymphoid response.
- extent of local tumour spread.
  - pTis   carcinoma in-situ.
  - pT1   tumour limited to gall bladder wall:
  -             a.   lamina propria.
  -             b.   muscularis.
  - pT2   tumour invades perimuscular connective tissue, no extension beyond serosa or into liver.
  - pT3   tumour perforates serosa (visceral peritoneum) and/or directly invades the liver and/or one other adjacent organ or structure, e.g., stomach, duodenum, colon, pancreas, omentum, extrahepatic bile ducts.
  - pT4   tumour invades main portal vein or hepatic artery, or invades two or more extra hepatic organs or structures.
- lymphovascular invasion – present/not present. Note perineural invasion.
- regional lymph nodes:
  - cystic duct node, pericholedochal, hilar, peripancreatic (head only), periduodenal, peri-portal, coeliac and superior mesenteric nodes.
  - pN0   no regional lymph node mestastasis.
  - pN1   regional lymph node metastasis.
- excision margins:
  - cystic duct limit of tumour and mucosal dysplasia clearance (mm)
  - adventitial margin of tumour clearance (mm)
  - hepatic and common bile duct margins of tumour clearance (mm).
- other pathology:
  - calculi, sclerosing cholangitis.

9 Liver

1. Anatomy

The liver, the largest gland in the body, is concerned with the production and secretion of bile and many metabolic functions crucial to normal homeostasis. The majority of it is surrounded by a peritonealised fibrous capsule and it is situated in the right upper quadrant of the abdomen for the most part under the cover of the ribs. It is divided into a large right and smaller left lobe by the attachment of the falciform ligament. The right lobe is further subdivided into the quadrate and caudate lobes by the gall bladder and the ligamentum teres (Figure 9.1). However, this is a purely anatomical subdivision as it has been found that the quadrate and caudate lobes are actually a functional part of the left lobe, i.e., they are supplied by the left hepatic artery and left hepatic duct. This has led to a different division of the liver into surgical lobes and segments (see below).

The hilum of the liver, or porta hepatis, is found on the infero-posterior surface with the lesser omentum attached to its margin. Emerging from and entering the porta hepatis (from posterior to anterior) are the portal vein, right and left branches of the hepatic artery, the right and left hepatic ducts and autonomic nerves.

Histologically, the liver is composed of lobules (Figure 9.1). Each lobule comprises a central vein (a tributary of the hepatic veins) with the portal tracts situated at the periphery. The portal tracts contain a branch of the hepatic artery, portal vein and bile duct. Each lobule is divided into triangular-shaped acini with terminal branches of the hepatic artery and portal vein at their bases and the central vein at the apex. The acinus is divided into three zones (zone three being the most remote from the blood supply). The liver cells (hepatocytes) are arranged in anastomosing cords, with those adjacent to the portal tract forming the limiting plate. Between the cords of liver cells are vascular channels (sinusoids) lined by a discontinuous layer of endothelial cells. These sinusoids carry blood (both arterial and portal) from the portal tract to the central vein. Channels (canaliculi) formed between adjacent hepatocytes conduct bile to the ducts in the portal tracts and then to the extrahepatic bile ducts and gall bladder.

Lymphovascular Supply

The liver receives 30% of its blood from the hepatic artery (oxygenated blood), the remaining 70% being supplied by the portal vein (venous blood rich in nutrients absorbed from the gut). The blood is conducted through the sinusoids from the portal tracts to the central veins which in turn drain into the hepatic veins and ultimately the inferior vena cava. Most of the lymphatics drain to nodes in the porta hepatis (hepatoduodenal ligament) and then pass to the coeliac nodes. A small number pass through the diaphragm into the posterior mediastinum.

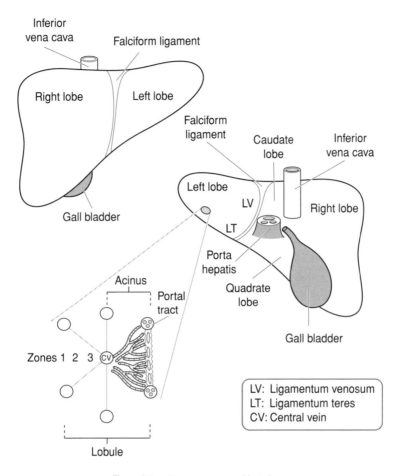

Figure 9.1.   Liver anatomy and histology.

2. Clinical Presentation

Patients with liver disease may be asymptomatic. The most common clinical sign is jaundice, although other stigmata of hepatocellular disease such as spider naevi, finger-clubbing, gynae-comastia, etc. may also be present. If the jaundice is obstructive then the patient will have dark urine and pale faeces. Weight loss, anorexia and anaemia may suggest an underlying malignancy. Fever and rigors may be seen if an abscess is present. Hepatomegaly (enlarged liver) may be encountered in numerous conditions including cirrhosis and malignancy.

A careful clinical history including medication, alcohol intake, travel and sexual practice is invaluable.

3. Clinical Investigations

- U&E – electrolyte imbalance may occur and hyponatraemia (low sodium) is a poor prognostic sign in liver failure.
- Liver function tests (LFTs) – these should include tests for liver secretory capacity (bilirubin, alkaline phosphatase and gamma glutamyl transferase (GGT)); synthetic capacity (albumin) and inflammation (aspartate aminotransferase (AST) and alanine aminotransferase (ALT)).
- Coagulation screen – measures clotting potential and as such is a test of hepatic function (synthesis of clotting factors).
- Serology – viral titres of hepatitis A, B and C.
- Autoimmune screen – anti-mitochondrial, anti-smooth muscle, anti-nuclear and membrane antibodies.
- Specific tests – serum iron, ferritin and TIBC (haemochromatosis); serum and urinary copper (Wilson's disease); serum alpha-1 antitrypsin (alpha-1 antitrypsin deficiency).
- Tumour markers – alpha fetoprotein (hepatocellular carcinoma); CEA (colorectal carcinoma).
- CXR – may detect primary lung tumour (which has metastasised to the liver).
- AXR – may show calcification around a hydatid cyst.
- USS – shows dimensions of intra- and extrahepatic bile ducts; useful in demonstrating both primary and metastatic tumours (colorectal metastases have a characteristic echogenic picture).
- CT scan – used to further define the nature and anatomical relationships of a lesion diagnosed by USS.
- Radio-isotope scanning – this provides information on the liver texture and is useful in diagnosing cirrhosis or multiple tumours (if > 2 cm). Tumours will have decreased uptake.
- Angiography – hepatic artery angiography can be used to delineate the vascular anatomy of a tumour prior to resection. It is the most sensitive method of diagnosing hepatocellular carcinoma and is useful in ensuring that a metastasis which is considered for resection is indeed a single deposit. It will also allow the extent of a vascular tumour to be mapped and, if indicated, embolised. An inferior venogram will establish if the inferior vena cava is involved by tumour prior to any resection.
- Peritoneal aspiration – may detect malignant cells in ascitic fluid.
- FNAC – percutaneous under USS/CT guidance.
- Needle core biopsy – Tru-cut needle biopsy under USS/CT guidance can be carried out on focal lesions which have given a poor yield on FNAC. A biopsy of "normal" parenchyma adjacent to the lesion will show the state of background liver disease which may provide a clue to diagnosis and, if severe, will rule out any attempt at resection. A needle core biopsy may also be performed on a suspicious lesion during laparotomy. Alternatively, diffuse medical liver conditions can be sampled percutaneously and blind by a Menghini needle.
- Staging laparoscopy with biopsy.

4. Pathological Conditions

Patients with liver disease may present with signs of liver failure or complications of it, e.g., oesophageal varices, or because of biochemically detected abnormal LFTs. The latter can indicate whether the pattern of damage is hepatic (parenchymal), extra-hepatic (obstructive) or mixed in nature. Hepatic assault is typified by viral hepatitis, alcohol or drug damage and extra-hepatic disease by duct obstruction due to stones or tumour, e.g., head of pancreas. Mixed biochemical profiles are not infrequently seen in these various disorders. Needle core biopsy is interpreted in close correlation with full clinical information that includes a detailed history and wide range of investigations (see above). Its aims are to distinguish between a surgical and medical cause for the damage, and in non-neoplastic conditions to assess the degree of necroinflammatory activity that is present and the repairative response of the liver to it. It also establishes a baseline against which subsequent treatment can be assessed or indicated, e.g., interferon therapy in chronic hepatitis. Liver damage has potential to resolve but if it is unresponsive to treatment or ongoing, a non-specific end-stage or cirrhotic pattern may be reached with few histological clues as to its aetiology. It is due to lobular damage and collapse of its framework with fibrous repair expanding and linking portal tracts with each other and the central veins. This micronodular (< 0.3 cm diameter) or macronodular pattern disturbs liver function and also its internal vascular relationships. As a consequence, liver failure (jaundice, anaemia, generalised oedema and ascites due to hypoalbuminaemia, hepatic encephalopathy) and portal venous hypertension with the risk of catastrophic haemorrhage from oesophagogastric varices, can ensue. In neoplasia or hepatic mass lesions the biopsy may be for diagnostic purposes to distinguish between hepatocellular carcinoma, metastatic carcinoma, malignant lymphoma and abscess, or for staging of known primary tumour elsewhere, e.g., colorectal carcinoma. The information accrued is then factored into future management decisions.

Non-neoplastic Conditions

Viral hepatitis: commonly hepatitis A, B, C or D. Hepatitis A (faeco-oral transmission) is usually of short duration, self-limiting without sequelae and not biopsied. Hepatitis B and C (transmission by blood, serum, secretions – hepatitis D is often a co-factor) are strongly associated with blood transfusion, sharps injuries and shared needles in drug abusers. Occasionally there is acute fulminant hepatitis but a significant minority go on to chronic carriage of viral antigen that can lead to chronic active hepatitis (> 6 months clinical duration) with eventual cirrhosis and hepatocellular carcinoma. Diagnosis is by positive serology matched to distinctive histological features (e.g., portal tract lymphoid follicles and bile duct damage in hepatitis C) which are also graded (the degree of necroinflammation) and staged (the absence or presence of fibrosis/cirrhosis) as a gauge of treatment response and evolution of disease. Tissue localisation of viral antigens can be demonstrated immunohistochemically or by in-situ hybridisation.

Alcohol (C_2H_5OH): chronic excess alcohol intake is a common aetiological factor in liver disease and is noted for variable individual susceptibility to it. Its hepatotoxic effect causes a wide range of changes including steatosis (fatty change), perivenular fibrosis, alcoholic hepatitis (lobular necroinflammation), Mallory's hyaline (tufts of intracytoplasmic intermediate filaments), cirrhosis and hepatocellular carcinoma. Abstinence short of the stage of cirrhosis leads to potential reversibility of damage. Similar morphological features are seen in NASH (non-alcoholic steatohepatitis) commonly associated with obesity, gut bypass procedures, diabetes and some drugs.

Drugs: the vast majority of drugs are metabolised in the liver and cause damage either due to excess dosage (actual, or apparent due to pre-existing decreased liver function) or individual idiosyncratic reaction to them. Various effects are seen with different agents: steatosis, cholestasis (commonest), granulomas, necrosis, hepatitis, veno-occlusion and peliosis (dilated blood channels). Location of damage varies within the acinar zones related to the blood supply and the particular agent involved. Diagnosis is strongly dependent on an appropriate clinical history and time scale of drug usage correlating with the damage. Common agents are: tricyclic antidepressants (chlorpromazine), methotrexate, NSAIDs, anaesthetic agents (halothane), antibiotics (tetracyclines, erythromycin) and paracetamol.

Autoimmune and cholangiodestructive diseases: characteristically in late-middle-aged females, chronic (lupoid) hepatitis is associated with a range of antinuclear and anti-smooth muscle antibodies and can be steroid-responsive. In this respect it is of paramount importance to separate it from an infective hepatitis in which steroids are contraindicated. Primary biliary cirrhosis, some cases of which overlap with autoimmune hepatitis, affects similar patients and is a non-suppurative, destructive, granulomatous disorder of bile ductules that leads to their disappearance (ductopaenia), fibrosis and ultimately cirrhosis. Serum IgM anti-mitochondrial antibody is typically elevated and progress can be gradual over a long time period, treatment being largely symptomatic to relieve hyperbilirubinaemia-related itch. Primary sclerosing cholangitis can affect intra- or extrahepatic bile ducts with a chronic inflammatory infiltrate and surrounding fibrosis leading to obstructive tapering of the ducts and their eventual disappearance. Diagnosis is by ERCP; there is a strong association with ulcerative colitis and predisposition to cholangiocarcinoma.

Systemic diseases: the liver can be involved in many other generalised conditions, e.g., diabetes, Crohn's disease, systemic vasculitis, amyloid (primary or secondary, e.g., due to rheumatoid arthritis) and hereditary disorders such as glycogen storage diseases, alpha-1 antitrypsin deficiency, cystic fibrosis, Wilson's disease (defect of copper metabolism) and haemochromatosis (defect of iron metabolism).

Focal mass lesions: these need to be distinguished radiologically and histocytologically from neoplastic conditions (see below) and include simple sporadic cysts (often biliary in origin), multiple simple cysts (polycystic disease of liver and kidneys), infective cysts, abscess, haemangioma and focal nodular hyperplasia. Abscess may arise from septicaemia, acute cholecystitis or portal pyaemia after perforated appendicitis or diverticulitis. Focal nodular hyperplasia is usually solitary in young-to-middle-aged women and has a central stellate fibrous scar containing proliferating bile ducts. It is considered to be a localised vascular abnormality, its main differential diagnosis being well-differentiated hepatocellular carcinoma. Bile duct adenoma and hamartoma (von Meyenberg complex) are usually encountered as small, pale, subcapsular nodules at laparotomy for bowel carcinoma and submitted as a wedge biopsy for frozen section queried as metastatic deposits.

Neoplastic Conditions

Adenoma: rare, causing acute abdominal presentation due to lesional haemorrhage in a middle-aged female with a history of oral contraception. Devoid of portal tracts or central veins within the nodule but preservation of the pericellular reticulin pattern and liver cell plates – these features help distinguish it from well-differentiated hepatocellular carcinoma.

Adenomatous hyperplastic or macroregenerative nodules: irregular nodules in background cirrhosis, 2–3 cm diameter with cytoarchitectural atypia and potentially premalignant.

Hepatocellular carcinoma: often in background cirrhosis and serum AFP is elevated in 25–40% of cases. Single, diffuse or multifocal, bile stained and prone to venous invasion with metastases to lung, adrenal gland and bone. The commonest patterns are trabecular, plate-like or sinusoidal comprising variably differentiated hepatoid cells.

A minority are encapsulated, pedunculated or in a younger patient fibrolamellar in type; these variants having a better prognosis than usual hepatoma.

Cholangiocarcinoma (intrahepatic): scirrhous, solitary or multifocal adenocarcinoma with a ductuloacinar pattern and predisposed to by primary sclerosing cholangitis, ulcerative colitis, liver fluke and biliary tree anomalies.

Metastatic carcinoma: commonly from gastrointestinal tract, lung and breast, there are some characteristic clues as to origin:

- colorectum – multiple, large nodules with central necrosis/umbilication, ± mucin ± calcification.
- gall bladder – bulk of disease centred on the gall bladder bed.

- lung – medium-sized nodules.
- stomach, breast – medium-sized nodules or diffuse cirrhotic-like pattern.

Note that carcinoma rarely metastases to a cirrhotic liver, i.e., the tumour is more likely to be primary.

Other cancers: malignant lymphoma (portal infiltrates or tumour nodules), leukaemia (sinusoidal infiltrate), angiosarcoma, epithelioid haemangioendothelioma.

Prognosis: in hepatocellular carcinoma this relates to size (> 5 cm), differentiation, encapsulation, multifocality, high serum AFP levels, vascular invasion and the presence of background cirrhosis (adverse). The majority die within several months of presentation and five-year survival is at most 5–10%. Chemotherapy is used palliatively. Small tumours, encapsulated, pedunculated and fibrolamellar variants are potentially curable by resection. Few patients with cholangiocarcinoma survive longer than 2–3 years due to late presentation and limited resectability. Solitary metastases, e.g., colorectal carcinoma or carcinoid tumour, can be resected to good effect.

5. Surgical Pathology Specimens – Clinical Aspects

Biopsy Specimens

FNAC and needle core biopsy can be carried out percutaneously either blind or preferably under radiological guidance, during laparoscopy, laparotomy or as a radiologically guided transvascular (vena cava) procedure. Coagulation status is checked prior to core biopsy to avoid risk of haemorrhage.

Resection Specimens

Neoplastic Lesions

The key to successful hepatic resection of malignant disease is careful patient selection. In general:

- A primary liver tumour may be considered for resection if it involves a single lobe and there is no invasion of the portal vein or inferior vena cava. There should be little evidence of cirrhosis in the surrounding liver.
- A solitary metastatic deposit (the vast majority of which will be from a primary colorectal carcinoma) localised to a single lobe may be considered for resection. There should be no evidence of metastatic spread elsewhere and the primary tumour should have been adequately excised.

Obviously, the background physiological state of the patient has to be taken into account before surgery is considered, i.e., resection is only justified in relatively young and medically fit individuals.

As was stated above the liver is divided into right and left "surgical lobes" which are different to the anatomical lobes. The surgical lobes are separated along a plane which extends from the gall bladder bed to the inferior vena cava – the main portal plane. The surgical lobes are then subdivided into eight segments – each segment is supplied by its own portal venous and hepatic arterial pedicle (Figure 9.2).

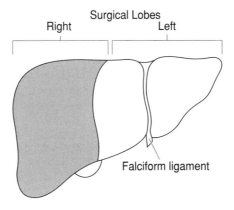

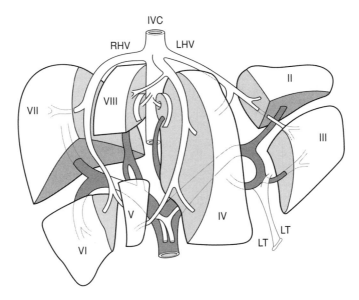

Figure 9.2.   (a) Surgical lobes of the liver. The surgical lobes of the liver compared with the usual anatomical division into left and right lobes by the falciform ligament. (b) Segments of the liver (after Couinard). IVC = inferior vena cava, RHV = right hepatic vein, LHV = left hepatic vein, MHV = middle hepatic vein, LT = ligamentum teres. Reproduced from Mann CV, Russell RCG, Williams, NS (eds.) Bailey & Love's short practice of surgery, 22nd edition. Chapman and Hall: London, 1995.

Major Liver Resection

An S-shaped right subcostal incision is used in all cases and once the abdomen is opened an initial laparotomy examination is done to ensure no other metastatic deposits are present. The definitive type of resection will depend on the site and extent of the tumour.

- *Right hepatectomy* – in this, the right surgical lobe is resected by transecting the liver through the main portal plane (main portal scissura). The cut surface of the residual liver is sprayed with thrombin glue to reduce postoperative blood loss and especially bile leakage.
- *Left hepatectomy* – this usually involves resection of the anatomical left lobe, the quadrate and caudate lobes (i.e., the left surgical lobe, although the caudate lobe may be left in situ). Again, the line of resection is the main portal plane.
- *Left lobectomy* – in this, the anatomical left lobe is resected by dividing the liver just to the left of the falciform ligament.
- *Extended right hepatectomy* – this involves the resection of the anatomical right lobe, i.e., the surgical right lobe plus the caudate and quadrate lobes. Again, the line of resection is just to the left of the falciform ligament
- *Extended left hepatectomy* – this is essentially a left hepatectomy which has been extended to also resect segments I, V and VIII.

As well as neoplastic conditions, major liver resection may also be used for other conditions such as trauma.

Segmental Liver Resection

Although major hepatic resection may be employed for large tumours, when a small tumour (either primary or secondary) occupies one or two segments, a segmental resection can be carried out. This removes a segment(s) of liver, which is supplied by its own vascular pedicle, and is therefore an anatomically based procedure. Whatever the segment to be resected, its vascular anatomy is delineated by intraoperative USS before dissection.

Segmental resection has several advantages over major resection; namely, as much functioning parenchyma is left as possible and the vascular supply to this is less likely to be compromised, there is reduced blood loss and the procedure is less likely to leave residual tumour.

If a metastatic deposit is single, small and superficial, a simple *wedge resection* using diathermy can be employed. This procedure may be performed during resection of the primary tumour, e.g., colorectal carcinoma, and sent for frozen section.

It is known that most metastatic tumours reach the liver by the portal circulation. However, the deposit itself gains its blood supply almost exclusively from hepatic arterial flow. Therefore, in inoperable metastatic disease, numerous techniques have been used to deliver chemotherapy directly into the hepatic arterial circulation:

- Infusion therapy – a catheter is passed percutaneously via the femoral artery.
- Implantable device – this can be placed at laparotomy and allows long-term infusion. An example of this technique is by using a *portacath*, which employs a self-sealing port which is placed subcutaneously and drugs can be injected into this at regular intervals. A catheter runs from the port to the hepatic artery.

Non-neoplastic Lesions – Liver Cysts

Liver cysts may be congenital or acquired (e.g., neoplastic, inflammatory/infective, traumatic, etc.). When surgery is to be carried out for a liver cyst an extensive preoperative clinical and radiological work-up is required to ascertain, as closely as possible, its aetiology. An initial thorough laparotomy examination is undertaken. For non-infective cysts, the cyst is opened and the contents aspirated and sent for cytological and microbiological examination. The cyst wall can then be excised using cautery if a neoplastic lesion is suspected. However, in non-neoplastic lesions (e.g., simple cyst) complete excision is not necessary and a large opening is made in the cyst to allow free drainage into the peritoneal cavity.

Hydatid cysts (*Echinococcus* tapeworm) may vary in size and situation within the liver. They may be excised without removing adjacent liver parenchyma (pericystectomy) or if the cysts are large or multiple, a segmental or major resection may be needed. When a pericystectomy is carried out and the cyst is opened, pads soaked in saline are packed around the cyst to prevent spillage of its contents into the peritoneal cavity.

For pyogenic abscess/cyst there are three main forms of treatment; long-term antibiotics, percutaneous drainage under radiological guidance and open surgical drainage. Percutaneous drainage is now by far the most popular method. However, if surgical drainage is employed the abscess is identified and separated from the peritoneal cavity by pads. The abscess contents are then aspirated and the cavity washed out. The cyst wall is then de-roofed to facilitate resolution. Pyogenic abscesses may also be treated by laparoscopic drainage.

Transplantation

The first successful human liver transplant was carried out in 1967 and today over 80% of recipients survive one year. Not only can adult livers be transplanted to adult recipients, but the shortage of donor organs has led to adult donor organs being transplanted to children. This is facilitated by resecting and transplanting only part of the donor liver, e.g., left liver (segments I–IV). General indications for transplantation are acute liver failure, end-stage chronic liver disease and neoplasms. Conditions encountered in the explant specimen can therefore be diverse including viral, autoimmune and alcoholic hepatitis; primary biliary and sclerosing cholangitis; end-stage cirrhosis and primary hepatocellular or cholangiocarcinoma.

6. Surgical Pathology Specimens – Laboratory Protocols

Biopsy Specimens

For needle core and wedge biopsy specimens see Gastrointestinal Specimens – General Comments (page 7).

Note that viral hepatitis is a category III pathogen – it should be submitted to the laboratory with an attached hazard of infection sticker and handled appropriately after 24–48 hours of thorough formalin fixation.

Routine histochemical stains that should be provided to help assess the degree of hepatic parenchymal loss, reticulin collapse/elaboration and fibrous distortion/replacement respectively, are PAS (± diastase), silver reticulin and Masson Trichrome. Haemochromatosis is diagnosed and graded by Perl's Prussian Blue or the dry-weight iron concentration is determined biochemically. Other stains are: rhodanine/Shikata's orcein for copper in Wilson's disease, primary biliary cirrhosis or chronic cholestatic disorders; PAS + diastase (globules in alpha-1 antitrypsin deficiency) and Congo Red (amyloid).

Needle cores may have an adherent fragment of skin if obtained percutaneously. They can also fragment in diseased liver with cirrhosis or tumour. Fatty liver is pale, haemochromatosis rusty. One aspect of a wedge biopsy is covered by peritonealised capsule and its cut margin is often frayed by diathermy. This margin should be painted and the wedge then cut into multiple vertical serial slices perpendicular to it.

Resection Specimens

Specimen

Liver resection is more commonly performed for a focal mass lesion such as a cyst, adenoma, focal nodular hyperplasia or metastatic colorectal carcinoma, and is, therefore, limited in extent, e.g., segmentectomy, lobectomy or partial hepatectomy. Other indications are major trauma and a small minority of resectable primary liver cancers. Specimen handling and reporting should document the nature of the abnormality, its extent, completeness of excision, vascular invasion and status of the background parenchyma. Total hepatectomy is encountered in transplantation surgery – aims are to identify the cause of hepatic failure, and for tumour to determine the stage and assess porta hepatis margins.

Initial Procedure

For partial resection

- weight (g) and measurements (cm) in each dimension.
- identify the capsular and cut parenchymal surfaces – the latter constitutes the surgical margin. Further orientation can only be given if marked appropriately by the submitting surgeon.
- paint the surgical margin and any areas of capsular bulging, retraction or reaction that might be related to an underlying mass lesion.
- serially section the liver perpendicular to the parenchymal resection margin at 0.5 cm intervals (Figure 9.3).
- photograph.

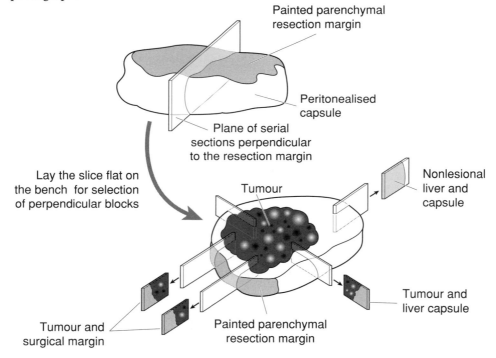

Figure 9.3.   Partial hepatectomy specimen.

- fixation by laying flat and immersion in 10% formalin for 36–48 hours.

Description

- note the number, size and distances (mm) to the capsule and surgical margin for each lesion.
- specific points are:
  - abscess – contents (pus: pyogenic/"anchovy sauce": amoebiasis), walled off, capsular reaction.
  - cyst – contents (fibrin, fluid (serous/mucoid)), wall (chitinous–hydatid).
  - trauma – capsular tear, subcapsular haemorrhage, parenchymal laceration.
  - tumour mass
    - edges: circumscribed/irregular/nodular/elevated.
    - central scar: focal nodular hyperplasia.
    - haemorrhage: haematoma, adenoma.
    - bile stained: hepatocellular carcinoma.
    - central necrosis/umbilication/mucinous/peripheral calcification: metastatic carcinoma.
- look for vascular invasion, e.g., thrombi in intrahepatic veins and/or any attached length of vena cava.
- nonlesional liver – fatty change/cholestasis/necrosis/cirrhosis/haemochromatosis.

Blocks for Histology (Figure 9.3)

- for abscess, cyst or trauma, four or five representative blocks of the wall, any capsular tear or haemorrhage and adjacent hepatic parenchyma are usually sufficient.
- for a tumour mass also sample a minimum of four or five representative blocks to demonstrate the lesion in relation to the capsule, surgical margin, uninvolved liver and any other relevant structures, e.g., veins. Additional blocks are taken as required, e.g., if in close proximity to the surgical margin. Sections from the periphery of a tumour are often more informative than from the centre as there is less necrosis with preservation of tumour tissue, and its interface with the parenchyma can be demonstrated.
- sample nonlesional liver.

For total hepatectomy specimens (Figure 9.4):
  - weigh (g) and measure (cm) in three dimensions.
  - if there is a previous diagnosis of hepatitis incise deeply at several points to ensure an adequate period (48–72 hours) of fixation prior to further handling.
  - identify the porta hepatis and transverse section its surgical margin to include the distal limit of the bile duct, hepatic artery and portal vein. Further transverse sections at mid-duct and hilar levels can be submitted.
  - count and sample all lymph nodes.
  - dissect off the gall bladder and routinely process if macroscopically normal.
  - section the liver in its long axis either side of the hilum.
  - sample representative blocks from the anatomical lobes and additionally as indicated by any mass lesion to demonstrate its relationship to the capsule, vessels and porta hepatis.
  - serially slice the rest of the liver to detect any further lesions and sample accordingly.

Histopathology Report

- tumour type – hepatocellular carcinoma/cholangiocarcinoma/metastatic carcinoma.
- tumour differentiation – well/moderate/poor.
- extent of local tumour spread (hepatocellular and intrahepatic cholangiocarcinoma)

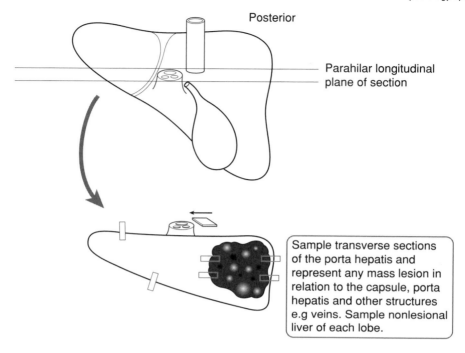

Posterior

Parahilar longitudinal plane of section

Sample transverse sections of the porta hepatis and represent any mass lesion in relation to the capsule, porta hepatis and other structures e.g veins. Sample nonlesional liver of each lobe.

Figure 9.4. Total hepatectomy specimen.

- pT1 solitary tumour without vascular invasion.
- pT2 solitary tumour with vascular invasion or multiple tumours, none more than 5 cm in greatest dimension.
- pT3 multiple tumours more than 5 cm or tumour involving a major branch of the portal or hepatic vein.
- pT4 tumour(s) with direct invasion of adjacent organs other than the gall bladder or with perforation of visceral peritoneum.
- lymphovascular invasion – present/not present. Note the propensity for hepatocellular carcinoma to invade portal tract veins, major branches of portal and hepatic veins and inferior vena cava. Cholangiocarcinoma typically shows perineural space invasion with spread to lymph nodes, lungs and peritoneum.
- regional lymph nodes: hilar (hepatoduodenal ligament), hepatic (along the proper hepatic artery), periportal (along the portal vein) and those along the abdominal inferior vena cava above the renal veins (except the inferior phrenic nodes).
  - pN0 no regional lymph node metastasis.
  - pN1 metastasis in regional lymph node(s).
- excision margins:
  - distances (mm) to the capsule and limits of excision of the hepatic parenchyma, bile ducts and major veins.
- other pathology:
  - hepatocellular carcinoma
  - hepatitis, cirrhosis (hepatitis/alcohol/haemochromatosis, etc.), adenomatous hyperplastic nodules, liver cell dysplasia.
  - cholangiocarcinoma
  - primary sclerosing cholangitis, ulcerative colitis, liver fluke, biliary tree anomaly.

10 Abdominal Wall, Umbilicus, Hernias, Omentum and Peritoneum

1. Anatomy

The anterior abdominal wall is formed by skin, fascia and striated muscles including rectus abdominus and the oblique muscles. The inguinal canal is an oblique passage through the groin area of the lower abdominal wall, and although present in both sexes, it is more prominent in the male, allowing structures to pass to and from the testis.

The umbilicus is present in the midline of the anterior abdominal wall and is a scar caused by the attachment of the umbilical cord, allowing blood vessels to pass to and from the foetus.

The greater omentum is a two-layered fold of visceral peritoneum that is attached to the greater curvature of the stomach and transverse colon. It hangs down between the coils of small intestine and the anterior abdominal wall. The omentum contains lymphoid aggregates which are thought to have an immunological function locally in the peritoneal cavity. The omentum provides a large area for electrolyte/fluid absorption and will also adhere to sites of inflammation/bleeding.

2. Clinical Presentation

Abdominal wall lesions present with a lump that may be associated with discomfort or discharge.

A hernia occurs when part or all of a viscus protrudes through the confines of the body cavity in which it is normally situated. It presents with a dull "dragging" sensation or palpable lump usually evident on coughing. Severe constant pain is a sign of impending strangulation and ischaemia of any omentum or small bowel contents which may also become obstructed.

Umbilical disease can present with a lump, discharge or inflammation (omphalitis) and infection leading to pain and abscess formation. Caput medussa results from dilatation of periumbilical veins secondary to increased portal venous pressure usually due to liver cirrhosis.

Omental disease is usually due to inflammation or malignancy in adjacent organs but primary disease can also lead to adhesions and small bowel obstruction; torsion produces nausea and vomiting, and tumour an abdominal mass.

3. Clinical Investigations

- FBP – elevated WCC in omphalitis.
- LFTs/liver biopsy – in patients with caput medussa.
- Pus swab – umbilical abscess/suppuration.
- AXR – dilated small bowel loops in obstructed hernia.
- Fistulogram – contrast may be passed into an umbilical fistula to show its origins and course.

- Herniography – this rarely used investigation involves injecting contrast into the peritoneal cavity. A plain AXR will then reveal the presence and position of a hernial sac.
- USS – useful in diagnosing a hernia and in distinguishing it from other groin conditions and in the investigation of tumours of the abdominal wall.
- CT/MRI scan – will outline tumours of the abdominal wall, and pelvic and abdominal tumours involving the omentum.
- FNA/needle core biopsy – used in the diagnosis of abdominal wall tumours.
- Laparoscopy and biopsy – useful in the investigation of omental lesions, particularly secondary tumours.

4. Pathological Conditions

Abdominal Wall and Umbilicus

Various conditions can affect the abdominal wall and result in both FNAC and histopathology specimens.

Secondary carcinoma: commonly due to either gastrointestinal or gynaecological cancer involvement, can be by direct spread at presentation or because of a subsequent metastatic recurrence. The former is not infrequently seen with a perforated bowel cancer and the inner layers of the abdominal wall may be dissected off separately or in continuity with it. The latter tends to be encountered as an intramural nodule or deposit with a previous history of bowel resection and is often amenable to diagnosis by clinical FNAC. Classically secondary carcinoma (colon, ovary, breast) can present as an umbilical deposit (Sister Mary Joseph's nodule) which is also a site for hernias, endometriosis or fistula due to persistence of an embryonic structure, e.g., the vitellointestinal duct or urachus. These result in umbilical protrusion, cyclical menstrual haemorrhage or serous discharge respectively. A persistent urachal remnant may be attached to the dome of the urinary bladder potentially acting as a source for internal hernia with bowel entrapment and ischaemia.

Abdominal fibromatosis ("desmoid tumour"): a locally infiltrative and recurrent form of fibromatosis typically in the anterior abdominal wall of a woman of childbearing age with a previous history of caesarean section. It has no potential to metastasise and may occasionally be associated with intestinal polyposis (Gardner's syndrome).

Amyloid: involvement of anterior abdominal wall subcutaneous fat in systemic amyloidosis allows a diagnosis to be made by needle aspiration or biopsy with smearing of fat onto glass slides for Congo Red staining.

Stomas: such as ileostomy or colostomy fashioned during a gastrointestinal surgical operation may subsequently be taken down as part of the planned procedure, or revised due to dysfunction. The latter can be due to ischaemia or mucosal prolapse with obstruction. Occasionally, secondary carcinoma involves the stomal site.

Hernias

External hernias involve protrusion of peritoneum ± omentum and bowel into the layers of the abdominal wall (particularly at the site of a previous surgical incision), inguinal or femoral canals. The hernial sac is usually thin walled comprising fibrous connective tissue lined by peritoneum. It may become irreducible and undergo secondary ischaemia of the contents and with ulceration and infection of the overlying skin. Internal hernias into anatomical spaces (e.g., the lesser omental sac) or across fibrous bands (congenital or acquired) may also obstruct and become ischaemic but are rare.

Omentum and Peritoneum

The omental fat and peritoneal serosa may be involved by various inflammatory and neoplastic disorders.

Inflammation: acute due to appendicitis or a perforated viscus (GU, diverticulitis), or granulomatous, e.g., tuberculosis, fungal peritonitis (chronic ambulatory peritoneal dialysis (CAPD)) or after previous surgery. CAPD can also be associated with the rare condition of fibrous or sclerosing peritonitis.

Infarction: spontaneous, idiopathic omental infarction in the right iliac fossa mimicking acute appendicitis (rare), or more commonly, infarction of an appendix epiploica (pericolonic fat tag) which may then undergo saponification and calcification. The latter are also seen as a consequence of acute pancreatitis or abdominal trauma. Omentum incarcerated within a hernial sac may also undergo ischaemia.

Keratin granulomas: an unusual finding most often related to treatment and follow-up of a previous gynaecological cancer, e.g., endometrioid adenocarcinoma of the uterus or vulval squamous carcinoma.

Peritoneal inclusion cysts: relatively common, solitary or multiple and should be distinguished from lymphangitic cysts (cytokeratin negative endothelial lining) and well-differentiated multicystic peritoneal mesothelioma. The latter is rare, occurring on the surfaces of the uterus, ovary, bladder, rectum and pouch of Douglas with potential for recurrence and invasion locally into retroperitoneum, bowel mesentery and wall. Some have a previous history of surgery, endometriosis or pelvic inflammatory disease.

Mesothelial proliferation: other mesothelial proliferations include:

- Mesothelial hyperplasia – commonly seen as a reactive phenomenon in omentum adherent to an inflammatory or neoplastic abdominopelvic lesion and within a hernia. Sometimes it is florid and distinction from mesothelioma can be difficult.
- Well-differentiated papillary peritoneal mesothelioma – rare, with most being an incidental finding at hysterectomy, usually localised and benign but occasionally diffuse.
- Diffuse malignant mesothelioma – epithelioid/sarcomatoid or mixed in pattern and a strong association with occupational asbestos exposure and spread from a primary pleural mesothelioma. Prognosis is poor with the majority of patients dying from their disease within months or 1–3 years. Of very limited suitability for resection.

Peritoneal serous epithelial proliferation: strongly associated with ovarian serous borderline tumours and either regarded as benign (endosalpingiosis), potentially progressive (invasive proliferating implants) or frankly malignant – primary peritoneal carcinoma. The former two conditions are microscopic findings while the latter is an ovarian serous-type adenocarcinoma with extensive peritoneal disease but minimal ovarian involvement.

Pseudomyxoma peritonei: characterised by filling of the peritoneal cavity with abundant mucin in which there is a component of either variably bland, atypical or frankly malignant epithelium. Prognosis is poor as it is refractory to treatment, slowly progressive and leads to bowel obstruction. There is a strong association with appendiceal and ovarian mucinous tumours and occasionally secondary colorectal or pancreaticobiliary neoplasms. Appendicectomy should be considered in the presence of bilateral cystic ovarian tumours associated with peritoneal disease.

Secondary adenocarcinoma: staging and therapy are considered:

- Staging – diagnosed either by peritoneal aspiration cytology, laparoscopic biopsy, or open biopsy with frozen section at exploratory laparotomy as a prequel to consideration of suitability for operative resection of an abdominopelvic cancer. Postoperative pathological staging of ovarian carcinoma also partly relates to the size (< or > 2 cm) of the peritoneal deposits – it requires removal of the primary ovarian lesion, biopsy of the contralateral ovary, omentum and peritoneum, and peritoneal washings for cytology if ascitic fluid is not present.

● Therapy – tumour debulking or cytoreductive surgery of extensive omental disease is an important initial step prior to adjuvant chemotherapy in ovarian and other abdominopelvic cancers.

Other cancers: these are rare, e.g., intra-abdominal desmoplastic small round cell tumour – divergent cellular differentiation, aggressive, pelvis and abdomen of young people.

5. Surgical Pathology Specimens – Clinical Aspects

Biopsy Specimens

Needle core biopsies of abdominal wall and umbilical tumours provide a diagnosis and allow future management to be planned. Laparoscopy and omental biopsy can be used as a staging investigation, and is particularly useful in gastric tumours and ovarian tumours/pseudomyxoma peritoneii.

Resection Specimens

Groin hernias – in uncomplicated groin hernias the principle of surgery is to reduce the hernia sac and repair the defect in the abdominal wall. This can be done by either suturing or introducing a prosthetic mesh. In complicated hernias in which the small bowel may be incarcerated, the hernia sac needs to be opened and the viability of the intestine assessed. If it is in question then a small-bowel resection may be required.

Abdominal wall tumours – primary abdominal wall tumours such as desmoid tumours are treated by wide excision. The excision usually entails excising the skin and rectus sheath, and may even extend down to the parietal peritoneum.

Umbilical lesions – primary tumours of the umbilicus, e.g., squamous carcinoma, are treated by excision of the umbilicus (omphalectomy), surrounding skin and full thickness of the peri-umbilical wall. If abscess formation occurs following umbilical infection this should be treated by incision and drainage. Omphalectomy may be required if infection is recurrent.

Omentectomy – this is a relatively straightforward procedure usually undertaken as part of more extensive surgery, e.g., during a gynaecological cancer operation for therapeutic cytore-duction and staging purposes. It involves ligation of the vessels along the greater curvature of the stomach and transverse colon with division of the omentum in this area.

6. Surgical Pathology Specimens – Laboratory Protocols

Abdominal Wall

Ranging from biopsy fragments taken at laparotomy to formal excision of an abnormal segment of tissue. Specimens from the inner aspect of the wall comprise rectus sheath muscle orientated along one edge to peritoneum and with distortion by the relevant pathological condition. External specimens are composed of skin, subcutaneous fat ± abdominal wall muscle and may also contain the umbilicus, a stoma or incisional hernia. Biopsy fragments are processed in the usual manner but larger specimens need to be individually described as to their constituent parts, their respective dimensions and the abnormalities that are present. These specimens are usually submitted already fixed in formalin.

Mass lesion (tumour, fibromatosis, endometriosis, abscess):

- maximum dimension (cm), edges (circumscribed/irregular), cut surface (mucinous/scirrhous/fibrotic/haemorrhage/pus), distances (mm) to the skin and nearest resection margin, involvement of skin (ulceration/tethering), subcutis, muscle or peritoneum.
- paint the deep and lateral resection margins.

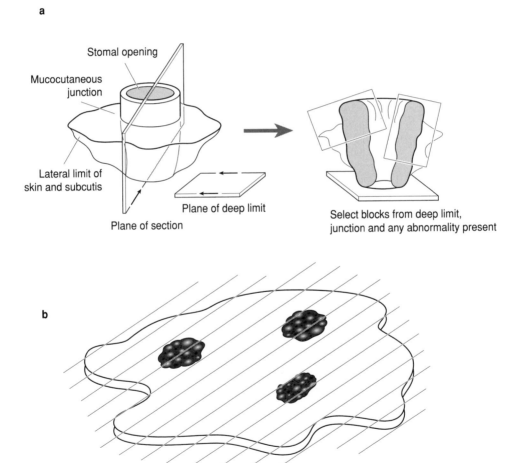

Figure 10.1.   **(a)** Sectioning of an abdominal wall mass, stoma (illustrated) or hernia. **(b)** Sectioning of omentum.

- serially section transversely at 3–4 mm intervals perpendicular to the skin or peritoneal surface.
- sample four or five representative blocks of the lesion showing its relationship to the various anatomical layers and resection margins. If close (< 0.5 cm) to a long-axis margin, obtain a longitudinal block to demonstrate this.

Stomas:

- note any mucosal prolapse, ulceration, ischaemia or tumour at the mucocutaneous junction, or bowel stricture – record their maximum dimensions (cm) and distances (cm) to the cutaneous, subcutaneous and proximal bowel resection limits.
- paint the deep and lateral resection margins.
- transverse section the proximal bowel resection limit.
- serially section the specimen transversely at 3–4 mm intervals perpendicular to the skin surface (Figure 10.1a).
- sample four or five representative blocks of the stomal junction/opening and any other relevant macroscopic abnormality.

Hernias

- note any surgical scars or ulceration of the skin, necrosis in the skin, subcutis, abdominal muscle, wall of the hernial sac or its contents.
- hernial sac – dimensions and wall thickness (cm).
- contents – omentum, bowel and their dimensions (cm).
- paint the deep and lateral resection margins.
- transverse section bowel resection limits, if present.
- sample four or five representative blocks of the hernial sac and its contents to demonstrate its relationship to the various anatomical layers and any abnormality that is present.

Omentum and Peritoneum

- laparoscopic biopsy fragments are processed in the usual manner and cut through multiple levels.
- omental specimens vary in size depending on whether the investigation is for diagnostic, staging or therapeutic purposes. Typically comprising lobulated fat or the omental curtain with a shaggy, lace-like appearance, weights vary from a few to several hundred grammes. Record the weight (g) and dimensions (cm).
- serially slices at 0.5 cm intervals and closely inspect (Figure 10.1b).
- note any macroscopic abnormalities – nature(abscess/fat necrosis/cysts/tumour), edge (circumscribed/irregular), consistency (cystic/fibrotic/mucoid/scirrhous), contents (serous fluid/lymph/mucin), number and the maximum dimension (cm).
- sample three representative blocks of macroscopically abnormal or unremarkable omental specimens.

Breast Specimens

TF Lioe

11. Breast

11 Breast

1. Anatomy

The mature adult breast is composed of fatty tissue and parenchyma in which terminal ductulo-lobular units of epithelium are surrounded by fibrous connective tissue stroma. There are about 15–25 lobes of parenchymatous elements associated with each of the lactiferous ducts which drain into the nipple. The presence of this functional lobar arrangement provides an anatomical framework for some surgical procedures such as major duct excision and quadrantectomy for cancer. The anatomical boundaries of the breast are not well defined except at the deep surface where the gland overlies the pectoralis fascia. The general topographical anatomy of the breast is illustrated in Figure 11.1

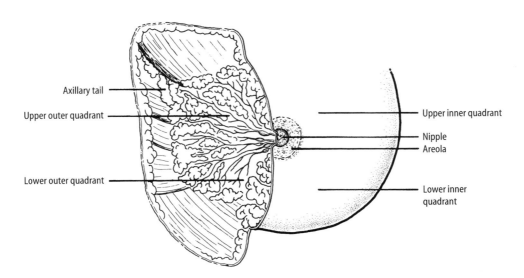

Figure 11.1. Topographical anatomy of the right breast. Reproduced with permission from Hermanek P, Hutter RVP, Sobin LH, Wagner G, Wittekind Ch (eds.). TNM Atlas: illustrated guide to the TNM/pTNM classification of malignant tumours, 4th edition. Springer-Verlag: Berlin and Heidelberg, 1997.

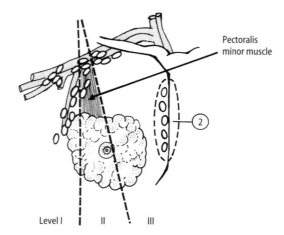

Figure 11.2. Breast: regional lymph nodes. Reproduced from Hermanek P, Hutter RVP, Sobin LH, Wagner G, Wittekind Ch (eds.). TNM Atlas: illustrated guide to the TNM/pTNM classification of malignant tumours, 4th edition. Springer-Verlag: Berlin and Heidelberg, 1997.

1. Axillary (ipsilateral): interpectoral (Rotter) nodes and lymph nodes along the axillary vein and its tributaries which may be divided into the following levels:
   i) *Level I* (low axilla): lymph nodes lateral to the lateral border of pectoralis minor muscle
   ii) *Level II* (mid-axilla): lymph nodes between the medial and lateral borders of the pectoralis minor muscle and the interpectoral (Rotter) lymph nodes
   iii) *Level III* (apical axilla): lymph nodes medial to the medial margin of the pectoralis minor muscle including those designated as subclavicular or apical

Note: Intramammary lymph nodes are coded as axillary lymph nodes

2. *Internal mammary* (ipsilateral): lymph nodes in the intercostal spaces along the edge of the sternum in the endothoracic fascia (2)

Any other lymph node metastasis is coded as a distant metastasis (M1), including supreclavicular, cervical or contralateral internal mammary lymph nodes

Lymphovascular Drainage

There are three routes of lymphatic drainage in the breast. The most important is to the axilla which receives 75% or more of the lymphatic flow to the axillary lymph nodes. These are located at various anatomical levels – Levels I, II and III (Figure 11.2.). Drainage via the internal lymphatics into the internal thoracic nodes comprises 25% or less of the lymph flow; the third and least important is to the posterior intercostal nodes where the ribs and vertebrae articulate.

2. Clinical Presentation

Symptomatic: patients commonly present with a palpable lump, breast pain, nipple discharge or rash. Breast pain is usually not associated with any significant pathology. Nipple discharge if bloody can be due to an intraduct proliferation which may require surgical excision (microdochectomy). Nipple rash may need to be biopsied to exclude Paget's disease. A palpable discrete lump can be cystic or solid. The majority of cystic lumps are benign simple cysts which can be drained by needle aspiration. Occasionally, cancerous lumps may have a cystic component which is usually bloody. Solid lumps are investigated by the triple assessment approach (see below) to provide a non-operative diagnosis of benignity or malignancy.

Screening: at present all women aged between 50 and 64 are invited to the National Health Service Breast Screening Programme, which initially involves mammography to screen out lesions that require further evaluation by the triple assessment approach such as a spiculate density or areas of microcalcification. Microcalcifications with no associated soft tissue abnormality may be the only sign of malignancy and is the mode of presentation of up to one third of cancers found at screening. Linear branching microcalcifications are usually associated with comedo ductal carcinoma in situ (DCIS) and have a higher predictive value for malignancy than non-linear irregular microcalcifications. Overall, the sensitivity of mammography is 85–90%.

3. Clinical Investigations

Clinical examination: symptomatic patients are referred to a dedicated Breast Clinic where they are assessed by a multidisciplinary team of specialists. The patient is usually first seen and examined by a breast surgeon who instigates further investigations where appropriate.

Radiological imaging: the patient normally has standard two-view mammography, i.e., craniocaudal and medio-lateral oblique views performed. Additional magnification views may be required to focus on a suspicious area and facilitate more detailed examination. The radiologist then decides if the lesion warrants further investigation by ultrasonography. Younger women with dense breast tissue are usually investigated by ultrasonography. Suspicious areas of microcalcification and parenchymal deformity are then aspirated and/or core biopsied.

Fine needle aspiration cytology (FNAC): this involves the insertion of a 23G needle into the lump. The needle is moved about within the lump and negative pressure is applied with the attached syringe on a holder. The procedure can be performed either by the clinician, radiologist or cytologist. The aspirated material is then smeared on glass slides, air dried and stained for immediate microscopic examination by the cytopathologist who will then indicate if the sample is adequate for diagnosis and if so whether the lesion is benign or malignant. Inadequate samples or aspirates with cellular features which are suspicious but not diagnostic of cancer may proceed to needle core or open biopsy. FNAC may need to be performed under radiological guidance in small or deep-seated lesions.

Needle core biopsy: this is performed with a wide-bore, spring-loaded device which requires local anaesthesia prior to the procedure. It can be done either with radiological guidance or freehand. The indications are to assess tumour invasion in a malignant aspirate especially in cases of microcalcification from screening patients, discordance between the triple assessment parameters, or to establish malignancy in cases of difficult or equivocal cytology such as a lobular or tubular carcinoma. In contrast to aspirate cytology, which allows immediate reporting, needle cores require overnight processing before a result is obtainable by histology.

Triple assessment approach: the above triple approach utilising the combination of clinical (surgical) examination, radiological imaging by X-ray and/or ultrasound and cytological assessment of aspirated material has been shown to be highly accurate in the preoperative diagnosis of breast cancer. This has superseded "frozen-section" examination of suspected breast cancers. Patients proven to have breast cancer by the triple assessment can then go on to a one-stage therapeutic procedure which is excision of the tumour together with axillary node dissection.

Open excision biopsy: in a small minority of cases, a non-operative diagnosis is not conclusive or malignancy cannot be excluded, hence an open biopsy is required for histological diagnosis.

Lesions like radial scars or papillary growths need formal histological assessment to exclude associated in-situ or invasive malignancy. Impalpable lesions and areas of microcalcification require radiological needle localisation to guide the surgeon to the area in question for adequate excision.

4. Pathological Conditions

Non-neoplastic Conditions

Fibroadenosis/fibrocystic changes: these are common in the breast and present as ill-defined masses or plaques. There is a varying degree of epithelial proliferation and hyperplasia, with or without cyst formation and associated apocrine metaplasia or sclerosing adenosis. Excision of these lesions sometimes occurs at the request of the patient despite a non-operative diagnosis of benignity by the triple assessment.

Cysts: simple cyst formation is very common and presents as a firm but fluctuant lump. Needle aspiration to dryness is usually all that is required.

Breast abscess: most commonly encountered in non-lactating premenopausal women in a subareolar location as a result of duct obstruction. It is usually diagnosed by FNAC and seldom requires surgical intervention unless there is failure to resolve.

Fat necrosis: this is most commonly seen in overweight women and those with pendulous breasts usually following a history of trauma. Clinically and radiologically, fat necrosis can mimic a carcinoma but can be distinguished by FNAC. However, an excision biopsy may be required if the lesion persists.

Duct ectasia: this is due to duct dilatation with filling of the duct lumen by amorphous material and there is accompanying chronic inflammation in the duct wall and periductal stroma. Nipple discharge is usually the first symptom but a worm-like palpable mass may form in the subareolar region in more advanced cases where there is periductal fibrosis. Excision of the area may be necessary to exclude DCIS.

Gynaecomastia: this is the most common clinical and pathological abnormality in the male breast. It is encountered in adolescent or adult males and is usually unilateral. In older men it may be due to certain drug usage such as digitalis, spironolactone and cimetidine. It forms a firm-to-rubbery plaque deep to the nipple. Patients with bilateral involvement tend to have diffuse lesions as compared to unilateral gynaecomastia which is more discrete. FNAC usually produces a low-to-moderately cellular specimen which may show a mild degree of nuclear atypia but the presence of bare nuclei should be reassuring. Excision of the lesion is most likely performed for cosmetic reasons. A small minority of cases is due to an underlying malignancy.

Reduction mammoplasty: bilateral reduction mammoplasty surgery may be performed on large pendulous breasts for physical, psychosexual or cosmetic reasons. Symmetrical volumes of fatty breast tissue are removed with overlying non-nipple-bearing skin. There is normally no significant pathology in the tissues.

Leakage from silicone implants: a fibrous capsule usually forms around a silicone implant but silicone may migrate into and through it. Rupture of the capsule can occur by accident, mammography or closed capsulotomy. Rupture of the silicone rubber envelope may occur asymptomatically and once outside the envelope, silicone can disperse through soft tissue, lymph nodes or the vasculature. Silicones are detected in the tissue as small round-to-irregular translucent droplets of amorphous refractile non-polarising material. Silicone leakage into the capsule is characterised by a typical microscopical appearance of oval-to-round holes partly filled with silicones. Giant cells of foreign body type may be found and granulomas as a reaction to silicone ("siliconomas") are seen after extracapsular rupture of an implant and after injection with silicone. Calcification of the capsule is common around implants which have been in situ for many years.

Neoplastic Conditions

Benign Tumours

Fibroadenoma: this is the commonest benign tumour of the breast, most often encountered in premenopausal women who present with a palpable, painless and mobile discrete lump. Non-operative diagnosis can be confidently made by the triple approach except in large lesions where excision may be advised to exclude a low-grade phyllodes tumour.

Proliferative lesions (radial scar/complex sclerosing lesion, intraduct papilloma, nipple adenoma, myoepithelioma): these lesions are due to epithelial proliferations of various complexities which can present as firm palpable masses. Mammography may show parenchymal deformity and foci of microcalcification, thus necessitating cytological assessment. The latter usually shows a highly cellular sample with some degree of nuclear atypia indicating either a core biopsy or local excision. Some of these lesions may harbour DCIS which can only be confirmed or discounted following histological examination.

Miscellaneous: rarely, benign lesions such as adenomas, hamartomas, fibromatosis or pseudoangiomatous stromal hyperplasia are encountered.

Malignant Tumours

Carcinoma in situ: carcinoma in situ is a proliferation of malignant epithelial cells within the ductulo-lobular system of the breast which on light microscopy shows no evidence of breaching the basement membrane to invade the adjacent stroma. There are two forms – ductal (DCIS) and lobular (LCIS) carcinoma in situ. LCIS cannot be diagnosed preoperatively and is seen incidentally on excision specimens as a marker for increased risk of developing malignancy. DCIS, on the other hand, is a heterogeneous group of pre-malignant lesions which are usually asymptomatic and impalpable but may be identifiable on mammography as foci of microcalcification. It can sometimes present as a mass lesion. Non-operative diagnosis of DCIS is based on FNAC and core biopsy. DCIS is categorised by the degree of nuclear pleomorphism as low, intermediate or high grade and by its architectural patterns – cribriform, solid, or micropapillary with or without comedo necrosis. DCIS with comedo necrosis is usually associated with dystrophic calcification and has a high nuclear grade. This sub-type has the highest risk of stromal invasion. The treatment of DCIS depends on the size and distribution of the lesion. Localised DCIS may be amenable to wide local excision while extensive disease requires a total mastectomy. Formal axillary dissection is usually not carried out. In cases of wide local excision, the specimen resection margins are carefully identified and labelled by an agreed protocol for close histological examination to assess completeness of surgical removal. Width of the excision margins around the tumour remains the most important factor in terms of risk of local recurrence and a minimum clearance of 10 mm should be achieved. All cases treated by breast-conserving surgery should have adjuvant radiotherapy.

Invasive carcinoma: breast carcinoma is a heterogeneous group of tumours with different morphological growth patterns which reflect the clinical behaviour and hence the prognosis. The most common form of invasive breast cancer is the ductal type, not otherwise specified, accounting for 75–80% of all breast cancers. This tumour type is diagnosed by exclusion of other specific types, viz. lobular, colloid or mucoid, tubular, medullary and cribriform. Invasive lobular carcinoma is the next most common tumour type, forming about 10–15% of cases. Tumours of mixed ductal and specific types are also encountered. Some of the specific tumour types such as colloid, tubular and medullary have a better prognosis as they are less aggressive. Not infrequently, breast cancer may be multifocal (within the same quadrant) or multicentric (involving other quadrants) and in some cases bilateral. Breast cancers are graded 1, 2 or 3 depending on the degree of diffferentiation (see below), which has been shown to correlate with biological behaviour. The tumour size, type, grade, presence or absence of lymphovascular invasion and nodal status are pathological prognostic factors determining adjuvant therapy and outcome for the patient. Certain biological markers such as oestrogen and Her2/neu receptor status can predict tumour response to hormonal or cytotoxic therapy respectively.

Paget's disease of the nipple: Paget's disease of the nipple is characterised by infiltration of malignant ductal epithelial cells into the epidermis of the nipple–areolar complex. Clinically, it presents as an itchy and scaly rash which may be mistaken for eczema but gradually gives rise to ulceration, crusting and bloody nipple discharge in advanced cases. Of breast cancers, 1–2% have associated Paget's disease. In patients presenting with features of Paget's disease without a clinically palpable mass, high nuclear grade DCIS is nearly always detected in the large subareolar lactiferous ducts and up to 40% will have an occult invasive tumour within the breast. An excision biopsy of the nipple is performed to confirm Paget's disease and treatment is usually by mastectomy.

Phyllodes tumour (cystosarcoma phyllodes): this is a tumour of fibro-epithelial origin usually seen in older women compared to those with a fibroadenoma. These tumours average 4–5 cm in size and have a history of rapid growth. Radiology reveals a lobulated or rounded solid mass. FNAC usually produces a highly cellular aspirate composed of epithelium and stroma, features which overlap with a fibroadenoma hence making distinction between the two difficult. However, stromal fragments which are densely cellular may suggest a phyllodes tumour and taking the patient's age and size of lesion into account, an excision biopsy would be indicated in these circumstances. The biological behaviour of these neoplasms is unpredictable. Towards the benign end of the spectrum they may locally recur if incompletely excised (a 10 mm margin should be achieved) but tumours with sarcomatous transformation will metastasise by the haematogenous route.

Mesenchymal tumours: malignant mesenchymal tumours such as angiosarcoma, malignant fibrous histiocytoma, leiomyosarcoma, liposarcoma are all rare and have to be distinguised from a metaplastic carcinoma or sarcomatous transformation in a phyllodes tumour.

Metastatic tumours: occasionally metastases from other primary sites may present as breast lumps such as melanoma, lymphoma, small cell lung carcinoma and gastro-intestinal adenocarcinoma. Some of these cases may be diagnosable preoperatively by FNAC.

Treatment and prognosis: the mainstay of treatment for breast cancer is surgery (with a 5 mm minimum tumour clearance of excision margins) followed by hormonal or chemotherapy where appropriate. Radiotherapy may be indicated to prevent local recurrence. In a small number of cases, neo-adjuvant therapy is instituted if the cancer is large and advanced or if surgery is contraindicated due to poor general health. Hormonal treatment is determined by oestrogen and progestogen receptor status as assayed by immunohistochemistry. Chemotherapy is usually indicated in high-grade and node-positive cancers particularly in the younger patient. Her2/neu receptor status is assessed either by immunohistochemistry or flourescent in-situ hybridisation technique as a predictive factor for patients with distant disease relapse who may respond to Herceptin therapy.

The single most important prognostic factor in breast cancer is nodal involvement at time of diagnosis. However, the five-year survival rate has also been shown to correlate with histological tumour type and the Nottingham Prognostic Index (see below).

Excellent prognosis tumour types with a five-year survival of greater than 80% include tubular, mucinous, cribriform and tubulolobular carcinoma. Good prognosis types with 60–80% five-year survival include mixed ductal NST/special type, tubular mixed and alveolar lobular variant. Intermediate prognosis (50–60% five-year survival) types include classical lobular, medullary and invasive papillary. Those with poor prognosis (< 50% five-year survival) are ductal NST, ductal and lobular mixed, pleomorphic lobular and metaplastic carcinoma.

5. Surgical Pathology Specimens – Clinical Aspects

Biopsy Specimens

Needle core biopsy: this is performed in cases of equivocal cytology for carcinoma, to assess stromal invasion in cases of DCIS and suspicious microcalcifications, and for grading and receptor status immunohistochemical studies in advanced cancer requiring neo-adjuvant therapy. Usually up to six cores of tissue, particularly for DCIS and microcalcifications, are taken with a 19G needle mounted on a spring-loaded gun under radiological guidance to yield 2–3 cm-long worm-like samples. They are X-rayed prior to fixing in formalin in cases of microcalcification to ascertain that the right area has been sampled.

Needle localisation biopsy: in cases where the non-operative diagnosis by FNAC and/or core biopsy is inconclusive, a diagnostic biopsy is required for histological assessment. The majority of these cases are from screening and involve foci of microcalcification of radiological concern. Some cases of stromal or parenchymal deformity, even though they have been proven to be malignant by FNAC or core biopsy, also require needle localisation (by stereotaxis or ultrasound) because they are impalpable and this assists the surgeon in removing the appropriate area.

Nipple biopsy: this is done either as a small wedge or punch biopsy of the nipple skin to confirm or exclude Paget's disease.

Microdochectomy: also known as main duct excision for cases of persistent nipple discharge or an intraductal epithelial growth which may have been suggested on smear cytology of the discharge material.

Resection Specimens and the Types of Surgery

Surgical treatment for localised breast cancer: most patients with breast cancer will have a combination of local treatment to control local disease and systemic treatment to manage metastatic disease. Local treatment consists of surgery and radiotherapy. Surgery can be an excision of the cancer with surrounding normal breast tissue (breast-conserving surgery) or a mastectomy. Axillary lymph node dissection is usually carried out at the same time for staging and prognostic purposes and for oncological management decisions in terms of adjuvant therapy. Certain clinico-pathological factors influence the selection for breast-conserving surgery or mastectomy depending on the likelihood of local recurrence after the former. These include the site and size of tumour, extent of DCIS, multifocal or multicentric disease, incomplete initial excision and the age of the patient. All patients treated with breast-conserving surgery should have adjuvant radiotherapy and also those with tumour involvement of the pectoralis major following mastectomy.

Breast-conserving surgery (BCS): BCS may consist of removal of the tumour with a 1 cm margin of normal tissue (wide local excision) or a more extensive excision of a whole quadrant of the breast (quadrantectomy). This comprises a cylinder of tissue taken from the skin superficially to the pectoralis fascia at the deep aspect. A partial mastectomy involves removal of the tumour with surrounding breast tissue and an ellipse of non-nipple-bearing skin. Small and impalpable cancers often detected by screening are usually localised radiologically by a guide wire prior to surgery to assist the surgeon in excising the appropriate area. The single most important factor predicting local recurrence following BCS is completeness of excision. Invasive or in-situ disease at the resection margins increases local recurrence by a factor of 3.4. An extensive in-situ component increases local recurrence only when margins are involved. The presence of tumour lymphovascular invasion (LVI) doubles the local recurrence rate and Grade I tumours are less likely to recur locally compared to higher grade tumours. Some of these factors are only fully appreciated after detailed histological assessment and subsequent conversion to mastectomy is not an infrequent occurrence. Clinically, breast cancers which are suitable for treatment by breast conservation include a single clinical and mammographic lesion, tumour < 3 cm in diameter or > 3 cm in large breasts and with no sign of local advancement (i.e., no extensive nodal involvement or metastases).

Cavity shavings: these are additional portions of breast tissue submitted separately as shavings from the cavity after excision of the tumour when the surgeon assesses that he/she does not have clear margins following the initial excision. They are labelled accordingly as to site, viz. medial, lateral, superior, inferior, deep or superficial.

Mastectomy: about a third of localised breast cancers are unsuitable for BCS and will require a total mastectomy. However, some patients who are suitable for BCS may also choose to have a mastectomy. Mastectomy removes the breast tissue with overlying skin including the nipple while the chest wall muscles are left intact. Patients who are best treated by mastectomy include those with multifocal disease, extensive in-situ component, centrally situated cancers, tumours > 4 cm in diameter or for whom BCS would produce an unacceptable cosmetic result. A subcutaneous mastectomy involves the removal of all breast tissue including the nipple–areolar complex but retaining the skin usually as part of a breast reconstruction procedure.

Axillary node surgery: axillary node dissection is performed in conjunction with BCS or mastectomy for prognostic/staging and therapeutic purposes. This can take the form of either node sampling or more commonly node clearance. Axillary node sampling is for staging purposes only and involves sampling three or four Level I nodes. However, in axillary node clearance (ANC) the axilla is formally dissected out and nodes from Levels I, II and III are retrieved for histological assessment and this usually totals between 20 and 40 nodes.

Sentinel node biopsy: approximately two-thirds of symptomatic and the majority of screening breast cancers are node negative. Axillary surgery in these cases would not be indicated if it could be predicted so as to avoid any risk of morbidity such as arm pain and lymphoedema. Lymphatic mapping and sentinel node biopsy is a new minimally invasive technique to identify patients with axillary node involvement. The sentinel node is defined as the first node to receive drainage from the tumour and is identified by injecting a vital blue dye, a radiocolloid or both around the area of the tumour just prior to surgery. A small incision is made in the axilla and a hand-held gamma probe or direct visual inspection used to identify the radioactive node or blue-stained lymphatic channels leading to a blue lymph node. The node is then excised and undergoes detailed histological examination which can involve multiple slices, section levels and the use of immunohistochemistry. Studies have reported identification of the sentinel node in more than 95% of breast cancer patients with a false negative rate for prediction of axillary nodal metastases of less than 5%.

6. Surgical Pathology Specimens – Laboratory Protocols

Biopsy Specimens

Needle core and nipple biopsies: these are counted, measured (mm), processed whole and cut through multiple levels. Nipple ellipses may need initial bisection depending on size.

Main duct excision specimens: these are weighed, measured and externally painted then serially and transversely sliced to look for any intraluminal papillary growths. Multiple slices are processed for histology.

Benign biopsies: excision of preoperatively proven benign lesions such as fibroadenoma are routinely weighed, measured and painted and representative tissue blocks taken for histology.

Needle localisation biopsy specimens: these are treated as resection specimens (see below).

Resection Specimens

Specimen Types

1. Total mastectomy ± ANC.
2. Breast-conserving surgery – wide local excision, quadrantectomy, partial mastectomy ± ANC.
3. Needle localisation biopsy –   for microcalcification
                                                       for parenchymal deformity.

Specimens submitted fresh to the laboratory that have a clearly palpable lesion can be initially incised following painting of excision margins and prior to thorough formalin fixation (24–48 hours). This allows sampling for consented research and optimal tumour fixation.

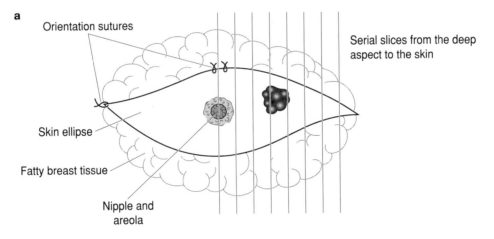

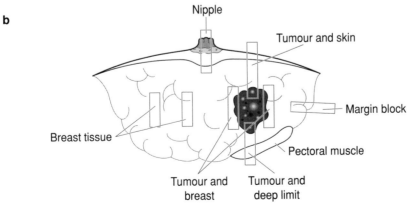

Figure 11.3. Blocking mastectomy/quadrantectomy specimens.

Impalpable and localisation specimens are not incised prior to fixation as this may distort the lesion, precluding accurate assessment of histological appearances and relationship to the margins, compounded by leaching of the paint onto the cut surface.

Initial Procedure

Mastectomy (total/partial) and quadrantectomy specimens:

- obtain all relevant histories of preoperative investigative procedures, e.g., FNAC, cores biopsy, etc. especially in cases of multifocal disease.
- weigh (g) and measure (cm) the specimen. Measure any ellipse of skin and note the presence or absence of the nipple–areolar complex and orientation sutures. Note the laterality (right or left).
- differentially paint all margins using artists' pigments or similar dyes according to an agreed protocol.
- serially slice transversely at 0.5–1cm intervals (Figure 11.3a) from the deep aspect to the skin using it as a spine to hold the specimen together.
- identify invasive tumour or DCIS areas (oozes toothpaste-like material in comedo type) and measure the largest diameter (mm).
- measure distances (mm) of the tumour edge to the excision margins.

Needle localisation and wide local excision specimens:

- obtain all relevant histories of preoperative investigative procedures, e.g., FNAC, cores biopsy, etc.
- make sure that laterality is stated (left or right) and orientation sutures are correctly placed before commencing. Note any accompanying specimen radiograph (obligatory for localisation specimens) and the presence and location of any guide wire(s).

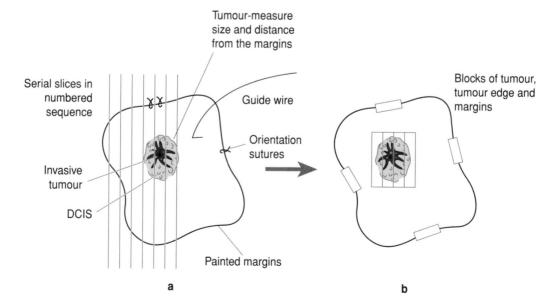

Tumour-measure size and distance from the margins

Serial slices in numbered sequence

Guide wire

Blocks of tumour, tumour edge and margins

Orientation sutures

Invasive tumour

DCIS

Painted margins

a   b

Figure 11.4. Blocking a breast localisation/wide local excision specimen.

- orientate the specimen with sutures or surgical clips as per protocol agreed with the surgeon (e.g., long suture for lateral margin, dark suture for deep, etc.).
- differentially paint all margins using artists' pigments according to an agreed protocol.
- serially slice the specimen at 0.3 cm intervals (Figure11.4a), lay out and number the slices in sequence. Inspect with reference to the radiograph and guide wire tip (if applicable) and note any macroscopic lesion(s).
- needle localisation specimens for microcalcification may show no obvious abnormality grossly. The laid out and numbered tissue slices should be X-rayed by a Faxitron machine to help locate the area(s) in question for block selection. If an X-ray facility is not available, block especially fibrous parenchyma rather than fatty tissue. Small specimens less than 20 grams, however, may be processed in their entirety.
- stromal deformity and mass lesions are identified grossly, the size and distances to the excision margins are measured.
- cavity shavings from various margins are weighed, painted and labelled accordingly before submitting for processing.

Description

- measure tumour size (mm) and note multifocal disease.
- measure distances (mm) of tumour to the margins.
- note the tissue block where the guide wire tip is in localisation specimens, that orientation sutures are in place correctly or if some sutures have fallen out.
- note the character of tumour (scirrhous, mucoid), edge (circumscribed, irregular), etc.
- note the character of surrounding breast tissue, and presence of skin, nipple, skeletal muscle at the deep aspect.

Table 11.1. Histological grading of invasive breast carcinoma

Three parameters are assessed and scored as follows:			
1. Tubule formation			Score
majority of tumour (> 75%)			1
moderate (10–75%)			2
little or none (< 10%)			3
2. Nuclear pleomorphism			
regular,uniform nuclei			1
larger, irregular nuclei			2
marked variation in size and shape (± multiple nucleoli)			3
3. Mitotic count (per 10 high-power fields – related to the objective field diameter)			
Leitz Diaplan	Leitz Ortholux	Nikon Labophot	
× 40 obj.	× 25 obj.	× 40 obj.	
0–11	0–9	0–5	1
12–22	10–19	6–10	2
> 22	> 19	> 10	3
Total score	Grade		Differentiation
3–5	I		well
6–7	II		moderate
8–9	III		poor

Blocks for Histology (Figures 11.3b, 11.4b)

- sample tumour, tumour edge, and tumour and nearest margin(s) (minimum 4–5 blocks).
- sample areas suspicious of DCIS.
- sample surrounding breast tissue (2 blocks).
- sample the nipple in mastectomy specimens and tumour-involved skin or muscle.
- in completion mastectomy specimens, sample cavity wall (3–4 blocks).
- count and sample all axillary lymph nodes and label separately where indicated (levels I, II and III).
- a representative complete section of any grossly involved lymph node is adequate.
- lymph nodes over 5 mm in maximum size should be sliced at approximately 3 mm intervals perpendicular to the long axis.

Histopathology Report

- type and side of specimen.
- specimen size: dimensions (cm), weight (g).
- tumour type.
- tumour grade : I, II, III (see Table 11.1 for grading system).
- DCIS present: no, yes (within/around/away from tumour).
- DCIS type.
- DCIS nuclear grade (low, intermediate, high).
- size of invasive component (cm).
- size of DCIS.
- size of invasive + DCIS.
- nearest margin: medial, lateral, inferior, superior, deep, superficial (skin).
- distance from margin: invasive/DCIS.
- lymphovascular invasion: not seen/present within or outside tumour.
- axillary nodal status: Levels I, II and III number of nodes and number involved by metastases.
- extranodal tumour deposits: yes/no.
- Paget's disease of nipple: yes/no.
- skin involvment by tumour: yes/no.
- TNM staging
  - pTis carcinoma in situ, Paget's with no tumour.
  - pT1 tumour ≤ 20 mm.
    T1 mic ≤ 1 mm.
    T1 a 1 mm < tumour ≤ 5 mm.
    T1 b 5 mm < tumour ≤ 10 mm.
    T1 c 10 mm < tumour ≤ 20 mm.
  - pT2 20 mm < tumour ≤ 50 mm.
  - pT3 tumour > 50 mm.
  - pT4 tumour of any size with direct extension to chest wall (ribs, intercostal muscles, serratus anterior but not pectoral muscle) or skin.
    (a) chest wall.
    (b) oedema including peau d'orange, skin ulceration or satellite nodules in the same breast.
    (c) a and b.
    (d) inflammatory carcinoma – sore red breast due to tumour involvement of dermal lymphatics.
  - pNx nodes cannot be assessed (not removed/previously removed).
  - pN0 no regional lymph node metastasis.
  - pN1 mi micrometastasis (> 0.2 mm but < 2 mm in greatest dimension).
  - pN1a metastasis in 1–3 ipsilateral axillary lymph node(s) (movable).

- pN1b internal mammary nodes with micrometastasis detected by sentinel node dissection but not clinically apparent.
- pN1c a + b.
- pN2a metastasis in 4–9 ipsilateral axillary nodes (fixed).
- pN2b metastasis in clinically apparent internal mammary nodes in the absence of axillary node involvement.
- pN3a metastasis in 10 or more ipsilateral axillary nodes, or ipsilateral infraclavicular nodes.
- pN3b internal mammary nodes with axillary node involvement.
- pN3c supraclavicular node metastasis.
- Prognosis
  - Nottingham Prognostic Index (NPI)
    - < 3.4 good prognosis, 85% five-year survival.
    - 3.4–5.4 intermediate prognosis, 68% five-year survival.
    - > 5.4 poor prognosis, 21% five-year survival.
  - NPI = 0.2 × tumour size(cm) + tumour grade + nodal score.
  - Nodal score – 1 node negative.
                  2 1–3 low axillary nodes involved.
                  3 4 or more nodes/apical node involved.
- Predictive factors.
  - Hormone receptor status – Oestrogen (ER) and Progesterone (PR) receptors.
  - Oncogene receptor status Her 2/Neu/C-erb B2.

- For scoring methods, see Tables 11.2 and 11.3.

Table 11.2.   Quick score method for immunohistochemical detection of ER status

Score for proportion of cells staining	Score for staining intensity
0. no nuclear staining 1. < 1% nuclei staining 2. 1–10% nuclei staining 3. 10–33% nuclei staining 4. 33–66% nuclei staining 5. 66–100% nuclei staining	0. no staining 1. weak staining 2. moderate staining 3. strong staining

Adding the two scores together gives a maximum score of 8. Data so far suggests that with this scoring system, response to hormonal therapy correlates with the following cut-off values:
    score 0 indicates hormonal therapy will definitely not work
    score 2–3 indicates a small (20%) chance of treatment response
    score 4–6 indicates an even (50%) chance of response
    score 7–8 indicates a good (75%) chance of response
Where PR content has also been determined, hormonal therapy is thought worthwhile in patients with low ER but high PR .

Table 11.3.   Scoring method for Her2/neu oncogene overexpression by immunohistochemistry

0: no cytoplasmic staining	Her2 negative
1+: weak cytoplasmic staining	Her2 negative
2+: moderate cytoplasmic staining	Her2 status equivocal, for *FISH testing
3+: strong cytoplasmic staining	Her2 positive

* Fluorescent in-situ hybridization.
Her2 positive cases for anti-HER2 therapy.

Head and Neck Specimens

Séamus S Napier with clinical comments by David S Brooker, Derek J Gordon, Richard W Kendrick, William J Primrose and Colin FJ Russell

Nasal Cavities and Paranasal Sinuses

1. Anatomy

The external nose contains the right and left nostrils (or nares), each communicating with the nasal cavities via a slight dilatation just inside the nostril called the nasal vestibule. Bone from the frontal, maxillary and nasal bones supports the upper one-third of the external nose while cartilage supports the lower two-thirds.

Each nasal cavity extends posteriorly from just behind the nasal vestibule, through the opening called the anterior choana, to communicate with the nasopharynx via the posterior choana. They are separated by the nasal septum, which is composed of bone posteriorly and cartilage anteriorly. Each nasal cavity has a roof, a floor, a medial (or septal) wall and a lateral wall (Figure 12.1). The roof of the nose is closely related to the frontal sinuses, the anterior cranial fossa, the ethmoidal sinuses and the sphenoidal sinus. The floor of the nose is closely related to the anterior maxillary teeth and the vault of the palate, while the medial wall represents the nasal septum. The lateral wall of the nose is complex and bears three (occasionally four) horizontal projections called turbinates or conchae, the superior turbinate being the smallest and the inferior turbinate the largest. The passageway of the nasal cavity below and lateral to each of the turbinates is called the superior, middle and inferior meatus respectively; above and behind the superior turbinate

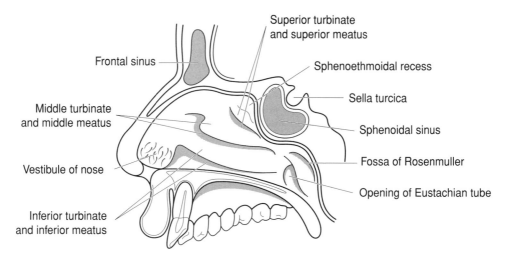

Figure 12.1. Right lateral wall of nasal cavity.

143

lies the sphenoethmoidal recess. The paranasal sinuses open onto the lateral wall of the nasal cavity, as does the nasolacrimal duct, so that disease affecting this region of the nose can obstruct the drainage of secretions and present as sinusitis.

Each nasal cavity is divided into functional areas, reflected in the nature of the epithelial lining. The nasal vestibule is lined by skin and contains many short hairs that help to filter particles from the inspired air. The olfactory area, concerned with the sense of smell, is restricted to the upper part of the nasal cavity and is centred on the cribriform plate of the ethmoid bone, the adjacent part of the nasal septum and the superior turbinate. The rest of the nasal cavity is lined by respiratory mucosa, the function of which is to warm and humidify the air and to trap particulate material. The complex architecture of the lateral wall of the nasal cavities facilitates this process by increasing the surface area and the turbulence of the airflow.

The paranasal sinuses are extensions of the nasal cavities and represent air-filled spaces in the skull bones lined by respiratory mucosa (Figure 12.2). They are usually absent or poorly developed at birth but enlarge most during the eruption of the permanent teeth and after puberty. They are located in the frontal, ethmoidal, sphenoidal and maxillary bones as paired structures about the midline but tend to be considered from a pathophysiological perspective into anterior and posterior groups. The anterior group comprises the frontal sinus, the anterior and middle ethmoidal sinuses and the maxillary sinus, all opening into the middle meatus, while the posterior ethmoidal sinuses and the sphenoidal sinus represent the posterior group and drain into the superior meatus and the sphenoethmoidal recess respectively. The nasolacrimal duct opens into the inferior meatus anteriorly.

The frontal sinuses lie between the outer and inner tables of the frontal bone and are closely related to the anterior cranial fossa. Disease in the frontal sinus is often associated with intracranial complications. The ethmoidal sinuses number between 3 and 18 and consist of a labyrinth

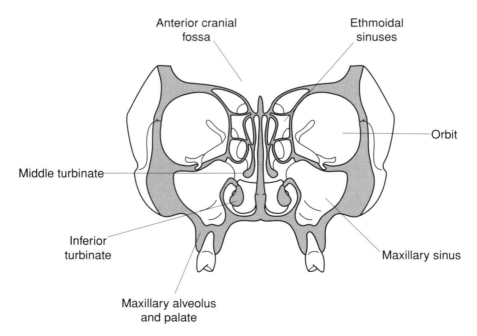

Figure 12.2. Ethmoidal sinuses and maxillary sinuses. Coronal view of nasal cavities at level of first molar tooth showing maxillary and ethmoidal sinuses.

of thin-walled bony cavities between the upper part of the nasal cavity and the orbits. The pathway for drainage of the frontal sinus passes through the anterior ethmoidal sinus group and may be impeded by disease in this area. The sphenoidal sinuses lie within the body of the sphenoid bone posterior to the upper part of the nasal cavity. Adjacent structures such as the optic chiasma, pituitary gland, internal carotid artery and cavernous sinus may be affected by disease of the sphenoidal sinuses. The maxillary sinus is the largest of the paranasal sinuses and is closely related to the posterior maxillary teeth, the floor of the orbit, the inferior portion of the lateral wall of the nose and the pterygoid plates of the sphenoid bone.

Lymphovascular Drainage

Lymphatics from the external nose and anterior nasal cavity, together with those from the skin of the mid-portion of the face, drain to Level I lymph nodes in the submandibular region. The rest of the nasal cavity and the paranasal sinuses drain to Level II lymph nodes in the upper part of the deep cervical chain (Figure 19.1), sometimes via the retropharyngeal nodes.

2. Clinical Presentation

Disease affecting the nose presents with unilateral or bilateral nasal obstruction, rhinorrhoea (watering of the nose), epistaxis (bleeding), facial pain, facial swelling, epiphora (watering of the eye) or proptosis (bulging outward of the eye). Deafness or otitis media may be due to obstruction of the opening of the Eustachian tube in the nasopharynx by extension of a nasal tumour.

3. Clinical Investigations

Direct visualisation of the nasal cavities is performed using a speculum for the anterior aspect or a postnasal mirror for the posterior portion. Endonasal endoscopy is the preferred method for sampling tissue from the nose and nasal sinuses. Plain radiographs of the nose and sinuses may demonstrate bone destruction, soft tissue mass or fluid levels although these are more accurately determined by CT and MRI scanning.

Markedly elevated erythrocyte sedimentation rates (ESR) and titres of "cytoplasmic" anti-neutrophil cytoplasmic antibodies (cANCA) are helpful adjuncts to diagnosis in the so-called "Lethal Midline Granuloma" syndrome, a collection of diseases characterised by progressive destruction of the nose and sinuses. These tests help distinguish principally between Wegener's granulomatosis and T-cell/natural killer cell lymphoma.

4. Pathological Conditions

Non-neoplastic Conditions

Sinusitis: acute infections are usually bacterial and often follow the common cold. Empyema or mucocoele may result if the draining of the secretions is obstructed. Chronic sinusitis follows acute sinusitis and may be associated with obstruction (e.g., by polyp or tumour) or immune compromise. Maxillary sinusitis may occur alone or may be associated with involvement of frontal and/or ethmoidal sinuses. Most cases respond to antibiotics and topical medications to improve drainage. Functional endoscopic sinus surgery (FESS) is the commonest surgical management of recurrent sinusitis; opening of the ostio-meatal complex under the middle turbinate or removal of pneumatised middle turbinates (concha bullosa) or nasal polyps will improve physiological drainage and allow biopsy sampling.

Pain of dental origin can mimic maxillary sinusitis and vice versa. Extraction of upper premolar or molar teeth may damage the floor of the maxillary sinus and result in an oroantral fistula through the socket.

Inflammatory polyps: a frequent complication of long-standing rhinitis, often but not exclusively allergic in origin. Often multiple and bilateral, they are a cause of sinusitis and nasal obstruction. Histologically, there is abundant myxoid or oedematous stroma covered by respiratory epithelium; ulceration and/or squamous metaplasia are common in larger polyps where they contact the nasal walls. The antrochoanal polyp is an uncommon large single inflammatory polyp that arises in the maxillary sinus and extends into the nasal cavity, presenting at the posterior choana. Nasal polyps in children are often associated with cystic fibrosis.

Wegener's granulomatosis: an uncommon systemic disorder characterised by necrotising granulomatous inflammation and vasculitis that usually presents in the upper respiratory tract, lungs and/or kidneys. Symptoms can be non-specific (malaise, pyrexia) or related to the anatomical sites involved; in the nose it may manifest as sinusitis, rhinorrhoea, epistaxis or nasal obstruction. Rarely are the classical features present in nasal biopsies; diagnosis requires a high index of suspicion and careful clinicopathological correlation. ESR and cANCA titres are useful in confirming the diagnosis, although a negative cANCA does not exclude Wegener's granulomatosis. A distinctive form of small multinucleate giant cell with clumped smudged nuclei, foci of granular collagen necrosis and neutrophil microabscesses are characteristic if underrecognised features.

Other non-neoplastic conditions that may affect the nose and sinuses include fungal infections (chronic non-invasive colonisation by *Aspergillus*, acute fulminant or angioinvasive aspergillosis, allergic fungal sinusitis), pyogenic granuloma, haemangioma and other vascular malformations, lymphoid hyperplasia, glial heterotopia and hairy polyp.

Neoplastic Conditions

Benign tumours: sinonasal papillomas are uncommon but are the most frequent benign neoplasms, subdivided into fungiform, inverted and cylindrical cell types. They occur twice as often in males as in females and affect adults aged between 30 and 60 years. They are usually unilateral lesions but may be multiple or multifocal. *Inverted papillomas* are the commonest form, found on the lateral nasal wall and sinuses. They have an endophytic growth pattern and are composed of thick non-keratinising "transitional" epithelium within oedematous stroma. *Fungiform papillomas* are exophytic lesions composed of transitional epithelium supported by fibrovascular stroma, found exclusively on the nasal septum. *Cylindrical cell papillomas* are rare. They are similar in distribution and appearance to inverted papillomas but are composed of tall columnar (cylindrical) oncocytic cells.

Other benign neoplasms include pleomorphic adenoma, solitary fibrous tumour, haemangiopericytoma, nasopharyngeal (juvenile) angiofibroma, sinus osteoma, meningioma, teratoma and paraganglioma.

Sinonasal cancer: the maxillary sinus is the commonest site for sinonasal malignancy and is usually either squamous cell carcinoma or adenocarcinoma in type. The nasal cavity is the second commonest site and is affected by a broad spectrum of lesions but tumours of the sphenoidal and frontal sinuses are rare. Risk factors include tobacco use, exposure to hard and soft wood dusts, nickel and irradiation.

Squamous cell carcinoma: the vast majority of malignant tumours of the mucosal lining of the nasal cavities and sinuses are classified as squamous cell carcinoma. The maxillary or ethmoid sinuses are the commonest sites but the nasal vestibule or septum can be affected. Many tumours have a "transitional cell" pattern, similar to that seen in inverted papillomas but exhibiting pleomorphism, necrosis and a broad, pushing invasive front. The term "non-keratinising squamous cell carcinoma" can be used but a spectrum of changes including the presence of single cell infiltration and/or abundant keratinisation may be seen, sometimes making distinction from the usual type of squamous cell carcinoma impossible.

Salivary gland-type adenocarcinoma: the second commonest type of malignant tumour with adenoid cystic carcinoma the pattern most often encountered.

Intestinal-type sinonasal adenocarcinoma: adenocarcinoma exhibiting the differentiation pattern of large or small intestinal mucosa, with or without cytological atypia. Strongly associated with hard wood dusts (males, ethmoidal sinuses) but may occur sporadically (females, maxillary sinus). Commonest pattern mimics colonic adenocarcinoma – metastasis needs to be excluded. Mucinous tumours with signet ring cells are rare.

Malignant lymphoma: all types of non-Hodgkin's lymphoma may affect the sinonasal region either as a site of origin or as part of disseminated disease; diffuse large B-cell lymphoma is the commonest. T-cell and natural killer cell lymphomas often demonstrate a striking tendency for vascular involvement, sometimes with bizarre acute ischaemic changes, such as tooth exfoliation and bone necrosis. The tumour cells may be small, large or intermediate in size; the admixture of other inflammatory cells masks the neoplastic component by mimicking an inflammatory condition such as infection or Wegener's granulomatosis.

Others: Low-grade sinonasal adenocarcinoma, olfactory neuroblastoma, malignant melanoma, small cell neuroendocrine carcinoma, sinonasal undifferentiated carcinoma, rhabdomyosarcoma, chondrosarcoma and chordoma are all uncommon.

Prognosis: outcome depends on the histological type of tumour as well as the extent of spread. Most lesions are advanced at presentation although lymph node metastasis with carcinomas is relatively infrequent. Local recurrence is a common problem in spite of radical surgery and radiotherapy. Melanomas, small cell neuroendocrine carcinomas and sinonasal undifferentiated carcinomas are particularly aggressive but five-year survival is the norm with adenoid cystic carcinomas. In certain subtypes, such as intestinal-type sinonasal adenocarcinoma and olfactory neuroblastoma, grading based on the degree of differentiation is important in that low-grade lesions do well while high-grade lesions do badly. Around 20% five-year survival is customary.

5. Surgical Pathology Specimens – Clinical Aspects

Biopsy Specimens

Rigid or fibre optic endoscopy is the usual method of sampling lesions in the nose and paranasal sinuses. When malignant disease is suspected, detailed examination and large biopsy samples are best obtained with this technique under general anaesthesia, as it avoids contaminating skin with tumour and compromising later definitive surgical procedures. Benign tumours such as nasal papillomas may be resected using endoscopic laser surgery but tend to be delivered as small fragments.

Resection Specimens

Excision specimens of nasal septum are easily delivered intact via a lateral rhinotomy incision. Medial maxillectomy is the commonest surgical procedure for low-grade tumours of the lateral aspect of the nasal cavity and/or maxillary, ethmoid and frontal sinuses. Resection specimens tend to be fragmented because of the fragile nature of the bone; in these cases, precise interpretation of surgical margins requires orientation of the tissue samples by the surgeon. Alternatively, separate biopsy samples of critical or suspicious areas may be taken after clearance of tumour and submitted separately. Palatal fenestration is recommended for low maxillary sinus tumours involving the oral cavity; definite or possible involvement of the posterior wall of the maxillary sinus requires maxillectomy. Prosthetic rehabilitation with an obturator constructed around an upper denture provides optimal functional and aesthetic results and allows good visualisation of the wound postoperatively, facilitating re-biopsy of suspicious areas.

Craniofacial resection describes a surgical approach through both the anterior skull and the mid-face performed for tumours of the frontal or ethmoid sinus that extend into the anterior cranial fossa. Total ethmoidectomy, nasal exenteration, maxillectomy and orbital exenteration can be performed if necessary.

Involvement of the orbital floor or medial wall is an important nodal point in the management of sinonasal tumours. Breach of the bony wall or involvement of periosteum by tumour may necessitate clearance or exenteration of the orbit.

Concomitant neck dissections are usually not indicated unless there is proven metastatic disease.

6. Surgical Pathology Specimens – Laboratory Aspects

Biopsy Specimens

Usually as small samples from open biopsies or core needle specimens, free-floating in formalin. Measure in three dimensions or length of core and submit in total. Specimens containing bone require decalcification and can be recognised by their tendency to sink rapidly in the fixative.

Resection Specimens

Septal Excision, Medial Maxillectomy and Craniofacial Resection Specimens

Most septal excision and medial maxillectomy specimens are for the less extensive or less locally aggressive neoplastic diseases, such as inverted nasal papilloma, olfactory neuroblastoma and even malignant melanoma. They are usually received as multiple fragments of mucosa with underlying bone and/or cartilage. In medial maxillectomy specimens, at least the inferior turbinate is included but, depending on tumour location, all turbinates may be represented.

Most craniofacial resection specimens are for extensive or locally aggressive neoplastic diseases of the frontal or ethmoid sinuses, where a curative outcome is expected. As such, they will represent composites of septal excision, medial maxillectomy, maxillectomy and skull base excisions. They are usually received intact or as two or three large fragments. They are handled as if they represented an extended medial maxillectomy specimen (see Chapter 14). Invasion into dura is an ominous finding.

Samples of critical or clinically suspicious margins taken at clearance of tumour should be submitted separately and handled as biopsy specimens.

Initial Procedure

- if intact, orientate the specimen and ink its margins.
- otherwise, if a larger specimen is submitted, ink its margins. A line of ink drawn across medium-sized fragments can aid orientation after microscopic examination and assist assessment of margins.

- slice the larger pieces into 0.4 cm-thick slices transversely, using a band saw or equivalent.
- measurements:
  - if intact, dimensions (cm).
  - if fragmented, number of fragments, total weight (g) and dimensions of largest specimen (cm).
  - tumour:
    - size (cm).
    - number of fragments consisting of tumour.
    - distance to closest surgical margins (cm).

Description

- tumour:
  - size, shape and colour.
  - presence of necrosis.
  - if fragmented, number of fragments containing tumour.
- adjacent mucosa:
  - colour and consistency.
  - presence of other lesions.
- other: lymph nodes, neck dissection

Maxillectomy Specimens

See Maxilla, Mandible and Teeth (Chapter 14).

Blocks for Histology

In cases of neoplastic disease, the histology should represent the tumour, its relationship to the adjacent mucosa and underlying bone or cartilage. Focal abnormalities of mucosa need to be sampled.

- three blocks of tumour to illustrate the interface with adjacent normal tissues.
- three blocks of adjacent mucosa.
- closest deep surgical margin.
- samples of other lesions, e.g., nodules or polyps.
- in intact specimens, sample the mucosal margins before sawing the bone and submit separately (reduces contamination of the margins). Cut with a sharp blade firmly down to bone and use a flat blunt instrument to dissect mucosa free from the bone.
- in intact specimens, saw the bone into 0.5 cm slices in the transverse plane (vertical plane in vivo).
- if fragmented, bread-slice larger specimens and submit as labelled blocks. Microscopic analysis may allow reconstruction and useful assessment of margins.

Histopathology Report

Final reports of sinonasal specimens should include details on:

- the specimen type and side.
- if fragmented, the number of fragments and the size of the largest.
- the type, subtype and grade of tumour present:
  - sinonasal papilloma variants.
  - squamous cell carcinoma and variants.

- – low-grade adenocarcinoma.
- – intestinal-type adenocarcinoma.
- – lymphoma.
- – the macroscopic size of tumour.
- – the presence or absence of invasion of bone.
- – the distance of tumour from the nearest margin.
- – the presence or absence of vascular invasion.
- – the presence or absence of dural invasion (if craniofacial resection).
- – other pathology such as radiation injury.

● TNM: classification of tumour spread

Maxillary sinus

- – pT1   mucosa.
- – pT2   bone erosion/destruction, hard palate, middle nasal meatus.
- – pT3   posterior bony wall maxillary sinus, subcutaneous tissues, floor/medial wall of orbit, pterygoid fossa, ethmoid sinus.
- – pT4a   anterior orbit, cheek skin, pterygoid plates, infratemporal fossa, cribriform plate, sphenoid/frontal sinus.
- – pT4b   orbital apex, dura, brain, middle cranial fossa, cranial nerves other than V2, nasopharynx, clivus.

Nasal cavity and ethmoid sinus

- – pT1   one subsite.
- – pT2   two subsites or adjacent nasoethmoidal site.
- – pT3   medial wall/floor orbit, maxillary sinus, palate, cribriform plate.
- – pT4a   anterior orbit, skin of nose/cheek, anterior cranial fossa (minimal), infratemporal fossa, pterygoid plates, sphenoid/frontal sinus.
- – pT4b   orbital apex, dura, brain, middle cranial fossa, cranial nerves other than V2, nasopharynx, clivus.

All sites: regional lymph nodes

pN0   no regional node metastasis.
pN1   metastasis in a ipsilateral single $\leq$ 3 cm.
pN2   metastasis in:
    a.   ipsilateral single > 3 to 6 cm.
    b.   ipsilateral multiple $\leq$ 6 cm.
    c.   bilateral contralateral $\leq$ 6 cm.
pN3   metastasis in a lymph node > 6 cm.

13 Lips, Mouth and Tongue

1. Anatomy

The mouth extends from the lips and cheeks to the oropharyngeal isthmus at the palatoglossal fold. It comprises a number of subsites, which can be divided into three functional types although the microscopic structure of each varies subtly from one region to the next. "Masticatory mucosa" is found on the maxillary and mandibular gingivae, the hard palate and on the dorsum of the tongue. It is bound tightly to underlying tissue and covered by keratotic, relatively thick, stratified squamous epithelium to withstand the trauma of chewing. In contrast, "lining mucosa" is elastic and is present on the inner aspect of the lips, on the buccal mucosae and their respective upper and lower sulci, the ventral surface of the tongue and the floor of the mouth. It is covered by relatively thin, stratified squamous epithelium supported by loosely textured fibrovascular connective tissue (Figures 13.1 and 13.2). "Specialised mucosa" refers to the taste buds.

The lips are composed of skin and mucosa around the opening to the mouth. They contain the orbicularis oris, fibrofatty tissue and many minor salivary glands. Upper and lower lips join at the buccal commissure (angle of the mouth). The mucosa of the lips begins at the vermilion border

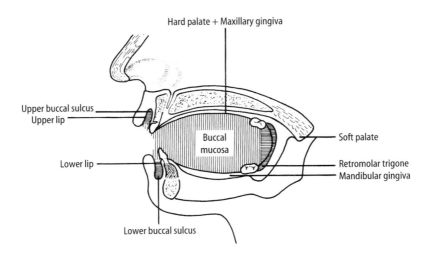

Figure 13.1. Mucosal subsites of lips and oral cavity. Reproduced from Hermanek P, Hutter RVP, Sobin LH, Wagner G, Wittekind Ch (eds.). TNM Atlas: illustrated guide to the TNM/pTNM classification of malignant tumours, 4th edition. Springer-Verlag: Berlin and Heidelberg, 1997.

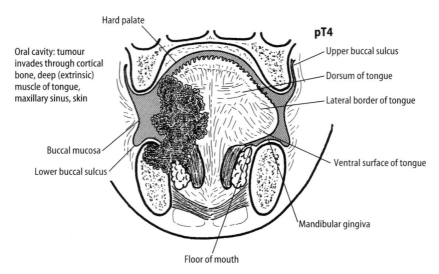

Figure 13.2. Mucosal subsites of tongue and floor of mouth demonstrating pT4 tumour of tongue. Reproduced from Hermanek P, Hutter RVP, Sobin LH, Wagner G, Wittekind Ch (eds.). TNM Atlas: illustrated guide to the TNM/pTNM classification of malignant tumours, 4th edition. Springer-Verlag: Berlin and Heidelberg, 1997.

with skin and extends across the free surface into the oral cavity proper. The cheeks are continuations of the lips; the skin forms most of the facial skin while the buccal mucosa is continuous through the upper and lower sulci with the gingivae and with the soft palate/oropharynx. Buccinator is the principle muscle of the cheek; it is perforated opposite the upper second molar tooth by the parotid duct. Many minor salivary glands lie between the muscle layer and the mucosa while the facial (or buccal) lymph node lies external to buccinator below the level of the occlusal plane.

The gingival margin has a scalloped outline as it encircles the teeth, forming the interdental papilla between adjacent teeth. Behind the last molar tooth on each side of the mandible, the gingiva forms a flat triangular region known as the retromolar trigone (or retromolar pad). The hard palate is formed mostly by the palatine processes of the maxillary bones and is covered by mucosa continuous with the upper gingivae. In the midline of the palate anteriorly just behind the incisor teeth, there is a small mucosal elevation called the incisive papilla. In the anterior palate the mucosa forms four or five transverse ridges called rugae while posteriorly it is smooth. Small numbers of minor salivary glands are present in the hard palate posteriorly and laterally close to the alveolar processes of the maxilla. The hard palate is continuous posteriorly with the soft palate, a mobile flap of mucosa, striated muscle and fibrofatty tissue separating the nasopharynx from the oropharynx.

The floor of the mouth is a horseshoe-shaped region between the tongue, the mandible and mylohyoid. It contains the sublingual salivary glands, the submandibular ducts, the lingual nerves and some of the extrinsic muscles of the tongue. Right and left submandibular ducts converge on the lingual frenulum, a midline fold running from the ventral surface of the tongue to the gingiva behind the lower central incisor teeth, forming a mucosal papilla in the floor of mouth approximately 1 cm posterior to the lingual gingiva.

The tongue is divided into two parts by a V-shaped groove called the sulcus terminalis; the anterior two-thirds lies within the oral cavity and the posterior one-third (the base) lies within the oropharynx. The anterior two-thirds is divided into:

Dorsal surface – the superior surface. It is covered by enumerable filiform papillae; between 30 and 50 dispersed fungiform papillae measuring approximately 1 mm in diameter and between 8 and 12 circumvallate papillae, measuring between 3 and 4 mm in diameter located in a line just anterior to the sulcus terminalis. The fungiform and circumvallate papillae bear taste buds.

Ventral surface – the inferior aspect. It has a smooth surface, merging with the floor of the mouth.

Lateral border – the side of the tongue. It extends from the tip to the palatoglossal arch (anterior pillar of the fauces).

The posterior one-third of the tongue has a cobblestone surface due to the accumulation of lymphoid tissue from the lingual tonsil. No papillae are present although taste buds may be numerous. The mucosa is contiguous with the palatine tonsils laterally and the vallecula of the epiglottis posteriorly.

The tongue is divided into right and left halves by a median fibrous septum, which is attached inferiorly to the hyoid bone. The muscles of the tongue are divided into the intrinsic group and the extrinsic group. The extrinsic group represents genioglossus, hyoglossus, stylogossus and palatoglossus, having attachments outside the tongue and considered important in the staging of malignant tumours; involvement of the extrinsic muscles by tumour signifies pT4 staging (Figure 13.2).

Lymphovascular Drainage

The face, oral tissues and tongue possess many lymphatic channels and display a variable pattern of lymphatic drainage. In general, the tissues of the anterior face and lips drain to lymph nodes in the submental and submandibular regions. The tissues of the lateral face, eyelids and anterior portion of the scalp and external ear drain to lymph nodes around the parotid region. The tissues of the posterior scalp and behind the ear tend to drain to retroauricular and suboccipital lymph nodes. These superficial lymph node groups ultimately drain to lymph nodes in the deep cervical chain situated around the internal jugular vein (Figure 19.1).

Within the oral cavity, the tissues of the palatal gingiva, hard palate and soft palate drain to retropharyngeal lymph nodes or directly to lymph nodes in the deep cervical chain. The tissues of the floor of the mouth and those of the lingual gingiva drain to nodes in the submental and submandibular regions, and ultimately to lymph nodes in the deep cervical chain.

There is much subregional variability in the lymphatic drainage of the tongue influenced by the presence of the median septum. Malignant tumour drains to ipsilateral lymph nodes in the deep cervical chain but contralateral node involvement should be considered with lesions at the tip of the tongue, lesions that cross the midline or involve the median fibrous septum and lesions in the posterior one-third.

2. Clinical Presentation

Disease affecting the mouth and tongue may be clinically silent or may present as a mass lesion, an ulcer, a white/red patch or with a painful/burning sensation often on eating hot or spicy foods. Pain is a rare presenting feature of malignancy, which is usually asymptomatic until advanced.

3. Clinical Investigations

The ease with which the oral cavity can be examined by direct visualization facilitates preoperative diagnosis and reduces the need for complex investigative procedures. Nevertheless, haematological investigations are often useful to determine haemoglobin levels, red blood cell indices, serum ferritin, vitamin B_{12} and folate levels.

Identification of pathological forms of *Candida* species can be achieved by direct visualization of Periodic acid/Schiff-stained smears sampled directly from affected mucosa. Precise sub-classification can be performed following culture of swabs or an oral saline rinse, the latter also providing a quantitative measure of oral fungal load.

Biopsy techniques are used frequently to sample mucosal abnormalities. The value of direct and indirect immunofluorescence should not be underestimated in blistering and/or ulcerating conditions. Endoscopy of the upper aerodigestive tract is performed prior to surgery for malignant disease to identify occult second primary neoplasms.

Fine Needle Aspiration Cytology (FNAC) can provide additional information to facilitate the resolution of a differential diagnosis of submucosal masses; cytology brushes can be used but interpretation of atypia in mucosal samples can be problematic.

Plain radiographs may detect a concurrent odontogenic or bony lesion and will often identify gross bone destruction by mucosal cancers. CT and MRI scanning are essential in planning surgery by indicating the depth of the tumour and detecting other changes in the neck. CT has less motion artefact and is good for bone detail while MRI gives superior soft tissue contrast without dental amalgam artefact or exposure to ionising radiation.

4. Pathological Conditions

Non-neoplastic Conditions

The oral mucosa is affected by a bewildering number of non-neoplastic conditions that are the subject of many textbooks. These are divided according to their clinical presentation as either lumps, ulcers or white/red patches.

Lumps: most discrete mass lesions of the oral mucosa represent forms of fibrous tissue overgrowth (fibroepithelial polyp) as a consequence of low-grade chronic trauma. The term fibrous epulis is reserved for lesions on the gums while those associated with dentures can be described as denture-induced hyperplasia. Mucous extravasation cysts and mucous retention cysts arise from small salivary glands within the submucosal tissues. Vascular anomalies, such as haemangioma and lymphangioma, can affect any oral site. Giant cell epulis (or peripheral giant cell granuloma) usually arises from the gum anterior to the premolar region, presumably as a response to irritational stimuli, but such lesions in older patients may be a manifestation of hyperparathyroidism.

Persistent diffuse swellings of the oral mucosa are much rarer and most represent vascular anomalies (such as haemangioma or lymphangioma) present since birth. Causes of intermittent diffuse swelling of the oral mucosa are orofacial granulomatosis (sometimes a manifestation of Crohn's disease) or angioedema, a selective deficiency of components of the complement system.

Ulcers: common on the lining mucosa and tongue and are often due to trauma from teeth, dentures or foodstuffs. Recurrent aphthous ulceration is characterised by crops of ulcers on the lining mucosa of young patients that heal spontaneously over a two-week period but recur. Three clinical subtypes are recognised: minor (ulcers 2–4 mm in diameter), major (single ulcer at least 10 mm in diameter, located posteriorly in the mouth that heals slowly) and herpetiform (a very rare type, usually close to the front of the mouth, composed of minute coalescing ulcers). Around 20% of patients with recurrent aphthous ulcers may suffer from a haematological deficiency due to a systemic disorder but most patients are otherwise healthy. Drugs can produce ulcers through either topical or systemic effects. Vesiculobullous disorders, such as erythema multiforme, pemphigus vulgaris and mucous membrane pemphigoid, are more likely to present with ulcers than with intact blisters because of the relative fragility of the oral mucosa compared to skin. Squamous cell carcinoma may often present as a non-healing ulcer.

White/red patches: the oral mucosa may become white due to accumulation of keratin or epithelial hyperplasia and may become red because of epithelial atrophy, increased vascularity or inflammation. Physical stimuli such as friction from teeth or dentures or through the use of tobacco can produce an irritational keratosis on any part of the oral mucosa, most often lining mucosa. "Chevron" parakeratosis and melanin incontinence point to tobacco-related lesions. Lichen planus/lichenoid reaction occurs commonly on the lining mucosa and dorsum of tongue as white striae or papules against a red background. Erosive forms are characterised by ulceration. Some lesions are a consequence of systemic drug therapy or as a response to amalgam restorations in adjacent teeth. Geographic tongue is characterised by irregular areas of mucosal erosion affecting the dorsal surface. Central areas of atrophy are outlined by a narrow peripheral zone of white mucosa and may be accompanied by deep fissuring of the tongue. The pattern of atrophic and white areas changes gradually, affected areas returning to normal and new lesions developing. *Candida* may affect the oral mucosa and may present as red or white lesions. Candidal infection is often a marker of underlying disease ("disease of the diseased") although a number of local factors can precipitate candidal infection, particularly smoking, xerostomia, high carbohydrate diet and topical steroid application. Furthermore, any mucosal lesion can be secondarily infected by *Candida*. A small proportion of white/red lesions of oral mucosa may ultimately develop squamous cell carcinoma, although it is not possible to predict which lesions will develop malignancy and when such an event might occur. Most authorities consider the presence of dysplasia in these potentially malignant lesions to be a worrying sign although there are significant problems with inter- and intra-observer variability in the assessment of dysplasia. Furthermore, approximately 50% of cases will never develop a tumour within the lifetime of the patient. Careful correlation of clinical, histopathological and other laboratory data are required to establish a precise diagnosis of oral white/red lesions.

Neoplastic Conditions

Benign tumours: squamous cell papilloma commonly occurs on the lips, cheeks and tongue and is often associated with viral warts on the hands. Neurilemmoma, neurofibroma and the granular cell tumour are not infrequently encountered. Lipoma presents as a mucosal polyp, clinically similar to a fibroepithelial polyp. Benign tumours of salivary gland origin arise in the upper lip and in the palate, usually at the junction between the hard and soft palates, the commonest of which is the pleomorphic adenoma. Benign salivary tumours are rare in the tongue and floor of mouth; most salivary tumours in the lower parts of the oral cavity are adenocarcinomas.

Malignant tumours: as at other sites in the upper aerodigestive tract, tobacco and alcohol use are the major risk factors for oral cancers. Their effects are related to dose and duration of use; together they have a multiplicative rather than additive effect. Recent interest has focussed on the role of viruses in oral malignancy. Certain forms of Human Papillomavirus have been detected in a proportion of tumours but their precise role in oncogenesis is unclear.

Squamous epithelial dysplasia: a rare finding; most lesions of the oral mucosa are not dysplastic. As with invasive tumours, epithelial dysplasia is strongly associated with tobacco smoking and alcohol use but paradoxically lesions arising in patients who do not use tobacco are most likely to develop carcinoma. In contrast to the cervix with which it has often – probably erroneously – been compared, oral dysplastic lesions are frequently hyperkeratotic with varying degrees of epithelial hyperplasia and/or atrophy. The grade of dysplasia can vary from mild to severe. Development of invasive squamous cell carcinoma seems to occur more frequently with increasing degrees of cytological disturbance (less than 5% for non-dysplastic lesions and low-grade dysplasia; around 50% for high-grade dysplasia) but there are no agreed criteria for grading or recognisable features of prognosis. Identifying high-grade dysplasia highlights the considerable risk of synchronous or metachronous squamous cell carcinoma but other factors such as site and the clinical appearance of the lesions need to be considered. Conservative surgery or ablative therapy (e.g., by laser or photodynamic therapy) will often be attempted but the effects of treatment are difficult to evaluate.

Intraoral squamous cell carcinoma: accounts for over 85% of primary malignant tumours in the mouth. Males are affected at least twice as often than females and most patients are aged between 40 and 60 years. Smoking and alcohol use are the main risk factors. The commonest intraoral sites are the lateral border/ventral surface of the anterior two-thirds of tongue (35%) and the floor of mouth (20%), followed by the mandibular gingiva/retromolar trigone, soft palate, buccal mucosa/buccal commissure and hard palate/maxillary gingiva. Tumours of the tongue and floor of the mouth tend to metastasise frequently to neck nodes – up to 30% of patients with carcinoma of the tongue and floor of mouth who have clinically negative necks will have metastatic disease. Tumours of the hard palate rarely involve nodes.

Histological and reportedly prognostic variants of squamous cell carcinoma include verrucous carcinoma, papillary squamous cell carcinoma (better than usual type), spindle cell squamous cell carcinoma, adenoid squamous cell carcinoma (same prognosis), basaloid squamous cell carcinoma and adenosquamous cell carcinoma (worse prognosis).

Prognosis: outcome for patients with intraoral squamous cell carcinoma depends on the precise anatomical site within the mouth (the further back in the mouth, the worse the outcome), the size of the tumour and the presence of regional nodal metastasis. Lymph node metastasis is the most significant factor in determining prognosis; extracapsular spread from affected nodes is also an indicator of limited prognosis, with increased risk of recurrence in the neck and of distant spread. The size and anatomical site of the tumour affects the ability to achieve surgical clearance with the risk of local recurrence but the pattern of tumour invasion is probably the most significant factor in determining lymph node metastasis. As with all upper aerodigestive tract malignancies, co-morbidity from cardiovascular and respiratory disease due to the effects of age, tobacco and alcohol use is a major adverse factor in survival.

Five-year survival with node-negative tongue carcinomas is approximately 50% falling to around 20% for patients with large tumours and positive nodes.

Squamous cell carcinoma of the lip: arising on the vermilion border of the lower lip although a few are seen on the upper lip. Probably represents a cutaneous rather than intraoral malignancy, as it is associated with long solar exposure. Less than 20% involve lymph nodes. Easily amenable to early detection and surgical excision, the five-year survival is in excess of 80%.

Squamous cell carcinoma involving either upper or lower lip but arising within the oral cavity (e.g., from the buccal commissure) is a true intraoral cancer, strongly associated with tobacco use. There is a greater likelihood of nodal metastasis but the prognosis is still reasonably good in comparison with similar lesions at other intraoral sites.

Other malignant tumours in the oral cavity include malignant lymphoma (usually a deposit of disseminated nodal disease), salivary gland types of adenocarcinoma, malignant melanoma (palate and maxillary gingiva), rhabdomyosarcoma (around the soft palate), and Kaposi's sarcoma (junction of hard and soft palate). The oral mucosa may be involved by direct spread from a malignant tumour in the minor salivary glands or from the nasal cavity/maxillary sinus.

5. Surgical Pathology Specimens – Clinical Aspects

Biopsy Specimens

Most oral biopsy specimens represent cold knife samples of an incisional or excisional nature. These are usually taken under direct vision and are repaired with either resorbable or nonresorbable sutures. Punch biopsies are rarely employed because of the difficulty in achieving a satisfactory repair.

Biopsy Technique

An ellipse of mucosa is removed with the scalpel blade with ideal minimal dimensions of 10×6 mm and tissue to a depth of 3 mm. The area sampled is selected to represent the most significant area of the lesion and to include the interface with adjacent normal tissues. It is a common misconception that the normal tissue is required to allow comparison with the diseased areas; rather the presence of normal tissue facilitates biopsy handling in that a stabilizing suture may be placed through the normal tissue without distorting the abnormal tissue. The tissue is placed in a fixative or onto orientation filter paper. The wound is repaired with sutures.

Resection Specimens

The type of surgical procedure for tumours of the lips and oral cavity depends on the precise location of the tumour, its T-stage, the presence of nodal disease, concurrent second primary lesions and the health of the patient.

Adequate local clearance with preservation of function is the aim with surgical treatment for intraoral cancers; large defects are repaired with microvascularised free-tissue flaps. A margin of 10 mm is the ideal but anatomical constraints and the large size of some of the tumours mean that surgical clearance is often restricted to 2 or 3 mm. In addition, extensive areas of abnormal mucosa are often present around the tumours.

Small superficial tumours of the tip or lateral border of the tongue can be treated by local "wedge" excision although formal hemiglossectomy is preferable for deeply infiltrative lesions. Subtotal or total glossectomy is performed for large tumours invading widely across the midline fibrous septum, involving the extrinsic muscles or affecting the posterior one-third.

The ipsilateral sublingual gland is usually included with resections of anterior floor of mouth mucosa; both sublingual glands are included for midline lesions. Partial glossectomy will be included with resections for tumours of the anterior floor of the mouth that spread into the tongue. Likewise, with tumours encroaching on the gingiva, compromised mucosa from the lower alveolus will be resected.

Resection may be restricted to the alveolar mucosa for superficial tumours of the upper and lower gingiva but larger tumours often require extensive resection. For example, a widely infiltrative carcinoma of the retromolar trigone may require removal of a portion of lower alveolar mucosa and bone, lingual sulcus, posterior buccal mucosa with lower and upper sulci, the posterior portion of the upper alveolar mucosa, the tonsillar bed and part of the soft palate. Part of the posterior tongue may also be included.

A full-thickness wedge excision of lip (V-shaped or W-shaped) is the commonest treatment for squamous cell carcinoma of the lip. To limit the development of new lesions, in-continuity mucosal "shave" excision of adjacent mucosal changes on the vermilion border is more often than not carried out at the same time.

When tumour encroaches on the periosteum at any intraoral site, the decision to resect bone depends on whether or not there has been previous radiotherapy to the jaw, the precise anatomical relationship of tumour and bone and how easily the periosteum dissects from the bone. The clinical extent of disease is almost always greater than that detected radiographically but the periosteum offers a considerable barrier to bone invasion and the usual pathway for direct spread into the jawbone is from the alveolar crest rather than through the cortical plate. In the non-irradiated jawbone with no bone erosion, there is no need to resect bone if tumour-bearing periosteum elevates easily. With radiographic bone destruction, marginal mandibulectomy (rim resection) or segmental mandibulectomy (hemimandibulectomy) is performed. Where there is radiation injury to the bone, this periosteal barrier is lost and direct spread through the cortical bone is more likely, warranting bone removal.

Ideally, where there is proven or a high likelihood of regional lymph node metastasis, an in-continuity neck dissection is performed.

6. Surgical Pathology Specimens – Laboratory Protocols

Biopsy Specimens

Usually one fragment is present free-floating in formalin although several specimens may be taken simultaneously. Portions of stabilising sutures may be present, usually located anteriorly. The surgeon only includes them to reduce artefacts of tissue handling when transferred to the container; rarely are they of significance.

- measure.
- place in cassette; if very small wrap in moist filter paper.
- mark for levels and D/PAS particularly if the sample represents a white/red patch or where a candidal infection is suspected.
- orientate the specimen at the embedding stage to facilitate microscopic assessment.

Resection Specimens

Major Resection Specimens

The vast majority of lip and oral mucosal resections are for neoplastic disease, although some smaller specimens will represent local excisions of non-healing traumatic ulcers where there is a low index of suspicion. Resections of larger lesions may include mucosa from adjacent sites as well as bone from the mandible or maxillary alveolus. Orientation of large resection specimens is generally easy because specific anatomical landmarks are discernible but smaller local excisions may be difficult.

Initial Procedure

- orientate the specimen(s) using the anatomical or surgeon's landmarks.
- ink only critical mucosal and deep resection margins. For glossectomy specimens and resections of retromolar trigone, the critical margins are usually the posterior limits with the lingual sulcus/tonsillar bed. In the tongue, tumour can unexpectedly involve the deep medial margin inferiorly and posteriorly in the floor of mouth/oropharynx by sarcolemmal spread of tumour along intrinsic muscle bundles in the tongue. To facilitate assessment of possible bone involvement, the periosteal limits of alveolar mucosa not in continuity with the underlying bone should be inked.
- with large or complex specimens or those with in-continuity resections of bone, e.g., resections of the retromolar trigone, sample the mucosal limits first by taking radial blocks (Figure 13.3).
- cut the specimen into 4mm-thick slices transversely (in the anatomical vertical plane).
- measurements:
  - dimensions of mucosa, deeper tissue and other components, e.g., bone (cm).

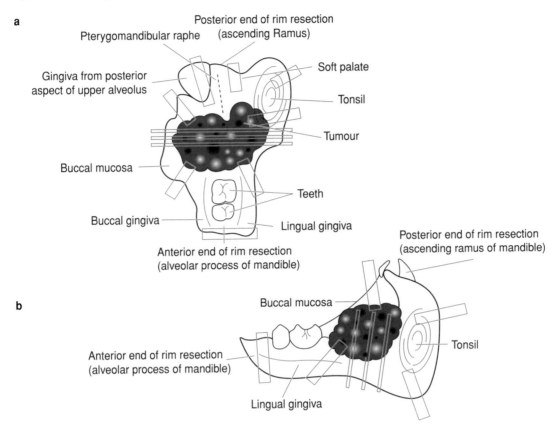

a

Posterior end of rim resection
(ascending Ramus)

Pterygomandibular raphe

Gingiva from posterior
aspect of upper alveolus

Soft palate

Tonsil

Tumour

Buccal mucosa

Teeth

Buccal gingiva

Lingual gingiva

Anterior end of rim resection
(alveolar process of mandible)

Posterior end of rim resection
(ascending ramus of mandible)

b

Buccal mucosa

Tonsil

Anterior end of rim resection
(alveolar process of mandible)

Lingual gingiva

Figure 13.3. Resection of right retromolar trigone with rim resection of mandible. Suggested siting and orientation of tissue blocks for resection of retromolar trigone. (**a**) View from above. (**b**) View from lingual aspect.

–   tumour   anteroposterior length × width (cm).
                 maximum depth (cm) from reconstructed mucosal surface.
                 distances to closest mucosal and deep surgical margins (cm).
–   mucosal abnormalities (cm).

Description

● tumour   plaque-like/ulcerated/fungating: usual type SCC.
             warty: well-differentiated SCC, verrucous carcinoma.
             polypoid: spindle cell SCC.
● mucosa   white/thickened: in-situ lesions.
● extent   document local spread, e.g., to salivary gland, tonsil, bone.
● other   neck dissection, mandibular bone.

Blocks for Histology

The histology should represent the deepest extent of the tumour, the relationship to the surface, mucosal and deep soft tissue margins and changes in adjacent oral mucosa (Figures 13.3 and 13.4).

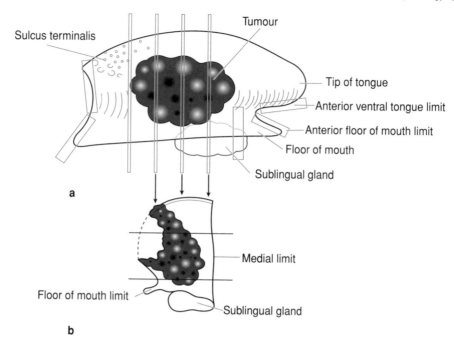

Figure 13.4. Right hemiglossectomy specimen. Suggested siting of blocks for hemiglossectomy specimen. (**a**) Lateral view. (**b**) View of transverse slice.

- at least one block of tumour per centimetre of maximum dimension.
- mucosal surgical margins, particularly the floor of the mouth, retromolar region and soft palate where the incidence of dysplasia is highest.
- deep surgical margins, particularly posterior and inferomedial margins.
- proximal lingual nerve, if present.
- adjacent uninvolved mucosa and associated tissue, e.g., sublingual gland.

Histopathology Report

Final reports of oral mucosal resection specimens should include details on:

- the specimen type, side and tissues present.
- the type of tumour present:
  - squamous cell carcinoma NOS.
  - SCC variants include basaloid, adenosquamous, spindle cell, verrucous adenocarcinoma (salivary gland types).
- the grade of tumour assessed at the invasive front.
- cohesive or non-cohesive patterns (more metastasis with non-cohesive).
- the extent of local spread.
- the distance of tumour from the nearest mucosal margin.
- the distance of the tumour from the nearest deep margin.
- intravascular and/or perineural spread.

If other specimens are attached as an in-continuity dissection (e.g., oropharyngeal mucosa, neck dissection, bone, etc.), these can be cut separately in the usual fashion.

Wedge Resection Specimens of Lip

Initial Procedure

- orientate the specimen.
- ink the deep and lateral resection margins.
- slice the specimen parasagitally so that the blocks contain both skin and intraoral mucosa, including the lateral shave excisions of vermilion border if present.
- if the tumour lies within 2 mm of a lateral limit, take a vertical block through the lateral limit block to illustrate the relationship of tumour to the surgical margin.
- measurements:
  - length of the lip along the vermilion border and height (cm).
  - tumour   length × width (cm).
             maximum depth from reconstructed mucosal surface (cm).
             distances to closest mucosal and deep surgical margins (cm).
- mucosal abnormalities.

Description

- tumour   plaque-like/ulcerated/fungating: usual type SCC.
                warty: well-differentiated SCC.
- mucosa   white/thickened/ulcerated: in-situ lesions.
- extent   spread into muscle.

Blocks for Histology

The histology should represent the deepest extent of the tumour, the relationship to the cutaneous, mucosal and deep soft tissue margins and changes in adjacent vermilion border mucosa and skin (Figure 13.5).

- at least one block of tumour per centimetre of maximum dimension.
- if lateral shave excisions of vermilion border are present, take one block from the cutaneous to mucosal aspects at the junction with the wedge and one transverse block of the lateral limit of each shave. If greater than 2 cm in length, take one additional block for every centimetre.
- cutaneous, mucosal and deep surgical margins.
- samples of other lesions not already represented, e.g., mucosal white areas or ulcers.

Histopathology Report

Final reports of lip resection specimens should include details on:

- the specimen type, size and side.
- the type of tumour present:
  - squamous cell carcinoma NOS.
  - adenocarcinoma (salivary gland types).
- the grade of tumour assessed at invasive front.
- the extent of local spread.
- the distance of tumour from the nearest lateral mucosal margin.

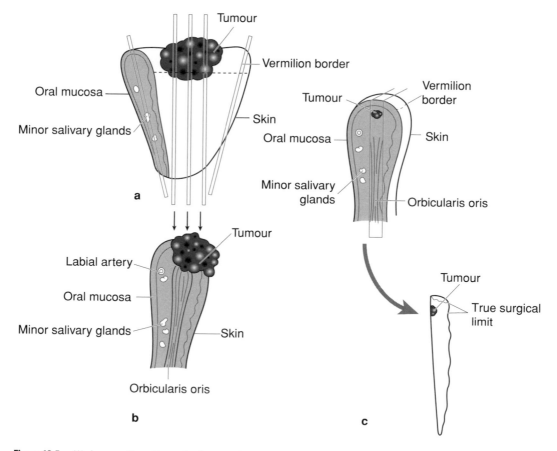

Figure 13.5. Wedge resection of lower lip. Suggested siting and orientation of blocks for wedge resection of lip. (**a**) View from in front. (**b**) Outline of central block(s). (**c**) Selection of transverse limits if original limit blocks contain tumour.

- the distance of the tumour from the nearest deep margin.
- intravascular and/or perineural spread.
- other pathology such as solar damage, dysplasia or radiation injury.

- TNM classification of tumour spread lip and oral cavity

    pTis   carcinoma in situ.
    pT1   tumour ≤ 2 cm in greatest dimension.
    pT2   tumour > 2 cm but ≤ 4 cm in greatest dimension.
    pT3   tumour > 4 cm in greatest dimension.
    pT4   Lip: tumour invades adjacent structures, e.g., through cortical bone, inferior alveolar nerve, floor of mouth, skin of face.
           Oral cavity: tumour invades adjacent structures, e.g., through cortical bone, into deep (extrinsic) muscle of tongue, maxillary sinus, skin.

Regional lymph nodes

pN0   no regional node metastasis.
pN1   metastasis in a ipsilateral single ≤ 3 cm.
pN2   metastasis in:
    a. ipsilateral single > 3 to 6 cm.
    b. ipsilateral multiple ≤ 6 cm.
    c. bilateral, contralateral ≤ 6 cm.
pN3   metastasis in a lymph node > 6 cm.

14

Maxilla, Mandible and Teeth

1. Anatomy

Detailed consideration of all craniofacial bones is impossible in a text of this sort but by focussing on the maxilla and mandible alone, this chapter offers a view of the processes affecting facial bones as a whole and how specimens derived from them might be handled.

The maxilla is the largest bone of the upper facial skeleton and houses the maxillary sinus. It articulates with a large number of other bones, relating to a number of clinically important anatomical areas, including the nasal cavity, the pterygomaxillary space, the infratemporal fossa and the orbit. It is composed of a body and four processes, namely alveolar, frontal, nasal and zygomatic processes. The *body of the maxilla* is pyramidal in shape with four surfaces, namely anterior, nasal, orbital and posterior (or infratemporal) surfaces. The *anterior surface* extends from the alveolar process of the upper anterior teeth below to the infraorbital margin, while the *orbital surface* forms the floor of the orbit. The *nasal surface* articulates with the ethmoid, lacrimal and palatine bones and the inferior turbinate to complete the lateral nasal and medial orbital walls. The *infratemporal surface* is convex and projects posteriorly and laterally.

The *upper alveolar process* projects from the inferior aspect of the maxilla and contains the sockets of the maxillary teeth. The roots of teeth posterior to the first premolar may be intimately related to the maxillary sinus; teeth and sinus may each become involved in diseases originating in the other. The slightly thickened posterior end of the alveolar process is called the maxillary tuberosity. The *frontal process* projects superiorly between the nasal and lacrimal bones, articulating with the frontal bone and contributing to the medial wall of the nasal cavity. The *palatine process* projects medially from the inferior aspect of the maxilla and forms most of the palatal vault and the nasal floor. The *zygomatic process* is a pyramidal projection from the lateral aspect of the maxilla where anterior, infratemporal and orbital surfaces converge, articulating with the zygomatic bone.

The mandible is composed of an arched *body*, which runs posteriorly on each side to attach to the flat *ramus*. The body of the mandible has an external surface, an internal surface, an upper border and a lower border. The *lower border* is rounded and well defined, outlining the profile of the lower jaw. The *external surface* bears the mental foramen between the premolar roots. The *internal surface* of the body is indented by the sublingual and submandibular glands. The superior border, more usually referred to as the *lower alveolar ridge*, contains the sockets of the mandibular teeth. The posterior aspect of the body joins the ramus behind the last molar tooth. The anterior surface of the ramus extending from the abrupt change in angulation of the bone is called the *ascending ramus* while the area around the junction of the body and ramus is called the *angle*. The coronoid process extends upwards and slightly forwards from the anterosuperior aspect of the ramus and bears the attachment of temporalis. The condylar process extends upwards and posteriorly from the posterior aspect of the ramus and bears the knuckle-shaped articulating *condylar head* on the narrow *condylar neck*. The *sigmoid notch* lies between these two processes. Near the centre of the medial surface of the ramus lies the mandibular foramen, where the inferior alveolar branch of the mandibular nerve and its accompanying vessels enter the mandible. The lateral and medial surfaces of the mandible bear several shallow fossae and roughened elevations corresponding to the attachments of muscles both of facial expression and of mastication.

Each fully developed tooth is composed predominantly of dentine. The *crown*, the portion visible within the mouth, is covered by a layer of hard translucent enamel while a thin layer of bone-like substance called cementum covers the conical *root*, which may be single or multiple. The crown and root join at a slight narrowing called the *cervical margin*. The dentine encloses a central cavity called the *pulp canal*; the portion towards the crown is dilated to form the *pulp chamber*, while the pulp canal narrows at the end of the root, the *apex*, into an *apical foramen*. The pulp chamber and canal contain the neurovascular supply to the tooth, passing through the apical foramen. The tooth is suspended in the alveolar bone by the periodontal membrane, composed of thick bundles of collagenous tissue running between the cementum and the bone. At the cervical margin, the periodontal ligament merges with the gingival mucosa; a narrow sleeve of epithelium continuous with the gingiva called the *epithelial attachment* surrounds the cervical margin.

The crown of each tooth has five surfaces. The biting surface is called the *occlusal* surface; on incisor teeth, this is termed the incisal edge. The surface closest to the tooth in front is called the *mesial* surface; that closest to the tooth behind is called the *distal* surface. The surface lying closest to the cheek is called the *buccal* surface (or the *labial* surface on anterior teeth); the surface lying closest to the tongue is called the *lingual* surface (or the *palatal* surface on upper teeth). Incisor teeth have a relatively broad crown with flattened edge for cutting food, while canine teeth have a single point or *cusp*. Premolar teeth have two cusps on the occlusal surface, one buccal and one lingual, while molars have four or five cusps.

There are 20 deciduous (or milk) teeth in the primary dentition – two incisors, a canine and two molars in each quadrant of the jaw. The teeth of the primary dentition begin their development in the first trimester of pregnancy as epithelial ingrowths from the lining of the oral cavity. The epithelial component of the tooth bud forms the enamel while the mesenchymal element gives rise to the remaining parts of the tooth. The crown of the tooth forms first but the root only forms after the crown is complete; root development is closely linked with eruption into the mouth. The deciduous incisors begin to appear in the mouth at around six months of age, usually the central before the lateral, followed by the first deciduous molar at around 12 months. The deciduous canine appears around 18 months and finally the second deciduous molar at around 24 months of age. The precise timing of eruption into the mouth is variable although the sequence is relatively unchanging and lower teeth tend to appear before the uppers.

There are 32 teeth in the permanent or secondary dentition – two incisors, a canine, two premolars and three molars in each quadrant of the jaw. There is an ordered pattern of replacement of the deciduous dentition by the permanent dentition. Beginning around six years of age, the first permanent molar erupts distal to the second deciduous molar, soon followed by shedding and replacement of the incisors. The deciduous molars are replaced by the premolars, while the eruption of the permanent canines straddles the eruption of the second permanent molar with the upper canine appearing latest, usually around 13 years of age. The process ends with the eruption of the third permanent molar or *wisdom tooth* around 18 years.

Lymphovascular Drainage

Lymph drainage of the teeth and jawbones corresponds to that of the regional cutaneous and mucosal sites, leading ultimately to the deep cervical chain (Figure 19.1).

2. Clinical Presentation

The maxilla and mandible are more usually affected by disease arising from closely related structures such as the teeth, oral mucosa and salivary glands and, in the case of the maxilla, the maxillary sinus, the orbit or the infratemporal fossa, rather than from primary bone disease. Many of these conditions are described elsewhere; primary diseases of the odontogenic apparatus and jawbones will be considered here.

Disease of the teeth presents as pain, mobility or swelling although some conditions are detected as incidental findings at radiographic examination. Caries and periodontal disease are painless until advanced destruction of tissue has occurred. A draining sinus opening onto mucosa or facial skin may accompany dental abscesses but others may present with soft tissue swelling of the face and other signs of spreading infection. Gingival bleeding is often the only sign of chronic marginal periodontal disease until increased tooth mobility or the drainage of pus from between gingiva and tooth occur. Developmental cysts, odontogenic hamartomas and neoplasms are often painless but may present with bony swelling, facial asymmetry or a failure of teeth to erupt. Discolouration of teeth, rapid wear or abnormal morphology are features of the hereditary developmental tooth disorders such as dentinogenesis imperfecta or amelogenesis imperfecta; usually all the teeth will be affected.

Primary disease of the jawbones presents as bony swellings that may or may not involve overlying mucosa or adjacent teeth.

3. Clinical Investigations

Vitality testing, using the cooling effect of evaporation of ethyl chloride or small electric currents, can assess the health of the pulpal tissues. Tenderness to percussion (TTP) indicates involvement of periodontal tissues. Probing the junction between tooth and gum can assess the depth and extent of periodontal destruction, the presence of bleeding signifying active inflammation. Mobility is assessed in terms of buccolingual and vertical movement and is due to destruction of periodontal support, perhaps as a result of periodontal disease or because of an adjacent cyst or tumour.

Plain radiographs are essential for the assessment of intrabony cystic lesions, particularly to determine the size, outline (unilocular or multilocular) and bone–lesion interface (sclerotic and well-defined implies a slow-growing lesion; ill-defined suggests a rapidly growing destructive lesion). CT scanning particularly with 3D-reconstruction is useful for large lesions and for assessing relationships with adjacent anatomical structures. MR images are not good at penetrating bone.

4. Pathological Conditions

Non-neoplastic Conditions

Radicular cyst (also known as *apical periodontal cyst, dental cyst*), *apical granuloma* and *chronic dental abscess*: these inflammatory lesions form a spectrum of changes related to the apical region of a non-vital tooth (usually a consequence of dental caries), with considerable overlap in clinical, radiological and pathological findings. Granulomas tend to be smaller (< 10 mm), have a sparser inflammatory cell infiltrate and show less-active inflammation than radicular cysts. Very large radiolucencies tend to be cysts rather than abscesses, although they may be infected. Very common, 70% of jaw cysts; 60% occur in maxilla; all ages but rare in children and with deciduous teeth. Arise when the contents of the necrotic pulp canal leak out of the apical foramina and set up an inflammatory reaction at the apex. The persistent inflammatory stimulus induces granulation tissue formation to help wall off the necrotic debris. Epithelial rests around the root ("cell rests of Malassez") proliferate, initially as complex strands and arcades then as a well-defined lining; when present the epithelium allows the term radicular cyst to be used. Cysts enlarge by a hydrostatic mechanism – the high protein content of the inflammatory exudate in the lumen draws water into the cyst while the lack of lymphatics in the wall prevents it draining away – producing a rounded radiolucency usually with a sclerotic border. May resorb the apical portion of the tooth. Most are located apically but 10% are seen in lateral relationship (accessory apical foramina). Treatment usually involves endodontic therapy (root canal treatment), apicectomy (removing the apical 2 mm of the tooth root via a surgical approach and sealing off the pulp canal) or removal of the tooth. Recurrence is uncommon but relates to a failure to control the contents of the pulp canal.

Dentigerous cyst (follicular cyst): a developmental cyst that surrounds the crown of an unerupted tooth and is attached at the cervical region. Common, 15% of jaw cysts; often in younger patients but not exclusively; usually seen in the upper canine, lower second premolar and third molar regions. Well-defined radiolucency, unilocular in form with a sclerotic border surrounding the crown of an unerupted tooth (so-called "dentigerous relationship"). May resorb roots of adjacent teeth. Develops from the dental follicle surrounding the crown of the unerupted tooth but through an unknown mechanism. Enlargement is by hydrostatic mechanisms but what generates the forces is not clear. Has a thin fibrous wall, minimal inflammatory cell infiltrate (if any) and a thin lining of stratified squamous epithelium. Treatment requires removal of the unerupted tooth, the cyst being delivered at the same time. Recurrence is rare.

Odontogenic keratocyst: a developmental cyst characterised by a distinctive lining of keratinising stratified squamous epithelium and a marked tendency for recurrence. Common, about 10% of jaw cysts; all ages, any site (but especially near angle of mandible) – "any cyst in the jaw can be a keratocyst". Well-defined radiolucency, often multilocular in form with a sclerotic border, which may be in dentigerous relationship. May resorb roots of adjacent teeth. Histology shows a thin lining of highly organised keratinising stratified squamous epithelium, which has a prominent palisaded basal layer. Daughter cysts within the wall are common. Derived from primordial dental structures, the epithelium has an active growth potential of its own, unlike that of radicular cysts and dentigerous cysts. Probably enlarges by epithelial growth; epithelium proliferates between trabeculae of bone where it accumulates fluid and keratin in the centre. This infiltrative growth pattern produces a multilocular radiolucency, in contrast to the ovoid or circular unilocular lesion of expansile cysts like the radicular cyst. Recurrences (20%) are due to small pieces of lining and/or daughter cysts that remain following curettage. Large cysts are treated by marsupialisation and packing; over time the cyst shrinks in size and may disappear completely. A small proportion of patients with keratocysts, particularly those aged under 18 years, have Gorlin's syndrome (many stigmata, including multiple synchronous and metachronous keratocysts, skeletal abnormalities especially of skull form, ribs and vertebrae, multiple basal cell carcinomas).

Other cysts: a large variety of cysts can occur in the jaws. Some will be developmental cysts unrelated to teeth (nasopalatine duct cyst, nasolabial cyst, dermoid cyst), others will be associated intimately with the odontogenic apparatus and will be developmental (lateral periodontal cyst, gingival cyst of adults, glandular odontogenic cyst) or inflammatory in nature (paradental cyst). In addition, samples from a periodontal pocket or inflamed dental follicle can mimic cystic lesions. Of these only the glandular odontogenic cyst is likely to recur because of the presence of daughter cysts in its wall.

Neoplastic Conditions

Odontogenic neoplasms and hamartomas provide a bewildering array of complex histological patterns although they are relatively uncommon clinical problems. Classification is based on resemblance to normal tooth formation. Most are benign or self-limiting and can be managed in a similar semiconservative fashion. Of the many different types, only ameloblastoma and odontome are common.

Ameloblastoma: the commonest odontogenic neoplasm, accounting for 1% of all jaw tumours. Usually found in the mandible, especially near the angle (60%), although up to 20% arise in the maxilla. Peak in fourth and fifth decades, but all ages affected. X-rays usually show multilocular radiolucency, often in dentigerous relationship; erosion of the lingual cortex or lower border is a characteristic sign; roots can be resorbed. The tumour may be solid, cystic or microcystic; in solid areas the histology is characteristic but can be very subtle in more cystic areas. Peripheral tall columnar ameloblast-like cells with polarised hyperchromatic oval nuclei and clear cytoplasm ("piano keyboard") surrounding more centrally placed cells resembling stellate reticulum. The tumour grows by epithelial proliferation and infiltrates along the soft tissues between bone trabeculae, usually extending far beyond the radiographic margins. Recurrence is inevitable if not resected completely. Multiple recurrences run the risk of soft tissue involvement (especially into the parapharyngeal spaces) and dissemination of tumour into lungs and lymph nodes.

There are many different histological subtypes: follicular, plexiform, acanthomatous, desmoplastic, granular cell, etc., which probably have no real clinical significance. Two variants have a better prognosis – the unicystic ameloblastoma and the extraosseous ameloblastoma.

Unicystic ameloblastoma: younger patients (teens/early twenties), predominantly in the lower third molar region: associated with unerupted tooth in dentigerous relationship. A single large cystic cavity is lined by epithelium that is not always typical of ameloblastoma; sometimes there is epithelial proliferation into the wall or as a luminal polyp. On account of the subtle character of the epithelium, diagnosis is easily missed. Fortunately, this type of ameloblastoma usually responds to thorough curettage and does not always require resection.

Extraosseous ameloblastoma: less than 5% of ameloblastomas arise in gingival soft tissue alone without bone involvement where they may resemble a fibrous epulis. Histologically fairly typical of ameloblastoma, less radical surgery is required than their intraosseous cousins; nevertheless cortical bone may have to be removed from the deep aspect of the tumour to ensure clearance.

Odontome: hamartomatous malformation forming distinct tooth-like structures (*compound*), disorganised masses of dentine, enamel, cementum (*complex*) or any combination of the two forms. Commonly identified in teenagers or young adults. Most are small, are related to the permanent dentition and are discovered accidentally when an unerupted tooth is being investigated; larger ones may produce bony expansion. X-rays show dense radio-opaque masses surrounded by a well-defined radiolucent zone; lesions in younger patients may have large radiolucent portions. Complex odontomes are seen most often in the posterior segments; compound odontomes in the anterior segments (especially maxilla). Multiple odontomes suggest Gardner's syndrome. Histologically they are composed predominantly of dentine with varying amounts of enamel, cementum and other soft tissue components typical of the odontogenic apparatus. Less well-developed forms have abundant pulpal and ameloblastic areas and can resemble other types of odontogenic tumour (e.g., ameloblastic fibroma, ameloblastic fibro-odontoma) while odontomes may be associated with other odontogenic tumours such as the calcifying odontogenic cyst.

Other rarer benign tumours or hamartomatous lesions include calcifying epithelial odontogenic tumour of Pindborg, adenomatoid odontogenic tumour, calcifying odontogenic cyst, ameloblastic fibroma, odontogenic fibromyxoma, cementoblastoma. Many will display speckled calcification on X-ray, differentiating them from cysts.

Malignant tumours: involvement of the jawbones by malignant tumour is usually a consequence of direct spread into the bone from mucosal or salivary lesions, although a number of primary bone and soft tissue sarcomas can arise in the jaws. Malignant tumours of the odontogenic apparatus are rare and are usually only diagnosed histologically although pain, paraesthesia, rapid growth, mucosal fixation or ulceration may be present. Radiographs may show irregular bone destruction.

They include: malignant ameloblastoma/ameloblastic carcinoma, clear cell odontogenic tumour, carcinoma arising in an odontogenic cyst (any type of odontogenic cyst and usually squamous cell carcinoma), primary intra-osseous carcinoma and odontogenic sarcomas, the latter being very rare. Overall, they tend to be low-grade malignancies, although recurrences and metastasis complicate some cases.

5. Surgical Pathology Specimens – Clinical Aspects

Biopsy Specimens

The vast majority of teeth are removed because of dental caries or periodontal disease and are not submitted for histological examination unless there are unusual clinical or radiological findings. Teeth adjacent to cystic lesions are removed either as part of the treatment for the lesion (e.g., the unerupted tooth associated with a dentigerous cyst) or because they cannot be restored to useful function (e.g., a tooth whose roots have been extensively resorbed by a keratocyst). Where a primary neoplastic lesion is suspected, teeth may be removed to provide access to underlying lesional tissue via the socket. Teeth may be submitted whole or as fragments; deeply buried unerupted teeth are most likely to be divided by the surgeon prior to removal.

Apicectomy is the removal of a short portion of the tooth root apex to control persistent periapical infection not responsive to non-surgical endodontic procedures. A flap of mucosa and associated periosteum is reflected to expose the area, the apical portion of the tooth is removed with a drill and the pulp canal opening sealed usually with amalgam. Soft tissues associated with periapical infection are removed en passant; most will represent a radicular cyst, apical granuloma or chronic dental abscess. Other benign-looking odontogenic lesions, such as small cysts or odontomes, will be accessed in a similar fashion, shelled out and the cavity curetted. The resulting specimens are usually submitted in total. Very large cystic lesions tend to be marsupialised rather than removed in total because of the risk of fracture or iatrogenic injury to nerves. A portion of the lining will be sampled, primarily to detect ameloblastoma, which requires more radical surgery than a keratocyst.

The close proximity of important anatomical structures in the jaws means that biopsy samples of primary bone lesions tend to be small. Benign-looking lesions will be removed in total, often as fragments, while suspected malignancies will be sampled to avoid compromising later definitive surgery. Accurate histological assessment often requires demonstration of the interface with normal bone so, in the mandible in particular, it is important to avoid sampling only the cortical bone. Access to lesional tissue is achieved either by reflecting a mucoperiosteal flap or extracting teeth in the region and using the sockets to expose the lesion. Biopsies are taken either as curettings or intact pieces removed with a drill or chisel.

Resection Specimens

Resection specimens of maxilla for neoplastic processes include maxillary alveolectomy, palatal fenestration (also known as partial maxillectomy), maxillectomy (also known as hemimaxillectomy) and radical maxillectomy (also known as extended maxillectomy). *Maxillary alveolectomy* is indicated when a small tumour of the alveolar mucosa encroaches on or invades for a short distance into the bone. The resection lies within the alveolar process and does not involve the maxillary sinus. *Palatal fenestration* is performed for relatively localised tumours of the upper alveolar mucosa or floor of the maxillary sinus. The specimen comprises a portion of unilateral maxillary alveolar bone and alveolar mucosa, the opposing mucosa on the floor of maxillary sinus with a minimum of the medial and lateral sinus walls. Tissue from the upper buccal sulcus and a portion of the palatal vault may be included. *Maxillectomy* is indicated for larger tumours of the maxillary sinus and mouth that involve all or part of the maxillary sinus. There are a number of modifications but the specimen includes all of the maxillary alveolar bone from the midline to the tuberosity, bone from the lateral and medial walls of the maxillary sinus are included at least to the level of the zygomatic buttress. The orbital floor may be included or left intact. *Radical maxillectomy* is indicated for tumours extending beyond the confines of the maxillary sinus into adjacent sites. The specimen includes the orbital floor, orbital contents or pterygoid plates and muscles with the maxillectomy.

Resection specimens of mandible for neoplastic processes include rim resection (also known as marginal mandibulectomy) and hemimandibulectomy (also known as segmental mandibulectomy). *Rim resection* is performed for tumours of the lower alveolus or floor of mouth mucosa where there is minimal invasion of bone. If teeth are present the line of excision passes below their apices, often including the inferior alveolar canal. If the ascending ramus is involved, the excision line may include the coronoid process. *Hemimandibulectomy* is indicated for extension of mucosal tumour into the cancellous bone of the body of the mandible either from the alveolar aspect or from the buccal or lingual cortical plates such that preservation of sufficient bone at the lower border to prevent stress fracture cannot be achieved. Reconstruction is facilitated by preserving as much bone as possible, consistent with clearance. However, if there is a risk of perineural spread of tumour within the mandible, a block of bone containing the entire inferior alveolar canal is excised from lingula to mental foramen. Ameloblastomas and other locally aggressive odontogenic tumours in the mandible usually require hemimandibulectomy; there is little risk of perineural spread so the excision can be less radical.

6. Surgical Pathology Specimens – Laboratory Aspects

Biopsy Specimens

Teeth

Should be received in formalin. Identify tooth (e.g., upper left second premolar or lower right second deciduous molar). Note the presence of caries or restoration, root resorption or attached soft tissue. Sample the soft tissue and process in the usual manner.

For an intrinsic developmental disorder of dental hard tissue (e.g., dentinogenesis imperfecta) submit for preparation of undemineralised 50-micron slice through the buccolingual plane of the tooth.

If no such intrinsic abnormality is suspected, decalcify in 5% formic acid. End point can be tested radiographically or with ammonia water. When negative, bisect molars in the mesio-distal plane; others in the buccolingual plane. Demineralise further briefly (2 or 3 days) then process and embed as normal. Sections should demonstrate pulpal tissue in pulp chamber and root canal as well as the interface between pulp and dentine.

Jaw Cysts

Usually as fragments free floating in formalin; record number of pieces and dimensions of largest. Submit small specimens in total; if large, submit representative slices.

NB: Small pieces of tooth root and/or bone are frequently included. Test carefully; specimens with hard tissue tend to sink quickly in the fixative.

Jaw Bone Biopsies

Usually as fragments in formalin; record number of pieces and dimensions of largest. If small, submit in total for decalcification; otherwise submit representative samples.

Resection Specimens

Specimen

Most maxillary and mandibular resections are for tumour arising in adjacent structures, although some will be for bone or odontogenic lesions or reactive conditions, such as osteoradionecrosis. Rim resections of alveolar bone will usually be accompanied by definitive resection of a mucosal tumour.

Hemimandibulectomy and Maxillectomy Specimens

Procedure

- radiograph the specimen.
- ink only the critical external periosteal limit and associated soft tissue limits around the tumour, usually posteriorly and superiorly.
- measurements:
  - anteroposterior length (cm) along lower border (hemimandibulectomy) or along alveolar process to tuberosity (maxillectomy).
  - maximum bone height (cm) of ramus (hemimandibulectomy) or of nasal aspect (maxillectomy).
  - associated soft tissue elements (e.g., oral mucosa, pterygoid muscles, orbital contents).
  - tumour maximum dimensions (cm).
  - distance to closest mucosal and deep soft tissue limits (cm).
  - distance to nearest anterior or posterior bone limit (cm).
- sample the mucosal and deep surgical margins as "radial" sections before sawing the bone and submit separately (reduces contamination of the margins). Cut with a sharp blade firmly down to bone and use a flat blunt instrument to dissect mucoperiosteum free from the bone in the way one might peel an orange (Figure 13.3).
- sample soft tissue elements of mucosal tumour prior to sawing the bone unless the tumour is very small (see next section)
- saw the bone into 0.5 cm slices in buccolingual plane (vertical plane passing between crowns of adjacent teeth).

Rim Resections of Alveolus

Procedure

- ink the external periosteal limit along one aspect to aid orientation of subsequent histological sections.
- measurements:
  - anteroposterior length (cm) along alveolus.
  - maximum bone height (cm).
  - associated soft tissue elements (e.g., mucosa) in the usual fashion.

- saw the bone into 0.5 cm slices in the buccolingual plane (vertical plane passing between crowns of adjacent teeth). If the attached mucosal tumour is larger than 1 cm diameter, sample tumour and margins in the usual fashion prior to sawing the bone.
- if the attached mucosal tumour is smaller than 1 cm diameter, saw the bone into 0.5 cm slices in the buccolingual plane (vertical plane passing between crowns of adjacent teeth) without disturbing the soft tissue.

Description

- tumour: solid, cystic or both solid and cystic.
             circumscribed or infiltrative.
             arising in bone or extension from adjacent structures.
- adjacent bone: periosteal reaction? osteomyelitis?
- mucosa: origin of tumour or secondarily involved?
- other: associated soft tissue elements (e.g., oral mucosa) in the usual fashion.

Blocks for histology

The histology should represent the tumour, its deepest extent, the relationship to the bony, mucosal and deep soft tissue margins and changes in adjacent tissues (Figures 13.3, 14.1 and 14.2).

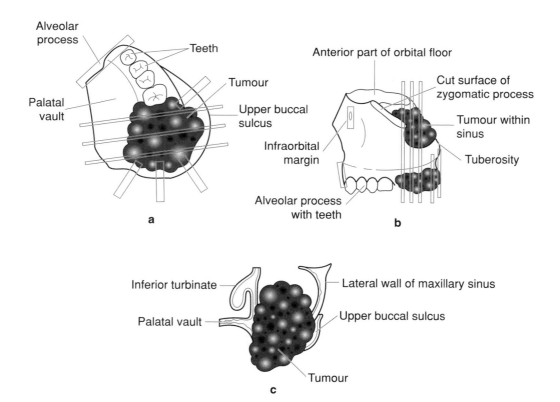

Figure 14.1.   Left maxillectomy specimen for carcinoma. Suggested siting and orientation of tissue blocks for maxillectomy specimens. (**a**) View of palatal aspect. (**b**) View from lateral aspect. (**c**) View of transverse cut surface.

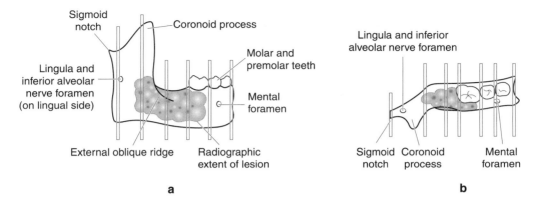

Figure 14.2. Right hemimandibulectomy for ameloblastoma. Suggested siting and orientation of tissue blocks for hemi-mandibulectomy for ameloblastoma or other intrabony tumour. (**a**) View from lateral aspect. (**b**) View from above.

- at least one block of tumour per centimetre diameter.
- abnormal areas of distant bone or mucosa.
- anterior and posterior surgical bone margins as transverse sections.
- mucosal and deep soft tissue and neurovascular surgical margins.

If other specimens are attached as an "in-continuity dissection" (e.g., mucosa, skin, lymph nodes, etc.), these can be cut separately in the usual fashion.

Histopathology report

- Final jawbone resection reports should include details on:
  - the specimen type.
  - the type of tumour present (and grade, if relevant).
  - the extent of spread.
  - the distance of tumour from the nearest cutaneous/mucosal margin.
  - the distance of tumour from the nearest deep soft tissue margin.
  - the distance of tumour from the nearest bone margin.

15

Pharynx and Larynx

1. Anatomy

The pharynx connects the nasal cavities and mouth with the larynx and oesophagus. It is divided into three functional parts, namely the nasopharynx, the oropharynx and the hypopharynx (Figure 15.1).

The *nasopharynx* lies behind the nasal cavities and above the level of the soft palate. The roof and posterior wall relate closely to the skull base and the first cervical vertebra. The lateral wall is an extension of fascia from the skull base called the *pharyngobasilar fascia*. The *Eustachian tube* opens into the lateral wall of the nasopharynx just behind and at approximately the same level as the inferior turbinate. It is lined by respiratory mucosa with accessory mucous glands, particularly numerous around the opening of the Eustachian tube. The slight depression posterior to the opening of the Eustachian tube is called the *fossa of Rosenmüller* (or *pharyngeal recess*). The *oropharynx* extends from the soft palate into the depth of the *vallecula*, the gutter between the posterior tongue and the epiglottis. The *tonsillar fossa* lies in the lateral aspect, between the palatoglossal and palatopharyngeal folds. The *hypopharynx* extends from the upper border of the epiglottis to the lower border of the cricoid cartilage. A narrow recess termed the *piriform fossa* lies on each side of the larynx between the aryepiglottic fold and the thyroid cartilage. Together with the oropharynx, it is lined by stratified squamous epithelium and contains accessory mucous glands (Figure 15.1).

A ring of lymphoid tissue surrounds the opening of the pharynx, comprising the pharyngeal tonsil (or adenoid), the palatine tonsils and the lingual tonsil. The adenoid lies on the posterior wall of the nasopharynx in the midline between the posterior edge of the nasal septum and the openings of right and left Eustachian tubes. The palatine tonsils each lie in their tonsillar fossa. This group of lymphoid aggregates is collectively described as *Waldeyer's ring*.

The larynx lies between the posterior one-third of the tongue superiorly and the trachea inferiorly. It is composed of three large midline cartilages – the epiglottis, the thyroid and the cricoid – with the smaller paired arytenoid cartilages. Other smaller paired cartilages are present, the corniculate and cuneiform cartilages, that are of lesser importance in surgical practice.

The *cricoid cartilage* is the most inferior of the laryngeal cartilages but is the cornerstone of the larynx. It is shaped like a signet ring, with the broadest part, the lamina, located posteriorly and the narrower arch continuous anteriorly encircling the opening to the trachea. It is connected to the highest tracheal cartilage by the cricotracheal ligament. The *thyroid cartilage* overlaps outside the cricoid cartilage. It is composed of two quadrangular laminae that join in the midline anteriorly (forming the laryngeal prominence or "Adam's apple") and diverge posteriorly, ending as two slender processes, a larger superior cornu and a smaller inferior cornu. It is attached to the cricoid by the cricothyroid membrane and to the hyoid bone above by the thyrohyoid membrane. The *epiglottis* is a thin leaf-shaped cartilage, attached at its inferior aspect to the inner

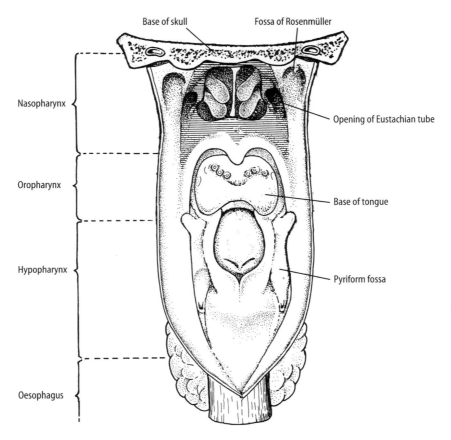

Figure 15.1.   Anatomy of the pharynx. View of pharynx opened from behind to reveal major subdivisions and anatomical land-marks of the pharynx. Reproduced from Hermanek P, Hutter RVP, Sobin LH, Wagner G, Wittekind Ch (eds.). TNM Atlas: illustrated guide to the TNM/pTNM classification of malignant tumours, 4th edition. Springer-Verlag: Berlin and Heidelberg, 1997.

surface of the thyroid cartilage just below where the thyroid laminae join anteriorly and extending superiorly and posteriorly to overhang the inlet to the larynx. The whole assembly is suspended from the hyoid bone by the thyrohyoid and hyoepiglottic membranes (Figure 15.2).

Right and left *arytenoid cartilages* are smaller than the epiglottis, thyroid and cricoid cartilages and are pyramidal in shape. They sit on top of the cricoid lamina, just lateral to the midline and are overlapped outside by the thyroid laminae. They each possess a muscular process (posteriorly and laterally), a vocal process (anteriorly) and an apex (superiorly and posteriorly). Extending anteriorly from the vocal process of each arytenoid to the inner surface of the thyroid cartilage is the vocal ligament. Each vocal ligament forms the basis of the *vocal cord*. A complex arrangement of extrinsic and intrinsic muscles coordinates the movements of the larynx and its constituent cartilages.

The surface anatomy of the larynx is defined by three sets of prominent mucosal folds – the aryepiglottic folds, the vestibular folds and the vocal cords. The *aryepiglottic folds* sweep upwards and laterally from the arytenoid cartilages posteriorly to the tip of the epiglottis, encircling the

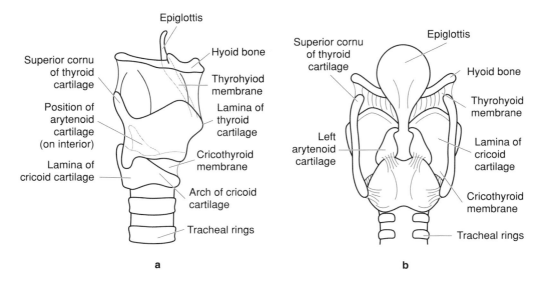

Figure 15.2.   The laryngeal cartilages. (**a**) View from the right lateral aspect. (**b**) View from the posterior aspect.

inlet to the larynx and representing the border between larynx and hypopharynx. The *vestibular folds* (or *false cords*) lie just above the vocal cords and run in the horizontal plane parallel to the vocal cords, separated from them by a shallow pouch called the *vestibule* (or *ventricle*). The larynx is divided into three regions – supraglottic, glottic and subglottic – according to their relationship with the vocal folds. The glottic region corresponds to the region of the vocal cords, while supraglottic and subglottic regions lie above and below respectively (Figure 15.3). A number of compartments are present within the larynx that can influence the spread of tumours. The *preepiglottic space* lies outside the larynx between the tongue, the hyoid bone and the epiglottis while the *supraglottic space* lies just below the mucosa of the supraglottic larynx from epiglottis to the false cords, these spaces communicating through fenestrations in the epiglottis. The *paraglottic space* lies between the vocal ligament and the lamina of the thyroid cartilage and communicates superiorly with the pre-epiglottic and supraglottic spaces. *Reinke's space* is restricted to the submucosa of the vocal cord, communicating with the paraglottic space and the *subglottic space*, the latter extending submucosally from the vocal cord into the trachea.

The larynx is covered almost entirely by respiratory mucosa with many seromucinous accessory glands in the submucosal tissues, particularly around the epiglottis and the vestibule. In contrast, the vocal cords are covered instead by stratified squamous epithelium with only a minimum of connective tissue around the vocal ligaments in which few (if any) lymphatic channels are found.

Lymphovascular Drainage

Lymph vessels from the nasopharynx, oropharynx, hypopharynx and the tonsils drain to Level II nodes in the upper deep cervical chain either directly or via the retropharyngeal groups (Figure 19.1). Bilateral drainage is common with nasopharyngeal, hypopharyngeal and laryngeal lesions.

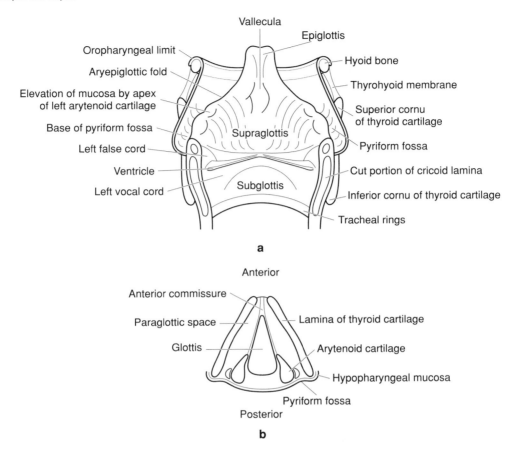

Figure 15.3. Laryngectomy specimen. (**a**) Idealised view of laryngectomy specimen opened from posterior. (**b**) Coronal section through larynx at level of vocal cords.

2. Clinical Presentation

Disease at any site in the pharynx can present with dysphagia (difficulty swallowing), dysphonia (change in voice quality), otalgia (earache), cranial nerve palsies or cervical lymphadenopathy. In the nasopharynx, tumours may evoke deafness, otitis media, epistaxis (nose bleeds), nasal obstruction or palsy of cranial nerves (especially II–VI, IX, X, XII) while those in the oropharynx usually present with sore throat or dysphagia. Hypopharyngeal masses may cause dysphagia or signs of laryngeal involvement, such as hoarseness or a whistling sound during inspiration (stridor).

Patients with laryngeal disease may present with alterations in the voice, particularly hoarseness or stridor.

3. Clinical Investigations

The nasopharynx can be inspected using a post-nasal mirror placed behind the soft palate but biopsy specimens are usually obtained with either rigid or flexible endoscopes. The hypopharynx and larynx can be inspected by indirect visualisation using a laryngeal mirror held against the soft palate or a fibre optic endoscope passed through an anaesthetised nose. Biopsies can be readily obtained under general anaesthesia using a laryngoscope and operating microscope. Endoscopy of the upper aerodigestive tract is performed prior to surgery for malignant disease to identify occult second primary neoplasms.

Serological studies for Epstein–Barr virus antigens are useful in nasopharyngeal carcinoma both in assessing the effects of therapy and in detecting recurrence. Baseline function of the thyroid gland should be determined prior to radical surgery or radiotherapy to the neck.

Ultrasonography has proved useful in evaluation of lymphadenopathy and in guidance of needles for FNA and core needle biopsy.

Barium studies are performed in cases of dysphagia and to assess swallowing function prior to treatment for malignant disease. Chest radiographs may identify a concurrent bronchial or lung lesion. CT and MRI scanning are essential in planning surgery by indicating the depth of the tumour and detecting other changes in the neck. CT has less motion artefact and is good for bone detail while MRI gives superior soft tissue contrast without dental amalgam artefact or exposure to ionising radiation.

FNA is essential in assessing patients presenting with cervical lymphadenopathy, particularly when there is a high probability of malignant disease.

4. Pathological Conditions

Non-neoplastic Conditions

Polyps and nodules: mucosal polyps are uncommonly detected in the nasopharynx and oropharynx and are likely to represent florid lymphoid proliferations in association with adenoid or tonsillar enlargement. Localised thickenings of the vocal cords usually arise at the junction of the anterior and middle one-thirds and may be unilateral or bilateral. They are due to trauma or voice abuse (hence the alternative term *singer's node*) but are also associated with smoking. Nodules are broadly based sessile lesions that are usually bilateral and arise in females while the pedunculated polyps are unilateral and predominate in males. Myxoid degeneration of Reinke's space (*Reinke's oedema*) arises in older females, affects both cords along their length and is associated with smoking and not voice abuse. All are characterised by mild hyperplasia of the stratified squamous epithelium, accumulation of myxoid matrix in the lamina propria, increased vascularity and fibrin deposition. Similar lesions may arise in the myxoedema of hypothyroidism. *Contact granuloma* or *contact ulcer* occurs posteriorly between the vocal processes of the arytenoid cartilages and consists of granulation tissue and ulcer slough; voice abuse and recent laryngeal intubation are common causes. *Amyloid* may present with laryngeal nodules or diffuse submucosal thickening but usually affects the ventricle or false cords; only rarely is there associated systemic amyloidosis. *Post-radiation spindle cell nodules* can mimic spindle cell carcinoma.

Cysts: tonsillar cysts arise in the oropharynx and hypopharynx. They represent accessory tonsillar tissue and are composed of a crypt of stratified squamous epithelium distended by squames and abundant lymphoid tissue in the wall. Laryngeal cysts may contain mucus or air. Mucus-filled cysts are the commonest and usually represent mucous retention cysts of the accessory glands in the supraglottic larynx, usually the ventricle or false cords. They are lined by ductal epithelium. Laryngocoeles and saccular cysts are both due to obstruction of the saccule in the laryngeal ventricle, the former containing air and the latter mucus. Both are lined by respiratory epithelium.

Tonsillar enlargement: tonsillitis is a common disorder of childhood characterised by frequent episodes of sore throat, dysphagia and otitis media. Although it tends to resolve with age, persistent exacerbations may be treated by tonsillectomy with or without concomitant adenoidectomy. Tonsils may be removed in adults for chronic tonsillitis or if a neoplasm is suspected, particularly if there is asymmetrical or unilateral enlargement. Lymphoid follicles with well-formed germinal centres are seen; there may be fibrosis. Actinomyces colonies (*sulphur granules*) may be present within the crypts. Florid tonsillar follicular hyperplasia may occur bilaterally in HIV infection.

Neoplastic Conditions

Benign tumours: Human Papillomavirus-associated squamous papillomas arise in the larynx either in children under five years of age with equal gender mix (*juvenile-onset laryngeal papillomatosis*) or in adults over 20 years of age, mostly in males (*adult-onset laryngeal papillomatosis*). The lesions in juvenile-onset laryngeal papillomatosis are multiple and affect the entire laryngeal mucosa. They may require repeated endoscopic laser de-bulking for airway obstruction; resolution usually occurs in adolescence but a small proportion of cases persist and may even spread into the trachea and bronchi. Adult-onset laryngeal papillomas are fewer in number and relatively easily excised although multiple lesions are more likely to recur. Histologically, hyperplastic stratified squamous epithelium covers well-formed fibrovascular papillary cores, sometimes with abundant koilocyte-like cells. Cytological atypia is absent or minimal. Development of malignancy is a rare event; these patients usually have been exposed to other factors known to be associated with laryngeal squamous cell carcinoma (radiation, tobacco use).

Nasopharyngeal (juvenile) angiofibroma: an uncommon lesion found only in teenage and young adult males. Arises in the roof of the nasal cavity posteriorly and grows into the nasopharynx; presents with unilateral nasal obstruction and epistaxis. A well-circumscribed mass, it has a fibrous cut surface and is characterised by irregular branching dilated vascular channels with partially muscularised walls. Plump spindle cells and mast cells are present in the stroma.

Other benign tumours that arise uncommonly in the pharynx and larynx include salivary gland adenomas (e.g., pleomorphic adenoma), neural tumours (e.g., neurilemmoma, neurofibroma, granular cell tumour), carcinoid tumour, paraganglioma (from paraganglia in the supraglottic or less often the subglottic larynx).

Malignant tumours: tobacco and alcohol use are the major risk factors for oropharyngeal, hypopharyngeal and laryngeal cancers. Their effects are related to dose and duration of use; together they have a multiplicative rather than additive effect. Glottic carcinomas are strongly linked to tobacco use and less associated with alcohol. Post cricoid carcinoma is associated with Patterson Brown–Kelly syndrome (Plummer–Vinson syndrome – Northern European females, iron deficiency anaemia, achlorhydria and upper oesophageal web) and with alcohol. Approximately 10% of patients with Patterson Brown–Kelly syndrome will develop post cricoid carcinoma. Recent interest has focussed on the role of viruses in pharyngeal and laryngeal malignancy. Human Papillomaviruses have been detected in a proportion of tumours, especially laryngeal carcinoma arising against a background of papillomatosis and tonsillar squamous cell carcinoma. Epstein–Barr virus is strongly associated with nasopharyngeal carcinoma, which is also associated with consumption of dietary nitrosamines and smoking.

Squamous epithelial dysplasia: An uncommon clinical problem on its own – most often seen adjacent to established tumours – although the more hyperplastic and/or keratotic lesions can present because of alterations in voice quality. Strongly associated with tobacco smoking. Characterised histologically by hyperkeratosis, epithelial hyperplasia and/or atrophy with varying grades of dysplasia. Development of invasive squamous cell carcinoma occurs more frequently with increasing degrees of cytological disturbance (less than 5% for non-dysplastic lesions and mild/low-grade dysplasia; around 15% for high-grade dysplasia) but the effects of treatment are difficult to evaluate. A number of classification systems have been proposed each with slightly differing terminology but all suffer problems of reliability. Identifying high-grade dysplasia highlights the considerable risk of synchronous or metachronous squamous cell carcinoma and should trigger further conservative surgery or ablative therapy (e.g., by laser) to the lesion.

Squamous cell carcinoma: accounts for approximately 90% of primary malignant tumours in the larynx, oropharynx and hypopharynx. Males are affected at least five times more often than females and most patients are aged between 40 and 60 years. In the oropharynx, squamous cell carcinoma most commonly arises in the posterior one-third of the tongue and tonsil. Tumours of the posterior tongue tend to be very large at presentation; tonsillar tumours are often occult, presenting with nodal metastasis. Most cases of hypopharyngeal squamous cell carcinoma arise in the pyriform fossa (75%) or the posterior pharyngeal wall (20%).

The commonest site of laryngeal squamous cell carcinoma is the glottis (75%) followed by the supraglottic larynx (15–20%) while subglottic tumours account for less than 5% of cases. Glottic tumours tend to be small and localised while supraglottic and subglottic tumours tend to be large with nodal metastasis in over 50% of cases.

Histological and reportedly prognostic variants of squamous cell carcinoma include verrucous carcinoma, papillary squamous cell carcinoma (better than usual type), spindle cell squamous cell carcinoma, adenoid squamous cell carcinoma (same prognosis), basaloid squamous cell carcinoma and adenosquamous cell carcinoma (worse prognosis).

Nasopharyngeal carcinoma: has a striking geographic distribution, being commonest in Southern China. Males are affected more often than females but the disproportion is not as marked as at other sites in the head and neck. Incidence peaks between 40 and 60 years although occasionally adolescents and young adults may be affected. The fossa of Rosenmüller is the commonest site although there may be no obvious mucosal abnormality on inspection. There are a number of histological subtypes – keratinising squamous cell carcinoma and non-keratinising carcinoma, the latter being subdivided into differentiated and undifferentiated patterns. Two-thirds of cases will have involved regional lymph nodes at presentation. Similar tumours can arise at other sites in the pharynx but tend not to be associated with Epstein–Barr virus.

Other malignant tumours in the pharynx and larynx include sinonasal transitional cell carcinoma, salivary gland-type adenocarcinoma (especially adenoid cystic carcinoma, mucoepidermoid carcinoma), lymphoma (particularly in the tonsil; diffuse large B-cell type), malignant melanoma, neuroendocrine carcinomas (larynx; moderately and poorly differentiated), chondrosarcoma (larynx) and metastatic tumours.

Prognosis: The precise site within the pharynx and larynx has a major impact on prognosis, probably because of the mass effect and the density of lymphatic channels in the submucosal tissues. Tumour biology is certain to have some influence as well as the likely response to therapy. Glottic tumours usually affect the anterior portion of the vocal cords, presenting with hoarseness while still small. In contrast, supraglottic and hypopharyngeal tumours are often very large fungating masses with extensive submucosal spread at presentation. Lymph node metastasis is rare with glottic cancers – there are few lymphatics in the vocal cords – but up to two-thirds of hypopharyngeal tumours have bilateral nodal disease at presentation. The mucosal/submucosal spread of the tumour affects the ability to achieve surgical clearance but the depth of invasion is probably the most significant factor in determining lymph node metastasis. Lymph node metastasis at presentation halves the chances of survival and doubles the risk of distant metastasis. Extracapsular spread from affected nodes is also an indicator of limited prognosis, with increased risk of recurrence in the neck and of distant spread. The effects of age, tobacco and alcohol use influence patients' general health; co-morbidity from cardiovascular and respiratory disease is a major adverse factor in survival.

Five-year survival with small glottic carcinomas is in excess of 80%, falling to less than 20% for patients with large tumours.

With nasopharyngeal carcinoma, female patients, those aged less than 40 years at presentation and those with undifferentiated carcinoma have improved survival while patients with cranial nerve involvement, keratinising squamous cell carcinoma and positive nodes in the lower neck do less well. Five-year survival with nasopharyngeal carcinoma is approximately 60%, dependent on the response to radiotherapy.

5. Surgical Pathology Specimens – Clinical Aspects

Biopsy Specimens

Incisional biopsies in the upper aerodigestive tract are usually directed at a specific lesion located either by visualisation or by CT or MR imaging. "Blind" biopsies may be taken, particularly from the fossa of Rosenmüller, base of the tongue, pyriform fossa and palatine tonsil, in the search for an occult primary carcinoma. Superficial biopsies of tonsil may miss a small submucosal tumour; tonsillectomy is preferred. Biopsies of pharyngeal and laryngeal lesions are usually taken at endoscopy with punch or cup forceps. While usually sufficient, it is sometimes difficult to make a histological diagnosis of malignancy as the specimens tend to be superficial, and submucosal tumours or the invasive components of well-differentiated squamous carcinoma may not be represented.

Resection Specimens

In general, tonsillectomy specimens are only submitted in cases of unilateral enlargement or where malignancy is suspected; specimens from children for repeated infective episodes or airway obstruction rarely require histological evaluation. In cases of metastatic squamous cell carcinoma to a cervical lymph node, the ipsilateral tonsil is removed when clinical and radiological evaluation fails to locate a primary lesion.

The type of surgical procedure for tumours of oropharynx, hypopharynx and larynx depends on the precise location of the tumour, its T-stage, the presence of nodal disease, concurrent second primary lesions and the health of the patient. The surgical clearance possible is limited by the anatomy and is in the region of a few millimetres at best.

In general, T1 and T2 glottic and supraglottic tumours without neck node metastasis are best managed either with radiotherapy or conservative surgery in the first instance. Laser resection using the operating microscope is becoming more widely used for glottic and supraglottic lesions. T3 glottic tumours with stridor are often managed with total laryngectomy but radiotherapy is an option if disease is limited and there is no stridor.

Total laryngectomy is the operation of choice in cases of radiotherapy failure, bulky T3 and T4 lesions, subglottic tumours and cord immobility and post-radiation perichondritis ("crippled larynx"). The ipsilateral lobe of thyroid is included when there is a likelihood of extralaryngeal spread in the subglottic region. The larynx will be included in major resections of hypopharynx.

Partial laryngectomy procedures can be divided into supraglottic laryngectomy and vertical hemilaryngectomy. Supraglottic laryngectomy removes the upper part of the larynx to the level of the ventricle, preserving the glottis while vertical hemilaryngectomy removes the vocal cord and false cord on one side. These operations are less commonly performed nowadays but may be indicated for small-volume T2 and T3 tumours. They can be combined with neck dissection procedures. Intraoperative frozen section analysis is essential to ensure clear margins in these conservative procedures.

Pharyngectomy with laryngectomy or pharyngolaryngooesophagectomy are the commonest operations for T2–T4 hypopharyngeal tumours, the defects being repaired by free jejunal transfer and gastric transposition respectively. T1 hypopharyngeal tumours can be resected endoscopically, especially lesions on the posterior wall. Lesions of the pyriform fossa may require partial pharyngectomy with laryngectomy.

6. Surgical Pathology Specimens – Laboratory Aspects

Biopsy Specimens

Usually one fragment is present free-floating in formalin although several specimens may be taken simultaneously.

- *measure*
    - place in cassette; if very small wrap in moist filter paper.
    - mark for levels.
    - orientate the specimen at the embedding stage to facilitate microscopic assessment.

Resection Specimens

Tonsillectomy and Adenoidectomy Specimens

Specimen

Most tonsillectomy specimens are submitted for exclusion of neoplastic disease in cases of tonsillar asymmetry or cervical lymphadenopathy. Specimens of oropharyngeal mucosa, posterior tongue or neck dissection may be attached.

Procedure
- orientate the tonsil(s).
- ink the deep resection margins.
- cut the tonsil into 4mm thick slices transversely.
- measurements:
    - dimensions of tonsil (cm).
    - dimensions of oropharyngeal mucosa, if present.
    - tumour   length × width (cm).
                maximum depth (cm).
                distances to closest mucosal and deep surgical margins (cm).
                mucosal abnormalities.

Description
    - tumour   infiltrative/occult: usual type SCC.
                bulky/fleshy: lymphoma.

- mucosa   white/thickened: in-situ lesions.
- extent   confined to tonsil or spread into adjacent soft tissues.

Blocks for histology

The histology should represent the deepest extent of the tumour, the relationship to the surface, mucosal and deep soft tissue margins and changes in adjacent tonsillar tissue. If tumour is not seen macroscopically in cases of proven nodal metastasis, submit in total.

- at least one block of tumour per centimetre of maximum dimension.
- mucosal and deep surgical margins.
- adjacent uninvolved tonsil.

Histopathology report

Final reports of tonsillectomy specimens should include details on:

- the specimen side.
- the type of tumour present:
    - squamous cell carcinoma NOS.
    - SCC variants include basaloid, adenosquamous, spindle cell, verrucous adenocarcinoma (salivary gland types).
    - neuroendocrine carcinomas.
    - lymphoma.
- the grade of tumour assessed at the invasive front:
    - cohesive or non-cohesive patterns (more metastasis with non-cohesive).
- the extent of local spread.
- the distance of tumour from the nearest mucosal margin.
- the distance of the tumour from the nearest deep margin.
- the presence of intravascular and perineural spread.

If other specimens are attached as an in-continuity dissection (e.g., oropharyngeal or lingual mucosa, neck dissection, etc.), these can be cut separately in the usual fashion.

Laryngectomy Specimens

Specimen

Most laryngectomy procedures are for neoplastic disease in the larynx although some will be required for hypopharyngeal tumours or because of post-radiation dysfunction. Specimens of neck dissection, hypopharyngeal resection, thyroidectomy, tracheostomy site or skin from neck may be attached.

Partial laryngectomy specimens are handled in a similar fashion but require orientation by the surgeon.

Procedure

- paint a vertical line of ink along one side of the larynx from epiglottis to tracheal limit to aid orientation and reconstruction after slicing.
- open the larynx vertically from behind with scissors and identify site of tumour.
- ink only the critical resection margins. This depends on the location and spread of the tumour, e.g., base of tongue and perihyoid soft tissues for anterior supraglottic lesions, lateral

pharyngeal wall for lateral supraglottic and pyriform fossa tumours, postcricoid region for large glottic or postcricoid tumours, lateral perithyroid region for subglottic tumours.
- dissect off the hyoid bone, strap muscles, thyroid, neck dissection, etc. Look out for extralaryngeal spread of tumour. Supraglottic tumours often spread out of the larynx via the thyrohyoid membrane and subglottic tumours via the cricothyroid membrane. Tumour will permeate directly through ossified cartilages more readily than through cartilage that is not ossified.
- cut the larynx into 4 mm-thick slices in the coronal plane (i.e., in the plane of the vocal cords) to provide "rings" of tissue, working from the lowermost aspect to the base of the epiglottis. This is easiest with a band saw or other heavy-duty slicing device.
- slice the remaining supraglottic portion parasagitally with a knife to define precisely the upper aspect of supraglottic lesions.
- measurements:
  - length of the larynx from superiorly to the inferior border of the cricoid (cm).
  - length of trachea (cm).
  - dimensions (cm) of mucosal defects and other specimens.
  - tumour   length × width (cm).
              maximum depth from reconstructed mucosal surface (cm).
              distances to closest mucosal and deep surgical margins (cm).
              mucosal abnormalities.

Description
- tumour   plaque-like/ulcerated/fungating: usual type SCC.
            warty: well-differentiated SCC, verrucous carcinoma.
            polypoid: spindle cell SCC.
- mucosa   white/thickened: in-situ lesions.
- extent   confined to larynx or spread through/between cartilages.
- other   tracheostomy, neck dissection, thyroid gland.

Blocks for histology
The histology should represent the deepest extent of the tumour, the relationship to the laryngeal cartilages, mucosal and deep soft tissue margins and changes in adjacent tissues (Figure 15.4).

- at least one block of tumour per centimetre of maximum dimension.
- mucosal and deep surgical margins.
- both vocal cords (individually identified) even if normal.
- samples of other lesions, e.g., mucosal white areas.
- tracheostomy site (if present).
- perilaryngeal lymph nodes not part of the neck dissection.

Histopathology report
Final reports of laryngectomy specimens should include details on:

- the specimen type
- the type of tumour present:
  - squamous cell carcinoma NOS.
  - SCC variants include basaloid, adenosquamous, spindle cell, verrucous adenocarcinoma (salivary gland types).
  - neuroendocrine carcinomas.

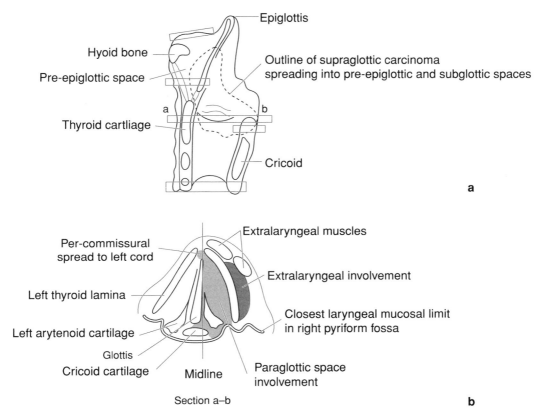

Figure 15.4.   Laryngectomy for supraglottic carcinoma with transglottic and extralaryngeal spread. Suggested siting and orientation of tissue blocks for laryngectomy specimen. (**a**) View from right lateral aspect. (**b**) Slice through vocal cords viewed from above.

- the grade of tumour assessed at the invasive front.
- cohesive or non-cohesive patterns (more metastasis with non-cohesive).
- the extent of local spread.
- the distance of tumour from the nearest mucosal margin.
- the distance of the tumour from the nearest deep margin.
- intravascular and/or perineural spread.
- involvement of perilaryngeal lymph nodes.
- other pathology such as dysplasia or radiation injury.

If other specimens are attached as an in-continuity dissection (e.g., neck dissection, thyroid gland, oesophagus, skin, etc.), these can be cut separately in the usual fashion.

Pharyngectomy Specimens

Specimen

Most pharyngectomy procedures are for neoplastic disease in the pharynx although some will be required for large laryngeal tumours. Specimens of neck dissection, laryngectomy, oesophagectomy, thyroidectomy, tracheostomy site or skin from neck may be attached.

Procedure

- open the pharynx longitudinally with scissors and identify site of tumour.
- ink the external and mucosal resection margins.
- slice into 4 mm-thick slices transversely.
- measurements:
  - length and width of specimen (cm).
  - maximum thickness (cm).
  - dimensions (cm) of mucosal defects and other specimens.
  - tumour   length × width (cm).
            maximum depth from reconstructed mucosal surface (cm).
            distances to closest mucosal and deep surgical margins (cm).
            mucosal abnormalities.

Description

- tumour   plaque-like/ulcerated/fungating: usual type SCC.
              warty: well-differentiated SC, verrucous carcinoma.
              polypoid: spindle cell SCC.
- mucosa   white/thickened: in-situ lesions.
- extent   confined to pharynx or spread to adjacent structures.
- other   neck dissection, oesophagectomy, thyroid gland.

Blocks for histology

The histology should represent the deepest extent of the tumour, the relationship to the adjacent structures or organs, mucosal and deep soft tissue margins and changes in adjacent tissues.

- at least one block of tumour per centimetre of maximum dimension.
- mucosal and deep surgical margins.
- samples of other lesions, e.g., mucosal white areas.

Histopathology report

Final reports of pharyngectomy specimens should include details on:

- the specimen type.
- the type of tumour present:
  - squamous cell carcinoma NOS.
  - SCC variants include basaloid, adenosquamous, spindle cell, verrucous adenocarcinoma (salivary gland types).
- the grade of tumour assessed at the invasive front.
- cohesive or non-cohesive patterns (more metastasis with non-cohesive).
- the extent of local spread.
- the distance of tumour from the nearest mucosal margin.
- the distance of the tumour from the nearest deep margin.
- intravascular and/or perineural spread.
- involvement of peripharyngeal lymph nodes.
- other pathology such as dysplasia or radiation injury.

If other specimens are attached as an in-continuity dissection (e.g., neck dissection, thyroid gland, oesophagus, skin, etc.), these can be cut separately in the usual fashion.

- TNM classification of tumour spread larynx:

  pTis   carcinoma in situ.
  pT1*   tumour confined to one subsite*, normal cord mobility.
  pT2*   tumour invades more than one subsite*, impaired cord mobility.
  pT3   tumour confined to larynx, fixation of 1 or 2 cords.
  pT4   tumour through thyroid cartilage and/or extends beyond larynx to, e.g., trachea, soft
         tissues of neck, thyroid, oesophagus.
* Exact details depends on whether tumour site is supraglottic, glottic or subglottic.

Regional lymph nodes:

  pN0   no regional lymph nodes involved.
  pN1   metastasis in ipsilateral single node ≤ 3 cm diameter.
  pN2   metastasis in:
         a. ipsilateral single > 3 to 6 cm.
         b. ipsilateral multiple ≤ 6 cm.
         c. bilateral, contralateral ≤ 6 cm.
  pN3   metastasis in a lymph node > 6 cm diameter.

TNM classification of tumour spread pharynx
  Oro-(hypopharynx):

  pT1   tumour ≤ 2 cm in greatest dimension (hypopharynx – and limited to one subsite).
  pT2   2 cm < tumour ≤ 4 cm in greatest dimension (hypopharynx – and more than one
         subsite).
  pT3   tumour > 4 cm in greatest dimension (hypopharynx – or with fixation of hemilarynx).
  pT4   tumour invades adjacent structures, e.g., pterygoid muscles, mandible, hard palate,
         deep muscle of tongue, larynx (hypopharynx – thyroid/cricoid cartilage, carotid
         artery, soft tissues of neck, pre-vertebral fascia/muscles, thyroid and/or oesophagus).

Nasopharynx:

  pT1   tumour confined to nasopharynx.
  pT2   tumour into oropharynx and/or nasal fossa.
  pT3   tumour into bone and/or nasal sinuses.
  pT4   intracranial extension and/or cranial nerves, hypopharynx, orbit.

Regional lymph nodes
  Oro- and hypopharynx:

  pN0   no regional lymph nodes involved.
  pN1   metastasis in ipsilateral single node ≤ 3 cm diameter.
  pN2   metastasis in:
         a. ipsilateral single > 3 to 6 cm.
         b. ipsilateral multiple ≤ 6 cm.
         c. bilateral, contralateral ≤ 6 cm.
  pN3   metastasis in a lymph node > 6 cm diameter.

Nasopharynx:

  pN1   unilateral nodal metastasis ≤ 6 cm, above supraclavicular fossa.
  pN2   bilateral nodal metastasis ≤ 6 cm, above supraclavicular fossa.
  pN3   metastasis in nodes > 6 cm or in supraclavicular fossa.

16

Salivary Glands

1. Anatomy

There are three paired major salivary glands – the parotid gland, the submandibular gland and the sublingual gland – as well as a multitude of minor salivary glands (Figure 19.1).

The *parotid gland* is the largest, weighing between 15 and 30 g. It is roughly pyramidal in shape, lying in front of and below the ear in the space between anterior aspect of sternocleidomastoid and the ramus of the mandible, projecting anteriorly onto the external surface of the masseter muscle for a variable distance. The lateral surface lies just below the skin and is roughly triangular in shape with its base superiorly close to the zygomatic arch and its apex (or *tail*) in the upper part of the neck. Medially, the gland extends into the infratemporal fossa, where it is closely related to the pharynx, the carotid sheath and the styloid complex. It is traversed by the facial nerve, entering on the posteromedial surface at the stylomastoid foramen and running forwards to the anterior surface on the outer aspect of the mandible, dividing into five terminal branches within the gland. The duct, "Stenson's duct", runs anteriorly across masseter to pierce buccinator and open opposite the upper second molar tooth. Accessory parotid gland tissue may be present on the masseter between the duct and the zygomatic arch. The gland contains serous acinar components divided into lobules, varying amounts of fat with a few mucinous or sebaceous elements.

The *submandibular gland* weighs between 7 and 15 g and occupies most of the submandibular triangle. It straddles the posterior border of mylohyoid; the larger superficial lobe lies just deep to the skin near the angle of the mandible while the smaller deep lobe lies inside the mouth between the tongue, mandible and the sublingual gland. Posteromedially it is separated from the pharynx by the styloid complex, glossopharyngeal nerve and hypoglossal nerve. The duct, "Wharton's duct", begins as tiny branches in the superficial lobe and runs posteriorly, emerging from the anterior aspect of the deep lobe. It runs through the sublingual space to open into the anterior floor of mouth at the sublingual papilla. The lobules of the submandibular gland are populated mostly by serous cells with lesser mucinous elements.

The *sublingual gland* is the smallest of the major salivary glands and weighs between 1.5 and 4 g. It lies in the floor of mouth between the mucosa, mylohyoid, the mandible and its fellow on the other side. Numerous tiny ducts ("Rivinus' ducts") drain directly into the floor of mouth but there may also be a larger common sublingual duct ("Bartholin's duct") that drains into the submandibular duct near its opening. It is predominantly mucinous in type with lesser serous elements.

Hundreds of *minor salivary glands* are dispersed in the submucosal tissues throughout the mouth and oropharynx. They are not found in the anterior hard palate or the attached gingiva except in the retromolar regions of the mandible. Each minor gland measures between 1 and 5 mm in diameter and they are usually not palpable clinically except in the lips. Most are innominate but for two sets of glands in the tongue, namely the glands of von Ebner around the circumvallate papillae and the glands of Blandin and Nunn in the ventral surface near the tip. Most minor glands are mucinous in type although the glands of von Ebner are serous.

Similar glands are located in the nasal mucosa, nasopharynx, larynx and hypopharynx but are referred to as "accessory glands" rather than salivary glands.

Lymphovascular Drainage

Lymph nodes are found in intraglandular, intracapsular and extraglandular locations in the parotid region. They drain the tissues of the scalp and lateral face and ultimately empty into the lymph nodes of the deep cervical chain. Small numbers of lymph nodes are located close to the submandibular gland but intraglandular and intracapsular nodes are rare. Tissues of the lower lip, tongue and anterior floor of the mouth (including the sublingual gland) drain through these nodes, communicating with those elsewhere in the deep cervical chain (Figure 19.1).

2. Clinical Presentation

Disease affecting the salivary glands will present with enlargement (that may or may not be painful) or as a consequence of dysfunction, usually hypofunction.

Enlargement can affect both major and minor glands and may be episodic or persistent. In the major glands, episodic swellings, worse at meal times and accompanied by pain, are due to obstruction of outflow by intraluminal sialoliths or mucous plugs. Symptoms and signs of ascending infection by pyogenic bacteria may also be present. Extrinsic pressure on the duct system, e.g., by tumours, can present with obstruction. The submandibular gland is most often affected by obstruction, the parotid gland less so.

Persistent localised swellings in the major glands are likely to represent a primary salivary gland neoplasm or lymph node disease. Most major gland tumours arise in the parotid gland and over 80% are benign lesions. From a surgical standpoint, the parotid gland is divided into superficial and deep lobes by the plane of the facial nerve as it traverses the gland. Most tumours arise in the superficial lobe and will present as facial swellings while deep-lobe lesions may present medially as parapharyngeal swellings or as a diffuse enlargement of the parotid region. Around 10% of salivary gland neoplasms arise in the submandibular gland around half of which will be malignant; sublingual gland tumours are very rare and almost always malignant. Motor or sensory nerve dysfunction or pain are sinister findings with a localised swelling in a major salivary gland and often signify malignancy.

Bilateral or multi-gland diffuse swellings point to a systemic process such as sarcoidosis, sialosis or autoimmune phenomena (myoepithelial sialadenitis or HIV).

Minor salivary gland swellings present as submucosal masses. Cystic lesions in young patients located towards the front of the mouth, particularly in the lower lip, will be mucous extravasation cysts; those cystic lesions towards the back of the mouth in older patients are likely to represent retention cysts although some will turn out to be cystic tumours. Neoplasms of the minor salivary glands have an overall benign-to-malignant ratio of 1:1 but tumours of the palate and upper lip are much more likely to be benign than malignant while the converse is true of tumours in the tongue, floor of the mouth and retromolar pad.

Hypofunction usually manifests as xerostomia although some of those who complain of a dry mouth will have perceived rather than real salivary dysfunction. Common causes of xerostomia include drug effects, post-radiotherapy changes and autoimmune disease and, less often, endocrine disturbances.

3. Clinical Investigations

Ultrasonography can provide useful information about swellings in the major salivary glands, particularly with cystic lesions. Plain radiography may identify sialoliths while sialography with injection of contrast media will outline the duct system. The relationship of tumour and the adjacent tissues can be evaluated with CT scanning and MR imaging, the differential weighting of MRI images often allowing better visualisation of the tumour–tissue interface. Assessment of the status of the neck nodes can be performed at the same time.

Stimulated parotid salivary flow rates are assessed in cases of xerostomia and can indicate the presence of organic disease. Serological investigations can assist with the diagnosis of viral infections and with diseases of autoimmune pathogenesis.

Fine needle aspiration cytology has greatly facilitated the management of patients with major salivary gland swellings. Definitive diagnosis of primary salivary gland disease can be difficult but FNA can be used to identify cases where open biopsy might not be advantageous, e.g., if metastatic deposit of squamous cell carcinoma in a juxtasalivary lymph node were suspected.

Open biopsies of major glands carry risks of nerve damage and salivary fistula formation; core needle biopsies can provide a preoperative diagnosis but suffer the same sampling problems as FNA. Incisional biopsies of minor salivary gland lesions are rarely performed because most of the lesions are relatively small and are either entirely innocent lesions or of low-grade malignancy. In either case, optimum results are provided by complete but non-mutilating excision at the first attempt. Diagnostic biopsies of large malignant minor gland lesions can assist the planning of a more radical excision by providing an estimate of tumour type and/or grade.

4. Pathological Conditions

Non-neoplastic Conditions

Cysts: common in minor glands, particularly in the lower lip. "*Mucocele*" is a non-specific clinical term used to mean "a localised collection of mucin" and may represent a mucous extravasation cyst, mucous retention cyst or cystic tumour. *Mucous extravasation cyst* arises when an excretory duct is ruptured; saliva escapes into the tissues, where it evokes a low-grade inflammatory reaction and is walled off by granulation tissue. May arise as a larger lesion from the sublingual gland when the term "ranula" refers to its resemblance to the belly of a frog. *Mucous retention cyst* occurs when an excretory duct becomes obstructed but is not ruptured. The duct becomes distended and forms the wall of the cyst so an epithelial lining is present.

Salivary duct obstruction: due to calculus formation, duct stricture, mucous plugs or external pressure on the duct system and is often accompanied by ascending bacterial sialadenitis. Calculi represent foci of dystrophic calcification occurring in the duct system. Occurring in the submandibular gland in 80% of cases, they may be intraglandular or extraglandular but lie in the duct system. The rest are found in the parotid, usually outside the main body of the gland, and in the minor glands. Duct stricture, mucous plugs and external pressure on the duct can be difficult to locate without sialography. The changes are often mild; the severity of the obstructive symptoms is inversely proportional to the degree of tissue destruction. If the gland is smaller than normal, it will be fibrotic and contain a stone. Histologically, there is ductal dilation, marked periductal and interlobular fibrosis, focal acinar atrophy and a focal moderate chronic inflammatory cell infiltrate. Respiratory metaplasia is seen in the duct system; there may be squamous metaplasia of the epithelium in contact with the stone. If the gland is relatively unremarkable macroscopically, there will be no stone and the microscopic changes will be subtle.

Sjögren's syndrome: a clinical condition characterised by xerostomia and xerophthalmia (dry mouth and eyes). Secondary Sjogren's syndrome refers to the changes arising in association with a systemic connective tissue disease (such as rheumatoid arthritis) while in primary Sjogren's syndrome there is no connective tissue disease. Mostly females (9F:1M), peak 30–40 years. Histologically there is marked lymphocytic infiltration of the major glands (T-cells mostly with occasional B-cells) causing acinar destruction. Proliferation of the ductal cells gives the ducts a solid appearance (known as epithelial–myoepithelial islands). There is little fibrosis. These appearances are called "myoepithelial sialadenitis" (MESA) or "benign lymphoepithelial lesion". Seen best in the parotid, but submandibular gland also affected. Minor glands show similar features, but usually to a lesser degree – myoepithelial islands are not encountered in minor glands. There may be blastic transformation of the B-cells beginning around the ducts and gradually extending outward into the parenchyma, giving rise to a slowly progressive low-grade non-Hodgkin's lymphoma (MAL Toma). Some authorities believe that the so-called "MESA" should be regarded as a low-grade lymphoma from the outset. Overall, 10% develop lymphoma of major salivary glands; the risk is greater with primary Sjogren's syndrome.

Neoplastic Conditions

Pleomorphic salivary adenoma: the commonest tumour with peak prevalence in second and third decades but occurs in all ages even in the newborn. Common in the parotid, palate and upper lip. Histologically, "pleomorphic" describes the architecture not the nuclear morphology. There is an incomplete capsule, a mixture of ducts, sheets of epithelium and myxoid matrix that may in areas resemble cartilage. Locally, recurrence may follow incomplete excision, especially if "shelled out" or if the capsule ruptures. Malignancy can occur in a pleomorphic adenoma but usually only after many years. Rare examples can metastasise to lymph nodes, lung, liver or bone. This so-called *(benign) metastasising pleomorphic adenoma* resembles the usual variant although there is usually a history of previous surgery suggesting vascular implantation as a major factor.

Warthin's tumour: occurs at the lower pole of parotid and may be bilateral. More often seen in males and usually older patients. Never in a minor gland and rare in submandibular gland. Probably represents a form of epithelial proliferation of entrapped epithelial elements in a lymph node. Histologically, very distinctive with multiple papillary projections of altered ductal epithelium into cystic spaces containing debris. Many lymphocytes in the stroma with germinal centres, hence the older term "papillary cystadenoma lymphomatosum". Benign; behaves like a lymph node in that other tumours may metastasise to a Warthin's tumour.

A number of other benign tumours can arise in the salivary glands. The term "monomorphic adenoma" has been abandoned since any salivary adenoma that is not a pleomorphic adenoma is a monomorphic adenoma. All are uncommon and include basal cell adenoma, canalicular adenoma, myoepithelioma (a variant of pleomorphic adenoma), oncocytoma and a variety of ductal papillomas and sebaceous adenomas.

Malignant tumours: are relatively uncommon. There are many different types, most are low grade although some are aggressive malignancies that metastasise widely. Males and females are affected equally; there is a wide age range, peak prevalence in 40–50 years but tumours in elderly patients are often high-grade cancers. Most patients have no known risk factors although increased incidence of salivary gland malignancy can follow head and neck irradiation or a long-standing untreated/recurrent benign tumour (e.g., pleomorphic adenoma). Infection by Epstein–Barr virus is linked with lymphoepithelial carcinoma in the Inuit.

Adenoid cystic carcinoma: common in the parotid gland and in minor glands, especially in the palate. Clinically, it is often very subtle; minor gland lesions are soft diffuse and purple mimicking a dental abscess while parotid lesions produce unusual signs like pain, facial paralysis or trismus before there is a palpable mass. Histologically, it has a classical "Swiss cheese" appearance with cribriform clusters of small darkly staining epithelial cells without much nuclear pleomorphism, mitotic activity or necrosis. Up to half display perineural invasion but this is only significant if it extends beyond the invasive front. Local spread is often extensive; because the tumour evokes no response from the tissues through which it infiltrates, it extends for considerable distances beyond what is identified clinically as the edge. Survival for 10 years is common but patients are often troubled by persistent local disease. Metastasis is via haematogenous routes (e.g., to lung) rather than to nodes.

Mucoepidermoid carcinoma: common in minor glands, especially in the palate, and the parotid gland. It is the commonest salivary tumour in children. Histologically, a mixture of goblet cells, squamous cells and other populations such as intermediate cells or clear cells; may be solid, cystic or both. Histology is little guide to prognosis although tumours with a poor prognosis tend to be large, solid rather than cystic, predominantly epidermoid in type, are infiltrative and cytologically pleomorphic with necrosis and many mitotic figures. Only 10% metastasise, usually after multiple recurrences or if cytologically aggressive and usually to nodes.

Acinic cell carcinoma: uncommon in minor glands; 95% occur in the parotid gland. Histologically, lobulated masses of benign-looking epithelial cells with abundant cytoplasm resembling the serous cells of salivary gland. Populations of other cells are present in varying proportions, e.g., clear cells, cells with vacuolated cytoplasm, ductal cells and/or cells of non-specific glandular type. Low-grade malignancy with nodal metastasis late (especially after recurrences rather than at presentation) in 10%.

Polymorphous low-grade adenocarcinoma: only found in minor salivary glands. Characterised by variable morphological patterns (papillae, cysts, solid areas, cribriform areas, tubular/ductal areas), cytological uniformity (cells often have clear nuclei) and indolent behaviour. Perineural and perivascular whorling is a characteristic feature. Can recur locally if incompletely excised; spread to regional nodes in 10%.

Carcinoma ex pleomorphic adenoma: malignant change may occur in pleomorphic adenoma but usually only in long-standing lesions in major glands. However, being increasingly recognised in minor glands, sometimes without the long history. Rapid enlargement of a long-standing lump, pain or VII nerve palsy and fixation to skin or deeper structures are common findings. Histologically, the commonest finding is a poorly differentiated adenocarcinoma overrunning an old pleomorphic adenoma. Often, there is a mixture of different salivary type carcinomas. Survival is related to the type of the carcinomatous component and the extent of invasion beyond the capsule of the pleomorphic adenoma, so that the prognosis for some patients with minimally invasive and/or histologically low-grade lesions might not be so bad.

Other salivary gland malignancies include epithelial–myoepithelial carcinoma, basal cell adenocarcinoma, hyalinising clear cell carcinoma and MALT lymphoma (low grade), myoepithelial carcinoma (intermediate grade), salivary duct carcinoma, adenocarcinoma NOS, small cell undifferentiated (neuroendocrine) carcinoma, lymphoepithelial carcinoma and primary squamous cell carcinoma (all high grade). Metastatic tumours are not rare in the parotid region; nodal deposits usually derive from squamous cell carcinoma or malignant melanoma in the scalp or facial skin while intraparenchymal deposits usually represent haematogenous dissemination of tumour from sites outside the head and neck.

5. Surgical Pathology Specimens – Clinical Aspects

Biopsy Specimens

Salivary cysts are generally dissected intact from the surrounding tissues together with adjacent minor salivary glands that may have been damaged by the procedure. Cyst rupture is only problematical if the lesion is a cystic tumour. Ranulas are usually marsupialised although recurrent or "plunging" types are treated by excision in continuity with the sublingual gland.

Open biopsies of minor salivary gland tumours are uncommon because precise interpretation of limited samples of large neoplasms is difficult and most tumour types can be managed with clearance by local excision. Core needle biopsies of parotid gland or less frequently submandibular gland tumours may be necessary for deep-lobe tumours where malignancy is suspected but FNA inconclusive.

Where Sjögren's syndrome is suspected, sampling of minor salivary glands is preferable to open biopsy of the parotid or submandibular glands.

Resection Specimens

Surgical resections of parotid glands are classified according to their relationship with the facial nerve. *Superficial parotidectomy* is performed for tumours lying lateral to the plane of the facial nerve as it courses through the gland. If the tumour lies in contact with but does not infiltrate branches of the facial nerve, it is dissected clear with preservation of the nerve. If infiltrated by malignant tumour, the nerve may be sacrificed and repaired with a graft from the nearby greater auricular nerve if a curative (rather than palliative) procedure is anticipated. *Extracapsular resection* can be performed when the tumour is small or lies distant to the nerve. The surgeon dissects external to the tumour capsule with preservation of the nerve; although conservative of glandular tissue, there is considerable risk of capsular rupture. Total parotidectomy procedures are divided into nerve-preserving and nerve-sacrificing types. *Total parotidectomy with nerve preservation* is performed for deep-lobe tumours that can be dissected clear of the nerve. The superficial lobe is removed initially to identify, dissect and preserve the nerve before removing the deep lobe. *Total parotidectomy with nerve sacrifice* (radical parotidectomy) is warranted for curative excision of clinically malignant tumours of either lobe that infiltrate the nerve. Nerve grafting may be performed if the proximal and distal stumps are free of tumour. Occasionally, access to a deep-lobe tumour is obtained via a median mandibulotomy procedure (splitting the mandible and reflecting the ipsilateral hemimandible laterally to expose the parapharyngeal space); the superficial lobe is conserved.

The submandibular and sublingual glands are removed in their entirety. If tumour is encountered in the deep lobe of the submandibular gland, the dissection can be continued anteriorly into the floor of mouth, including the sublingual gland and all of Wharton's duct, if required. En-bloc resection of either gland with adjacent tissues as required is performed for widely infiltrating malignant tumours.

6. Surgical Pathology Specimens – Laboratory Aspects

Small Biopsy Specimens of Minor Glands

Excisions of mucoceles:

- A single tissue nodule free-floating in fixative, non-orientated. Usually less than 20 mm in diameter and may include overlying mucosa. Adjacent minor glands may be present. Measure. Bisect; submit in total.

- Specimens from marsupialised ranulas represent floor-of-mouth mucosa. Measure as a mucosal specimen, bisect and submit in total.

Sampling of minor glands for xerostomia:

- Several small tissue nodules free-floating in fixative, non-orientated. Count number of glands (minimum of six glands recommended for useful assessment of focal lymphocytic sialadenitis). Measure largest in three dimensions; submit in total.

Resection Specimens

Specimen

Parotidectomy

Most superficial and total parotidectomy specimens are submitted for neoplastic conditions although less often the gland may be removed because of persistent infections. In total parotidectomy specimens where the facial nerve has been preserved, the superficial and deep lobes will be separate.

Submandibulectomy

Most submandibulectomy specimens are removed for calculus/obstructive sialadenitis.

Procedure

- orientate the specimen. The medial aspect is usually the most critical margin. The surgeon should give some indications on the request form but it can still be difficult particularly with fragmented specimens. Superficial parotidectomy specimens usually resemble an isosceles triangle; the smoothest surface will represent the superficial aspect and the shortest side the superior aspect of the gland. The markings of the mandibular ramus and/or mastoid process may be present. If separate from the superficial portion, the deep lobe may be impossible to orientate. The superficial lobe of the submandibular gland has a smooth capsular surface while the irregular edge and the indentation of mylohyoid identify the deep aspect.
- ink sparingly and allow to dry fully – gelatinous pleomorphic adenomas often separate easily from the thin capsule and overrun of ink will overestimate involvement of the surgical limits.
- measurements:
    - dimensions of specimen(s) (cm).
    - weight(s) (g).
    - dimensions of tumour (cm).
    - distance to closest margin.

Description

- tumour   location (deep lobe or superficial lobe).
    consistency of tumour (solid/cystic; gelatinous, fleshy, firm).
    interface with adjacent parenchyma (encapsulated, circumscribed or infiltrative margin).
    if encapsulated, proportion of capsule exposed on outer surface of specimen.
- gland   parenchyma – normal, fibrotic or fatty.
- other   note the presence of stones and lymph nodes.

Blocks for histology

- one block per centimetre diameter of tumour.
- closest margin.
- adjacent uninvolved parenchyma.
- lymph nodes.

Minor Gland Excisions for Tumour

Fifty per cent of minor gland lesions will be malignant although most of these will be of low histological grade. Usually received as free-floating specimens in formalin.

Procedure

- orientate the specimen. The deep aspect is usually the most critical margin. The surgeon should give some indications on the request form as to laterality and anterior–posterior orientation but it can still be difficult particularly with specimens from lip or buccal mucosa. The colour and texture of the mucosa from the hard palate may help orientate palatal resections.
- ink sparingly and allow to dry fully.
- measurements:
    - dimensions of mucosa and depth of specimen (cm).
    - dimensions of tumour (cm).
    - distance to closest mucosal and deep margins (cm).

Description

- tumour   location.
                       consistency of tumour (solid/cystic; gelatinous, fleshy, firm).
                       interface with adjacent parenchyma (encapsulated, circumscribed or infiltrative margin).
- mucosa   intact or ulcerated?
- other   appearances of adjacent minor glands and neurovascular bundles.

Blocks for histology

The histology should represent the deepest extent of the tumour, the relationship to the adjacent structures or organs, mucosal and deep soft tissue margins and changes in adjacent tissues (Figure 16.1).

- one block per centimetre diameter of tumour.
- closest mucosal margin (if appropriate).
- closest deep margin.
- adjacent uninvolved mucosa and glands.
- proximal (and distal, if relevant) nerve limits.

Histopathology report

Final reports of resection specimens of tumour should include details on:

- the specimen type.
- the type of tumour present (and grade if relevant).

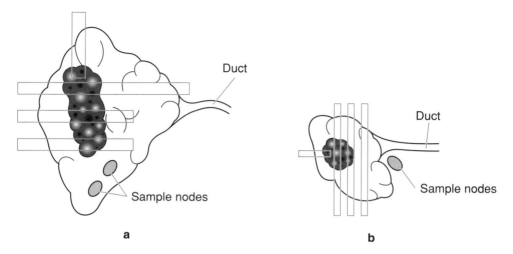

Figure 16.1. Resection of parotid and submandibular salivary glands. Recommended siting and orientation of blocks for resection of parotid (**a**) and submandibular (**b**) glands.

- the distance of the tumour from the nearest cutaneous/mucosal margin (if appropriate).
- the distance of the tumour from the nearest deep margin.
- the presence or absence of perineural and vascular invasion.
- the presence or absence of lymph node metastasis (if appropriate).

- TNM classification of tumour spread of salivary glands:

    pT1   tumour ≤ 2 cm, without extraparenchymal extension*.
    pT2   tumour < 2 to ≤ 4 cm, without extraparenchymal extension*.
    pT3   tumour > 4 cm, and/or extraparenchymal extension*.
    pT4   tumour invades skin, mandible, ear canal, facial nerve base of skull, pterygoid plates
           or encases carotid artery.
    * Extraparenchymal extension is clinical or macroscopic evidence of invasion of soft tissues
    or nerve, except those listed under pT4. Microscopic evidence alone is not sufficient.

Regional lymph nodes:

    pN0   no regional lymph nodes involved.
    pN1   metastasis in ipsilateral single node ≤ 3 cm diameter.
    pN2   metastasis in:
           a. ipsilateral single > 3 to 6 cm.
           b. ipsilateral multiple ≤ 6 cm.
           c. bilateral, contralateral ≤ 6 cm.
    pN3   metastasis in a lymph node > 6 cm diameter.

17

Thyroid Gland

1. Anatomy

The thyroid gland lies in the lower part of the anterior neck, partly enveloping the larynx and upper trachea (Figure 17.1). It is composed of right and left *lobes*, interconnected by a narrower *isthmus*, from which may occasionally arise the *pyramidal lobe*. The entire gland normally weighs 15–30 g, each roughly conical lobe measuring approximately $4 \times 3 \times 2$ cm. The lower pole of each lobe is usually located at the level of the third or fourth tracheal cartilage with the upper pole ascending and diverging laterally to lie close to the superior aspect of the lamina of the thyroid cartilage. Medially, each thyroid lobe is related to the thyroid cartilage, the cricoid cartilage and the upper tracheal cartilages, anteriorly to the strap muscles of the neck and posterolaterally to the carotid sheath. The isthmus is variable in size, usually measuring about 1 cm in length and width and lies over the trachea inferior to the cricoid cartilage. The pyramidal lobe, when present, ascends from the isthmus along the line of the thyroglossal duct and probably represents colonisation of that embryonic structure by thyroid cells during the descent of the developing organ in early life from the foramen caecum in the tongue.

Histologically, the thyroid gland is composed of follicles of cuboidal epithelial cells surrounding eosinophilic colloid, arranged in small pear-shaped lobules supported by delicate fibrovascular stroma. C-cells that secrete calcitonin are dispersed throughout the gland singly or in small clusters but are most numerous around the junction of the upper and middle one-third of the lateral lobes. They are usually inconspicuous on routine stains but can be identified with immunohistochemical stains lying within the follicles. Other lesser components of the thyroid gland include solid cell nests (remnants of the ultimobranchial body), thymic tissue and paraganglia; occasionally parathyroid glands may become incorporated within the thyroid.

Lymphovascular Drainage

The rich lymphatic supply of the thyroid gland drains to lymph nodes in the central and lateral compartments of the neck, located in pretracheal, paratracheal, prelaryngeal, retropharyngeal and retro-oesophageal sites and in the deep cervical chain (Figure 19.1).

2. Clinical Presentation

Disease affecting the thyroid gland can present as enlargement (called *goitre*) that may be diffuse or nodular or as a consequence of hormonal imbalance; rarely there may be pain. Hypothyroidism is characterised by lethargy, mental slowness or depression, intolerance of cold or weight gain

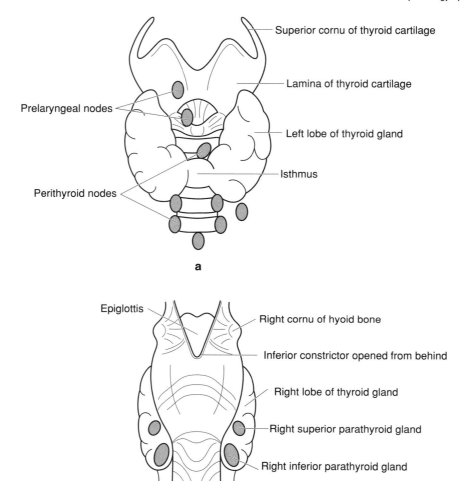

Figure 17.1. Thyroid gland and parathyroid glands. **a**. View of thyroid gland from anterior aspect to show relation to larynx and regional lymph nodes. **b**. View of thyroid gland from posterior aspect to show location of parathyroid glands.

while thyrotoxicosis manifests as intolerance of heat, excessive sweating, weight loss in spite of increased appetite, anxiety, tiredness and occasionally cardiac arrhythmias.

Tumours of the thyroid gland usually present with a solitary nodule with normal thyroid function although some tumours can secrete hormones. Occasionally metastasis to cervical lymph nodes or bone may represent the initial symptom of differentiated thyroid cancer. High-grade cancers can present with hoarseness, dysphagia or difficulty breathing.

3. Clinical Investigations

Thyroid function is routinely assessed by measuring blood levels of thyroid stimulating hormone (TSH) and, if appropriate, the levels of thyroxine and triiodothyronine in patients with thyroid gland disease, including those with neoplastic conditions. Occasionally calcitonin levels are measured. Elevated plasma thyroglobulin (and calcitonin in medullary thyroid carcinoma) following ablative therapy for malignant disease can indicate recurrence or metastasis. Autoantibodies to thyroglobulin, microsomal antigen and the TSH receptor may also be evaluated.

Ultrasonography is helpful in distinguishing a solitary nodule from a multinodular goitre with a so-called dominant nodule but cannot differentiate benign from malignant disease. Plain radiographs of the neck and chest may demonstrate deviation of the trachea, mediastinal expansion or lymphadenopathy although they are more accurately determined by CT and MRI scanning. Scintiscanning, particularly with Iodine-123 rather than Technetium-99m, can determine the functional status of the tissue. Functioning or "hot" nodules are very unlikely to be malignant.

FNA is the investigation of choice for thyroid enlargement, particularly for solitary nodules in euthyroid patients or when there is a history of a rapidly growing mass with airway obstruction. A definitive diagnosis is often possible with FNA, although the distinction between a cellular colloid nodule, follicular adenoma and a follicular carcinoma is generally impossible.

Assessment of vocal cord function is important in the clinical assessment of patients with goitre; vocal cord paralysis is a sinister finding.

4. Pathological Conditions

Non-neoplastic Conditions

Graves' disease: the commonest cause of hyperthyroidism and is characterised by thyrotoxicosis, a diffuse goitre, ocular signs and pretibial myxoedema. It affects females much more often than males and usually presents between the ages of 20 and 40 years. It is an autoimmune disease; the thyrotoxicosis is due to activation of the TSH receptor when the autoantibodies bind to it. Typically, the gland is symmetrically and diffusely enlarged, weighing between 50 and 150 g. Histologically the lobular architecture is preserved. There is reduced colloid in the small irregular follicles, which are lined by tall active-looking columnar cells. Simple non-branching papillary infoldings are often present.

Hashimoto's thyroiditis: a common cause of hypothyroidism and is characterised by hypothyroidism and firm diffuse goitre. It affects females much more often than males and usually presents between the ages of 30 and 50 years. It is an autoimmune disease; the hypothyroidism is probably due to a combination of inactivation of the TSH receptor by autoantibodies and destruction of functioning gland. A proportion of patients may be euthyroid or hyperthyroid at presentation but hypothyroidism is inevitable. The gland is symmetrically and diffusely enlarged, weighing between 50 and 100 g. Histologically there is diffuse lymphoplasmacytic infiltration with germinal centre formation. The follicles are small and sparse with reduced or absent colloid. Hürthle cell change is widespread. A rare variant shows much fibrosis, affecting older patients and often males.

Multinodular goitre: a common cause of thyroid gland enlargement. Probably the end result of persistent stimulation of the glandular epithelium to proliferate and synthesise colloid through the TSH negative feedback loop, due to dietary deficiency of iodine, ingested *goitrogens* that interfere with the availability of iodine or an enzymatic defect, alone or in combination. Patients are generally euthyroid but, when severe, hypothyroidism will result; occasionally late-stage disease will be associated with a mild degree of hyperthyroidism (Plummer's disease). Congenital enzymatic deficiencies (*dyshormonogenic goitre*) present in early childhood, marked dietary iodine deficiency or goitrogen ingestion is seen in certain geographical regions (*endemic goitre*) affecting adolescents, while sporadic (or *non-endemic*) goitre is rarely detected until much later in life. Initially in all forms there is a simple diffuse goitre but gradually the gland becomes nodular as a consequence of follicle rupture, inflammation and fibrosis with re-epithelialisation due to the persistent stimulation. Macroscopically, multinodular goitres are characterised by massive enlargement of the gland with heterogeneous nodularity, histology revealing follicles distended by colloid, old and recent haemorrhage and irregular areas of scarring with calcification.

Others: ectopic or accessory thyroid gland tissue, multifocal granulomatous thyroiditis (due to vigorous palpation of the gland), tuberculosis, sarcoidosis, de Quervain's thyroiditis, radiation changes, Reidel's thyroiditis (a form of systemic fibrosing disorder).

Neoplastic Conditions

Follicular adenoma: expansile round lesion 1–3 cm in diameter with thin complete capsule. Soft and fleshy, pale or brown in colour; haemorrhage, fibrosis, cyst formation or calcification may be present. Uniform pattern of growth; follicles of similar sizes (in contrast to hyperplastic nodules). Embryonal, microfollicular, normofollicular or macrofollicular subtypes. No invasion of capsule. Variants include Hürthle cell adenoma and hyalinising trabecular adenoma.

Thyroid cancer: Risk factors for thyroid carcinoma include irradiation (particularly in first two decades of life), underlying thyroid disease (especially Hashimoto's thyroiditis), family history of thyroid cancer including rare inherited syndromes such as Multiple Endocrine Neoplasia syndromes 2A and 2B, or non-MEN familial medullary thyroid carcinoma.

Thyroid carcinomas are classified into three broad types "differentiated thyroid cancer", medullary thyroid carcinoma and anaplastic carcinoma. *Differentiated thyroid cancer* encompasses papillary carcinoma, follicular carcinoma and their variants.

Papillary carcinoma: commonest thyroid malignancy, F: M = 3:1, 20–50 years. A few cases arise against a background of familial adenomatous polyposis syndromes. Very variable macroscopic appearances from tiny grey–white foci to tumours replacing the entire gland, but many are 2–3 cm diameter, white, firm, granular, infiltrative masses. Cystic degeneration is common, especially in nodal metastases. Has characteristic nuclear features of enlargement, optical clarity, grooving and cytoplasmic pseudoinclusions. True papillary processes with fibrovascular cores are common but not required for the diagnosis. Psammoma bodies are seen in 50%. Multiple foci of papillary carcinoma are found in both lobes in 20% of cases, probably representing intraglandular lymphatic metastases.

Histological and prognostic variants of papillary carcinoma include macrofollicular, oncocytic, solid (similar prognosis to the usual type), columnar cell, dedifferentiated, diffuse follicular, diffuse sclerosing, tall cell, (worse prognosis), and micropapillary, encapsulated, follicular (better prognosis).

Follicular carcinoma: second commonest thyroid malignancy accounting for 15% of primary tumours, 30–60 years, F: M = 3:1. Similar macroscopic features to follicular adenomas but the capsule is thicker. Key diagnostic features are capsular and vascular invasion. Tumours exhibiting a few foci of capsular invasion but no vascular invasion rarely metastasise and are described as minimally invasive. Those with multiple areas of capsular invasion and vascular invasion are termed "widely invasive follicular carcinoma", may metastasise to bone and lung and have a variable prognosis. Oncocytic (or Hürthle) cell carcinoma, a variant of follicular carcinoma, tends to have a less good prognosis.

Patients with differentiated thyroid cancer are stratified according to a number of factors related to the risk of recurrence or metastasis, summarised by the acronym GASH (gender age stage histology). See Table 17.1.

Medullary carcinoma: a neuroendocrine malignancy with a pattern of C-cell differentiation accounting for 5–10% of thyroid neoplasms. About 25% of cases of medullary thyroid carcinoma are familial and arise against a background of Multiple Endocrine Neoplasia syndromes 2A and 2B or as a pure familial form but most are sporadic. Macroscopically, it is tan-coloured or pink, may feel soft and is usually well circumscribed or even occasionally encapsulated. There are a number of histological patterns (solid, nested, follicular, trabecular) and cell types (spindle, clear, granular); amyloid is present in 80%. Metastasis to regional lymph nodes occurs particularly with larger tumours and spread to lung, liver or bone may occur. The prognosis is linked to stage; involvement of soft tissues in the neck and regional nodes usually indicate reduced survival.

Anaplastic carcinoma: a rare thyroid malignancy that arises in older patients. Presents as a rapidly enlarging mass (may be history of goitre or a pre-existing nodule) with hoarseness, dyspnoea or dysphagia. Very large, pale, fleshy tumour that infiltrates widely in the neck; may have foci of haemorrhage and necrosis. There are three histological patterns – a squamoid type, a spindle cell type and a giant cell type – but there is marked nuclear pleomorphism and a high mitotic count; vascular invasion is usually present. The prognosis is poor, most patients die from local tumour growth in spite of external beam radiotherapy. Metastasis occurs frequently in regional lymph nodes and beyond.

Primary malignant lymphoma: a rare neoplasm in the thyroid gland (1–2%), presenting in elderly patients with a rapidly enlarging mass, stridor and dysphagia. There is a strong association with pre-existing Hashimoto's thyroiditis (MALToma). The tumour is large, replaces much of the thyroid gland and is usually of diffuse, large B-cell type (although other types may occur). The tumour cells infiltrate between follicles, produce lymphoepithelial lesions and extend into the perithyroid soft tissues. In contrast to anaplastic carcinoma, it responds well to radiotherapy and chemotherapy, although the long-term prognosis depends on the stage.

Others: insular carcinoma, "pure" squamous cell carcinoma, paraganglioma, small cell neuroendocrine carcinoma, sarcoma, thymic tumours, carcinomas showing thymus-like differentiation (CASTLE), mucoepidermoid carcinoma, metastatic carcinoma.

Table 17.1. GASH risk assessment of patients with differentiated thyroid cancers

Risk category	Criteria
Low-risk patients	Females less than 45 years of age
High-risk patients	All patients under 16 years of age
	All males
	Females over 45 years of age
Low-risk tumours	Papillary carcinoma less than 1 cm in diameter
	Minimally invasive follicular carcinoma less than 1 cm in diameter
High-risk tumours	Papillary or follicular carcinoma greater than 1 cm in diameter
	Multifocal neoplasms
	Metastasis to regional nodes or beyond

5. Surgical Pathology Specimens – Clinical Aspects

Biopsy Specimens

Open incisional biopsy is rarely performed on the thyroid gland. Core needle biopsy can provide a tissue diagnosis where the differential diagnosis rests between anaplastic carcinoma and malignant lymphoma. Very occasionally, incisional biopsy and intraoperative frozen section assessment may be required when an inoperable thyroid mass is encountered.

Resection Specimens

Traditionally, when surgery is advised in Graves' disease, subtotal thyroidectomy has been carried out although, because of recurrent hyperthyroidism in 5–10% of cases, there is an increasing tendency to perform total thyroidectomy. On the few occasions when operation is required for aesthetics and/or obstructive symptoms in Hashimoto's thyroiditis, total thyroidectomy is the operation of choice. Likewise, total thyroidectomy may be required for patients with multinodular goitre because of goitre size and/or compressive symptoms; if unilateral, lobectomy may suffice.

Total lobectomy with resection of the isthmus in continuity represents the minimum appropriate surgical procedure in any patient with a solitary thyroid nodule, particularly when there is suspicion either on clinical grounds or FNA that a malignancy is present. When a firm preoperative diagnosis of differentiated thyroid malignancy is made, total or "near-total" thyroidectomy is performed. This initial operation will represent adequate surgery for follicular adenomas, the low-risk papillary carcinomas and minimally invasive follicular carcinomas. Completion total thyroidectomy is preferred for high-risk tumours in high-risk patients. The intermediate group of low-risk patients with high-risk tumours or high-risk patients with low-risk tumours can be managed by either total thyroidectomy or lobectomy. Extensive differentiated thyroid carcinomas involving adjacent viscera may require laryngectomy, tracheal resection and pharyngectomy.

Medullary thyroid carcinoma is treated by total thyroidectomy.

Neck dissection is performed in differentiated and medullary tumours if there is clinically palpable nodal metastasis. Occasionally nodes from Level VI are removed even if there is no suspicion of metastasis.

6. Surgical Pathology Specimens – Laboratory Aspects

Biopsy Specimens

Usually as small samples from open biopsies or core needle specimens, free-floating in formalin. Measure in three dimensions or length of core and submit in total.

Resection Specimens

Specimen

Most thyroid resections are performed for neoplastic disease, to prevent recurrence in Graves' disease or to relieve compressive symptoms from multinodular goitre or Hashimoto's thyroiditis.

Some lobectomy specimens will represent diagnostic procedures for suspicious lesions with equivocal FNA findings. Only occasionally will specimens of neck dissection be included.

Initial procedure

- orientate the specimen, if possible.
- search for parathyroid glands.
- ink the external resection margins.
- slice into 4mm thick slices transversely in the coronal plane.
- measurements:
  - weight of specimen (g).
  - dimensions of specimen (cm).
  - tumour size (cm).
  - distance to closest surgical margins (cm).

Description

- tumour   number of tumour deposits.
                  size, shape and colour.
                  solid or cystic or both.
                  encapsulated or infiltrative.
- capsule   present or absent.
                  thick or thin.
                  regular or irregular.
                  intact or breached by tumour.
- adjacent gland outer surface: smooth or roughened/breached by tumour.
                  colour and consistency.
                  presence or absence of nodules.
- others   lymph nodes, neck dissection, parathyroid gland.

Blocks for histology

In cases of neoplastic disease, the histology should represent the tumour, its relationship to its own capsule (if any), the capsule of the thyroid gland and adjacent structures (Figure 17.2). Focal abnormalities of the thyroid parenchyma need to be sampled as do adjacent lymph nodes and the parathyroid glands.

In inflammatory or diffuse reactive disease, representative samples of gland and capsule are required.

Macroscopically encapsulated neoplastic disease:

- for tumours up to 5 cm in diameter, submit total circumference, the blocks illustrating the interface of tumour, capsule and adjacent gland.
- for tumours greater than 5 cm in diameter, submit one additional block of tumour per centimetre diameter, blocks illustrating the interface of tumour, capsule and adjacent gland.
- closest surgical margin.
- samples of other lesions, e.g., nodules or fibrous areas.
- parathyroid gland(s).
- perithyroid lymph node(s).

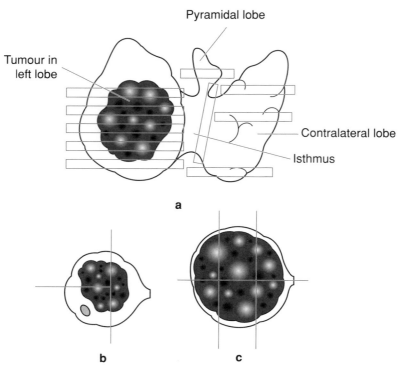

Figure 17.2. Total thyroidectomy specimen. **a**. Recommended block selection to include isthmus, pyramidal lobe and contralateral lobe if present. Tissue block composites depend on the size of the tumour. **b**. Small. **c**. Large. Include other nodules.

Macroscopically invasive neoplastic disease:

- three blocks of tumour to illustrate interface with adjacent normal tissues.
- three blocks of adjacent gland.
- closest surgical margin.
- samples of other lesions, e.g., nodules or fibrous areas.
- parathyroid gland(s).
- perithyroid lymph node(s).

Multinodular disease:

- one block from each nodule up to a maximum of five blocks.
- for dominant nodules, submit one additional block of tumour per centimetre diameter, the blocks illustrating the interface of nodule and adjacent gland.

Inflammatory disease:

- submit three representative blocks from each lobe and one block from the isthmus if present.

Histopathology report

Final reports of thyroid specimens should include details on:

- the specimen type, side, size (cm) and weight (g)
- the type and subtype of tumour present, if any:
  - follicular adenoma.
  - papillary carcinoma and variants.
  - follicular carcinoma and variants.
  - medullary carcinoma.
  - anaplastic carcinoma.
  - lymphoma.
- the macroscopic size of tumour and degree of encapsulation.
- the presence or absence of invasion of the capsule and surrounding tissues.
- the distance of tumour from the nearest margin.
- the presence or absence of vascular invasion.
- involvement of perithyroid lymph nodes.
- other pathology such as Hashimoto's thyroiditis or radiation injury.

If other specimens are attached as an in-continuity dissection (e.g., neck dissection), these can be handled separately in the usual fashion.

- TNM classification of tumour spread of thyroid gland.

  Papillary, follicular and medullary carcinoma.

  pT1   tumour $\leq$ 2 cm, intrathyroidal.
  pT2   tumour > 2 to $\leq$ 4 cm, intrathyroidal.
  pT3   tumour > 4 cm, or minimal extrathyroidal extension.
  pT4   tumour extends beyond thyroid capsule with invasion of:
      a.   subcutaneous tissues, larynx, trachea, oesophagus, recurrent laryngeal nerve.
      b.   prevertebral fascia, mediastinal vessels, carotid artery.

Anaplastic/undifferentiated carcinoma (both considered pT4).

  pT4a   tumour limited to thyroid*.
  pT4b   tumour beyond thyroid capsule[+.]
              considered surgically resectable* and unresectable[+].

Regional lymph nodes.

  pN0   no regional lymph nodes involved.
  pN1a   metastasis in Level VI lymph node.
  pN1b   metastasis in other regional lymph node(s).

18 Parathyroid Glands

1. Anatomy

There are usually four parathyroid glands, arranged as superior and inferior pairs on either side of the midline closely related to the thyroid gland (Figure 17.1). These tan-coloured oval structures each normally measure 4–6 mm in maximum dimension and weigh around 50 mg. The superior parathyroid gland (derived from the fourth pharyngeal pouch) is fairly constant in position and lies on the posteromedial aspect of the superior thyroid pole. A few superior parathyroid glands are located medial to the upper pole or in the retropharyngeal or retro-oesophageal space. The inferior parathyroid glands, derived from the third pharyngeal pouch are less constant in location, although they tend to be symmetrical bilaterally. Over half are found around the inferior pole of the thyroid lobe although other common locations include the thymus or high up on the anterior aspects of the thyroid lobe. Occasionally they may be located in the mediastinum or rarely in association with the roots of the great vessels.

Lymphovascular Drainage

The rich lymphatic supply of the parathyroid glands drains with that of the thyroid gland to lymph nodes in the anterior and lateral neck, located in deep cervical chain as well as in pretracheal, paratracheal, prelaryngeal, retropharyngeal and retro-oesophageal sites (Figure 19.1).

2. Clinical Presentation

Disease affecting the parathyroid glands usually presents as a consequence of altered function. Hyperparathyroidism describes an altered metabolic state due to increased secretion of parathyroid hormone (parathormone). Rarely seen nowadays is the full spectrum of "bones, stones, groans and moans"; biochemical investigation of non-specific complaints such as profound tiredness, nausea or thirst is the usual method of diagnosis although a small proportion of cases are detected during investigation of patients with organ-specific complaints. *Primary hyperparathyroidism* is due to an increased secretion of parathormone from one or more of the parathyroid glands, usually caused by an adenoma. *Secondary hyperparathyroidism* is due to the physiological response of the four parathyroid glands to persistent hypocalcaemia, usually renal failure, malabsorption syndromes or Vitamin D deficiency. *Tertiary hyperparathyroidism* is a result of persistent autonomous hypersecretion of parathormone in long-standing secondary hyperparathyroidism following correction of the hypocalcaemia.

Hypoparathyroidism is a result of reduced secretion of parathormone and is characterised by neuromuscular excitability. Rapid onset of hypoparathyroidism, e.g., following surgery to the neck, results in muscular tetany and paraesthesia while an insidious onset, such as with autoimmune disease, may induce mucocutaneous candidosis, cataracts and basal ganglia changes as well.

Pseudohypoparathyroidism refers to a rare inherited defect of parathyroid hormone receptor function in peripheral tissue characterised by insensitivity to circulating parathormone; the glands are hyperplastic.

3. Clinical Investigations

Biochemical tests are the mainstay of the diagnosis of parathyroid gland disease. In conjunction with the clinical history and physical examination, relative plasma concentrations of calcium, inorganic phosphate levels and parathormone allow classification of hyperparathyroidism as primary, secondary or tertiary. Alkaline phosphatase levels are elevated when there is increased osteoblastic activity as a result of bone resorption and stimulation of osteoblastic activity. Evaluation of autoantibodies is useful when autoimmune-associated hypoparathyroidism is suspected.

Chest radiographs are helpful in excluding a paraneoplastic effect of bronchogenic carcinoma as a cause for the hyperparathyroidism. CT and MRI scanning may locate enlarged parathyroid glands in the neck but currently the most reliable method is technetium-labelled isotope scintigraphy.

4. Pathological Conditions

Non-neoplastic Conditions

Primary chief cell hyperplasia: usually accounts for 10% of cases of primary hyperparathyroidism but is also seen against a background of secondary hyperparathyroidism. About 25% of cases of primary chief cell hyperplasia are familial and arise in Multiple Endocrine Neoplasia syndromes 1 and 2 or as an isolated familial form, but most are sporadic. The four parathyroid glands are symmetrically enlarged in around 50% of patients while the asymmetric enlargement of the remainder mimics parathyroid adenoma (*pseudoadenomatous hyperplasia*). Microscopically, the glands contain numerous chief cells in diffuse sheets or as nodules with oncocytes; transitional forms also present. Mitotic figures may be present. Intraglandular adipocyte numbers are usually much reduced, although rarely the fat cells may be abundant (*lipohyperplasia*). Cystic change may occur in very large glands. Distinction from adenoma formation can be difficult but the enlargement of multiple glands is usually diagnostic.

Primary clear cell hyperplasia: the four parathyroid glands are markedly enlarged, particularly the superior glands. The chief cells are arranged in small nests and have profoundly clear cytoplasm ("water-clear" cells). There is usually marked hypercalcaemia but water-clear cell hyperplasia is not MEN-associated.

Secondary parathyroid hyperplasia: very similar appearances to primary chief cell hyperplasia but there tends to be symmetrical enlargement, particularly in the early stages. Early changes include loss of the intraglandular adipocytes with conspicuous nests of chief cells but in long-standing cases the glands usually have a marked nodular pattern. Oncocytes may be prominent in established cases; cystic change and fibrosis may develop.

Cysts: usually arise due to degenerative changes in an adenoma or hyperplastic parathyroid gland but some are developmental anomalies of the third and fourth branchial arches. Cystic degeneration in an adenomatous or hyperplastic gland is usually associated with hyperparathyroidism; typical chief cells line the fibrous wall of the cyst. Developmental cysts tend not to be functional and are usually associated with the inferior parathyroid glands; these cysts are lined by respiratory or cuboidal epithelium with parathyroid cells in the fibrous wall.

Neoplastic Conditions

Adenoma: a benign tumour of the parathyroid glands with a gender ratio of 3F:1M, mostly affecting patients aged 40–60 years. Very rarely may arise in Multiple Endocrine Neoplasia syndromes 1 and 2. Usually only one gland is affected and it may be located either in the neck or at an ectopic site. Usually a tan-coloured circumscribed nodule; large tumours may be cystic. Microscopically, it is composed of chief cells in cords and nests with occasional gland-like structures; neoplastic chief cells are larger than their normal counterparts. Variable numbers of oncocytic cells are present in clusters. Nuclear pleomorphism is common and is probably a degenerative phenomenon. Fibrosis is not common but may be present if there has been previous haemorrhage. Correlation of surgical and pathological findings is required to distinguish adenoma from hyperplasia; the presence of one enlarged gland usually signifies an adenoma. A rim of compressed normal or atrophic parathyroid tissue may be seen in around 50% of cases but is less commonly seen in larger lesions.

"*Double adenoma*": very rare and requires the presence of two enlarged glands (each weighing more than 70 mg) and two normal-sized glands; MEN 1 syndrome; may be impossible to distinguish from hyperplasia.

Variants include microadenoma (< 6 mm diameter), oncocytic adenoma, lipoadenoma.

Carcinoma: a rare cause of primary hyperparathyroidism. Patients are usually older than those with adenomas and often have very high levels of parathormone secretion. Usually pale, solid tumour; may be encapsulated but often infiltrates adjacent soft tissues. Microscopically, the lesion is composed of chief cells arranged in a solid or trabecular pattern with thick fibrous bands, numerous mitotic figures and capsular invasion but these changes may also be present in a proportion of adenomas. Invasion of nerves, blood vessels and adjacent soft tissues are more reliable features of malignancy. Local recurrence and hypercalcaemia are the main problems; metastasis to lymph nodes or to lung and liver occur in a third of cases.

5. Surgical Pathology Specimens – Clinical Aspects

Biopsy Specimens

Incisional biopsy is rarely performed for parathyroid disease although intraoperative frozen section analysis is required to establish that parathyroid tissue has been removed rather than a thyroid nodule or small lymph node.

Resection Specimens

Surgical exploration of the neck and parathyroidectomy is curative in most cases of primary and tertiary hyperparathyroidism. In primary hyperparathyroidism, it is usual for both parathyroid glands from the affected side to be removed to facilitate distinction between hyperplasia and adenoma. Subtotal parathyroidectomy is the treatment of choice for hyperplasia and for tertiary hyperparathyroidism. Approximately 100 mg of parathyroid tissue is left in the neck or transplanted into the patient's forearm.

Parathyroid carcinoma is usually diagnosed after excision of the affected gland. Recurrent disease is treated by en-bloc resection and removal of the ipsilateral lobe of thyroid gland. Neck dissection is usually performed only if there is clinically palpable nodal metastasis.

6. Surgical Pathology Specimens – Laboratory Aspects

Resection Specimens

Specimen

Most parathyroid resection procedures are performed for neoplastic disease or for primary or tertiary hyperplasia. Only when recurrent primary carcinomas are being resected will specimens of neck dissection be included.

Initial Procedure

- in cases of known or suspected parathyroid carcinoma, ink the external resection margins.
- remove the surrounding fat.
- slice into 4 mm-thick slices transversely in the coronal plane. If less than 5 mm in maximum dimension, submit in total.
- measurements (after the removal of the periglandular fat):
    - weight of specimen to three decimal places (g).
    - dimensions of specimen (cm).
    - tumour: size (cm).

Description

- tumour: size and colour.
  solid or cystic.
  encapsulated or infiltrative.
- adjacent gland: compressed rim of normal or suppressed parathyroid gland.
- other: neck dissection, thyroid gland resection; presence of other parathyroid glands.

Blocks for histology

The histology should represent the abnormal parathyroid tissue, its relationship to its capsule (if any) and adjacent parathyroid gland parenchyma.

Submit each parathyroid gland in total (maximum of three blocks for markedly enlarged glands).

Histopathology report

Final reports of parathyroid specimens should include details on:

- the specimen location (right/left, superior/inferior), size and weight.
- the type of tumour present, if any.
- the macroscopic size of tumour and degree of encapsulation.
- the presence or absence of invasion of capsule and surrounding tissues.
- the distance of tumour from the nearest margin.
- the presence or absence of vascular invasion.

If other specimens are attached as an in-continuity dissection (e.g., neck dissection), these can be handled separately in the usual fashion.

19 Neck – Cysts, Tumours and Dissections

1. Anatomy

The neck extends from the lower border of the mandible and the base of the skull superiorly to the thoracic inlet at the level of the clavicles inferiorly. Within this area are contained pharynx, larynx and oesophagus, submandibular and the tail of the parotid salivary glands, bones, skeletal muscles, nerves, blood vessels, lymph nodes and the thyroid and parathyroid glands. The side of the neck is divided by the sternocleidomastoid muscle, which passes obliquely across the neck from the sternum and clavicle below to the mastoid process and occipital bone above. The area in front of this muscle is called the *anterior triangle* and extends to the anterior midline of the neck. The area behind the muscle is called the *posterior triangle* and extends to the anterior margin of trapezius muscle behind (Figure 19.1).

The anterior triangle is divided into:

- The submental triangle, which lies between the anterior belly of digastric, the mandible and the body of the hyoid bone.
- The digastric triangle, which lies between the anterior and posterior bellies of digastric below and the lower border of the mandible above.
- The carotid triangle, which lies between the superior belly of the omohyoid, the anterior border of sternocleidomastoid and the stylohyoid and posterior belly of digastric muscle superiorly.
- The muscular triangle, which extends from the hyoid bone to the sternum and is limited posteriorly by the superior belly of omohyoid.

The posterior triangle of the neck is divided into:

- The occipital triangle lying between the anterior border of trapezius, the posterior border of sternocleidomastoid and the inferior belly of omohyoid below.
- The supraclavicular triangle lies between the inferior belly of omohyoid, the clavicle and the lower part of the posterior border of sternocleidomastoid.

Lymphovascular Drainage

The neck contains many lymph nodes subdivided into groups and located both superficially and deep within the neck. While individual nodes can be described with reference to adjacent anatomic structures it is common practice, particularly in oncology, to divide the node groupings in the neck into six levels (Figure 19.2).

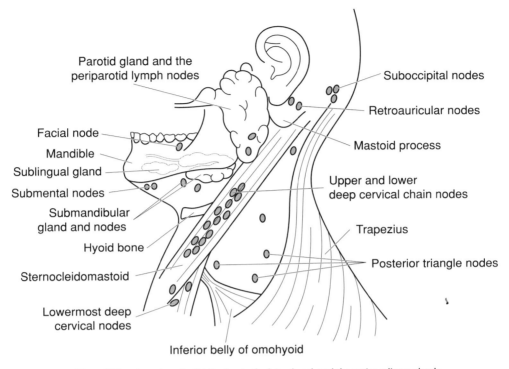

Figure 19.1. Lymph node distribution in the lateral neck and the major salivary glands.

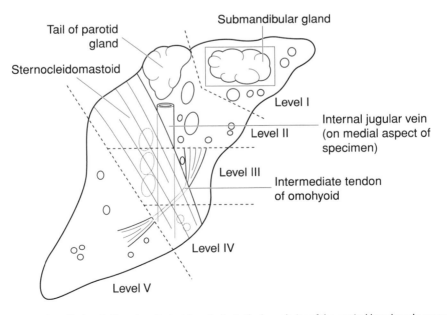

Figure 19.2. Right radical neck dissection. Dashed lines indicate the boundaries of the cervical lymph node groups.

Level I:

This group consists of the nodes within the submental and digastric triangles and is also known as the submandibular group. In practice, the submandibular salivary gland is included in the specimen when lymph nodes in this level are resected.

Level II:

Level II nodes represent the upper jugular group and consist of the nodes around the upper third of the internal jugular vein (IJV) and the adjacent spinal accessory (XIth) nerve. They extend from the level of the carotid bifurcation (approximating to the superior border of the thyroid cartilage) to the base of the skull. The posterior boundary of this group is the posterior border of the sternocleidomastoid muscle and the anterior boundary is the lateral border of the sternohyoid muscle. The tail of the parotid gland is often included when nodes from this group are resected.

Level III:

This group of lymph nodes corresponds to the middle jugular group and consists of lymph nodes located around the middle third of the IJV. They extend from the carotid bifurcation to the intermediate tendon of omohyoid, where it crosses the IJV. The posterior boundary is the posterior border of the sternocleidomastoid muscle and the anterior boundary is the lateral border of the sternohyoid muscle.

Level IV:

This group of lymph nodes, also known as the lower jugular group, consists of nodes located around the lower third of the IJV extending from the intermediate tendon of omohyoid where it crosses the IJV to the clavicle below. The posterior boundary is the posterior border of the sternocleidomastoid muscle while the anterior boundary is the lateral border of the sternohyoid muscle. Lymph nodes within Levels II, III and IV correspond to the jugular group or deep cervical chain of lymph nodes. They tend to be regarded as subdivisions of a functional unit rather than as distinct groups in their own right.

Level V:

Lymph nodes in this group, also known as the posterior triangle group, comprise the lymph nodes located along the lower half of the spinal accessory (XIth) nerve and represent the lymph nodes in the occipital triangle. The anterior boundary is the posterior border of the sternocleidomastoid muscle, the posterior boundary is the anterior border of trapezius with the clavicle below.

Level VI:

Lymph nodes in this group, also known as the anterior compartment group, comprise the nodes surrounding the midline structures of the neck extending from the level of the hyoid bone above to the suprasternal notch below. On each side, the lateral boundary is the medial border of the carotid sheath. Individual groups of lymph nodes within this compartment are the perithyroid nodes, the paratracheal nodes and the precricoid nodes.

Other groups of lymph nodes within the neck are also recognized and include the suboccipital, periparotid, retropharyngeal groups and the buccal lymph node.

2. Clinical Presentation

Lesions in the neck usually present as swellings and may be associated with any of the major anatomical structures in the region, in particular lymph nodes, thyroid gland and salivary glands or from other tissues such as skin, blood or lymphatic vessels, nerves or fat. Disease affecting lymph nodes usually presents as enlargement, either a single lymph node or several nodes, unilaterally or bilaterally. The nodes may be tender or painless and vary in consistency from soft to firm, rubbery or hard. In young patients cervical lymphadenopathy is usually due to a reactive process but a neoplasm is more likely in older patients. Malignant lymphoma commonly presents as cervical lymphadenopathy; metastatic deposits in cervical lymph nodes may be the presenting feature of tumours in the posterior tongue, nasopharynx, tonsil, larynx or thyroid gland. Metastases in cervical lymph nodes usually derive from primary lesions above the level of the clavicles although 10% will arise from distant sites, such as lung, stomach or testis. Cystic lesions in young patients are usually due to developmental abnormalities, such as thyroglossal duct cysts or branchial cysts while those in adults are most likely to represent metastasis to a lymph node in which there is cystic degeneration. Sinuses opening onto the skin surface may arise from thyroglossal duct cyst or branchial cyst lesions or infective lesions, e.g., related to the mandibular teeth.

3. Clinical Investigations

Swellings in the neck require thorough clinical evaluation to determine the tissue or organ affected, whether the enlargement is solid or cystic and whether or not adjacent tissues are involved. Movement on swallowing tends to point to an intimate relationship with the hyoid bone or thyroid gland while pulsation or the detection of a *bruit* indicates association with or origin from major vascular structures. Tumours may involve adjacent nerves producing characteristic patterns of paralysis or altered sensation, such as Horner's syndrome or Trotter's syndrome. Ultrasound investigation is helpful in identification of cystic lesions and can provide information on the presence of other lesions in adjacent organs without the risks of ionising radiation. Plain radiographs of the facial bones or sinuses may reveal clinically undetected lesions while barium studies are useful in visualising pharyngeal diverticula or in tracking developmental sinuses or fistulae. CT scanning and MR imaging can determine the consistency of the lesion, identify enlarged lymph nodes and detect the presence of occult primary tumours in clinically silent anatomical sites. Scintiscans may be required if neoplastic or developmental lesions of the thyroid gland are suspected. Angiography will demonstrate the presence of a significant vascular component within a lesion and its relationship to adjacent vascular structures. Fine needle aspiration cytology has greatly facilitated the investigation of neck lumps in recent years. Even if characteristic features allowing diagnosis are not present, FNA can distinguish cases where open biopsy can be performed effectively; ultrasound guidance allows precise sampling of deeply placed lesions. Endoscopic examination of the nasal cavities, pharynx, larynx, oesophagus and bronchi under general anaesthesia with biopsy is commonly performed prior to definitive surgery for squamous cell carcinoma of the upper aerodigestive tract; an occult second primary tumour can occur in up to 10% of cases.

4. Pathological Conditions

A wide variety of diseases can account for enlargement of cervical lymph nodes. These may be reactive or neoplastic, they may be a consequence of local or systemic conditions and may or may not have a known cause. Conditions not related primarily to reactive disorders of lymph nodes or malignant lymphomas are discussed below.

Non-neoplastic Conditions

Thyroglossal duct cyst: probably the commonest developmental neck cyst, due to failure of the embryonic thyroglossal duct (extending from the posterior tongue into the neck) to atrophy.

Midline in 90%, below hyoid in 70%; associated with a sinus in 40% of cases. Lined by squamous and/or respiratory epithelium; less than half contain thyroid follicles; may represent the patient's only functioning thyroid tissue.

Branchial cleft cyst: derived from remnants of the embryonic branchial apparatus following incomplete obliteration of the branchial pouches; the most common form is believed to derive from the second branchial pouch. Cyst lies in the lateral neck near the angle of the jaw at the anterior border of sternocleidomastoid; the sinus may open onto the skin at the junction of the middle one-third and lower one-third while the tract follows the carotid sheath and may fistulate into tonsillar fossa. Lined by squamous epithelium with reactive lymphoid tissue in the wall; 10% contain respiratory epithelium.

Miscellaneous lesions: other developmental cysts in the neck include dermoid cyst (often extending into the neck from the sublingual region), cervical thymic cyst and cervical bronchial cyst. The "plunging ranula" is a mucous extravasation cyst from the sublingual gland that extends into the neck through mylohyoid. Cutaneous and subcutaneous haemangiomas are relatively common but do not differ from their counterparts elsewhere. Lymphangiomas are uncommon in the neck but usually arise low in the posterior triangle. Lesions composed of very dilated vessels can be termed cystic hygroma, although all forms are more usually described as "lymphatic malformations".

Neoplastic Conditions

Metastatic malignant tumour in cervical lymph nodes: metastasis to regional lymph nodes from primary tumours elsewhere in the head and neck is common, particularly with mucosal squamous cell carcinoma, cutaneous malignant melanoma and thyroid gland carcinoma. The frequency of lymph node involvement and the distribution of metastatic deposits vary with the site and type of the primary tumour. For example, nasopharyngeal carcinoma often involves multiple nodes throughout the neck while squamous cell carcinoma of the lower lip rarely spreads to nodes and then usually only as a single deposit in Level I. Tumours of the anterior two-thirds of the tongue generally metastasise to one or two ipsilateral Level II/III nodes while carcinomas from the posterior one-third of the tongue, hypopharynx or larynx can involve several nodes on both sides of the neck. Cervical lymph node metastasis is not just reserved for head and neck primaries; tumours of lung or upper gastrointestinal tract can occasionally spread to nodes in the supraclavicular region. Lymph node metastasis may be detected either at the time of presentation with the primary lesion or after initial therapy although in about one-third of patients, the cervical lymph node deposit is the presenting feature. Usually the primary tumour is located following clinical/endoscopic examination or imaging but may not be found in 10% of cases. Over 80% of occult primary tumours presenting with cervical metastasis are located in the head and neck, especially nasopharynx, posterior one-third of the tongue, tonsil, hypopharynx and thyroid gland. Adverse prognostic features can vary with the type of tumour but include the presence of multiple tumour deposits particularly in Levels IV and V, extracapsular spread into adjacent tissues, involvement of extranodal lymphatic channels and tumour involvement of surgical margins.

Paraganglioma: an uncommon neuroendocrine tumour arising at sites of autonomic paraganglia within the head and neck. Commonest in the bifurcation of the common carotid artery (carotid body paraganglioma or *chemodactoma*); others include the superior bulb of the jugular vein (*glomus jugulare*), the promontory of the middle ear (*glomus tympanicum*), the ganglion nodosum of the vagus nerve and the larynx. Carotid body paraganglioma affects males and females equally although the others are more common in females. Usually adults; 10% bilateral or multicentric, 10% familial or associated with syndromes such as neurofibromatosis or Multiple

Endocrine Neoplasia syndrome; 10% recur; 10% malignant. Slowly growing painless mass; may evoke neural symptoms such as hoarseness, conductive deafness or an intracranial mass effect. Characteristic histology of discrete cell nests (*Zellballen*) of polygonal endocrine chief cells and spindle-shaped neural sustentacular cells. Neither nuclear pleomorphism nor the presence of mitotic figures signify malignancy; rather markedly infiltrative growth pattern and/or metastasis required. The intimate relationship to adjacent vital structures makes wide excision impossible with recurrence likely.

5. Surgical Pathology Specimens – Clinical Aspects

Biopsy Specimens

A lymph node in the neck may be excised for histopathological assessment when persistently enlarged and when there is no clear reactive cause. In most cases, FNA has indicated the presence of a lymphoproliferative disorder that might represent lymphoma. Exclusion of metastatic squamous cell carcinoma is important; definitive treatment of the neck following such inadvertent open biopsy with possible skin contamination is more extensive than might otherwise be required.

Resection Specimens

Excision of a thyroglossal duct cyst requires clearance of the entire thyroglossal tract from the base of tongue to the isthmus of the thyroid and perhaps beyond; the central portion of the hyoid bone may be included. The risk of recurrence of the cyst is much reduced by this procedure.

Treatment of a branchial cyst requires removal of the entire lesion; fibrosis following infection and intimate relationships to carotid sheath and a number of large nerves in the neck makes the procedure difficult.

Neck dissection is either elective (clinically negative neck) or therapeutic (known metastasis). Justification for an *elective neck dissection* rests on three observations: occult disease will develop into clinically evident disease, sometimes inoperable when eventually detected; there is a risk of distant metastasis with untreated occult neck metastasis; and additional histological information of prognostic value may be gained. Arguments against elective neck dissection include unnecessary treatment when there is a low risk of metastasis and significant morbidity and a risk of mortality in elective surgery. The decision to perform an elective neck dissection is based on a risk of metastasis of more than 20%, whether or not the neck nodes can be easily assessed clinically, the availability of the patient for close follow-up and the fitness of the patient for surgery. Sentinel node sampling is being developed as a technique to identify occult metastasis but requires considerable pathological expertise for accurate interpretation. Elective irradiation of the neck may be an acceptable alternative to a "watch and wait" policy.

Usually, the less extensive neck dissection procedures are the operations of choice in the clinically negative neck. The choice depends on the nature and site of the primary tumour and the expected pattern of nodal spread. Nodes in Levels I–IV are removed for oral and oropharyngeal tumours, Levels II and III for laryngeal and hypopharyngeal tumours but elective dissection is rare for thyroid carcinomas. Bilateral dissection may be indicated if the primary tumour crosses the midline.

The rationale of *therapeutic neck dissection* is the clearance of disease with preservation of function. Classical radical neck dissection is performed for nodal metastasis > 6 cm in diameter, multiple large metastatic deposits in several levels, recurrent disease following neck irradiation, gross extranodal spread involving the skull base and skin involvement. Other so-called functional dissections may be performed to preserve the spinal accessory nerve, sternocleidomastoid and internal jugular vein, consistent with achieving clearance.

Two or more positive nodes following histological examination of the specimen and/or the presence of extracapsular spread merit postoperative radiotherapy.

6. Surgical Pathology Specimens – Laboratory Aspects

Biopsy Specimens

Thyroglossal duct cysts:
Usually as a single strip of fibrous tissue with or without a nodule surrounded by fat free-floating in fixative, non-orientated; the body of the hyoid may be present. Measure in three dimensions. If 10 mm in length or less, submit in total. If larger, block serially and submit representative samples.

Branchial cleft cysts:
Usually as a single cystic nodule surrounded by fat free-floating in fixative, non-orientated. A sample of adjacent lymph nodes may be present. Measure in three dimensions. If 10 mm in diameter or less, submit in total. If larger, block serially and submit representative samples.

Resection Specimens

Resections of Carotid Body Paraganglioma

Usually received as non-orientated soft tissue mass in formalin. Larger specimens may be fragmented.

Procedure

- ink the external limits of the specimen.
- measurements:
  - dimensions of specimen (cm).
  - weight (g).
  - tumour maximum dimensions (cm).
  - distance to closest soft tissue limits.

Description

- tumour   colour; areas of haemorrhage or necrosis (preoperative embolisation?). circumscribed, encapsulated or infiltrative margin?
- other   vessels or nerves identifiable?

Blocks for histology

- the histology should represent the tumour and the relationship to the margins, vessels and/or nerves.
- section the specimen into 4 mm-thick slices and sample the tumour and margins.

- select at least one block of tumour per cm diameter to represent the various morphological patterns present.

Histopathology report

Final paraganglioma reports should include details on:

- the type of tumour present.
- the nature of the tumour–tissue interface.
- the relationship to major vessels and nerves.
- the distance of tumour from the nearest margin.

Neck Dissection Specimens

The vast majority of neck dissection specimens are submitted for neoplastic conditions although occasionally nodes from Level I may be removed to facilitate access to vessels for microvascular anastomosis during reconstructive jaw surgery. Neck dissection specimens may be classified as "comprehensive" neck dissection specimens (radical or modified radical neck dissections) or selective neck dissection specimens (e.g., suprahyoid or supraomohyoid neck dissection specimens). These are listed in Table 19.1.

Initial Procedure

- orientate the specimen. The surgeon should give some indications on the request form but it can still be difficult particularly with selective dissections, for example, of Levels II and III only. Figure 19.2 and the following anatomical landmarks may assist:
  - the superior aspect: submandibular gland, mandibular periosteum, tail of parotid gland, posterior belly of digastric.
  - the inferior aspect: intermediate tendon of omohyoid where it crosses the IJV; the fatty tissues from the posterior triangle region (Level V) tend to be bulkier inferiorly.
  - the medial aspect: the IJV running inferiorly and slightly anteriorly.
  - the lateral aspect: skin, platysma, sternocleidomastoid.
- open the IJV longitudinally, if present, to view its luminal aspect. Extracapsular spread from a tumour deposit is easily identified at this time as a white area in the wall of the IJV and

Table 19.1. Categories and components of neck dissection specimens

Neck Dissection Specimens	Lymph Node Groups	Other Structures Present
Comprehensive		
Radical	Levels I–V	SCM, IJV and XIth nerve
Modified Radical	Levels I–V	Variable; one or all will be lacking
Extended Radical	Levels I–V	Other lymph node groups or non-lymphatic structures
Selective		
Suprahyoid	Levels I–II	Variable, one or all will be lacking
Supraomohyoid	Levels I–III	Variable, one or all will be lacking
Anterolateral Neck	Levels II–IV	Variable, one or all will be lacking
Posterolateral Neck	Levels II–V and suboccipital nodes	Variable, one or all will be lacking
Anterior compartment	Level VI	Variable, one or all will be lacking

may indicate the location of the closest medial deep surgical margin. The involvement of the lumen of the vein by tumour is not considered an independent risk factor in survival.

- dissect off the muscles. Start with platysma, then sternocleidomastoid. The presence and extent of extracapsular spread approaching the lateral deep surgical margin can be easily detected at this stage. Then remove mylohyoid, digastric, etc. Leave omohyoid attached (if present) to mark the junction of Levels III and IV. Reducing the bulk of the specimen improves the detection of smaller nodes.
- divide the specimen into the respective node levels (Levels I–V) as detailed above. The precise anatomical boundaries of the various node groups are lost during the operation, particularly if the specimen is distorted during removal but precise distinction is usually not critical.
- separate the submandibular gland from Level I nodes, by dissecting along the plane of the capsule. Separate the tail of the parotid gland from the Level II nodes.
- harvest the nodes from each of the tissue portions. Remove palpable nodes intact with scissors. These should be bisected along the long axis or sliced serially, depending on size. Slice the remaining tissue into 4 mm slices. Palpate slices for smaller nodes as usual.

Measurements:
- length of IJV, if present (cm).
- dimensions (cm) of tumour deposits (NB: not the size of the node).
- if a tumour mass of several matted nodes is present, record its maximum dimensions. Micrometastasis (< 0.2 cm) is recorded as nodal involvement but its precise significance is unclear.
- distance to nearest deep surgical margin (usually medial).

Blocks for histology

- for large nodes, submit one representative slice; for smaller nodes, submit in total. Remember to keep the nodes from each level separate.
- one block of each of the following is recommended unless involved by tumour:
  - the submandibular and parotid glands.
  - the closest medial and lateral deep surgical margins.
- if other specimens are attached to the neck as an "in-continuity dissection" (e.g., skin, mandible, oral mucosa, thyroid gland, larynx or pharynx), these can be cut separately in the usual fashion.

Histopathology report

Final neck dissection reports should include details on:

- the specimen type.
- the type and grade of tumour present.
- the number of lymph nodes recovered from each level.
- the number of positive lymph nodes in each level.
- the location of the largest tumour metastasis and its dimensions.
- the presence or absence of extracapsular spread and the levels involved.
- the distance of the tumour from the nearest deep margin.

Eye, Muscle and Nerve Specimens

Roy W Lyness

Eye, Muscle and Nerve Specimens
(including rectal biopsy for Hirschsprung's disease)

1. Anatomy

The adult eye measures approximately $23 \times 23 \times 24$ mm (Figure 20.1). The anterior aspect (*cornea*) is transparent, allowing light to enter and be focussed by the crystalline *lens* before being picked up by the photosensitive *retina* and converted into electrical impulses which are transmitted to the brain by the *optic nerve*.

The surface of the cornea is protected by the *eyelids* and lubricated by the *lacrimal gland*, which produces tears. The tears flow over the eye keeping the surface moist and are collected at the *caruncle* where they drain via the *naso-lacrimal duct*.

The amount of light admitted to the eye is controlled by the *pupil* rooted in the *ciliary body*, which controls the focusing of the *lens* and the production of aqueous humor that fills the *anterior chamber*, draining to the systemic circulation (conjunctival veins) via the *trabecular meshwork* in the *filtration angle* and *Schlemm's canal*.

The *posterior chamber* contains gelatinous material known as *vitreous humor*.

The eye is "inflated" by systemic blood pressure within the capillary meshwork that is the *choroid*, which also contains the nerve supply to the ciliary body and pupil. Blood pressure is responsible for the tension or firmness of the eye. Take away the blood pressure and the eye will become soft. The choroid is covered on the external surface by the *sclera* to which the *extra-ocular muscles* are attached in order to move the eye.

2. Eyelids

The ophthalmic surgeon's most common biopsy is the eyelid. To most intents and purposes the laboratory management is that of a biopsy of skin. However, the problem for the ophthalmologist is gaining adequate clearance for malignant lesions as a wide excision of a lid lesion may deprive the patient of sufficient lid cover for the eye resulting in a lack of lubrication and protection from abrasion and infection. To this end, marking the orientation of the specimen and the limits of excision is of great importance.

It is best practice that the surgeon draws a diagram of the area and marks the lateral or medial, superior or inferior margins of the biopsy specimen with sutures and records the marks made on the diagram. The deep limit can be marked with dye in the laboratory.

The most common tumours of the eyelid are basal cell carcinoma and squamous cell carcinoma. Other tumours to be considered are malignant melanoma, sebaceous gland tumour and Merkel cell carcinoma. In some oculo-plastic operations a series of biopsies from the margins of excision may be sent to the laboratory for frozen section and report, in order to ascertain whether or not excision of a malignant lesion is complete. This is difficult work, relying on cooperation between surgeon and the laboratory to identify correctly the orientation of the specimens.

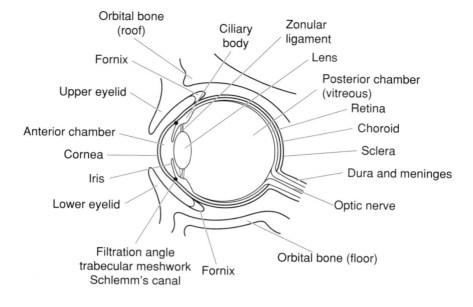

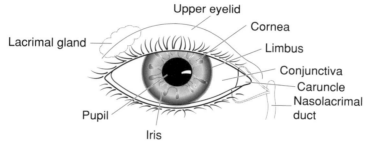

Figure 20.1.   Anatomy of the eye.

The gamut of benign tumours include: squamous papillomas, keratoses, naevi, inclusion cysts, chalazion and molluscum contagiosum.

The eyelid biopsy is often a wedge resection of the lid. A central section through the eyelid to ascertain the deep limit of excision and a superior or inferior limit of excision are taken. The lateral blocks are cut through from the lateral or medial aspect towards the centre. This allows all six limits of excision to be judged (Figure 20.2).

3. Conjunctiva

The conjunctiva is covered by specialised squamous epithelium containing mucus-secreting cells. The specialised epithelium is on the posterior aspect of the eyelids and covers the eye to the limbus, where it becomes entirely squamous epithelium to cover the cornea.

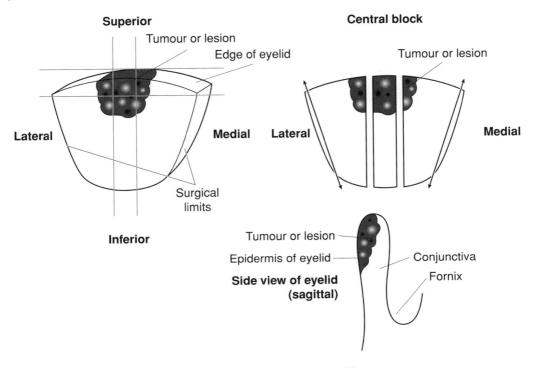

Figure 20.2. Wedge resection of eyelid.

The common lesions of the conjunctiva are:

1. *Degenerative:* pinguecula,
    pterygium.
2. *Pigmented:* naevi,
    malignant melanoma,
    extrinsic, e.g., injury.
3. *Inflammatory:* not usually biopsied but may be scraped for diagnosis of trachoma or other
    parasite infection.
4. *Malignancy:* basal cell carcinoma,
    squamous cell carcinoma,
    malignant melanoma.

The purpose of conjunctival biopsies is usually diagnostic ± cosmesis. As with eyelid biopsies, an assessment of the limits of excision may be of importance but usually the presence of infiltrating tumour in a biopsy from the fornix of the conjunctiva is sufficient justification for more radical treatment.

4. Cornea

Corneal "scrapes" of ulcerating lesions may be sent to microbiologists in order to identify organisms by direct microscopy and culture. Bacterial infections, fungi and Acanthamoeba may be identified this way. Occasionally the edge of a corneal ulcer may be submitted to the laboratory for histology as the lesion is resisting antibiotic therapy. These small biopsies are submitted whole and examined through levels. Using special stains, fungi (usually *Aspergillus* but occasionally *Fusarium* or *Penicillium*) or Acanthamoeba may be identified. It is unusual to find bacteria due to the therapeutic measures taken.

Corneal "buttons", as they are known in the trade, are submitted to the laboratory for evaluation of and corroboration of clinical diagnoses. They should be measured for maximum diameter and described grossly for evidence of ulceration, scarring, transparency/opacity and abnormal pigmentation.

Using a long sharp blade (e.g., disposable microtome blade) the cornea is cut across the ulcer, the pigmentation or maximum opacity so as to leave roughly three-fifths of the lesion for processing and a reserve of two-fifths of the lesion for other investigations, e.g., electron microscopy. Care has to be taken to avoid artefacted abrasion or removal of the squamous epithelium covering the cornea or the posterior layer of endothelial cells.

Histological sections are cut and stained with H+E. In essence, there are two main types of histology:

1. *Inflamed/scarred* – indicating an ongoing or previous infection or ulcer.
2. *Non-inflamed* – indicating a congenital dystrophy or abnormality, e.g., keratoconus, Fuch's dystrophy.

It may be that a congenital abnormality such as keratoconus will result in ulceration and scarring but most dystrophies have little evidence of inflammation or vascularisation.

Electron microscopy may have to be used to differentiate between some of the more obscure lesions affecting the cornea.

5. Iris

Small biopsies of the iris may be taken to confirm and/or treat a clinical diagnosis of *malignant melanoma*.

Pigmented lesions of the iris are most often *benign naevi*. However, serial clinical observations may identify lesions that are growing rapidly, particularly when they involve the filtration angle, have an irregular pattern of growth and show changes in pigmentation.

In the laboratory, one uses a dissecting microscope to attempt to orientate the small specimen especially if the operative procedure has been a sector iridectomy where the root of the iris (filtration angle, adjacent cornea/sclera and ciliary body) is included. This is especially important as the presence of infiltration of the trabecular meshwork and *Schlemm's canal* by tumour is an indicator of a poor prognosis.

6. Orbit

Biopsies of the orbit are of two types:

1. Where the clinicians believe they can gain access to the pathology via Tenon's capsule and take a pinch from the subjacent tissue. These are often unsatisfactory.

2. Where, after clinical and radiological evaluation, a formal biopsy for diagnosis and/or treatment is made, often involving a lateral orbitotomy (cutting bone at the side of the orbit) to gain access to the lesion deep within the orbit or in the cone formed by the extra-ocular muscles.

Lesions of the orbit present clinically as proptosis (eye coming forward) with varying degrees of squint, double vision and discomfort.

As this is a tricky site for surgery, patients are often referred to specialist ophthalmic surgeons and centres with their attendant pathological facilities.

Patients require a complete clinical examination and evaluation as often clues to the cause of the proptosis may be found as a result of detecting the presence of tumour elsewhere, e.g., lobular breast carcinoma, prostate carcinoma, lymphoma, von Recklinghausens syndrome. Equally, blood biochemistry (thyrotoxicosis, tumour markers), serology (systemic lupus erythematosus, Wegener's granulomatosis) and radiology (e.g., bony sclerosis versus bony erosion, presence or absence of calcification, e.g., meningioma, varix within a tumour mass), CT scanning and MRI are valuable.

The process of clinical evaluation is important as ideally surgeons attempt to remove only small resectable primary tumours, e.g., cavernous haemangioma, pleomorphic adenoma of the lacrimal gland, while avoiding irresectable malignancies and metastatic tumours.

In the laboratory, the investigation of biopsies is the same as from anywhere else in the body with the following caution. Biopsies of inflammatory lesions should be investigated thoroughly as missing an infective lesion (fungus, tuberculosis) may result in a patient being treated inappropriately with steroids, exacerbating the condition. Similarly, confusion between chronic inflammatory lesions and the usual low-grade lymphomas seen in the orbit is made more likely by the often miserly and inadequate biopsies of the orbital fat taken via Tenon's capsule.

7. Lacrimal Apparatus

This consists of a lacrimal gland situated in the superolateral aspect of the orbit, making tears which are drained via the punctum to the naso-lacrimal duct in the nasopharynx. The gland measures approximately 1–1.5 cm in diameter, has a histological appearance similar to the salivary glands and is subject to a similar spectrum of pathological lesions.

The two main tumours of the lacrimal gland are *pleomorphic adenoma* and *adenoid cystic carcinoma*. Pleomorphic adenoma is benign, occurring in middle age with a tendency to recur if inadequately excised. It causes painless proptosis and has bony sclerosis on X-ray. Adenoid cystic carcinoma occurs in a younger age group, infiltrates local structures causing painful proptosis as it has an affinity for nerves and erodes the surrounding orbital bone.

Both require complete excision for adequate therapy, pleomorphic adenoma being usually amenable to lateral orbitotomy in the first instance but may require more drastic action as the recurring tumour infiltrates between the two bony tables of the skull, causing serious problems of tumour control. Adenoid cystic tumour may require oculo-plastic surgery to gain adequate control of the disease.

For the laboratory, besides diagnosing the lesion, it is important to be able to identify the limits of excision and comment on their involvement or otherwise by the tumour.

Tumours of the naso-lacrimal ducts include benign polyps and malignancies common to the nasal sinuses and upper respiratory tract. The clinical presentation is epiphoria as the tears are unable to drain via the duct, overflowing the eyelid. Laboratory management is as always in ENT cases, which is to diagnose the nature of the lesion and if malignant, detail the adequacy of the excision (see exenteration later).

8. Eyes – Evisceration, Enucleation and Exenteration

There are three types of biopsy involving the eye or "globe" as it is called in ophthalmic pathology:

1. *Evisceration:* this is where the contents of the eye are removed via an incision around the limbus, taking iris, ciliary body, lens, vitreous, choroid and retina but leaving the sclera.
2. *Enucleation:* this is where the eye or globe is removed with a short piece of optic nerve.
3. *Exenteration:* this is where the eye, surrounding orbital contents, eyelids, naso-lacrimal apparatus ± orbital bone are removed.

There are three main reasons for removing an eye or its contents:

1. *Life-threatening conditions:* either pus or tumour.
2. *Pain:* usually absolute glaucoma with loss of vision.
3. *Cosmesis:* to remove an unsightly eye or to prevent facial asymmetry in young people around a collapsed micro-ophthalmic or expanding buphthalmic eye.

Evisceration

The dishevelled and disorganised contents of the eye are submitted in formalin fixative. If possible they should be examined grossly and, if recognisable, sorted into component parts. Calcified material (lens or remnants of osseous metaplasia in a phthisical eye) should be identified and processed via acid to avoid damage to microtome blades.

When examining the contents of the eye it is difficult to give a comprehensive account to validate the clinical history of the eye, and one is often reduced to noting the degree and type of the inflammatory process and, in the case of acute inflammation and pus, the presence of and type of organisms. Rarely is this procedure used to treat a tumour.

Enucleation

External Anatomy

It is necessary to confirm that the specimen is indeed the right or left eye as given on the histopathology request form. This is done by orientating the eye using the positions of the rectus muscle, tendons and the superior and inferior oblique extra-ocular muscles. The superior oblique muscle has a long string-like tendon inserting into the sclera lateral and slightly posterior to the superior rectus muscle and superior to the optic nerve. The inferior oblique muscle is fleshy and brown right up to the insertion into the globe and is situated lateral and inferior to the optic nerve. So the eyes should have the superior oblique muscle, optic nerve and inferior oblique muscles forming a triangle when viewed posteriorly (Figure 20.3).

Having orientated the eye, a systematic list of the external features is made. The normal diameter is 23–24 mm. Conditions such as glaucoma may thin the sclera causing herniations or staphylomata in areas of weakness. Otherwise there may be a slight increase in diameter as may also be seen in myopia. Examination of the cornea includes noting any surgical or traumatic incisions, sutures, opacities or pigmentation. Is the iris visible? Is it symmetrical, abnormally pigmented or deficient? If it is deficient, where on a clock face (12 o'clock = superior) and what size? Is there pus or proteinaceous fluid in the anterior chamber?

The conjunctiva and sclera are examined for abnormal pigment, incisions, or evidence of radiotherapy plaques or bands for the treatment of detached retina.

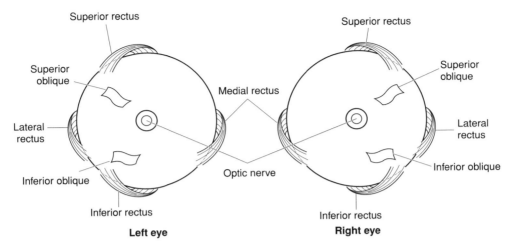

Figure 20.3.   Anatomical orientation of the eye. Landmarks on the eyes as viewed from the posterior aspect.

The optic nerve and scleral vessels are examined for evidence of tumour. After making these gross observations, it is advisable to photograph the external surfaces of the eye.

Laboratory Details

Fixation of the eye: Globes are usually fixed in formalin fixative. Prior to cutting, they are transferred to 95% alcohol as this "hardens" the sclera making it slightly easier to cut and improves the colour and presentation of the eye prior to photography.

Tools required: The best instrument to cut a globe is a long, very sharp thin blade. The idea is to get one long smooth cut that cuts the whole of the eye, rather than a series of sawing movements that disrupt the internal anatomy and make processing and sectioning difficult. A disposable microtome blade (10–15 cm) may be used but extreme care has to be taken to avoid spilling an innocent person's blood over the specimen.

Eyes opened and found to contain bone or calcified debris are gently decalcified in acid before finishing off the cutting. Eyes containing foreign bodies should have them removed carefully after noting and photographing their location.

Trans-illumination in eyes containing tumour: It may be possible to trans-illuminate the eye using a strong, narrow beam of light (usually fibre optic) in order to locate the mass. This is helpful in deciding how to cut and open the eye in order to have the classical section of central cornea, centre of pupil, lens, lesion and optic nerve.

Similarly, X-ray examination for bone or foreign bodies may be undertaken using needles on the external surface to help locate the lesion.

Techniques: (Figure 20.4) A thin section of the optic nerve is taken first and submitted for histology.

Vertical cuts to give calottes is the technique used when studying surgical lens extractions and the surgical site following a failure of or complications of cataract surgery. An implanted plastic lens may interfere with the smooth cutting of the blade and therefore should be anticipated.

Horizontal cuts give calottes which include cornea, centre of pupil, lens, lesion, macula and optic nerve. The inferior oblique helps one identify the posterior temporal sclera.

The calottes should be cut first 1 mm from the optic nerve proceeding anteriorly to cut the cornea about 2 mm medial to the limbus. The globe is placed on the cutting block and the

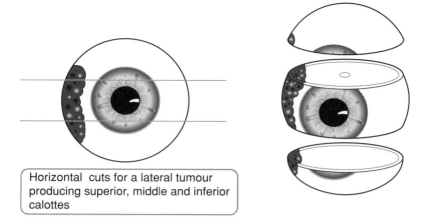

Horizontal cuts for a lateral tumour producing superior, middle and inferior calottes

Figure 20.4. Blocking an eye specimen.

procedure repeated on the other side of the optic nerve. Vertical cutting results in a nasal calotte, a central wedge-shaped block and a temporal calotte. These can be further examined under liquid to conserve the anatomy, keeping the retina in situ.

All blocks are examined, carefully noting

- the depth and contents of the anterior chamber.
- the presence or absence of the lens.
- the presence or absence of cataract, the vitreous (clear, gelatinous or turbid, the presence or absence of membranes).
- the retina, whether it is in situ or detached (a subretinal exudate indicates a true as opposed to artefactual retinal detachment).
- the presence or absence of recent/old haemorrhage in the vitreous or choroid.
- the thickness of the sclera.

Pathological Conditions

Tumours: There are two main tumours affecting the eye, *malignant melanoma* (presents from second decade to very elderly) and *retinoblastoma* (which presents in childhood). However, many other tumours have been described within the eye including adenomas and adenocarcinomas of the ciliary body epithelium, schwannomas, lymphomas, haemangiomas and metastatic tumours from lung, breast and stomach.

Malignant melanomas may occur anywhere in the uveal tract but are most commonly found in the choroid. They arise in the choroid, pushing Bruch's membrane over them until they perforate it causing the overlying retina to detach with consequent formation of a subretinal exudate. The tumour gains access to the venous side of the systemic circulation via the perforations of the sclera by the artery, vein and nerve bundles and may be seen causing black pigmentation in the region of the vortex veins. Alternatively, malignant melanomas may infiltrate the filtration angle of the anterior chamber en route to Schlemm's canal and the conjunctival veins. This causes abnormal pigmentation of the conjunctiva at the limbus. Uveal malignant melanoma classically metastasises to the liver.

Prognosis for these tumours depends on three major factors

1. Age at presentation: older is worse than young.
2. Site within the eye: posterior is better than equatorial, which is better than anterior where it quickly gains access to the venous side of the systemic circulation via Schlemm's canal.
3. Size of tumour (maximum diameter):
   - 15 mm poor prognosis,
   - 10 mm guarded prognosis,
   - 5 mm interesting, but not immediately lethal.

The size of tumour covers factors such as cell type, as small tumours tend to be spindle B cell type and the larger tumours have increasing numbers of epithelioid cells. Similarly, larger tumours tend to be exiting the eye via the sclera or Schlemm's canal.

TNM classification of tumour spread ciliary body and choroid malignant melanoma.

pT1   tumour ≤ 10 mm maximum diameter, ≤ 2.5 mm height*.
pT2   tumour > 10 to 16 mm maximum diameter, > 2.5 to 10 mm height*.
*   a   no extraocular extension.
     b   microscopic extraocular extension.
     c   gross extraocular extension.
pT3   tumour > 16 mm maximum diameter and/or 10 mm height.
pT4   pT3 with extraocular extension.
pN1   regional lymph node metastasis.

Retinoblastoma – two types:

1. Congenital: where both eyes ± the pineal gland are affected.
2. Sporadic: where one eye is affected and the patient carries a genetic risk for the next generation.

The tumour arises in one, two or all three of the layers of the retina forming retinoblasts which may infiltrate the overlying vitreous (endophytic) or the underlying subretinal space (exophytic). The tumour exits the eye via the optic nerve to the brain. It infiltrates the choroid if there has been damage to Bruch's membrane (usually following X-radiation treatment). From there it may metastasise systemically.
     Treatment of congenital retinoblastoma usually involves excising the worse eye and treating the better eye with collumated irradiation, hoping to conserve some function. For sporadic cases the affected eye is removed, hoping to avoid spread to the brain via the optic nerve.

TNM classification of tumour spread retinoblastoma

pT1   tumour confined to the retina, vitreous or subretinal space.
pT2   minimal invasion of optic nerve (not through lamina cribrosa) and choroid.
pT3   significant invasion of optic nerve (through lamina cribrosa but not to resection line) and choroid.
pT4   extraocular invasion.
pN1   regional lymph node metastasis.

Glaucoma: The main cause for enucleation is the painful blind eye. Such eyes usually have a long history of attending an ophthalmologist with episodes of therapy (medical and surgical) before opting for pain relief and pre-emptively preventing the eye from rupturing due to the increased intra-ocular pressure causing thinning and anaesthesia of the cornea.

Such eyes are cut and processed with attention to the clinical history in order to corroborate the clinical findings and demonstrate the cause of the open or closed angle glaucoma.

Inflammation: The eye is subject to endophthalmitis secondary to penetrating injuries or surgical procedures. This may be treated by steroids provided it is not infected. Infections – bacterial, fungal, helminthic (toxocariasis) and protozoal (toxoplasmosis) – cause a spectrum of acute to chronic inflammation. The presence of pus and the potential of infection to track to the CNS may necessitate evisceration or enucleation. Often the inflammation subsides but the resultant healing process precipitates detachment of the retina and glaucoma requiring enucleation of a painful blind eye.

Granulomatous inflammation affecting the choroid or sclera may be the result of sympathetic endophthalmitis, sarcoidosis, rheumatoid arthritis, Wegener's granulomatosis and the terminal stages of miliary TB.

Exenteration

Exenteration is carried out to gain control of a malignant tumour affecting the tissues around the eye, e.g., eyelids, orbital contents, nasal sinuses, palate, etc. Often there is no direct extension of the tumour into the eye and no evidence of tumour metastasis within the choroid. The object of the laboratory investigation is to determine whether or not the radical surgical excision of tissue from around the eye has removed the tumour with clear surgical margins and if the tumour is in the microvasculature leading to cervical lymph nodes.

Procedures

Radical dissections may come with many fragments including a dissection of the eye, eyelids and orbital contents. It is necessary to identify and orientate the components of the overall dissection in order to determine the surgical limits of excision.

For the central block of eye, eyelids and orbit, it is useful to mark the cut edges of the block of tissue with different dyes to ensure that the superior/inferior and medial/lateral limits are easily identified. The eye is orientated using the lids and caruncle to confirm the side from which it was taken according to the request form and the superior/inferior, medial/lateral limits. Any gross evidence of tumour should be accurately located and described.

Using the cornea and optic nerve as landmarks as described in the procedures for the enucleated globe, antero-posterior incisions are made on either side of the cornea and optic nerve to obtain a central block that should have lids, cornea, lens, vitreous, retina, choroid, sclera and optic nerve within surrounding tissues as a central block leaving medial and lateral calottes of eye and surrounding soft tissues. Further blocks may be cut to obtain medial and lateral limits of excision as required. These are often in a horizontal plane.

9. Muscle Biopsies

This is specialised work and should only be undertaken by laboratories and pathologists with experience of enzyme histochemistry and the evaluation of the results. Small muscle biopsies (other than for tumours) are taken from the belly of viable muscles in order to diagnose conditions causing muscle weakness. Biopsies should not be taken from extremely wasted muscles as only end-stage pathology rather than ongoing pathological changes will be demonstrated.

Conditions causing muscle weakness fall into three main categories:

1. Congenital disorders of muscle, i.e., biochemical abnormalities resulting in a dystrophy or myopathy.

2. Acquired disorders of muscle secondary to pathology of the nervous system.
3. Acquired disorders due to inflammation of muscle or the microvasculature.

As with all biopsies, a full history of the condition and clinical work-up is of importance to the pathologist.

Laboratory Techniques

Muscle biopsies are processed using frozen section techniques in order to enable histochemical methods of staining and morphometric evaluation of muscle fibre types, innervation and enzyme biochemistry. Muscle biopsies in formalin fixative and paraffin wax embedding are of limited use, allowing only evaluation of inflammatory conditions and confirming muscle wasting.

Orientation of the small muscle biopsy is of great importance. The classical histological section is a cross section of muscle fibres and fascicles. Longitudinal sections of muscle fibres are of limited use except when looking for neuro-muscular junctions.

It is necessary for the biopsy to be taken to the laboratory immediately following removal from the patient, so as to conserve the potential for enzyme histochemistry. If this is not possible then ammonium sulphate fixative solution may be used but this requires practice and familiarity by technicians and pathologists to ensure that the histochemical techniques work.

The biopsy is orientated to give a transverse section using a dissecting microscope. The biopsy is placed in O.C.T. on a small piece of cork and snap frozen in iso-pentane cooled in liquid nitrogen. The process of snap freezing is important as crystal artefacts will result if the freezing process is too slow. Transverse sections are cut and stored using a cryostat.

The standard histochemical stains, besides H+E, are ATPase and NADH to differentiate between muscle fibres, a modified Gomori to study mitochondria and a battery of other enzyme histochemical stains to study the biochemistry of the muscle including acid phosphatase, succinic dehydrogenase, cytochrome oxidase, phosphorylase. Immunocytochemical staining (e.g., Dystrophins 1–3, Merosin, Adhalin, Utrophin and Spectrin) is also being used to examine for and subtype muscle dystrophies.

10. Peripheral Nerves

A peripheral nerve biopsy may be taken to evaluate disorders causing peripheral weakness and/or loss of sensation when no central nervous system cause is implicated. Over the age of 45 years there is a gradual loss of peripheral nerve axons but the process may be accelerated by disease. Ordinarily, peripheral nerves have a process of degeneration and regeneration with wear and tear due to the vicissitudes of life. The process may be accelerated by disease. Most often the pathologist is seeking to determine the condition of the nerve, i.e., the number of axons relative to the patient's age, the condition of the myelin sheath and the presence or absence of any abnormal cellular or non-cellular infiltrate.

Peripheral nerve biopsies are placed in formalin fixative. In the laboratory they are orientated using a dissecting microscope as it is important to obtain the classical transverse section of the nerve which allows a relative count of the axons as well as staining for and evaluation of the myelin nerve sheaths. The nature of infiltrates may be determined using routine staining methods. Only very rarely is one asked to tease out the longitudinal axons in a biopsy for clinical purposes.

11. Colorectal Mucosal Biopsies for Hirschsprung's Disease

Pinch biopsies of colonic and rectal mucosa may be taken for the evaluation and determination of the severity and extent of Hirschsprung's disease in children. The innervation and motility of the gut can be determined using enzyme histochemistry for acetyl-cholinesterase activity. If there is no staining the bowel is innervated. Positive staining indicates an aganglionic or hypoganglionic area which results in a bowel stricture and constipation. Using a series of biopsies, the distribution of the hypoganglionic segments can be mapped out prior to surgical resection.

The pinch biopsies are taken by the clinician and taken immediately to the laboratory in order to conserve the enzyme activity. The biopsy is orientated in the laboratory using a dissecting microscope so as to give a classical section of mucosa with epithelium, lamina propria, muscularis mucosae and submucosal connective tissue from top to bottom. It is not necessary to see a full thickness of bowel wall as the enzyme technique evaluates the presence of autonomic innervation by testing for the presence of acetyl-cholinesterase, which breaks down the presence of acetyl-choline and by inference proves the presence of a nerve supply.

The orientated biopsy is placed in O.C.T. on a piece of cork and snap frozen in iso-pentane cooled in liquid nitrogen, so as to avoid ice crystal artefacts distorting the specimen if cooled too slowly.

Frozen sections are cut and conserved using a cryostat. The sections are stained for H+E in order to examine for ganglion cells from Meissner's plexus in the submucosa and acetyl-cholinesterase for the presence or absence of positive staining.

Gynaecological Specimens

W Glenn McCluggage

21 Ovary

1. Anatomy

The ovaries are paired structures lying in the right and left iliac fossae, on either side of the uterus attached to the posterior aspect of the broad ligaments (Figure 21.1). In the reproductive age group, each ovary is typically approximately 3 cm in maximum dimension, but the size may vary considerably. In the prepubertal and postmenopausal periods, the ovaries are usually smaller. Typically the ovary is ovoid in shape. The external surface may be smooth or convoluted, especially in the late reproductive period. The ovary contains an outer cortex and an inner medulla. Follicular structures, including cystic follicles, corpora lutea and corpora albicantia are usually visible on sectioning. A hilar region is also apparent. The ovary is covered by a layer of peritoneum, the mesovarium.

Lymphovascular Supply

The blood supply to the ovary is from the ovarian artery, a branch of the aorta. This courses along the surface of the ovary and anastomoses with the ovarian branch of the uterine artery. Subsidiary branches enter the ovarian hilus and then travel through the medulla and cortex, anastomosing to form capillary channels. Veins accompany the arteries and in the hilum form a plexus which drains into the ovarian vein. The ovarian veins course along the surface of the ovaries, the right draining into the inferior vena cava and the left into the left renal vein.

The ovarian lymphatics originate with the theca layers of the follicles and course through the ovarian stroma to form a hilar plexus. Eventually they accompany the ovarian vessels to drain into the upper para-aortic lymph nodes at the level of the lower pole of the kidney.

2. Clinical Presentation

Clinical features related to ovarian pathology are often non-specific and, in general with ovarian neoplasia, symptoms occur late in the course of the disease when the tumour has often spread beyond the ovary. Symptoms related to ovarian tumours include swelling or a feeling of fullness in the abdomen or pelvis, the presence of an abdominal mass, irregular uterine bleeding and abdominal or pelvic pain. There may be associated ascites, especially with ovarian malignancies, but also with some benign neoplasms such as fibromas. With ovarian endometriosis, pain and swelling may fluctuate depending on the stage of the menstrual cycle. In younger patients, ovarian pathology may be discovered during the course of investigations for infertility. Ovarian pathology may also be discovered incidentally during abdominal or pelvic imaging or as a result of an

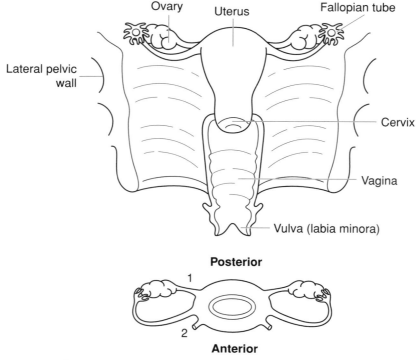

1. Ovarian ligament
2. Round ligament

Figure 21.1.   Overview of gynaecological anatomy. Based on Hermanek P, Hutter RVP, Sobin LH, Wagner G, Wittekind Ch (eds.). TNM Atlas: illustrated guide to the TNM/pTNM classification of malignant tumours, 4th edition. Springer-Verlag: Berlin and Heidelberg, 1997.

increased serum CA-125. Serum CA-125 measurements and abdominal ultrasound are currently being evaluated in screening programmes for ovarian cancer.

3. Clinical Investigations

Serum CA-125 measurements: an increase in serum CA-125 may be an indicator of ovarian malignancy. However, modest or even marked elevation of serum CA-125 may occur in many non-neoplastic diseases or non-ovarian neoplastic diseases, this serum marker being relatively non-specific. CA-125 is produced by mesothelial cells, and conditions which involve the peritoneal cavity with its lining of mesothelial cells are especially liable to result in an elevated serum CA-125. These conditions include ascites, endometriosis, peritoneal tuberculosis and disseminated non-ovarian neoplasms.

Abdominal USS and CT scan: in cases of ovarian neoplasia abdominal USS or CT scan often shows a complex ovarian mass with alternating solid and cystic areas. There may be coexistent ascites and an omental cake, indicating omental involvement by tumour. Unilocular or multilocular thin-walled cystic lesions often indicate benign neoplasms. CT scanning is often performed to stage ovarian neoplasia.

Peritoneal aspiration: aspiration of ascitic fluid and cytological examination may be performed in the investigation of ovarian neoplasia.

Laparoscopy: this may be indicated in certain conditions, e.g., suspected endometriosis. Biopsy can be performed at laparoscopy.

In patients with suspected ovarian neoplasia, a *risk-malignancy index* is calculated. This is a means of assessing the likelihood that an ovarian mass is malignant and takes into account the menopausal status (pre or post menopausal) of the patient, the ultrasound findings and the serum CA-125 measurement.

4. Pathological Conditions

Non-neoplastic Conditions

Follicular or functional cysts: these are extremely common and are secondary to an absence of the normal preovulatory luteinizing hormone surge that triggers ovulation. They are usually found in the reproductive age group and are generally asymptomatic although acute abdominal pain and bleeding into the peritoneal cavity may occur secondary to rupture. Follicular cysts may be multiple. In children they can be associated with sexual pseudoprecocity.

Grossly follicular cysts are usually thin walled and contain watery fluid. Histologically they are lined by granulosa or theca cells or a combination of both. These cell types are often luteinised.

Corpus luteum cyst: during the ovulatory cycle a corpus luteum is formed which, when fertilization does not occur, involutes. At the time of menstruation the centre of the corpus luteum is cystic and filled with blood. This is known as a cystic corpus luteum. When this cystic mass becomes greater than 3 cm in diameter, it is designated a corpus luteum cyst. These lesions are often asymptomatic but can be associated with menstrual irregularities. Rupture may result in pain and intra-abdominal haemorrhage.

Grossly a corpus luteum cyst is lobulated or well circumscribed. The wall is composed of luteinised granulosa cells and the lumen contains fresh or altered blood.

Polycystic ovarian disease: this disease is characterised by anovulation and the development of multiple follicular cysts within both ovaries. Often patients are infertile and have menstrual irregularities. Typically the ovaries are enlarged with multiple small cysts located just below the cortex. The outer cortex of the ovary is typically thickened. Histologically the cysts are usually lined by a thin layer of granulosa cells and a more prominent layer of lipid-laden theca interna cells.

Endometriosis: the ovary is the most common site of endometriosis, which is defined as the presence of endometrial tissue, usually both glands and stroma, outside the uterus. Most common in the reproductive age group, but occasionally encountered in postmenopausal women, the symptoms are protean and varied. Patients may present with a palpable abdominal mass, abdominal or pelvic pain, dysmenorrhoea, dyspareunia, irregular uterine bleeding or infertility.

Endometriosis within the ovary may take the form of an endometriotic cyst. These can be single or multiple and are often bilateral. They generally have a thick fibrous wall which is yellow to brown in colour with a ragged internal surface. The cyst contents are typically brown fluid which may be inspissated, giving rise to the term "chocolate cyst" of the ovary. Rarely, tumours can arise within ovarian endometriotic cysts and these usually take the form of a thickened area within the wall. Endometriosis within the ovary may also be non-cystic, appearing as small red, blue or brown spots. Often, endometriotic foci are not apparent to the naked eye.

Histologically, endometriosis is typically composed of endometrial glands and stroma. In some cases, one or both of these components may be absent, or obscured by a superimposed haemorrhagic, inflammatory or fibrotic process. Occasionally, all that remains is a fibrotic area containing haemosiderin or ceroid-laden macrophages. In such cases, a presumptive diagnosis of endometriosis may be made.

Simple cysts: simple benign cysts are common within the ovary. They cannot be classified into any specific type since the lining is attenuated or lost. Most are probably of epithelial origin, being lined by attenuated epithelial cells or of follicular origin lined by atrophic granulosa or theca cells. Immunohistochemistry for EMA. (epithelial cells positive) or α-inhibin (granulosa cells positive) assists in determining the origin of the cyst.

Stromal hyperplasia: this is relatively common in the perimenopausal or early postmenopausal age group. Both ovaries are enlarged, often only mildly so, by a nodular stromal proliferation. Usually the nodules are yellow to white in colour and they may be confluent. Histology confirms a nodular proliferation of stromal cells with scant cytoplasm. There may be androgenic or oestrogenic manifestations and, on occasions, associated endometrial hyperplasia or adenocarcinoma.

Stromal hyperthecosis: this rare condition is often associated with signs of hyperandrogenism. Oestrogenic manifestations, coexistent endometrial hyperplasia or adenocarcinoma may also occur. Typically, both ovaries are enlarged and yellow/white in colour with a vague nodular pattern. Histologically, there is usually accompanying stromal hyperplasia, but in addition luteinised stromal cells are present singly or in small groups.

Massive oedema: this is a rare cause of unilateral ovarian enlargement and is probably secondary to partial torsion of the ovary. Presentation is often with abdominal pain and a palpable ovarian mass. There may be evidence of androgen excess. On sectioning the ovary it is typically oedematous and pale in colour and watery fluid exudes from the cut surface. Histologically, there is separation of the stromal cells by oedema fluid which surrounds residual ovarian structures. Luteinised stromal cells may be present. The outer cortex is typically not oedematous but rather is composed of dense fibrous tissue.

Neoplastic Conditions

The ovary is unique in that an extremely wide range of neoplasms, both benign and malignant, may arise here. Primary tumours may be of surface epithelial, germ cell or sex cord-stromal derivation.

Benign tumours: may be of surface epithelial type (serous, mucinous or endometrioid cystadenoma/cystadenofibroma and Brenner tumour), germ cell type (e.g., benign cystic teratoma) or sex cord-stromal type (e.g., fibrothecoma). They can be solid or cystic or contain a mixture of solid and cystic components.

Malignant tumours: primary malignant ovarian neoplasms are of *surface epithelial, germ cell or sex cord-stromal type.* Surface epithelial tumours are most common and these are serous, mucinous, endometrioid, clear cell, transitional or undifferentiated carcinomas in type. Borderline neoplasms (tumours of low malignant potential) also occur and these may be one of any of the morphological subtypes described, most commonly serous or mucinous. These are neoplasms with malignant nuclear characteristics but in which there is no evidence of stromal invasion. Ovarian surface epithelial adenocarcinomas are most common in middle-aged and elderly women, in nulliparous women and those with an early menarche and late menopause. The oral contraceptive pill is protective. It has been suggested than women who are exposed to ovulation-inducing drugs are at increased risk of the development of ovarian carcinoma. Women with BRCA1 or BRCA2 gene mutations are at increased risk of the development of both ovarian and breast cancer. Outside BRCA1 and BRCA2 groups, there is a familial predisposition to the development of ovarian cancer. The risk of developing ovarian adenocarcinoma, especially of serous type, increases with the number of ovulations over a lifetime (incessant ovulation theory).

Repeated ovulation with disruption of the ovarian surface mesothelium is thought to result in the development of cortical inclusion cysts. The cells lining this are then under the influence of the ovarian stromal microenvironment and it is thought that this may result in the development of a neoplastic process.

Mucinous, endometrioid and clear cell adenocarcinomas may have an alternative pathogenesis. For example, K-ras mutations are found in mucinous adenocarcinomas and these may develop from pre-existing borderline mucinous neoplasms, unlike serous adenocarcinomas which are thought to arise de novo. Endometrioid and clear cell carcinomas can be associated with endometriosis in the ipsilateral or contralateral ovary or elsewhere in the pelvis, and it is clear that a proportion of these neoplasms arise from endometriosis, sometimes from atypical endometriosis. Since the preferred theory for the development of endometriosis is retrograde menstruation, it is interesting that tubal ligation is protective for the development of endometrioid and clear cell carcinomas but not for other morphological subtypes. Endometrioid neoplasms may coexist with similar tumours in the endometrium in up to 25% of cases. The ovary is a common site for metastatic carcinomas. The most common primary sites include colon, pancreas, biliary tree, stomach, breast and endometrium. Features favouring metastasis, but by no means specific for this, include bilaterality, the presence of nodular tumour deposits especially on the cortical surface of the ovary, extensive necrosis and vascular invasion.

Aetiological factors in the development of ovarian germ cell (e.g., immature teratoma, yolk sac tumour, dysgerminoma) and sex cord-stromal (e.g., Sertoli–Leydig tumours) neoplasms are not well known. Gonadoblastomas often occur in patients with underlying gonadal dysgenesis while sex cord-stromal tumour with annular tubules can be associated with Peutz–Jeghers syndrome. Sex cord-stromal neoplasms may cause oestrogenic or androgenic excess due to hormone elaboration. Occasionally this may result in endometrial hyperplasia or adenocarcinoma.

It should be stressed that a wide variety of other neoplasms, both benign and malignant, also arise within the ovary.

Treatment: treatment of malignant ovarian neoplasms is usually total abdominal hysterectomy and bilateral salpingo-oophorectomy. Omentectomy and peritoneal washings are usually performed as part of the staging procedure. Postoperative chemotherapy is often necessary, especially for tumours which have spread beyond the ovary or for tumours which are confined to the ovary but where the capsule is deficient and/or there is ascites or positive peritoneal washings. The FIGO staging system for ovarian cancer is used.

Prognosis: the prognosis of ovarian adenocarcinoma is generally poor, overall five-year survival being in the region of 30–40%. This is largely due to the fact that many carcinomas have spread beyond the ovary, and are FIGO stage III or IV. The prognosis for stage I tumours is generally good. Borderline epithelial neoplasms have an excellent prognosis, if adequately staged, and if there are no invasive peritoneal or omental implants.

Some ovarian sex cord-stromal neoplasms, e.g., granulosa cell tumours, exhibit a low-grade malignant behaviour with late recurrence or metastasis being a common feature. Many malignant germ cell tumours, especially those occurring in children or young adults, are highly aggressive but often respond well to modern chemotherapeutic regimens.

5. Surgical Pathology Specimens – Clinical Aspects

Biopsy Specimens

Fine needle aspiration (FNA) specimens of ovarian cystic lesions may be performed under ultrasound guidance (transvaginal or transabdominal) or at laparoscopy or laparotomy. Ovarian wedge biopsies are occasionally performed at diagnostic laparotomy for lower abdominal pain and core biopsies are carried out when it is unclear whether an ovarian mass is benign or malignant. Cystectomy with preservation of the residual ovary may be performed in patients in whom benign cystic lesions are suspected clinically.

Resection Specimens

In general, with the exception of young women, when a malignant ovarian tumour is suspected, total abdominal hysterectomy, bilateral salpingo-oophorectomy and omentectomy is performed. This is generally via an abdominal approach. Any ascitic or free peritoneal fluid is sent for cytological examination and if none is present peritoneal washings are performed. In young women with a clinically and/or radiologically malignant ovarian lesion, in whom preservation of fertility is desirable, unilateral salpingo-oophorectomy (usually with omentectomy) may be performed. This should be followed by discussion of the case and assessment of the need for further surgery at a multidisciplinary gynaecological oncology meeting. In occasional cases, where the presence of widespread disease precludes total tumour debulking, then only small fragments or a proportion of the tumour will be removed. Unilateral salpingo-oophorectomy may be performed when a benign ovarian neoplasm or a benign cyst is suspected. Prophylactic oophorectomies, usually with removal of the fallopian tubes, may be performed in those with a hereditary predisposition to developing ovarian cancer.

6. Surgical Pathology Specimens – Laboratory Protocols

Biopsy Specimens

FNA specimens are centrifuged and the specimens examined cytologically, usually with both Giemsa and Papanicolaou stains. Ovarian wedge biopsies are weighed and measured, sectioned thinly and examined intact. Core biopsies are examined intact, usually at multiple levels.

Resection Specimens

Initial Procedures and Description

- abrading the cortical surface should be avoided in order to preserve the mesothelial lining.
- each ovary is weighed (g) and measured in three dimensions (cm) and if necessary photographed. The presence of fallopian tubes is confirmed and they are measured.
- the cortical surfaces of the ovaries may be inked but in general this is not necessary.
- the cortical surface of each ovary is closely inspected around the whole circumference. The presence of obvious tumour deposits on the capsular surface or of papillary areas or capsular breach is noted. This is important since if a malignant tumour breaches the capsular surface it is at least stage IC. In many instances this is the cut-off for adjuvant chemotherapy.
- abnormal ovaries are serially sectioned at approximately 1 cm intervals. Note that large cystic lesions may contain abundant fluid which can exude under pressure. The characteristics of the fluid should be noted, e.g., serous, mucinous or bloody. Scissors can also be of use in opening and blocking cystic lesions.
- if the ovary is predominantly solid, the colour and consistency of the lesion is noted as is the presence or absence of areas of haemorrhage or necrosis.
- if the lesion is both solid and cystic, record the proportion of each.

- if the lesion is cystic, note whether the cyst is unilocular, multilocular or whether a main cyst is present together with multiple smaller daughter cysts. The presence of residual ovary is documented.
- with a cystic lesion, describe whether the internal surface of the cysts are smooth or whether they contain papillary projections.
- the presence of other elements within the lesion is recorded, e.g., hair and teeth in dermoid cysts.
- ovaries removed prophylactically in those with a hereditary predisposition to develop ovarian cancer are serially sectioned parallel to the short axis at 2–3 mm intervals. The presence of any gross abnormality is noted. The entire ovaries (and fallopian tubes) should be submitted for histological examination since very small neoplasms, which are not recognisable grossly, may be present.
- grossly normal ovaries removed during a hysterectomy for benign disease or for uterine or cervical neoplasms are bisected longitudinally and inspected.
- any paraovarian cystic or solid lesions should be treated in a similar way.
- omentum is weighed, measured in three dimensions (cm) and sectioned thinly. The presence of obvious tumour deposits, grittiness or areas of thickening or induration is noted.

Blocks for Histology (Figure 21.2)

- as stated previously, ovaries removed prophylactically in those with a hereditary predisposition to develop ovarian cancer are examined in their entirety.
- a single section through the long axis of the ovary suffices for grossly normal ovaries removed as part of a hysterectomy specimen for benign disease or uterine or cervical cancer.
- for suspected benign cystic lesions (thin-walled unilocular or multiloculated cysts) without thickenings or papillary excrescences on the external or internal surfaces, representative sampling suffices. With mucinous lesions, at least one block per cm is required as malignant areas may be focal and coexist with benign and borderline areas.
- for those lesions with papillary excrescences on the internal or external surface, multiple blocks are taken, especially from the papillary areas. This is important since these areas often represent borderline foci.
- for grossly malignant neoplasms, representative sections are taken, usually one section per cm of tumour.
- special attention should be given to the sampling of areas of capsular breach or infiltration by tumour.
- in neoplasms with a variegated appearance, grossly different areas are blocked.
- paraovarian lesions should be blocked similarly.
- representative sections of omentum are examined. If the omentum is grossly normal, three or four blocks suffice. Any tumour deposits or areas of thickening, grittiness or induration are preferentially sampled. If histological examination reveals implants or borderline lesions, then multiple additional sections may have to be examined.

Histopathology Report

- side of tumour – right/left or bilateral.
- dimensions of tumour – measure in three dimensions (cm).
- gross appearance – solid/cystic, colour and consistency, presence of haemorrhage or necrosis.
- tumour type – it is stressed that a wide range of benign and malignant tumours may arise within the ovary. The ovary is also a relatively common site for metastatic carcinomas.
- tumour differentiation – there is no universally agreed grading system for ovarian adenocarcinomas. Most systems use a combination of cytological and architectural features and

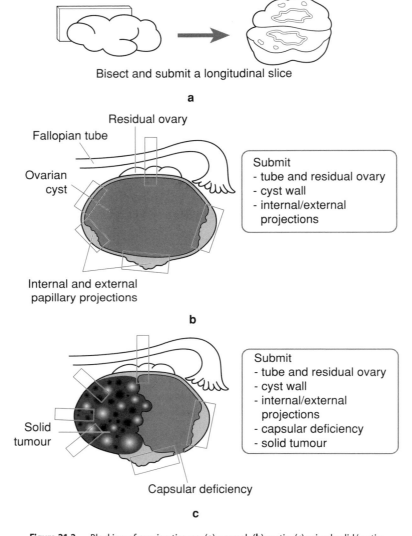

Figure 21.2. Blocking of ovarian tissues: (**a**) normal, (**b**) cystic, (**c**) mixed solid/cystic.

grade neoplasms as well, moderately or poorly differentiated. Clear cell carcinomas should be graded solely on the nuclear features.

- capsule – it should be stated whether the capsule is intact, deficient or breached by tumour.
- lymphovascular invasion – present/not present.
- lymph nodes – mention sites and presence or absence of tumour involvement.
- omentum – involved/not involved by tumour and size of tumour deposits (cm).
- other organs (fallopian tube, uterus, cervix) – involved/not involved by tumour.
- peritoneal washings/ascitic fluid – involved/not involved by tumour.

● other pathology – the presence of coexistent pathology should be mentioned. Endometrioid and clear cell carcinomas may arise in endometriosis.

FIGO/TNM Staging

pT1   growth limited to the ovaries:
    a. one ovary, capsule intact, no serosal disease or malignant cells in ascites or peritoneal washings.
    b. two ovaries, capsule intact, no serosal disease or malignant cells in ascites or peritoneal washings.
    c. one or both ovaries with any of: capsule rupture, serosal disease or malignant cells in ascites or peritoneal washings.

pT2   growth involving one or both ovaries with pelvic extension:
    a. uterus, tubes.
    b. other pelvic tissues.
    c. 2a or 2b plus malignant cells in ascites or peritoneal washings.

pT3   growth involving one or both ovaries with metastases to abdominal peritoneum, and/or regional nodes:
    a. microscopic peritoneal metastasis beyond pelvis.
    b. macroscopic peritoneal metastasis ≤ 2 cm in greatest dimension beyond pelvis.
    c. peritoneal metastasis > 2 cm in greatest dimension and/or regional lymph node metastasis (N1).

pT4/M1 growth involving one or both ovaries with distant metastases, e.g., liver parenchyma or positive pleural fluid cytology.

Regional nodes: obturator, common iliac, external iliac, lateral sacral, para-aortic, inguinal

pN0   no regional lymph node metastasis.
pN1   metastasis in regional lymph node(s).

22 Fallopian Tube

1. Anatomy

The fallopian tubes are paired structures which extend from the uterine cornu to the medial pole of the ovary. They are generally 8–12 cm in length. There are four segments to the fallopian tube, which from medial to lateral are the intramural segment, the isthmus, the ampulla and the infundibulum (Figure 22.1). The lateral aspect of the infundibulum is fimbriated and opens into the pelvic cavity. Microscopically, the fallopian tube consists of mucosa, submucosa, muscularis and serosa which is covered by a single layer of mesothelial cells.

Lymphovascular Supply

The fallopian tubes are supplied both by a branch of the ovarian artery and a branch of the uterine artery. The venous drainage is similar. The lymphatic channels draining the fallopian tube descend within the mesosalpinx behind the ovary where they form part of the subovarian plexus.

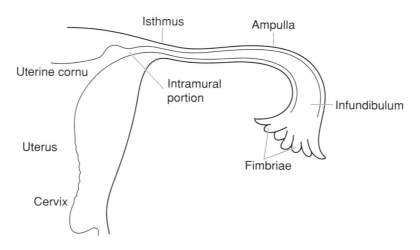

Figure 22.1. Fallopian tube anatomy.

2. Clinical Presentation

Most fallopian tubes submitted as surgical pathology specimens are a component of larger specimens and symptomatology specifically related to pathology in the fallopian tube is relatively rare. However, ectopic pregnancies occur in the fallopian tube and usually present with abdominal pain. If there is associated haemoperitoneum the pain is severe and associated with signs of peritonism. Other fallopian tube pathologies may result in abdominal pain or patients can present with infertility. With neoplasms or other pathological lesions causing enlargement of the fallopian tube there may be a palpable abdominal mass with or without associated ascites. Fallopian tube pathology is occasionally discovered incidentally during abdominal or pelvic imaging.

3. Clinical Investigations

- Serum CA-125 measurements: an increase in serum CA-125 may be found with primary fallopian tube carcinoma.
- Abdominal USS scan: ectopic pregnancies may be seen on ultrasound scan and there is usually a positive pregnancy test. Primary fallopian tube malignancies may also be identified on scanning as well as conditions such as hydrosalpinx or pyosalpinx.
- Laparoscopy: this is undertaken in order to directly visualise the fallopian tube.
- Fine needle aspiration cytology: this can be performed either at laparoscopy or under ultrasound guidance. Paratubal cysts or cystic lesions of the fallopian tube, such as hydrosalpinx, are especially liable to be aspirated.

4. Pathological Conditions

Non-neoplastic Conditions

Paratubal or fimbrial cysts: these are extremely common, especially paratubal cysts. They are thin-walled cysts usually containing serous fluid. They can be multiple and histologically are lined by a single layer of bland, usually ciliated, epithelial cells. The epithelial lining may be attenuated.

Hydrosalpinx and pyosalpinx: hydrosalpinx is dilatation of the fallopian tube. Although rarely of unknown aetiology, it is usually secondary to obstruction of the tube with subsequent dilatation. One of the most common causes is pelvic inflammatory disease. Other causes include endometriosis, tumour or a lesion within the uterus. Grossly, the fallopian tube is dilated, sometimes massively so. There may be associated haemorrhage within the lumen, resulting in haematosalpinx. With superimposed infection, pus can accumulate within the lumen and wall of the tube resulting in pyosalpinx. Histology shows marked dilatation of the lumen of the tube with oedema within the wall and numerous polymorphs in the case of pyosalpinx.

Ectopic pregnancy: with tubal ectopic pregnancies the fallopian tube is generally dilated, sometimes with an area of rupture. Sectioning the tube reveals blood clot and sometimes grossly visible placental tissue within the lumen. Histology shows blood clot, decidua, chorionic villi and a placental site reaction. Foetal parts may be identified.

Neoplastic Conditions

The fallopian tube is a relatively rare primary site of neoplastic lesions, both benign and malignant.

Benign tumours: benign tumours of the fallopian tube are rare. They include adenomatoid tumours which are usually firm grey–white or yellow, well circumscribed nodules that involve part of the wall of the tube. A variety of other benign neoplasms, similar to those found within the ovary, may rarely involve the fallopian tube.

Malignant tumours: primary malignant neoplasms of the fallopian tubes are rare with secondary involvement by ovarian or uterine carcinoma more common. Most are serous adenocarcinomas, similar to those which occur in the ovary, although a variety of other morphological subtypes have been described. Because of their rarity, little is known about the aetiological factors in the development of fallopian tube carcinoma. They usually occur in middle-aged or elderly women and are more common in nulliparous women. There is an increased incidence of fallopian tube malignancies in women with BRCA1 and BRCA2 mutations.

Treatment: treatment of malignant tubal neoplasms is usually total abdominal hysterectomy, bilateral salpingo-oophorectomy and omentectomy. Surgical staging is similar to that performed for ovarian cancer, including peritoneal washings. Postoperative chemotherapy is often necessary since tumours are frequently advanced.

Prognosis: the prognosis of fallopian tube carcinoma is generally poor and is related to the advanced tumour stage at presentation.

5. Surgical Pathology Specimens – Clinical Aspects

Biopsy Specimens

Segments of fallopian tube are removed during sterilisation procedures (tubal ligation) performed either via an open approach or at laparoscopy. Tubal or paratubal cysts may be aspirated at laparotomy or laparoscopy or under ultrasound guidance and the fluid sent for cytological examination. Such cysts may also be removed, leaving the fallopian tube intact.

Resection Specimens

Most fallopian tubes submitted for pathological examination are part of a TAH and BSO performed for either benign or malignant disease. Fallopian tube alone may be resected in tubal ectopic pregnancy or where benign cysts or indeterminate fallopian tube nodules are present. When a malignant neoplasm of the fallopian tube is suspected TAH and BSO is usually performed. Fallopian tubes may be removed prophylactically, along with the ovaries, in those with a hereditary predisposition to developing ovarian cancer, e.g., those with BRCA1 or BRCA2 gene mutations.

6. Surgical Pathology Specimens – Laboratory Protocols

Biopsy Specimens

FNA specimens are centrifuged and the specimens examined cytologically, usually with Giemsa and Papanicolaou stains. Tubal ligations are measured, the presence of any gross abnormality noted and a single transverse section is examined histologically to document that the fallopian tube is present.

Resection Specimens

Specimen

The specimen may consist of fallopian tube only or, more commonly, both fallopian tubes are present as part of a TAH and BSO.

Initial procedure and description

- the length (cm) of each fallopian tube is recorded.
- the presence or absence of a fimbriated end is noted.
- if a sterilization clip is present this is documented.
- note the presence of any gross external abnormality, such as cyst, nodule or tumour.
- if the fallopian tube is dilated, the diameter is measured.
- if necessary any gross lesion may be photographed.
- if tumour is present, note the presence or absence of serosal involvement or breach.
- if grossly normal, the fallopian tube is serially sectioned at 3–5 mm intervals.
- the presence of any gross abnormality seen on sectioning, e.g., luminal occlusion, pus, placental tissue or haemorrhage is noted.
- if an ectopic pregnancy is suspected, note the presence or absence of tubal rupture.
- if a tumour is present, the size in three dimensions (cm), the colour and consistency are noted as is the presence or absence of haemorrhage and necrosis.
- if a cyst is present, it is measured and documented as unilocular or multilocular. The relationship to the fallopian tube should be stated. The character of the internal and external surfaces is noted as is the consistency of the fluid.
- fallopian tubes removed prophylactically in those with a predisposition to developing ovarian cancer are serially sectioned transversely at 2–3 mm intervals. The entire fallopian tubes should be examined histologically since small neoplasms which are not visible grossly may be present.

Blocks for Histology

- as stated, fallopian tubes removed prophylactically in those with a hereditary predisposition to develop ovarian cancer should be examined in their entirety.
- a single transverse section is examined in cases of tubal ligation.
- if the fallopian tube is grossly normal, one or two transverse sections are examined in a single cassette.
- any gross lesion, e.g., cyst or nodule, is blocked to show its relationship to the tube.
- in cases of suspected ectopic pregnancy, several sections should be taken (Figure 22.2). Blood clot and placental tissue identified grossly are sampled as is any site of tubal rupture. A section should also be taken from an area of grossly normal proximal tube. If trophoblastic tissue is not identified in initial sections, then extra blocks are taken.
- for malignant fallopian tube neoplasms, at least one block per cm of tumour is submitted for histology. These are taken preferentially from any gross areas of serosal involvement to show the most extensive tumour infiltration. Blocks are also taken to demonstrate origin of the tumour from the fallopian tube. Blocks of uninvolved fallopian tube should also be submitted.
- in neoplasms with a variegated appearance, grossly different areas are blocked.

Histology Report

- side of tumour – right/left or bilateral.
- dimensions of tumour – measure in three dimensions (cm).

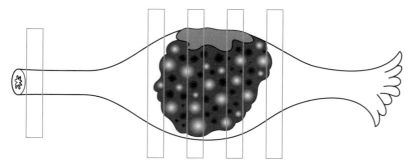

1. Proximal limit
2. Multiple transverse sections of the dilated tube, its contents and any areas of deficiency

Figure 22.2.   Blocking the fallopian tube in an ectopic pregnancy.

- gross appearance – solid/cystic, colour and consistency, presence of haemorrhage or necrosis.
- tumour type – most primary fallopian tube malignancies comprise serous adenocarcinomas.
- tumour differentiation – well, moderate or poorly differentiated.
- extent of local tumour spread – involvement of mucosa, submucosa, muscularis, serosa, surrounding structures.
- lymphovascular invasion – present/not present.
- lymph nodes – sites and presence or absence of tumour involvement.
- involvement of other organs, e.g., ovary, omentum.
- peritoneal washings/cystic fluid – involved/not involved by tumour.

FIGO/TNM Staging

pT1   tumour limited to the fallopian tube(s).
pT2   tumour involving tube(s) with pelvic extension.
pT3   tumour involving tube(s) with metastases to abdominal peritoneum, and/or regional nodes.
pT4   tumour involving tube(s) with distant metastases, e.g., liver parenchyma or positive pleural fluid cytology.

23 Uterus

1. Anatomy

The uterus is situated in the pelvic cavity between the rectum posteriorly and the urinary bladder anteriorly. The body of the uterus (uterine corpus) comprises the superior part and this is joined to the cervix, which comprises the inferior portion of the uterus (Figure 23.1). The length of the uterus varies widely depending on the parity and the menopausal status but generally ranges from 5–15 cm in those uteri which are not involved by any specific pathologic process. The weight of the uterus also varies widely between 20 and 120 g. Multigravid uteri are considerably larger than nulligravid uteri. The uterus is lined by an inner endometrium composed of endometrial glands and stroma. Most of the wall is composed of myometrial smooth muscle. The lumen of the uterus is connected to the lumen of the fallopian tubes. The part of the uterine body above the level of the

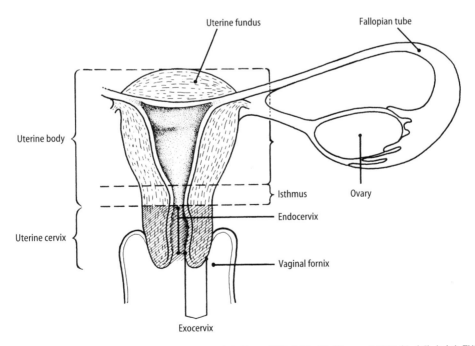

Figure 23.1. Uterine anatomy. Reproduced from Hermanek P, Hutter RVP, Sobin LH, Wagner G, Wittekind Ch (eds.). TNM Atlas: illustrated guide to the TNM/pTNM classification of malignant tumours, 4th edition. Springer-Verlag: Berlin and Heidelberg, 1997.

fallopian tubes is the fundus. The lower portion of the uterus which merges with the cervix is known as the isthmus. The anterior surface of the uterus is covered by peritoneum which reflects forwards onto the bladder. The peritoneal surface extends lower posteriorly before being reflected onto the rectosigmoid. The lower peritoneal reflection on the posterior aspect can be used as a means to distinguish the anterior and posterior surfaces of the uterus. The anterior and posterior peritoneal linings merge laterally to form the broad ligaments which extend to the pelvic side wall.

Lymphovascular Supply

The uterus is supplied by the uterine arteries. These are bilateral paired arteries which arise from the internal iliac arteries. The veins of the uterus drain into the uterovaginal venous plexus which is located within the broad ligament. These veins ultimately open into the internal iliac veins. Uterine lymphatics drain into the pelvic and peri-aortic lymph nodes (Figure 23.2).

2. Clinical Presentation

Clinical features related to uterine pathology are most commonly those of abnormal uterine bleeding. In premenopausal patients this may take the form of menorrhagia (heavy periods), dysmenorrhoea (painful periods) or a variety of other forms of abnormal uterine bleeding. In postmenopausal patients, the most common symptomatology is postmenopausal bleeding. This should always be taken seriously and uterine malignancy excluded. Other symptomatologies related to uterine pathology include a palpable abdominal or pelvic mass, pain within the pelvis or abdomen (often deep seated), a feeling of fullness within the abdomen and uterine prolapse. Uterine pathology may also be associated with symptoms such as constipation, urinary frequency or infertility.

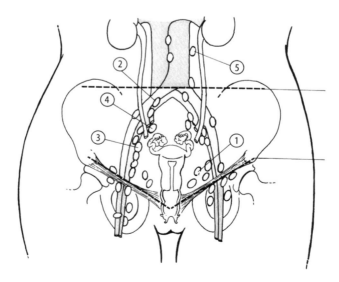

Figure 23.2. Uterus – regional lymph nodes. 1. Hypogastric internal iliac. 2. Comon iliac. 3. External iliac. 4. Lateral sacral. 5. Para-aortic. Reproduced from Hermanek P, Hutter RVP, Sobin LH, Wagner G, Wittekind Ch (eds.). TNM Atlas: illustrated guide to the TNM/pTNM classification of malignant tumours, 4th edition. Springer-Verlag: Berlin and Heidelberg, 1997.

3. Clinical Investigations

Ultrasound scan: transvaginal ultrasound scan is often performed in patients with abnormal uterine bleeding and other symptomatology related to the uterus. This may show focal lesions or diffuse thickening of the endometrium or myometrium. The endometrial thickness can be measured and related to the menopausal status of the patient.

Endometrial sampling: usually sampling of the endometrium to provide material for histology is necessary for a definitive pathological diagnosis, especially in cases of abnormal uterine bleeding such as postmenopausal bleeding. In some centres, endometrial brushings with cytological examination is carried out but this is rare. Previously, the most common means of sampling the endometrium was by dilatation and curettage (D & C). This requires a general anaesthetic and is performed as an inpatient procedure. However, pipelle endometrial biopsies can now be performed as an outpatient procedure without the need for a general anaesthetic. Histological sampling of the endometrium may also be performed in women who are being treated with tamoxifen or those who are infertile.

Hysteroscopy: in many cases, hysteroscopy with direct visualisation of the endometrium is performed and biopsies are taken at this procedure.

MRI scanning: in cases where endometrial sampling confirms a malignancy, radiological staging procedures are carried out and this usually comprises MRI scanning.

4. Pathological Conditions

Non-neoplastic Conditions

Cyclical or non-cyclical endometrium: endometrial sampling may reveal normal proliferative or secretory endometrium or postmenopausal atrophic endometrium. Endometrial appearances can also reflect the use of exogenous hormones or the presence of abnormal levels of endogenous hormones. Non-cyclical endometria may be a manifestation of conditions such as anovulatory cycles or luteal phase deficiency.

Endometrial polyps: endometrial polyps are benign endometrial lesions which often result in abnormal uterine bleeding and are most common postmenopausally. They may be single or multiple. They are often removed piecemeal and should be sampled in their entirety when small. With larger lesions selective pathological sampling is performed. Occasionally, carcinoma arises in a pre-existing polyp.

Endometritis: this is an inflammatory condition of the endometrium which may result in abnormal uterine bleeding. Generally, the presence of plasma cells is required for a definitive pathological diagnosis.

Products of conception: products of conception may be submitted for histological examination from therapeutic or spontaneous abortions.

Neoplastic Conditions

A range of benign and malignant neoplasms can involve both the endometrium and myometrium.

Endometrial hyperplasias: these are a spectrum of preneoplastic conditions which confer an increased risk of subsequent development of endometrial adenocarcinoma. The WHO classification of endometrial hyperplasias is used with hyperplasias categorised as simple or complex in type based on architectural features. These are further subdivided into typical and atypical forms, depending on the presence or absence of cytological atypia.

Endometrial carcinomas: a variety of different carcinomas may arise from the endometrium. There are two main types (type I and type II) although not all neoplasms fall neatly into either category. The prototype of *type I endometrial carcinoma is endometrioid adenocarcinoma* and *type II uterine serous carcinoma.* type I and type II neoplasms have different clinicopathologic characteristics, although it is emphasised that there may be overlap. In general, type II carcinomas behave in a much more aggressive manner. Endometrial carcinomas (especially type I) may be associated with obesity, hypertension and diabetes and with unopposed oestrogen hormone therapy. There may also be an association with oestrogen-secreting ovarian tumours, mainly those within the sex cord-stromal group. Endometrial carcinomas are more common in women of low-parity, high socio-economic status and in the postmenopausal age group. There is some evidence that continuous combined hormone replacement therapy may be protective against endometrial carcinoma. Occasionally, there is a familial predisposition to developing endometrial cancer. Endometrial carcinoma is the second most common neoplasm to arise in patients with hereditary nonpolyposis colorectal cancer.

Type I endometrial carcinomas usually arise in a background of endometrial hyperplasia. This association is not apparent with type II endometrial cancers, which arise within an atrophic endometrium from a precursor known as endometrial intraepithelial carcinoma (EIC).

Endometrial carcinomas may be polyploid in appearance and project into the endometrial cavity. Conversely, some tumours diffusely infiltrate the underlying myometrium.

Uterine smooth muscle tumours: uterine leiomyomas (fibroids) are one of the most common benign neoplasms to occur in women, especially within the reproductive and early post-menopausal age group. They are often multiple but may be solitary. Uterine leiomyomas can be submucosal, intramural or subserosal. Occasionally they may separate from the uterus and lie within the pelvic cavity, so-called parasitic leiomyomas. They are usually well circumscribed, white in colour with a typical firm whorled appearance and bulge above the surrounding myometrium. Degeneration may result in a variety of different gross appearances.

Adenomyosis: adenomyosis is a common condition characterised by extension of endometrial glands and stroma into the underlying myometrium. Usually this results in diffuse uterine enlargement although occasionally well-circumscribed nodular masses are formed, so-called adenomyomas. Typically, adenomyosis results in a trabeculated appearance to the myometrium because of the associated smooth-muscle hypertrophy around the pale or haemorrhagic adeno-myotic foci. Adenomyosis is most common in the reproductive age group and is thought to develop under oestrogenic influence. It is a common cause of irregular uterine bleeding.

Malignant uterine mesenchymal lesions: malignant uterine mesenchymal lesions comprise endometrial stromal sarcomas, leiomyosarcomas and undifferentiated uterine sarcomas. Endometrial stromal sarcomas usually cause diffuse uterine enlargement due to infiltration of the myometrium by irregular tongues of neoplastic endometrial stromal cells. There is often marked vascular permeation and the tumour may extend beyond the uterus. Leiomyosarcomas and undifferentiated uterine sarcomas are generally high-grade malignant neoplasms, usually comprising a dominant mass with or without satellite nodules. Grossly, areas of haemorrhage and necrosis are common.

Other uterine neoplasms: endometrial stromal nodules are benign, well-circumscribed proliferations of endometrial stroma. Histologically, they are identical to endometrial stromal sarcomas and are differentiated from the latter due to their circumscription and lack of infiltrative myometrial permeation or vascular invasion. They may involve both the endometrium and myometrium or may be predominantly located within the myometrium.

Uterine carcinosarcomas (Malignant Mixed Mullerian Tumours) are highly aggressive neoplasms composed of carcinomatous and sarcomatous elements. Although traditionally regarded as a subtype of uterine sarcoma there is now ample evidence that these are, in fact, metaplastic carcinomas. They are usually bulky neoplasms in elderly patients, often with a polyploid appearance and exhibiting deep myometrial infiltration and vascular invasion.

Treatment: treatment of malignant uterine lesions (carcinomas, sarcomas, carcinosarcomas) usually comprises total abdominal hysterectomy and bilateral salpingo-oophorectomy. Peritoneal washings are performed as part of the staging procedure. Lymph nodes may be sampled, especially when preoperative endometrial biopsy shows a high-grade endometrioid or serous carcinoma or when radiological investigations suggest deep myometrial invasion or extrauterine spread. Preoperative staging comprises MRI scanning to assess the extent of tumour spread. Postoperative radiotherapy or chemotherapy is often needed. This is especially so with high-grade or Type II endometrial carcinomas or where there is cervical involvement or deep myometrial penetration. The FIGO staging system for endometrial carcinoma is used. Occasionally with advanced tumours, surgical resection is not feasible and primary treatment is radiotherapy or chemotherapy. Adjuvant treatment of all malignancies should be discussed at a multidisciplinary gynaecological oncology meeting.

Uterine leiomyomas may be treated by total abdominal hysterectomy or, in those who wish to preserve their fertility, medical treatment or myomectomy (simple removal of the fibroids). Adenomyosis is often not expected clinically and is only diagnosed on a hysterectomy specimen performed for menorrhagia.

Troublesome menorrhagia can in most cases be managed by endometrial ablation (balloon dilatation, laser ablation or hysteroscopic resection) with resort to simple hysterectomy in a minority of cases with post-ablation recurrence of symptoms.

Prognosis: the prognosis of low-grade, early-stage (Stage Ia or Ib) endometrial adenocarcinoma of endometrioid type is excellent but overall survival decreases with increasing tumour stage. Prognosis is also poor with Type II endometrial adenocarcinomas, especially uterine serous carcinoma. Leiomyosarcoma, undifferentiated uterine sarcoma and carcinosarcoma usually have a poor prognosis, especially if large and of advanced stage. Endometrial stromal sarcomas are usually low-grade neoplasms. The overall prognosis is usually favourable although there is a significant risk of late recurrence after many years and subsequent metastasis with these tumours. Adjuvant progesterone therapy may be indicated, since these tumours may be hormone responsive.

5. Surgical Pathology Specimens – Clinical Aspects

Biopsy Specimens

Endometrium pipelle biopsies may be performed blind or under hysteroscopic visualisation. Endometrial dilatation and curettage (D & C) is performed under general anaesthetic. Tissue from therapeutic abortions (performed at D & C) or spontaneous abortions may also be received.

Resection Specimens

The endometrium and superficial myometrium may be removed as multiple chippings at transcervical resection of the endometrium (TCRE). Most uterine specimens comprise a hysterectomy, performed either abdominally or vaginally. Occasionally the cervix is left behind. This is known as a subtotal hysterectomy. The ovaries and fallopian tubes may also be removed with the uterus and cervix. If the uterus is being removed as part of a tumour operation then peritoneal washings should also be sent. Sometimes for uterine fibroids, myomectomy is performed where the fibroid is removed but the uterus is left in situ. A radical hysterectomy is often indicated for cervical cancer or for endometrial cancer involving the cervix. This also involves removing a segment of vagina and the parametrium on both lateral aspects of the uterus.

6. Surgical Pathology Specimens – Laboratory Protocols

Biopsy Specimens

Endometrial pipelle or curettage biopsies are weighed and processed intact for histopathogical examination. Very scanty pipelle samples may need to be filtered from the fixative. Similarly, TCRE chippings are weighed and all examined. If histology of these samples shows the presence of fat it may be omental in origin and implies potential perforation of the uterine wall. The clinician should be alerted without delay. For suspected products of conception, the specimen is weighed and the tissue is examined grossly with particular reference to the presence of blood clot, decidua, placental tissue and foetal parts. Small specimens can be examined in their entirety but with larger specimens representative sections are taken in order to confirm the presence of products of conception. When vesicles are identified, note their maximum diameter – if 2–3 mm or more this raises the possibility of a molar pregnancy and extensive sampling is required in order to confirm the presence of a hydatidiform mole and distinguish a partial from a complete mole. Flow cytometric examination or image cytometry of such specimens may be indicated since partial moles are often triploid whereas complete moles and hydropic abortions are usually diploid. A small minority of molar gestations leads to persistent trophoblastic disease and rarely choriocarcinoma or placental site trophoblastic tumour.

Resections Specimens

The uterus is usually removed together with the cervix as part of a hysterectomy. Occasionally the cervix is left in situ and a subtotal hysterectomy is performed. Myomectomies may also be performed, especially for uterine fibroids.

Initial procedure and description

- the specimen is weighed (g).
- the specimen is measured in three dimensions (cm), i.e., superior to inferior, medial to lateral, anterior to posterior.
- the specimen is orientated. The peritoneal reflection extends lower on the posterior aspect of the uterus than anteriorly.
- ovaries and tubes, if present, are inspected and dealt with as described previously.
- the presence of any external abnormality is noted, e.g., tumour infiltration, serosal adhesions.
- the os of the cervix and the uterine cavity are entered using a probe.
- cutting along the probe, the uterus is opened longitudinally either along the lateral axis or along the anteroposterior axis from the external os to the cornu.
- the nature of the endometrium is commented on. The thickness can be measured and the presence of tumour, polyp or any focal lesion described and measured (cm).
- the presence or absence of uterine fibroids is noted. These are counted and the dimensions of the largest stated. Usually, uterine fibroids have a typical white whorled appearance and bulge above the surrounding myometrium. The presence of any grossly abnormal areas such as haemorrhage, necrosis, calcification or cystic degeneration is recorded.
- any cervical abnormalities are noted as described in Chapter 24.
- if a tumour is present the dimensions are measured. If this comprises an endometrial carcinoma (usually known from a previous biopsy specimen) then the depth of myometrial invasion is ascertained (inner or outer half) as is the presence or absence of gross cervical involvement. Assessment of myometrial invasion can be difficult as these uteri are often atrophic with a thin, compressed myometrium. Look for pale tumour tissue disrupting the

intramyometrial line of vessels. Any obvious spread to the ovaries or fallopian tubes is documented.
- the presence of tumour infiltrating to the serosal surface of the uterus is also noted and in those tumours which do not extend to the serosal surface the minimum thickness of uninvolved myometrium is measured (mm).
- the presence of grossly visible foci of adenomyosis is recorded.
- the uterus is then sliced either transversely or longitudinally (depending on personal preference) at 3–5 mm intervals. During this procedure the presence of previously unidentified leiomyomas and the depth of invasion of endometrial carcinomas into the myometrium can be better assessed.
- photography may be undertaken.
- myomectomy specimens are enumerated, weighed, measured and described.

Blocks for histology

- when the hysterectomy was performed for benign disease, two representative sections showing the endometrial–myometrial junction and if possible the full wall thickness are examined. Two blocks of cervix showing the transformation zone (one from the anterior and one from the posterior lip) are also taken (Figure 23.3).
- when grossly visible adenomyosis is present this is sampled.
- if leiomyomas are present and these are grossly typical, one or two represenative sections suffice. If there are multiple leiomyomas, not all need to be examined microscopically.
- if there are areas of haemorrhage or necrosis within a leiomyoma or if any unusual gross findings are present, then extensive sampling should be undertaken, especially from the periphery of the lesion.
- with endometrial carcinomas, multiple sections are examined (Figure 23.4). They are taken to show the deepest point of myometrial infiltration, and also from uninvolved endometrium to assess the presence of coexistent hyperplasia.
- sections are taken from the cervix from any gross areas of cervical involvement. When this is not seen take three or four representative sections of the lower uterine segment and cervix.
- any grossly visible endometrial polyps are sampled.
- when there is a history of endometrial hyperplasia the endometrium should be examined in its entirety to assess the worst degree of hyperplasia and to evaluate the presence of a coexistent adenocarcinoma.
- ovaries and tubes, when grossly normal, are examined as per a benign protocol.
- any lymph nodes are examined in their entirety.

Histopathology report

- site of tumour within the uterus – fundus, body, lower uterine segment.
- size of tumour – measure in three dimensions (cm).
- gross appearance of tumour – polypoid or infiltrative. Colour and consistency. Presence or absence of haemorrhage and necrosis.
- tumour type – a variety of different adenocarcinomas arise in the endometrium. It is not acceptable to simply render a diagnosis of adenocarcinoma. The type of the adenocarcinoma should be stated.
- tumour differentiation – endometrial carcinomas of endometrioid and mucinous types are graded as Grade I–III (FIGO grading system). This depends on architectural and cytological features. Some of the special morphological subtypes such as uterine serous carcinoma and clear cell carcinoma are not graded since these are automatically high-grade tumours.

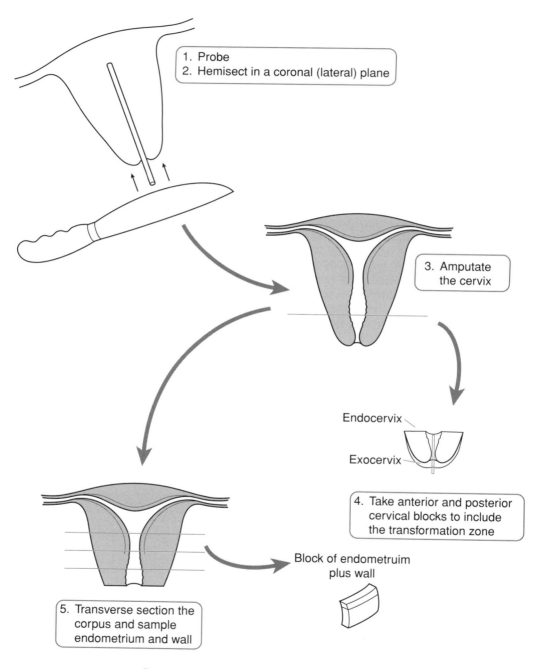

1. Probe
2. Hemisect in a coronal (lateral) plane

3. Amputate the cervix

Endocervix

Exocervix

4. Take anterior and posterior cervical blocks to include the transformation zone

Block of endometruim plus wall

5. Transverse section the corpus and sample endometrium and wall

Figure 23.3. Blocking a routine hysterectomy specimen.

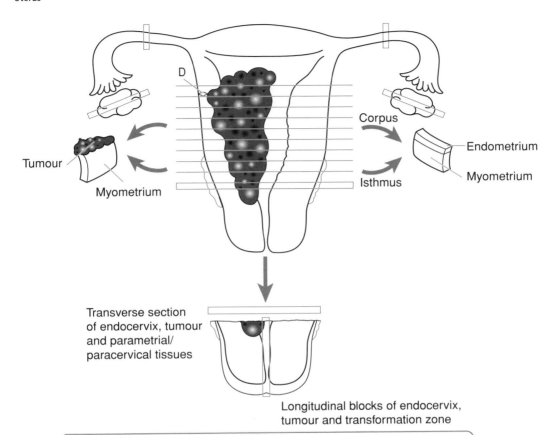

D

Corpus

Tumour

Myometrium

Endometrium

Isthmus

Myometrium

Transverse section
of endocervix, tumour
and parametrial/
paracervical tissues

Longitudinal blocks of endocervix,
tumour and transformation zone

1. Process adnexae
2. Probe and hemisect laterally
3. Amputate cervix and block
4. Transverse section corpus and isthmus
D = distance of deepest extent of tumour to nearest part of the serosa (mm)

Figure 23.4. Blocking a hysterectomy for uterine carcinoma.

- myometrial invasion – presence or absence of myometrial invasion. If present – confined to inner half or involves outer half.
- lymphovascular invasion – present/not present.
- lymph nodes – mention sites, number identified and presence or absence of tumour involvement.
- cervical involvement – presence or absence of involvement of the endocervical glands and stroma.
- serosal involvement – present/not present.
- measure minimum distance (mm) from the deepest point of myometrial infiltration by tumour to the serosa.
- surrounding endometrium – presence or absence and type of hyperplasia.

- other pathology – the presence of coexistent pathology should be mentioned.
- peritoneal washings – presence or absence of tumour cells.
- ovary and fallopian tube – presence or absence of tumour metastasis. Note that, especially with endometrioid tumours, synchronous neoplasms may be present within both the ovary and endometrium.

FIGO/TNM Staging

pTis carcinoma in situ.
pT1   tumour confined to the corpus:
    a.   limited to the endometrium,
    b.   invades less than half of the myometrium,
    c.   invades more than half of the myometrium.
pT2   tumour invades corpus and cervix:
    a.   endocervical glands only,
    b.   cervical stroma.
pT3   outside the uterus but not outside the true pelvis:
    a.   serosa and/or adnexae, and/or malignant cells in ascites/peritoneal washings,
    b.   vaginal disease (direct extension or metastasis).
pT4   extends outside the true pelvis or has obviously involved the mucosa of the bladder or rectum.

Regional nodes: pelvic (obturator and internal iliac), common and external iliac, parametrial, sacral and para-aortic.

pN0   no regional lymph nodes involved.
pN1   metastasis in regional lymph node(s).

24 Cervix

1. Anatomy

The cervix is joined to the body of the uterus and usually measures 2.5 to 3 cm in length. The bladder is situated anteriorly and is separated from the cervix by loose connective tissue. On the posterior aspect the upper cervix is covered by peritoneum. Part of the cervix lies within the vagina and is surrounded by a reflection of the vaginal wall called the fornix. The ectocervix (outer cervix) is covered by non-keratinising stratified squamous epithelium and the endocervix (inner cervix) is lined by a single layer of mucin-secreting epithelial cells. The junction between the two is known as the transformation zone (Figure 23.1).

Lymphovascular drainage

The blood supply to the cervix is from the uterine artery. As the uterine artery approaches the cervix it divides into ascending and descending branches. The descending branch supplies the cervix and upper vagina. The veins of the cervix drain to the uterovaginal plexus in the base of the broad ligament. Cervical lymphatics drain into small perforating lymphatic vessels which eventually leave the cervix via two main vessels which are closely opposed to the uterine arteries. These drain into pelvic lymph nodes. The pelvic lymph nodes which the cervical lymphatics drain into are the external iliac nodes, the internal iliac nodes and the common iliac nodes (Figure 24.1).

2. Clinical Presentation

A variety of dysplastic preinvasive lesions, of both squamous and glandular type, are commonly encountered within the cervix. These are usually picked up because of an abnormal cervical smear, performed in the United Kingdom as part of the NHS cervical screening programme. These abnormalities are often associated with and due to infection by human papilloma virus (HPV). Other symptoms related to cervical pathology include watery vaginal discharge and postcoital and intermenstrual bleeding. With advanced cervical tumours invading the bladder or rectum there may be urinary or bowel symptoms. Large tumours can protrude through the external cervical os into the vagina. Small cervical tumours may be asymptomatic. With advanced tumours the ureters can become obstructed with resultant hydronephrosis and renal failure – lymphoedema and deep venous thrombosis may also occur.

3. Clinical Investigations

Most preinvasive dysplastic lesions are picked up because of an abnormal cervical smear. When a significant cytological abnormality is identified patients are referred to a gynaecologist for

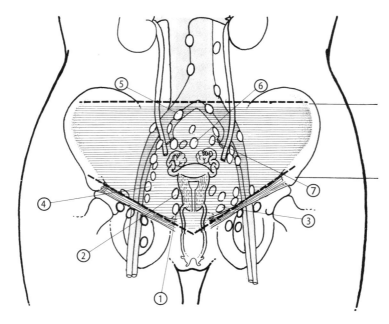

Figure 24.1.   Cervix – regional lymph nodes. 1. Paracervical nodes. 2. Parametrial nodes. 3. Hypogastric (internal iliac) including obdurator nodes. 4. External iliac nodes. 5. Common iliac nodes. 6. Presacral nodes. 7. Lateral sacral nodes. Reproduced from Hermanek P, Hutter RVP, Sobin LH, Wagner G, Wittekind Ch (eds.). TNM Atlas: illustrated guide to the TNM/pTNM classification of malignant tumours, 4th edition. Springer-Verlag: Berlin and Heidelberg, 1997.

colposcopy. This involves looking at the cervix under a special microscope (colposcope) and often taking a biopsy or performing local excision of an abnormal area of cervix (loop or cone biopsy). These areas are identified by their lack of uptake of iodine stain (acetowhite epithelium – AWE) and abnormal surface appearances (e.g., vascular punctation or a mosaic pattern). HPV testing may also be undertaken and involves molecular testing of material taken at a cervical smear. In patients with cervical discharge material may be sent for microbiological investigations. In cases of cervical tumour, radiological investigation, usually in the form of MRI, is carried out for staging purposes.

4. Pathological Conditions

Non-neoplastic Conditions

A variety of benign non-neoplastic conditions occur within the cervix. The chief importance of these is their potential for misdiagnosis as cervical intraepithelial neoplasia (CIN) or cervical glandular intraepithelial neoplasia (CGIN). These conditions include reserve cell hyperplasia, immature and mature squamous metaplasia, inflammatory induced atypia, tubal and tuboendometrial metaplasia, endometriosis and microglandular hyperplasia. Mesonephric remnants, when present within the cervix, may also lead to diagnostic problems.

Neoplastic Conditions

The two main malignant neoplasms to occur within the cervix are invasive squamous cell carcinoma and adenocarcinoma. Mainly due to the advent of organised screening programmes, precursor lesions (CIN and CGIN) are identified much more commonly by cytology and the incidence of invasive cervical tumours is decreasing.

Cervical Intraepithelial Neoplasia (CIN): CIN is the preferred designation in the UK for the spectrum of dysplastic preinvasive squamous lesions which are associated with an increased risk of the subsequent development of cervical squamous carcinoma. These usually arise at the transformation zone of the cervix and are divided into CINI, CINII and CINIII (previously known as mild, moderate and severe dysplasia respectively). Morphological changes associated with HPV infection are termed koilocytosis. In some countries koilocytosis and CINI are collectively termed low-grade squamous intraepithelial lesion (LSIL) while CINII and CINIII are designated high-grade squamous intraepithelial lesion (HSIL). The transition from CINI to CINIII may take many years and all grades of CIN may revert to normal, especially CINI. The aim of cervical screening is to pick these lesions up in the preinvasive stage. Treatment then reduces the risk of development of squamous carcinoma.

Cervical Glandular Intraepithelial Neoplasia (CGIN): similar to the situation with CIN, preinvasive glandular lesions may be encountered. These are much rarer than the corresponding squamous lesions and are less likely to be picked up on cytological examination. They often coexist with squamous lesions. In the UK the preferred designation is cervical glandular intraepithelial neoplasia (CGIN). These are divided into low-grade and high-grade CGIN. The WHO classification uses the terms glandular dysplasia (atypical hyperplasia) and adenocarcinoma in-situ, corresponding to low-grade and high-grade CGIN respectively. Many of these lesions are associated with HPV infection.

Invasive tumours: approximately 70–80% of invasive carcinomas of the cervix are squamous cell in type. Most of the remainder are adenocarcinomas. Rarer morphological subtypes include adenosquamous carcinoma and neuroendocrine small cell carcinoma. A variety of other malignant tumours occur within the cervix but these are rare.

The main risk factor in the development of both squamous carcinoma and adenocarcinoma of the cervix is infection with HPV. There may be an association with oral contraceptive use and cervical adenocarcinoma. Other factors implicated in the pathogenesis of cervical cancer, including early age at first intercourse, multiple sexual patterns, etc., are not independent of HPV infection. Smoking is also a risk factor for the development of cervical squamous carcinoma.

Treatment: following referral because of an abnormal cervical smear (or occasionally a clinically suspicious cervix or symptoms such as postcoital bleeding) colposcopic examination is performed. In general, low-grade lesions (koilocytosis and CINI) are treated by local ablative procedures or cytological follow-up while high-grade lesions (CIN II and CIN III) are treated by local excision. Usually this is in the form of diathermy large-loop excision of the transformation zone (LLETZ) of the cervix. Occasionally, cold-knife cone biopsies may be performed, especially if a small invasive carcinoma is suspected or if a cervical glandular lesion is suggested on cytology. With more advanced cervical tumours (usually greater than stage Ia) radical hysterectomy is usually carried out. This involves removing the uterus and cervix with a cuff of vagina. The surrounding parametrium on both sides is also removed and pelvic lymph nodes are sampled. The FIGO staging system for cervical cancer is used. With advanced cervical cancers the initial treatment may be radiotherapy or chemoradiation. This may be followed by salvage hysterectomy at a later date. Whether radiation or chemoradiation is given post surgery for cervical carcinomas depends on careful clinical and pathological staging.

Cone biopsies with careful assessment of margins and cytological follow-up may be performed in patients with early (stage Ia) tumours. Occasionally, in young patients with early stage Ib cancers (usually less than 2 cm) and who wish to preserve their fertility, a trachelectomy may be performed followed by the insertion of a suture into the cervix. Trachelectomy involves a local excision of the cervix with the surrounding parametrium. Pelvic lymph nodes are usually sampled laparoscopically during this procedure. Careful pathological examination is required to ascertain whether further, more radical, surgery is needed. All cases should be discussed at a multidisciplinary gynaecological oncology meeting.

Prognosis: following ablative or local excision of pre-malignant cervical lesions, close cytological follow up is carried out for a period of 5–10 years depending on the diagnosis.

The prognosis of invasive cervical cancers is largely dependent on the tumour stage. Micro-invasive carcinomas (variously defined as stage Ia1 or Ia2 carcinomas) have an excellent prognosis and these may be treated by conservative local excision therapies, usually in the form of loop or cone biopsies. The prognosis of more advanced cervical cancers, as already stated, largely depends on the stage of the tumour, especially the presence of extracervical spread, with an overall five-year survival of about 55%.

5. Surgical Pathology Specimens – Clinical Aspects

Biopsy Specimens

Many biopsy specimens of cervix submitted to the pathology laboratory comprise small punch biopsies performed at colposcopic examination. Cervical polyps are removed following direct visualisation of the cervix. Loop and cone biopsies are local excisions of the cervix, usually performed at colposcopic examination. Wedge biopsies are taken with grossly visible neoplasms, in order to confirm the presence of tumour.

Resection Specimens

In general, with the exception of young women who wish to preserve their fertility, surgical treatment of cervical carcinoma comprises radical hysterectomy with removal of pelvic lymph nodes. Occasionally, simple hysterectomy is performed in women with CIN or CGIN who have other benign uterine pathologies or symptoms related to the uterus or who do not wish to be subjected to regular cytological follow-up.

6. Surgical Pathology Specimens – Laboratory Protocols

Biopsy Specimens

Small cervical colposcopic punch biopsies are examined intact at multiple histological levels. Loop and cone biopsies are measured (each individual fragment is measured in three dimensions), carefully sectioned into multiple serial blocks (Figure 24.2) and the entire tissue examined histologically. Each block is routinely cut into a standard and deeper H and E sections. Further levels can be obtained if histology shows a suspicious area or incomplete correlation with the preceding cytology. Wedge biopsies are measured in three dimensions, sectioned thinly and examined in their entirety at multiple histological levels.

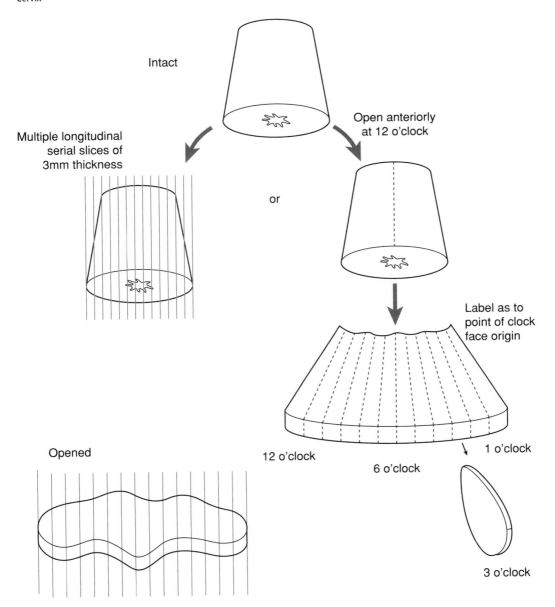

Intact

Open anteriorly
at 12 o'clock

Multiple longitudinal
serial slices of
3mm thickness

or

Label as to
point of clock
face origin

Opened

12 o'clock

6 o'clock

1 o'clock

3 o'clock

Figure 24.2.   Blocking a cervical cone or loop biopsy

Resection Specimens

In cases of cervical cancer (usually greater than stage Ia) the operation of choice is radical
hysterectomy together with pelvic lymph node sampling. Radical (Werdheim's) hysterectomy

involves removal of the uterus and cervix together with a cuff of vagina and the surrounding parametrium. Both ovaries and fallopian tubes are also usually removed although in young women they may be left behind in order that ova may be available for those who wish to have children.

A trachelectomy is performed in young women with cervical cancer who wish to preserve their fertility. This operation is usually undertaken for early stage Ib carcinomas, the carcinoma measuring less than 2 cm in maximum diameter. During the process of trachelectomy local excision of the cervix is undertaken together with the surrounding parametrium, and pelvic lymph nodes are sampled.

Sometimes, simple hysterectomy is carried out for extensive or recurrent CINIII, or in patients with CIN who are symptomatic for other reasons, e.g., dysfunctional uterine bleeding. No uterus should be dissected or reported without full knowledge of any prior endometrial sampling or cervical cytology results.

Procedure, description and blocks for histology in a radical hysterectomy (Figure 24.3)

- the specimen is weighed and the combined length of the uterus and cervix measured.
- the external surface of the uterus and cervix are carefully evaluated to ascertain whether there is any tumour infiltration.
- at this stage the serosal surface of the uterus and the external surface of the cervix together with the vaginal resection margin can be inked. Different colours of ink may be used to designate right and left lateral, anterior and posterior. Care should be taken so that the ink does not contaminate other surfaces, especially on sectioning.
- the vaginal limit is sectioned in its entirety and processed for histological examination. Scissors are useful for obtaining these blocks.
- the cervix is detached from the uterus by a complete transverse cut. A parallel slice from the proximal limit of the amputated cervix provides blocks of right and left parametrium, which should be inspected for the presence or absence of tumour and lymph nodes.
- the cervix is opened longitudinally and the presence of any gross tumour noted.
- if a tumour is apparent it is measured in three dimensions (cm) and its site stated (anterior, posterior, left lateral, right lateral, etc.).
- if a gross tumour is identified, representative longitudinal sections are examined, a minimum of one from each quadrant depending on the tumour location and distortion of the cervical anatomy. These are taken to show the deepest point of infiltration into the underlying cervical stroma and the relationship of the tumour to the closest margins. Blocks are labelled as to their site of origin.
- if no tumour is seen grossly then the entire cervix should be sectioned and examined histologically. Sections are labelled as to what part of the cervix they are taken from; e.g., 1 to 12 o'clock, with 12 being from the anterior lip of the cervix.
- two sections are taken from the lower uterine segment to assess the presence or absence of spread of tumour into the lower uterus.
- the uterus is carefully examined and if unremarkable sampled as per a benign protocol.
- the ovaries and tubes are carefully sectioned and if unremarkable sampled as per a benign protocol. It is usually convenient to dissect and block the adnexae prior to the handling of the main specimen.
- photography can be undertaken at any stage in the cutting process.
- lymph nodes are carefully sectioned and labelled as to their site of origin. These are usually dissected and submitted to the laboratory by the surgeon in separately labelled pots.

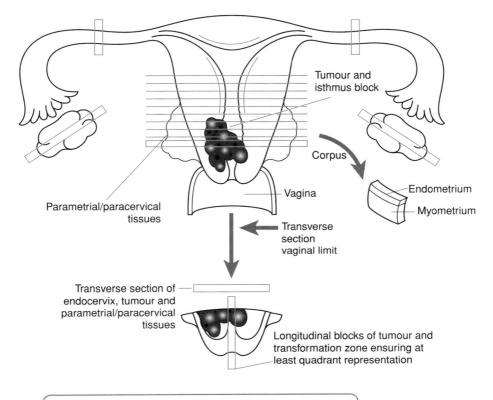

Figure 24.3.   Blocking a radical hysterectomy for cervical carcinoma.

Procedure for dealing with trachelectomy specimens

- the specimen is orientated, weighed and measured in three dimensions (cm).
- the parametrial surface is inked.
- the tissue is serially sliced longitudinally at 3–4 mm intervals and examined in its entirety.

Procedure for hysterectomy with CIN and CGIN

- the cervix is amputated and longitudinally sectioned to give good junctional zone representation. The number of blocks obtained depends on the local cervical anatomy and distortion/stenosis as a result of previous procedures, e.g., LLETZ. Block numbers may therefore range from three to four (quadrants) right up to twelve. They are labelled as to their site of origin. It is better to take fewer blocks with good junctional zone representation rather than many blocks with poor representation.

Histopathology report

- the number of blocks of tumour examined and the site of the tumour are stated.
- the tumour is measured in three dimensions (cm). If this is not possible grossly then it is done histologically. The maximum depth and length of invasion are measured on the slide. It should be remembered that there is a third dimension and this is calculated by taking into account the presence of tumour in adjacent tissue blocks. If a block is taken as measuring 3 mm in thickness then the total third dimension can be calculated on this basis.
- tumour type – most tumours within the cervix are either of squamous or glandular type.
- tumour differentiation – both squamous carcinomas and adenocarcinomas are classified as being well, moderately or poorly differentiated. For squamous carcinomas, the prognostic significance of grading is controversial. Squamous carcinomas can also be classified as large cell keratinising, large cell non-keratinising and small cell non-keratinising.
- the presence or absence of the following are noted:
  - adjacent CIN, CGIN or signs of HPV infection.
  - vaginal, paracervical or parametrial soft tissue tumour involvement.
  - tumour at the circumferential limit (state anterior, posterior, right or left lateral), or if clear, the minimum distance (mm) from it (Figure 24.4).
  - vaginal limit involvement.
  - lymphovascular permeation.
  - lymph node involvement (site, intraparenchymal or extracapsular spread).
  - response to preoperative chemoradiation.
  - uterine involvement, although this does not affect the staging of cervical cancer.
  - coexisting pathology in other organs, e.g., vaginal HPV or VAIN.
- for tumours confined to the cervix note the minimum distance (mm) from the tumour to the external cervical surface (Figure 24.4) and state which aspect of the cervix.
- when local excision is performed for a small invasive cancer, record the tumour distance (mm) to the ectocervical, endocervical and deep limits.

FIGO/TNM Staging

pTis carcinoma in situ (= CIN III or adenocarcinoma in situ/high-grade CGIN).
pT1 carcinoma confined to the uterus.
   1A   lesions detected only microscopically; maximum size 5 mm deep and 7 mm across; venous or lymphatic permeation does not alter the staging.
      1A1 $\leq$ 3 mm deep, $\leq$ 7 mm horizontal axis.
      1A2 3 mm < tumour depth $\leq$ 5 mm, $\leq$ 7 mm horizontal axis.
   1B   clinically apparent lesions confined to the cervix or preclinical lesions larger than stage 1A (occult carcinoma).
      1B1 clinical lesions no greater than 4 cm in size.
      1B2 clinical lesions greater than 4 cm in size.
pT2 invasive carcinoma extending beyond the uterus but has not reached either lateral pelvic wall. Involvement of upper two-thirds of vagina, but not lower third.
   a.   without parametrial invasion.
   b.   with parametrial invasion.
pT3 a.   invasive carcinoma extending to either lower third of vagina and/or
   b.   lateral pelvic wall and/or causes hydronephrosis/non-functioning kidney.
pT4 invasive carcinoma involving urinary bladder mucosa and/or rectum or extends beyond the true pelvis.

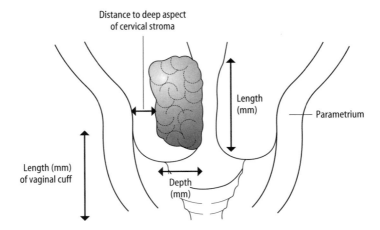

Width (mm) = sum of involved serial blocks of standard thickness
Tumour volume (mm^3) can be estimated by length x depth x width

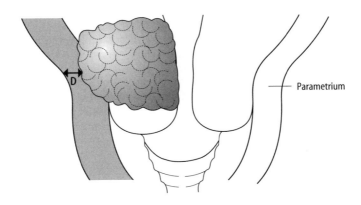

D = tumour distance (mm) to the Circumferential
Radial Margin (CRM) of excision of
the parametrium

Figure 24.4. Cervical carcinoma – tumour dimensions and margins. Reproduced from Allen DC. Histopathology Reporting: Guidelines for Surgical Cancer. Springer-Verlag: London, 2000.

Regional nodes: paracervical, parametrial, hypogastric (internal iliac, obturator), common and external iliac, presacral, lateral sacral.

pN0   no regional lymph nodes involved.
pN1   metastasis in regional lymph nodes(s).

25 Vagina

1. Anatomy

The vagina lies anterior to the rectum and posterior to the bladder. It measures 6–12 cm in length normally. The upper aspect terminates in a circular fold around the cervix to form the vaginal fornices. The vaginal surface is lined by non-keratinising stratified squamous epithelium and the wall comprises fibromuscular connective tissues (Figure 21.1).

Lymphovascular Supply

The descending branch of the uterine artery supplies the upper vagina. The lower vagina is supplied by branches of the internal pudendal artery. The veins of the vagina drain to the uterovaginal plexus, which eventually drains to the internal iliac veins.

The lymphovasular supply of the vagina is closely related to that of the cervix and vulva. Superiorly, lymphatics drain along the uterine artery into the external iliac lymph nodes. In the mid-vagina the lymphatic drainage terminates in the hypogastric nodes while the inferior aspect of the vagina terminates in the inguinal lymph nodes.

2. Clinical Presentation

Primary pathology of the vagina is relatively rare. Symptomatology related to primary vaginal disease may include a mass or feeling of discomfort, vaginal bleeding or discharge, dyspareunia (painful coitus) or postcoital bleeding. Occasionally, primary vaginal disease is discovered at colposcopic examination. Many of the signs and symptoms experienced by women with malignant vaginal lesions are similar to those encountered with cervical cancer.

3. Clinical Investigations

Usually, vaginal tumours can be directly visualised. Dysplastic squamous lesions (known as vaginal intraepithelial neoplasia, VAIN) may be seen at colposcopic examination. With suspected primary vaginal malignancies, pelvic MRI is used to assess the stage of the tumour and the presence or absence of pelvic or inguinal lymphadenopathy. Exfoliative cytology with microscopic examination of cells obtained by aspiration of the vaginal pool is occasionally used in the diagnosis of vaginal lesions, but this practice is not widespread.

4. Pathological Conditions

Non-neoplastic Conditions

Non-neoplastic vaginal lesions are uncommon. A variety of benign cysts may be encountered, usually involving the subepithelial tissues. These include epithelial inclusion cysts, mullerian derived cysts and mesonephric cysts. Fibroepithelial stromal polyps are relatively common. Grossly, these are polypoid lesions covered by unremarkable or hyperkeratotic surface squamous epithelium. Occasionally, following vaginal hysterectomy, the fallopian tube may prolapse and present as a nodule within the vagina. Vaginal granulation tissue may also occur post vaginal hysterectomy. Endometriosis occasionally presents within the vagina and macroscopically is seen as small haemorrhagic areas.

Neoplastic Conditions

Primary neoplastic conditions of the vagina are relatively rare.

Benign tumours: benign vaginal tumours include squamous papilloma and a variety of benign mesenchymal tumours, the commonest of which is leiomyoma.

Malignant tumours: the most common primary malignant tumour by far to arise within the vagina is squamous carcinoma. However, primary squamous carcinomas of the vagina are rare and much less common than spread from a primary tumour arising elsewhere, e.g., cervix, uterus, urinary bladder or rectum. If the tumour also involves the cervix then it is most likely to be of cervical origin. Pre-invasive vaginal squamous lesions also occur. They often coexist with CIN lesions within the cervix and with dysplastic lesions elsewhere in the lower female genital tract, e.g., vulva. They are categorised as vaginal intraepithelial neoplasia (VAIN) and graded I to III, similar to the grading system used for CIN. These may be identified at colposcopic examination during investigation of an abnormal cervical smear. Adenocarcinomas rarely arise as a primary lesion within the vagina. A type of vaginal adenocarcinoma (clear cell carcinoma) may be associated with in-utero exposure to diethylstilboestrol. Other malignant tumours of the vagina include adenosquamous carcinoma, malignant melanoma and a variety of malignant mesenchymal lesions. The aetiological factors in the pathogenesis of vaginal squamous carcinoma are broadly similar to those implicated in the pathogenesis of the corresponding cervical lesions. Previous pelvic irradiation and a history of preinvasive or invasive disease are predisposing factors to squamous carcinomas of the vagina.

Treatment: benign vaginal lesions such as cysts and fibroepithelial polyps are usually removed by biopsy. Benign mesenchymal tumours should be excised preferably with a rim of uninvolved tissue in order to avoid local recurrence. Surgical treatment of early-stage malignant vaginal tumours is radical hysterectomy. Further treatment, usually in the form of radiotherapy or chemoradiation, is then dependent on staging and these cases should be discussed at a multidisciplinary gynaecological oncology meeting. With advanced vaginal tumours, radiotherapy may be the initial treatment. Occasionally, recurrent vaginal tumour may be managed by vaginectomy (colpectomy).

Prognosis: the prognosis of malignant vaginal tumours largely depends on the FIGO staging. Tumours are staged by a combination of clinical and pathological parameters. Clinical assessment includes speculum examination, bimanual pelvic and rectal examinations, cystoscopy and proctosigmoidoscopy. Overall five-year survival is in the region of 40%. Other prognostic factors such as tumour grade, patient age and tumour localisation are of less prognostic significance.

5. Surgical Pathology Specimens – Clinical Aspects

Biopsy Specimens

Small benign polypoid lesions are often removed by biopsy following direct visualisation. In cases of suspected malignancy punch or wedge biopsies are performed to confirm the diagnosis. Cystic lesions and submucosal benign mesenchymal lesions are usually removed with a small rim of surrounding uninvolved tissue.

Resection Specimens

As already stated, in malignant vaginal disease the preferred surgical treatment is radical hysterectomy. This is similar to that performed for cervical cancer.

6. Surgical Pathology Specimens – Laboratory Protocols

Biopsy Specimens

Small biopsies are examined in their entirety. The number of biopsy fragments is counted and the entire specimen is submitted and examined at multiple levels.

Resection Specimens

Radical or Werdheim's hysterectomy involves removal of the uterus and cervix together with the upper vagina. This operation, which generally also involves pelvic lymphadenectomy, is usually performed for stage I disease located in the upper part of the vagina. Otherwise, many vaginal cancers are primarily treated by radiotherapy. Occasional vaginectomy (colpectomy) specimens are encountered.

Procedure and description for radical hysterectomy (Figure 25.1)

- the specimen is weighed (g) and the length of the uterus, cervix and vagina measured (cm). The serosal surface of the uterus and the external surface of the cervix and vagina are inked. Care should be taken so that the ink does not contaminate other surfaces.
- the distal vaginal limit is transversely sectioned in its entirety and processed for histological examination. Scissors are useful for obtaining these blocks.
- on opening the vagina the site of the tumour and its relationship to the cervix is assessed and described.
- the distance of tumour to the distal vaginal limit of excision is measured (cm).
- the tumour is carefully transversely sectioned and the minimum distance from tumour to the circumferential limit measured (mm). The nearest circumferential limit should be stated.
- the deep soft tissue paravaginal margin is sampled for histological examination.
- the presence or absence of cervical involvement is noted grossly.
- sections are taken from the cervix to show its relationship with the vaginal tumour if possible.
- the uterus is sampled as per a benign protocol.
- the ovaries and tubes, if present, are sampled as per a benign protocol. It is often convenient to do this prior to handling of the main specimen.

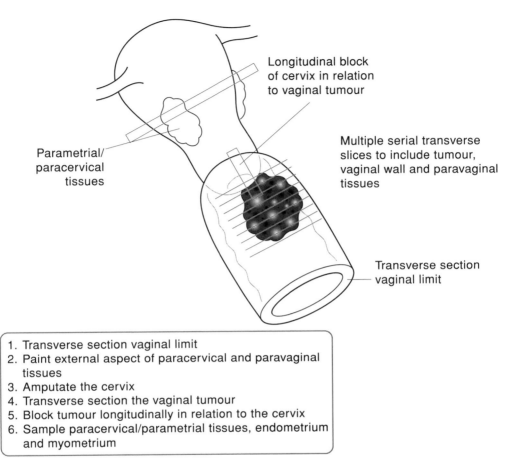

Longitudinal block
of cervix in relation
to vaginal tumour

Parametrial/
paracervical
tissues

Multiple serial transverse
slices to include tumour,
vaginal wall and paravaginal
tissues

Transverse section
vaginal limit

1. Transverse section vaginal limit
2. Paint external aspect of paracervical and paravaginal
   tissues
3. Amputate the cervix
4. Transverse section the vaginal tumour
5. Block tumour longitudinally in relation to the cervix
6. Sample paracervical/parametrial tissues, endometrium
   and myometrium

Figure 25.1.   Blocking a radical hysterectomy specimen for vaginal carcinoma.

- photography may be undertaken at any stage.
- colpectomy specimens: weigh, measure, paint externally, open longitudinally, describe the tumour (its dimensions and distance to the specimen limits), transverse section into multiple serial slices.

Blocks for histology (Figure 25.1)

- multiple representative blocks of tumour are submitted for histopathological examination. These may be taken either transversely or longitudinally but should show the relationship with both the cervix and the nearest circumferential margin.
- the vaginal distal limit is blocked in its entirety for histological examination.
- any lymph nodes submitted are sampled for histology and their site of origin noted.
- as already stated the uterus, ovaries and tubes are examined as per a benign protocol.

Histopathology report

- the site of the tumour (upper, mid or lower; anterior or posterior; left side or right side) within the vagina is stated.
- the tumour measurement is given in three dimensions (cm) if possible.
- tumour type – most tumours arising primary within the vagina are squamous carcinomas. Adenocarcinomas are rarer although they do occur. With an adenocarcinoma, secondary spread from elsewhere should always be excluded, e.g., bladder, uterus, rectum.
- tumour differentiation – squamous carcinomas and adenocarcinomas are classified as well, moderately or poorly differentiated.
- the presence or absence of the following are noted:
    - adjacent VAIN or signs of HPV infection.
    - lymphovascular permeation.
    - lymph node involvement (site, intraparenchymal or extracapsular spread).
    - VAIN or tumour at the distal vaginal limit, or if clear, the minimum distance (mm) from it.
    - paravaginal soft tissue extension.
    - tumour at the circumferential limit (state which one), or if clear, the minimum distance (mm) from it.
    - response to preoperative chemoradiation.
    - coexistent pathology in other organs, e.g., CIN.

FIGO/TNM Staging

pT1   tumour confined to the vagina.
pT2   tumour invades paravaginal tissues but does not extend to pelvic wall.
pT3   tumour extends to pelvic wall.
pT4   tumour invades mucosa of bladder or rectum, and/or extends beyond the true pelvis.

Regional nodes: upper two-thirds – pelvic nodes; lower third – inguinal nodes.

pN0   no regional lymph node metastasis.
pN1   metastasis in regional lymph node(s).

26 Vulva

1. Anatomy

The vulva is lined by skin. Posteriorly it is limited by the anus, laterally by the inguinal folds and anteriorly by the mons pubis. The hymen is the medial aspect of the vulva. The vulva comprises the outer hair-bearing labia majora and inner labia minora, the clitoris and the urethral meatus (Figure 26.1). Mucous glands, including Bartholin's glands, open into the vulva.

Lymphovascular Supply

The internal pudendal artery gives off a branch which provides part of the blood supply to the vulva, which is also contributed to by branches from the femoral artery. The venous drainage follows the arterial blood supply.

The lymphatic drainage of each side of the vulva is largely to the ipsilateral inguinal and femoral lymph nodes although some contralateral drainage occurs. Most of the lymphatic drainage is to

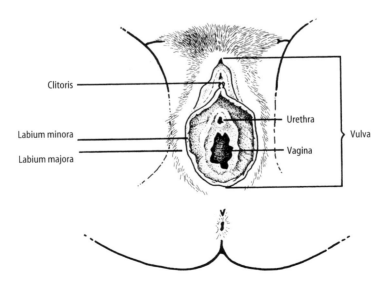

Figure 26.1. Vulval anatomy. Reproduced from Hermanek P, Hutter RVP, Sobin LH, Wagner G, Wittekind Ch (eds.). TNM Atlas: illustrated guide to the TNM/pTNM classification of malignant tumours, 4th edition. Springer-Verlag: Berlin and Heidelberg, 1997.

the superficial inguinal lymph nodes and therefore these are usually the first lymph nodes involved by metastatic tumour in vulval carcinoma. The lymphatic drainage from the clitoris and the midline perineal area is bilateral.

2. Clinical Presentation

The vulva may be involved by a variety of dermatological disorders. Often the main presenting symptom with these is itch (pruritis) or redness. Pre-invasive vulval squamous lesions (known as vulval intraepithelial neoplasia (VIN)) and vulval dystrophies commonly present in this way. Malignant lesions often present with a mass, itching, bleeding or an area of ulceration. There may also be discharge, dysuria (painful micturition) and a foul smell. The most common sites of tumours are the labia majora, the labia minora and clitoris in order of frequency. When tumour has spread to the inguinal lymph nodes a palpable mass may be present and this can ulcerate through the skin and discharge. Lymphoedema and deep venous thrombosis may occur with advanced tumours.

3. Clinical Investigations

Most benign dermatological disorders and VIN are diagnosed by a punch biopsy. Colposcopic examination may be used to directly visualise lesions. Radiological investigations are indicated in staging of vulval cancers in order to ascertain whether regional lymph nodes are enlarged. In some places exfoliative cytology has been applied to the evaluation of vulval lesions but this is not in widespread use. Fine needle aspiration biopsy is of value in assessing enlarged inguinal lymph nodes and confirming a diagnosis of metastatic cancer.

4. Pathological Conditions

Non-neoplastic Conditions

A variety of benign dermatoses may affect the vulval region as with other areas of skin. Non-neoplastic vulval dystrophies (although non-neoplastic they may be associated with vulval squamous carcinoma) comprise lichen sclerosis and squamous hyperplasia.

Neoplastic Conditions

Similar to the cervix, preinvasive dysplastic squamous lesions occur on the vulva. These are known as *vulval intraepithelial neoplasia (VIN)*. They are further categorised as VIN I, II or III. Most malignant tumours arising on the vulva are *squamous carcinomas*. Rarer primary tumours include basal cell carcinoma, adenocarcinoma, Paget's Disease, adenoid cystic carcinoma, small cell carcinoma, malignant melanoma and aggressive angiomyxoma. A variety of benign neoplasms, similar to those occurring elsewhere on the skin, can occur on the vulva.

Vulval intraepithelial neoplasia (VIN): VIN lesions are categorised as grade I to III. There are at least two clinicopathological types of VIN although there is some overlap. Bowenoid VIN occurs in a younger age group and is often associated with similar lesions in the cervix and elsewhere in the lower female genital tract and with HPV infection. Simplex or differentiated VIN may be associated with lichen sclerosis or squamous cell hyperplasia. It occurs in an older age group and is usually not associated with HPV infection or lesions elsewhere in the lower female genital tract.

Vulval squamous carcinoma: similar to the situation with VIN there are two well-defined clinicopathological types of vulval squamous carcinoma, although there is some overlap. The Bowenoid type occurs in a younger age group and is often associated with adjacent Bowenoid type of VIN III. There may be concurrent lesions elsewhere in the female genital tract and there is an association with HPV infection. The other type of invasive squamous carcinoma is usually not associated with VIN, although rarely there may be adjacent differentiated or simplex VIN. It occurs in an older age group and there is usually no association with HPV infection or with lesions elsewhere in the female genital tract.

Treatment: treatment of VIN is usually wide local excision with careful follow-up. There is a risk of multicentricity and the development of further lesions, especially with the Bowenoid type of VIN. Colposcopic examination may be useful in follow-up and patients with the Bowenoid type of VIN should be investigated for lesions elsewhere in the female genital tract, e.g., CIN. Especially when there are multiple lesions and where invasive carcinoma has been excluded by multiple biopsies, laser ablation and other local ablative techniques may be used for treatment of VIN. This preserves the normal vulval anatomy. With extensive VIN, total or partial vulvectomy may be necessary.

For early, low-stage carcinomas of the vulva the usual treatment is wide local excision with ipsilateral lymph node dissection. For very superficially invasive squamous carcinomas (less then 1 mm invasion) lymph node dissection may not be necessary. Local excision of a carcinoma can comprise *simple excision, hemivulvectomy or radical vulvectomy.* In those undergoing radical vulvectomy (usually with centrally located tumours) bilateral inguinal lymph node dissection is usually performed.

Prognosis: the prognosis of VIN is good and is largely determined by the risk of subsequent development of squamous carcinoma. Careful follow-up is therefore necessary. With very superficially invasive squamous carcinomas (less then 1 mm, stage Ia) the prognosis is extremely good and the risk of lymph node metastases is close to zero.

With invasive carcinomas of the vulva, survival is primarily related to the stage of the disease. The most important prognostic factor is the presence or absence of lymph node involvement. Patients with stage I carcinoma have a mean five-year survival of 85%. For stage IV tumours this drops to approximately 10%.

5. Surgical Pathology Specimens – Clinical Aspects

Biopsy Specimens

Small vulval punch biopsies are usually taken for confirmation of the presence of specific dermatoses, vulval dystrophies, VIN or invasive carcinomas.

Resection Specimens

Resections specimens are usually for VIN or tumours and include wide local excisions, hemivulvectomies and radical (total) vulvectomies. With a total vulvectomy all the perineum surrounding the vagina is removed. Inguinal lymph nodes from one or both sides are usually submitted with tumour resections.

6. Surgical Pathology Specimens – Laboratory Protocols

Biopsies Specimens

Small vulval punch biopsies are counted and examined in their entirety at multiple histological levels.

Resection Specimens

Wide local excisions

- these are treated like a skin ellipse. The deep and lateral margins are inked and representative blocks taken to show the lesion in relation to them. Especially with VIN, it may be difficult to assess the presence of a lesion grossly as this can be very subtle. The presence of a previous biopsy site may assist in this regard.

Hemivulvectomies and radical vulvectomies – procedure and description

- hemivulvectomies (or partial vulvectomies) require orientation by the surgeon. If this is not done it may be necessary to contact the surgeon before sectioning is performed.
- a total vulvectomy looks like an ellipse of skin with a central defect corresponding to the vaginal vault. The specimen is orientated. The clitoris is present superiorly and in the midline. The hair-bearing labia majora are present laterally. Inguinal fat, when present, is on the superior aspect of the specimen and to both sides (Figure 26.2).
- if a gross lesion is seen this may be photographed.
- the specimen is inked including the free lateral and deep margins.
- the length, width and depth of the specimen are measured (cm). Diagrams may be necessary and help in reporting.
- if inguinal fat is present on one or both sides this is carefully sectioned, looking for lymph nodes. These are separated and labelled as from the right or left side.
- the presence of any gross lesion is noted and measured in three dimensions (cm). The distances to the nearest resection margins are measured and detailed.
- the presence of any other smaller lesions is documented similar to the main lesion.

Blocks for histology (Figure 26.2)

- multiple blocks are taken of all lesions seen grossly.
- transverse blocks are taken to show the relationship of the lesion to the nearest margins including the lateral, deep and vaginal margins. The margins are labelled on the slide.
- also submit representative blocks of grossly normal skin.
- longitudinal sections of clitoris and any relevant lesion are taken.
- all lymph nodes are serially sectioned and completely submitted. The right and left sided lymph nodes are separated.

Histopathology report

- the site (right, left, labia majora/minora, clitoris) and gross characteristics of the tumour are stated, e.g., polypoid, ulcerated.

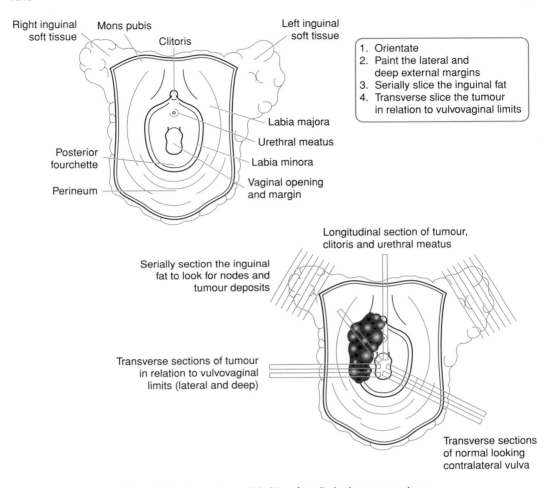

Right inguinal soft tissue
Mons pubis
Clitoris
Left inguinal soft tissue

1. Orientate
2. Paint the lateral and deep external margins
3. Serially slice the inguinal fat
4. Transverse slice the tumour in relation to vulvovaginal limits

Labia majora
Urethral meatus
Posterior fourchette
Labia minora
Perineum
Vaginal opening and margin

Longitudinal section of tumour, clitoris and urethral meatus

Serially section the inguinal fat to look for nodes and tumour deposits

Transverse sections of tumour in relation to vulvovaginal limits (lateral and deep)

Transverse sections of normal looking contralateral vulva

Figure 26.2.   Orientation and blocking of a radical vulvectomy specimen.

- tumour measurements – the width of tumour in two dimensions (cm) is given.
- tumour type – the vast majority of malignant tumours are squamous carcinomas although rarer morphological subtypes may occur.
- tumour differentiation – squamous carcinomas are classified as well, moderately or poorly differentiated.
- depth of invasion – the depth of invasion is measured from the epithelial–stromal junction of the adjacent most superficial dermal papilla to the deepest aspect of the tumour.
- the nature of the invasive component – whether the invasive squamous carcinoma is confluent or exhibits a "finger-like" growth pattern may be of prognostic importance.
- the presence or absence of the following are noted:
  - adjacent VIN (and its grade), signs of HPV infection or associated vulval dystrophy.
  - lymphovascular permeation.
  - lymph node involvement (site, number involved, intraparenchymal or extracapsular extension).

- VIN or tumour at the skin or vaginal margins, or, if clear, the minimum distance (mm) from them.
- tumour at the deep margin, or, if clear, the minimum distance (mm) from it.
- involvement of other structures such as the vagina or anus.

FIGO/TNM Staging

pTis   carcinoma in situ.
pT1   tumour confined to vulva/perineum ≤ 2 cm in greatest dimension.
    a.   stromal invasion ≤ 1 mm.
    b.   stromal invasion > 1 mm.
pT2   tumour confined to vulva/perineum > 2 cm in greatest dimension.
pT3   tumour invades lower urethra/vagina/anus.
pT4   tumour invades any of: bladder mucosa/rectal mucosa/upper urethral mucosa/pubic bone.

Regional nodes: femoral and inguinal.

pN0   no regional lymph node metastasis.
pN1   unilateral regional lymph node metastasis.
pN2   bilateral regional lymph node metastasis.

27 Placenta

1. Anatomy

The term or near-term placenta usually weighs between 400 and 500 g although there may be considerable variation. The placental tissue itself is composed of chorionic villi lined by cytotrophoblast and syncytiotrophoblastic cells. Underlying this is the chorionic plate and placental membranes into which is inserted the umbilical cord. The umbilical cord consists of two arteries and one vein embedded in a gelatinous matrix.

2. Clinical Presentation

In general, not all placentas are sent for pathological examination. There is a variety of indications for placental examination including gross placental abnormalities, foetal death, foetal physical abnormalities, multiple births and maternal problems such as hypertension and diabetes.

Procedure and description for dealing with placentas

- the placenta is weighed and measured in three dimensions (cm).
- the umbilical cord is measured and its insertion into the chorionic plate described (central, eccentric, marginal or velamentous [membranous]).
- the cord is sectioned and the number of blood vessels noted. The normal umbilical cord contains two arteries and one vein. A segment of umbilical cord greater than 5 cm above the placental insertion should be examined as below this the arteries may fuse. Single umbilical cord arteries are associated with a number of fetal abnormalities.
- note the following:
  - the presence of knots within the umbilical cord. If a true knot is present then differences in cord colour and diameter on either side of the knot are present.
  - the state of the maternal surface of the placenta, i.e., whether it is complete or ragged.
  - the state of the membranes, i.e., whether they are complete, ragged, translucent, opaque or dull (suggesting chorioamnionitis) or show meconium staining (this usually has a green colour). White or yellow nodules may indicate amnion nodosum.
- the placenta is carefully sectioned at 0.5–1 cm intervals and the presence of intervillous fibrin, infarcts (these appear as firm white or yellow areas), haematoma or any other focal lesion noted. The percentage of placenta involved by infarcts or haematoma is estimated.
- the presence of any other gross abnormality is described.
- in cases of suspected metabolic disease, the placenta may be sent to the laboratory unfixed and fresh tissue frozen.

Blocks for histology

- three representative sections of placental parenchyma.
- two cross sections of the umbilical cord.
- a membrane roll is prepared by cutting a long strip of membranes and leaving it attached to the placental disk. The membranes are then rolled around the disk and a cross-section is taken.
- any grossly abnormal area is sampled.

Histopathology report

- weight (g) and dimensions (cm) of placenta.
- length of umbilical cord (cm).
- number of vessels within umbilical cord.
- cord insertion – central, eccentric, marginal, velamentous (membranous).
- maternal surface – complete, ragged.
- membranes – complete, ragged, translucent, opaque.
- infarcts – percentage of placenta area involved.
- intervillous fibrin – extent.
- haematoma – volume or dimensions (cm).
- maturity and outline of placental chorionic villi – consistent with gestation, accelerated or delayed, hydropic or molar changes.
- villous oedema – none, mild, moderate, severe.
- chorioamnionitis – absent, present, severity of. It implies ascending genitourinary infection.
- funisitis (inflammation of the umbilical cord) – absent, present, severity of.
- villitis – absent, present, severity of. It implies transplacental maternal infection.
- viral inclusions – absent or present. Immunohistochemistry may be required to confirm and characterise.
- foetal blood vessels – normal, abnormal.
- description of any other gross lesion.

Multiple gestation placentas

Multiple gestation placentas may be of four types.

1. Diamnionic, dichorionic separated twin placentas. These are separated twin placentas. The discs are completely separate. Each placenta is described separately.
2. Diamnionic, dichorionic fused twin placentas.
3. Diamnionic, monochorionic, fused twin placentas.
   - In 2 and 3 there is a single placental disc with two umbilical cords. Common outer membranes are present.
4. Monoamniotic, monochorionic fused twin placentas.
   - There are two umbilical cords but no dividing membrane.

Dividing membranes comprise two amnions and either one or two intervening chorions. Monochorionic membranes (monozygotic identical twins) divide easily whereas dichorionic (from either monozygotic or dizygotic [fraternal] twins) are more opaque and difficult to separate. Membrane distribution is studied histologically from both a non-separated area and the T zone point of attachment to the foetal surface (Figure 27.1). Vascular anastomoses between the two sides are also sought – these can lead to discrepancies in size and viability of the foetuses.

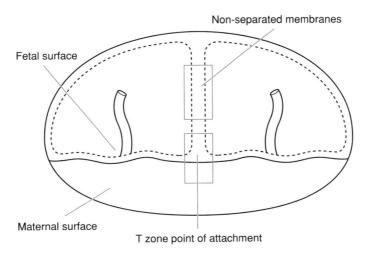

Non-separated membranes

Fetal surface

T zone point of attachment

Maternal surface

Figure 27.1.   Examination of membrane distribution in twin pregnancy.

Placenta creta

This may be subdivided into placenta accreta, placenta increta and placenta percreta. In placenta accreta there is undue adhesion to the myometrial placental bed of the uterus with no intervening decidual layer. In placenta increta anchoring chorionic villi penetrate deeply into the myometrium. With placenta percreta chorionic villi infiltrate right through the wall of the uterus. With these conditions there is a risk of failure of normal postpartum placental separation. With placenta percreta, there is a risk of potentially fatal uterine perforation and haemoperitoneum. All these conditions may be diffuse or focal and the depth of penetration may vary in different areas of the placental bed. They are characterised by no intervening decidua between the uterine bed and the chorionic villi. Predisposing factors include placenta praevia, previous Caesarian section and previous placental retention requiring manual removal. Management of the complications of placenta creta may require hysterectomy.

Urological Specimens

Declan M O'Rourke, Maurice B Loughrey

28

Kidney, Renal Pelvis and Ureter

1. Anatomy

The kidneys are situated in the retroperitoneum and lie between the upper border of the twelfth thoracic and third lumbar vertebrae. Each kidney has a convex lateral border and a concave medial border which merge at the poles (superior and inferior portions). Surrounding each organ is the fibrous renal capsule, which is loosely adherent to it. Adipose tissue (peri-renal fat) encases the capsule and is in turn surrounded by the Gerota's fascia, which secures the kidney to the posterior abdominal wall. Much of the medial border comprises an indentation – the hilum – through which the renal vessels, nerves, lymphatics and the renal pelvis enter or leave the renal sinus, the space enclosed by the renal parenchyma. The right kidney is usually slightly lower than the left on account of the liver. Each kidney is about 11–12 cm in length, 5–7.5 cm in breadth, and 2.5–3.5cm in thickness and weighs between 115 and 175 g (Figure 28.1). The persistence of distinct fetal lobes is common and is a normal anatomical variant.

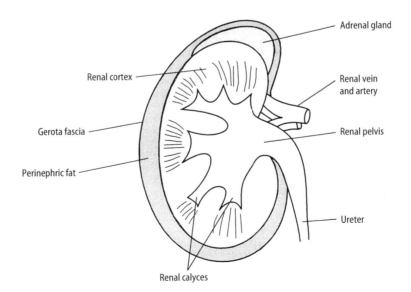

Figure 28.1. Anatomy of the kidney. Reproduced from Hermanek P, Hutter RVP, Sobin LH, Wagner G, Wittekind Ch (eds.). TNM Atlas: illustrated guide to the TNM/pTNM classification of malignant tumours, 4th edition. Springer-Verlag: Berlin and Heidelberg, 1997.

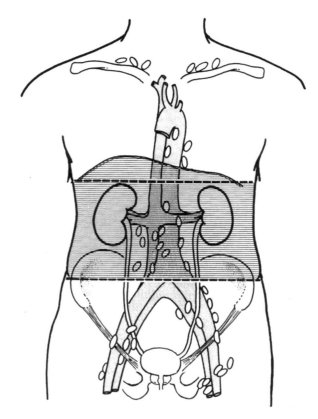

Figure 28.2. Kidney – regional lymph nodes. The regional lymph nodes are the hilar, abdominal para-aortic and paracaval nodes. Laterality does not affect the N categories. Reproduced from Hermanek P, Hutter RVP, Sobin LH, Wagner G, Wittekind Ch (eds.). TNM Atlas: illustrated guide to the TNM/pTNM classification of malignant tumours, 4th edition. Springer-Verlag: Berlin and Heidelberg, 1997.

The relative position of the main structures in the hilum is generally as follows: the vein is in front, the artery in the middle, and the ureter behind and directed downwards. The renal capsule is easily stripped off revealing a smooth and even surface. The parenchyma consists of cortex and medulla that are grossly distinct. The cortex forms a 1 cm layer beneath the renal capsule and extends down between the renal pyramids forming the columns of Bertin. The medulla consists of renal pyramids and is divided into an outer medulla and inner medulla or papilla. The papilla protrudes into the minor calyx. Its tip has between 20 and 70 openings of the papillary collecting ducts (Bellini's ducts).

The renal pelvis is the sac-like expansion of the upper ureter. Two or three major calyces extend from the pelvis and divide into minor calyces, into which the papillae protrude. The ureters measure approximately 30 cm in length equally divided between retroperitoneum and pelvis. They are usually placed on a level with the spinous process of the first lumbar vertebra and run downwards and medially in front of the psoas major and, entering the pelvis, reach the lateral angle of the bladder. Finally, the ureters run obliquely for about 2 cm through the wall of the bladder and open by slit-like apertures into the cavity at the lateral angles of the trigone. Owing to their oblique course, the upper and lower walls of the terminal portions of the ureters become closely applied to each other when the bladder is distended, and, acting as valves, prevent regurgitation of urine from the bladder.

Lymphovascular Drainage

There is a dual lymphatic drainage system. The major lymphatic drainage follows the blood vessels from the parenchyma to the renal sinus, then to the hilum, and terminating in the para-aortic lymph nodes. There is also a capsular lymphatic drainage from the superficial cortex extending from the capsule to the hilum and joining the major lymphatic flow. When tumour spreads from the kidney, it is initially to the hilar and then to the para-aortic lymph nodes (Figure 28.2).

2. Clinical Presentation

Presentations of medical renal diseases are best grouped as nephrotic syndrome, nephritic syndrome, acute renal failure and chronic renal failure. Nephrotic syndrome (NS) is defined as the excretion of more than 3.5 g protein/24 hours associated with hypoalbuminaemia, hypercholesterolaemia, and oedema. Nephritic syndrome is usually characterised by the relatively sudden onset of haematuria with RBC casts and proteinuria accompanied by hypertension, and a reduced glomerular filtration rate. Acute renal failure (ARF) is the loss of renal function occurring rapidly, usually over days. It is characterised by a rapid increase in creatinine and oliguria. Chronic renal failure (CRF) is the progressive loss of renal function, occurring over a period of several years as a result of glomerular or tubulo-interstitial pathology.

Diseases of the kidney and upper urinary tract present with a variety of symptoms including gross haematuria, loin pain, fever or a mass lesion. Causes can be divided generally into congenital (cysts, tumours) and acquired. Of the acquired group these include medical (acute and chronic pyelonephritis) and surgical (stones) causes.

Renal cell carcinoma may remain clinically occult for most of its course. The classic triad of flank pain, haematuria, and flank mass is infrequent (10%) and is indicative of advanced disease. Twenty-five to to 30% of patients are asymptomatic, and renal cell carcinoma is found on incidental radiological study. Other signs and symptoms include;

- weight loss (33%),
- fever (20%),
- hypertension (20%),
- hypercalcemia (5%).

Gross haematuria (67%) is the most common presenting symptom of renal pelvis and ureteric tumours. Pain is the next most common symptom, either in the flank or in conjunction with gross haematuria and, therefore, due to clot colic. Other presentations include pyuria, weight loss, anaemia, unexplained fever, hypertension, renal failure, and calculus disease.

3. Clinical Investigations

- Biochemical studies in medical renal disease (i.e., urea and electrolytes, creatinine clearance, 24-hour urinary protein, plasma protein electrophoresis and Bence Jones urinary protein).

- Intravenous urogram (IVU) – not frequently used in the initial evaluation of renal masses because of its low sensitivity and specificity.
- Intravenous pyelogram (IVP) – in PUJ obstruction reveals a delayed nephrogram that may persist for 24 hours or more. Ultrasound has superceded IVP in children.
- Retrograde pyelography – this tends to be used in two circumstances to confirm the presence of a constant filling defect, either in the ureter or renal pelvis, and to investigate patients with a non-functioning kidney.
- Cystoscopy and ureteropyeloscopy – this procedure is used increasingly for the diagnosis of upper tract urothelial tumours as biopsy forceps or cytology brushings can be used to collect tissue.
- Cytopathology – voided urine samples obtained for cytopathology lack sensitivity, especially for low-grade tumours, but this increases for higher-grade tumours, which tend to shed more tumour cells.
- Contrast-enhanced CT scanning – has become the imaging procedure of choice for diagnosis and staging of renal cell cancer. In most cases, CT imaging can differentiate cystic from solid masses and supplies information about lymph nodes, renal vein and inferior vena cava involvement.
- Ultrasonography – can be useful in evaluating questionable cystic renal lesions if CT imaging is inconclusive. Large papillary renal tumours are frequently undetectable by renal ultrasound.
- Renal arteriography – is not used in the evaluation of suspected renal mass as frequently now as it was in the past.
- MRI – useful in suspected inferior vena cava involvement.
- DMSA/DPTA scans for renal function (more use in paediatric nephrology).
- Doppler scans following renal transplantation to look at renal arterial and venous flow.

4. Pathological Conditions

Non-neoplastic Conditions

Renal stones: nephrolithiasis affects 2–10% of the population and symptoms (renal colic) arise as these calculi become impacted within the ureter as they pass toward the urinary bladder. Types of renal calculi include calcium stones (75%), magnesium ammonium phosphate stones (15%) and cystine stones (2%). Plain abdominal film may diagnose and locate the stone. Treatments include extracorporeal lithotripsy, ureteroscopy, percutaneous nephrolithotomy/nephrostomy, open nephrostomy and, less commonly, nephrectomy (chronic pain, large staghorn calculi, poorly functioning).

Chronic pyelonephritis: refers to renal injury induced by recurrent renal infection in patients with urinary tract obstruction, renal dysplasia, or, most commonly, vesicoureteral reflux (VUR). It is associated with progressive renal scarring, which can lead to end-stage renal disease (ESRD). Intravenous urogram establishes the diagnosis of pyelonephritis and nephrectomy is required in cases with significant morbidity or loss of function.

PUJ obstruction: one of the most common congenital abnormalities of the urinary tract and associated with a number of anomalies. The aetiologies are numerous and classified on an anatomic basis as either extrinsic (scars, VUR) or intrinsic (developmental). Treatment is primarily surgical (pyeloplasty) which now can be performed laparoscopically.

Hydronephrosis and hydroureter: common clinical conditions and major causes include calculi, reflux (children), prostate enlargement, pregnancy and cervical cancer. Although patients usually present with some signs or symptoms, hydronephrosis can be an incidental finding. Grossly, the pelvi-calyceal system is dilated with compression of the papillae and parenchymal thinning progressing to the point at which only a thin rim of parenchyma is present. Intravenous pyelogram (IVP) is probably the most useful imaging study for identifying both the presence and cause of hydronephrosis and hydroureter. Treatments include ureteral stenting, nephrostomy tube and ultimately may require nephrectomy for pain or loss of function.

Pyonephrosis: refers to infected purulent urine in an obstructed collecting system (e.g., stones, tumours, PUJ obstruction) and may develop from ascending infection of the urinary tract or the haematogenous spread of a bacterial pathogen. Similar to an abscess, it typically is associated with fever, chills and flank pain. The diagnosis is usually confirmed with ultrasound. This disorder is relatively uncommon and treatment options include percutaneous nephrostomy and antibiotic therapy. In cases with marked obstruction (± staghorn calculi) and loss of function, nephrectomy may be required.

Xanthogranulomatous pyelonephritis (XGP): a chronic inflammatory disorder of the kidney characterised by a mass originating in the renal parenchyma. It resembles a true neoplasm in terms of its radiographical appearance and ability to involve adjacent structures or organs. Occuring in late-middle-aged females, the exact aetiology of XGP is unknown, but it is generally accepted that the disease process requires long-term renal obstruction (stones, frequently of staghorn proportions) and infection (Proteus or Escherichia coli). The gross appearance of XGP is a mass of yellow tissue with regional necrosis and haemorrhage, superficially resembling that of a renal cell carcinoma. The pathognomonic microscopic feature is the lipid-laden "foamy" macrophage accompanied by both chronic- and acute-phase inflammatory cells. Nephrectomy is the treatment of choice.

Renal cysts: occur in one third of people older than 50 years. While the majority are simple cysts, renal cystic disease has multiple aetiologies. Broad categories of cystic disease include the following: congenital, genetic, acquired, cysts associated with systemic disease (Von Hippel–Lindau) and malignancy (renal cell carcinoma).

The most common larger cysts are acquired cysts, simple cysts, and cysts with ADPKD.

Autosomal dominant polycystic kidney disease (ADPKD): one of the most common inherited disorders in humans, and the most frequent genetic cause of renal failure in adults. ADPKD is a multisystem and progressive disorder characterised by formation and enlargement of cysts in the kidney and other organs (e.g., liver, pancreas, spleen). Clinical features usually begin in the third to fourth decade of life, with the major cause of morbidity progressive renal dysfunction resulting in grossly enlarged kidneys. The kidneys sometimes require removal when complicated by infection, haemorrhage or when they reach a huge size.

Congenital anomalies: anomalies in form, position, mass and number; parenchyma maldevelopment.

Vascular diseases: hypertension, thrombotic microangiopathy, renal artery stenosis, dissection and aneurysm, renal emboli and infarcts, renal atheroemboloism, renal vein thrombosis, vasculitis.

Miscellaneous: other tubulointerstitial diseases, malakoplakia, tuberculosis, metabolic and miscellaneous conditions.

Neoplastic Conditions

Adult Tumours

Benign

Oncocytoma: represents 4% of renal tumours and usually occurs in adults over 50 as an incidental finding. It has a benign behaviour if strict diagnostic criteria are followed. Grossly it is circumscribed, brown–yellow, with a stellate central scar in larger lesions. It may be bilateral or multifocal and can invade the renal capsule. Histologically it has a sheeted or nested pattern of uniform cells with intensely eosinophilic and coarse granular cytoplasm. Patterns not allowed include; papillary areas, clear/spindle cells and vascular or fat invasion.

Angiomyolipoma (AML): represents less than 1% of renal tumours. It is a benign neoplasm composed of blood vessels, smooth muscle and fat and has a characteristic radiological appearance. Usually only one large mass but multiple masses suggests associated tuberous sclerosis. Grossly red, grey–white and yellow it can invade local lymph nodes and renal vein even though benign. It is multiple in one third and bilateral in 15% of cases. It stains immunopositively for HMB 45 and melan-A. Generally asymptomatic, surgical removal is performed only when they exceed 4 cm due to the risk of rupture and haemorrhage.

Other benign tumours: Papillary adenoma, metanephric adenoma, adenofibroma and cystic nephroma represent other less common tumours.

Benign mesenchymal tumours: renomedullary interstitial cell tumour, adult mesoblastic nephroma, leiomyoma, haemangioma, lymphangioma, and solitary fibrous tumour.

Malignant Tumours

Renal cell carcinoma: more than 90% of tumours in the kidney which come to surgery are renal cell carcinomas and these cause approximately 2.4% of cancer deaths. The age is usually > 50 years old with a M:F ratio of 2:1. A number of cellular, environmental, genetic, and hormonal factors have been studied as possible causal factors including cigarette smoking, obesity, hypertension, unopposed oestrogen therapy, and occupational exposure to petroleum products, heavy metals, solvents and asbestos. The risk of renal cell carcinoma is increased with the abuse of phenacetin-containing analgesics, acquired cystic kidney disease associated with chronic renal insufficiency, renal dialysis, tuberous sclerosis, Von Hippel–Lindau disease and renal transplantation with its associated immunosuppression. Prognostic factors include nuclear grade, tumour size, stage and metastases. Treatment usually consists of radical nephrectomy with partial nephrectomy for small (< 4 cm – pT1a) peripheral tumours. Cure is possible even with extension into renal vein, inferior vena cava and right atrium. Chemotherapy is largely ineffective but interferon may be helpful. The overall five-year survival is 45% (all types), 70% if node-negative and 15% if there is renal vein or perinephric fat involvement. Excision of solitary metastases has been found to be effective.

Heidelberg/Rochester classification (1997):

- Clear cell carcinoma 75%.
- Chromophil carcinoma 10–15%.
- Chromophobe carcinoma 5%.
- Collecting duct carcinoma < 1%.
- Renal cell carcinoma, unclassified < 1%.

Renal cell carcinoma, clear cell type: derived from the proximal convoluted tubule, it accounts for 70% of renal tumours. Cytogenetic abnormality includes 3p deletion in 98% of cases and this is considered the initial mutation. It is characterised by a multinodular tumour mass with a predominantly yellow cut surface and additional brown and white foci. Most are solid, but some are composed of multiple cysts varying in size up to 2–3 cm in diameter. Histologically it has compact, tubulocystic, alveolar or rarely papillary architecture. The cells have clear cytoplasm (from glycogen/lipid) and distinct but delicate cell boundaries. A chicken wire/delicate vasculature is common.

Chromophil renal cell tumours: originate from the proximal or distal convoluted tubule and represent 15% of renal tumours. They are associated with multifocal adenomatous change in the adjacent kidney and are bilateral in 10%. Dialysis-related carcinomas are usually papillary.

Cytogenetic abnormalities include trisomy 7 and 17. The five-year survival is > 80%, which is better than clear cell independent of stage. As a rule, chromophil tumours have a papillary or tubulopapillary growth pattern which may appear solid when tightly packed or in undifferentiated areas. The papillary stalks are often expanded by collections of foamy macrophages and psammoma bodies are common. Immunohistochemistry shows positive cytokeratin 7 and variable vimentin staining. Basophilic and eosinophilic variants exist.

Chromophobe renal cell tumours: originate from the intercalated cells of cortical collecting ducts and represent 5% of renal tumours. They are slightly better in behaviour than clear cell when sorted by grade/stage. Cytogenetic studies show multiple monosomies. The cut surface of the fresh specimen appears homogeneously orange and turns tan or sandy after formalin fixation. Histology shows large cells with distinct cell borders and reticular cytoplasm. Some have a perinuclear halo or translucent zone. They are positive with Hale's colloidal iron, cytokeratin 7, EMA and vimentin. Differential diagnosis includes oncocytoma, eosinophilic papillary or clear cell carcinomas (all Hale's colloidal iron negative).

Collecting duct carcinomas: although rare (< 1%) these are usually large tumours located in the medulla or central parts of the kidney with extension into the perinephric fat and invasion of the renal pelvis. The white-coloured and firm cut surface is interspersed with foci of necrosis and the tumour often has an indistinct border with the surrounding kidney because it is infiltrative. Intra-renal satellite nodules and parenchymal infarction are common as a result of widespread angioinvasiveness. Regional spread with infiltration of the ipsilateral adrenal and lymph node metastases are common. The growth pattern is tubular combined with a microcystic and solid pattern associated with an intensive desmoplastic stromal reaction.

Renal cell carcinoma, unclassified: contains morphology not accepted in recognised categories with apparent composites of recognised types; sarcomatoid without recognisable epithelial elements; mucin-producing; mixtures of epithelial and stromal elements; and unrecognisable cell types.

Sarcomatoid carcinoma: 1% of renal tumours and not a distinct histological entity, but due to progressive transformation of different subtypes of renal cell carcinoma. However, most tumours are clear cell carcinomas since they are more common. It is very aggressive with a median survival of 19 months. Grossly it is fleshy, grey–white with infiltrative margins and composed of atypical spindle or tumour giant cells with marked nuclear pleomorphism. It must have an epithelial component (may need generous sampling) and should have sarcomatoid overgrowth of at least one low-power field. It is positive with cytokeratins (focal) and vimentin.

Urothelial carcinoma: upper tract urothelial tumours of the renal pelvis and ureters are relatively rare. Tumours of the renal pelvis account for approximately 10% of all renal tumours and 5% of all urothelial tumours. Ureteral tumours are even more uncommon. Transitional cell carcinoma (TCC) accounts for more than 90% of upper tract urothelial tumours. The mean age of occurrence is 65 years with a male-to-female ratio of 3:1. Aetiological factors are similar to those of bladder cancer. A majority are papillary or exophytic, distending and blocking the pelviureteric system, but if infiltrative the firm, grey–white tumour can involve renal parenchyma causing confusion with other renal cancers, in particular sarcomatoid carcinoma or collecting duct carcinoma. Squamous carcinoma and adenocarcinoma are rare but many form a component of high-grade TCC. The distribution of upper tract transitional cell carcinoma is: renal pelvis – 58%; ureter – 32% (73% of which are located in the distal ureter); both renal pelvis and ureter – 7% and bilateral involvement – 2–5%. Approximately 30–75% of patients also develop bladder tumours at some point in their cancer course.

Nephroureterectomy with excision of the bladder cuff is indicated in patients with renal pelvis TCC, regionally extensive disease, and high-grade or high-stage lesions. Segmental ureterectomy coupled with ureteral reimplantation is a procedure indicated for tumours located in the distal ureter. Renal-sparing surgery, including segmental ureterectomy and endoscopic therapy, is used in patients with small, lower-grade superficial lesions. This approach is used more frequently in patients with one kidney, bilateral disease and compromised renal function. Medical treatment of upper tract urothelial tumours involves the instillation of chemotherapeutic agents mitomycin C or bacille Calmette–Guérin (BCG). It is the most appropriate for patients with multiple superficial disease or carcinoma in situ who also have bilateral disease and/or limited renal function. This appears to be safe as adjuvant therapy, but its efficacy is not firmly established and should thus be considered second-line therapy. Only stage and age are significant prognostic factors and the five-year survival ranges from 91% for stage pT1 to 23% for pT3.

Other cancers: leiomyosarcoma, liposarcoma, haemangiopericytoma, malignant fibrous histiocytoma and metastatic neoplasms (melanoma, lung, other kidney, GIT, breast, ovary and testis).

Paediatric Tumours

Wilms' tumours: comprise more than 80% of renal tumours of childhood, usually in children 2 to 4 years old. There is a slight preponderance of females. Associations with congenital anomalies – cryptorchidism, hypospadias, other genital anomalies, hemihypertrophy, and aniridia – are well recognised. Wilms' tumours are usually large masses; more than 5 cm and solid. They are composed of variable admixtures of blastema, epithelium and stroma. The epithelial component usually consists of small tubules or cysts lined by primitive columnar or cuboidal cells. The stroma may differentiate along the lines of almost any type of soft tissue.

They are divided into two categories: favourable and unfavourable histology, based on the absence or presence of cellular anaplasia, which is found in approximately 6% of Wilms' tumours and can be associated with an adverse outcome. Thus, it is important to sample Wilms' tumour specimens extensively. The usual treatment approach in most patients is nephrectomy followed by chemotherapy (vincristine, dactinomycin, doxorubicin) with or without postoperative radiotherapy (> pT2). With current strategies, survival rates are approaching 90%.

Other paediatric renal tumours: cystic nephroma, mesoblastic nephroma, clear cell sarcoma of the kidney, rhabdoid tumour, metanephric adenofibroma, ossifying renal tumour of infancy, lymphangioma, intrarenal teratoma and uncommon tumours – renal cell carcinoma, lymphoreticular and haematopoietic tumours.

5. Surgical Pathology Specimens – Clinical Aspects

Biopsy Specimens

Fine needle aspiration cytology (FNAC): less often performed now but usually in association with a renal core biopsy in the investigation of a mass lesion.

Percutaneous needle biopsy: this is more often used in the investigation of medical renal disease but is also used for the evaluation of a renal mass. This technique obtains a core of fresh renal tissue using a biopsy gun under radiological (ultrasound or CT) guidance. Medical renal biopsies require special collection procedures and should be done only in centres with appropriate facilities and after consultation with the pathologist. Two to three cores are taken with fresh tissue for immunofluorescence (IF), fixed tissue for light microscopy (some laboratories use special fixatives, e.g., Bouins) and electron microscopy (3% glutaraldehyde). Surgical renal biopsies are routinely fixed in 10% formalin.

Indications for renal biopsy include glomerular haematuria, some cases of proteinuria, and suspected renal neoplasm and following renal transplantation to distinguish rejection from other causes of deterioration in renal function. Interpretation of findings requires expertise in the categorisation of glomerulonephritis and other glomerulopathies (e.g., diabetes mellitus, amyloid, hereditary renal disease), interstitial nephritis and renal vascular disease, monitoring transplant rejection, diagnosis of drug toxicity and systemic disease affecting the kidneys (e.g., vasculitis).

Open renal biopsy: performed under general anaesthesia if core biopsy is not possible and more often in the transplant situation (donor and recipient) when there is uncertainty about the state of the kidney. They often consist only of superficial cortex.

Pelvi-ureteric junction obstruction specimen: The specimen may be funnel shaped if unopened and triangular if opened. The length, diameter at both ends and thickness of the wall are measured and the presence and size of any strictures described. The specimen is opened along the main axis. The mucosal surface is examined for lesions and irregularities in texture. The outer surface is examined for mass lesions and fibrosis. Multiple sections taken along the long axis are submitted.

Resection Specimens

Simple nephrectomy, radical nephrectomy and partial nephrectomy. Laparoscopic nephrectomy is now feasible in experienced hands only.

Simple nephrectomy: is indicated in patients with an irreversibly damaged kidney because of symptomatic chronic infection, obstruction, calculus disease, or severe traumatic injury. It is also indicated to treat severe unilateral parenchymal damage from nephrosclerosis, pyelonephritis, reflux or congenital cystic dysplasia of the kidney.

Radical nephrectomy: is the treatment of choice for patients with renal cell carcinoma (RCC). Radical nephrectomy encompasses ligating the renal artery and vein, removing the kidney outside the Gerota's fascia, the ipsilateral adrenal gland, and performing a complete regional lymphadenectomy from the crus of the diaphragm to the aortic bifurcation. The surgical approach includes either a transperitoneal incision (extended or bilateral subcostal and thoracoabdominal) or an extraperitoneal incision, depending on the size and location of the tumour and the patient's condition. The surgical approach is guided more by individual preference than by necessity.

Removal of the adrenal gland has been advocated because the gland is enclosed within Gerota's fascia and because ipsilateral adrenal metastasis occurs in 2–10% of most reported series. The risk of adrenal metastasis is related to the malignant potential of the primary tumour, its size and position. Patients with large tumours or tumours high in the upper pole probably are better served by a standard radical nephrectomy that includes adrenalectomy.

The role of regional lymphadenectomy in patients with localised kidney cancer is controversial. Because no widely effective treatments are available for metastatic RCC, regional lymphadenectomy may benefit a small number of patients. Extensive nodal involvement is associated with a poor prognosis.

Partial nephrectomy (nephron-sparing surgery (NSS)): recent advances in preoperative staging, specifically modern imaging techniques, and improvements in surgical techniques have made nephron-sparing surgery (NSS) an attractive alternative to nephrectomy in select patients. It allows for optimal surgical treatment and, at the same time, obviates overtreatment and nephron loss when possible. Indications include synchronous bilateral tumours, tumours in a solitary kidney, or the presence of a poorly functional contralateral kidney (e.g., chronic pyelonephritis). Recently, indications for NSS for RCC have been expanded to include a normal contralateral kidney in younger patients with an incidental, localised, single, small (< 4 cm) RCC.

6. Surgical Pathology Specimens – Laboratory Protocols

Biopsy Specimens

Core needle biopsy (renal tumour): this is usually one or two cores which are counted, measured (mm) and processed for initial histological examination through three levels. Careful handling is necessary to avoid crush artefact. When sectioning levels, intervening stained sections may be usefully kept for ancillary immunohistochemical studies if required.

Closed core needle biopsy (medical renal) and open wedge biopsy (donor renal transplant): these small biopsies (10–15 mm long) are all handled in a similar fashion and embedded in total. A minimum of two core biopsies, each containing renal cortical tissue, is recommended to provide adequate material for light microscopy (LM), immunofluorescence (IF) and electron microscopy (EM). Using a microscope, renal tissue can easily be discriminated from fat or muscle. The cores are divided and in certain cases it is reasonable to omit IF or EM to save material for LM. If immediate transfer of biopsies cannot be accomplished, one unfixed portion for IF is sent in phosphate-buffered saline or on crushed ice and samples for LM and EM fixed immediately.

For LM, fixation in buffered formalin is common practice particularly if immunohistochemistry rather than immunofluorescence is required. Fixation with Bouin's fluid is also used for kidney biopsies due to a superior preservation of morphological details. For allograft biopsies and if diagnosis is urgently needed in native kidney biopsies, a frozen section or rapid embedding procedure should be available. Serial 2–3 μm sections are prepared for use in histological and immunohistochemical staining procedures. Stains employed include Haematoxylin and Eosin (H&E), Periodic–Acid–Schiff (PAS), Silver–Methenamine and the Masson trichrome stain.

Immunohistochemistry/Immunofluorescence: for native kidney biopsies the following antibodies should always be used: IgG, IgM, IgA, complement factors (C3, C4 and C1q) and fibrin. Additional antibodies can be necessary (kappa and lambda light chains for light chain deposition disease) and for allografts, antibodies against viral antigens and C4d (humoral rejection). EM has an important diagnostic role in more than 50% of cases and is essential for a correct diagnosis in up to 25%.

Resection Specimens

These specimens include radical nephrectomy, nephroureterectomy, ureterectomy, simple nephrectomy, partial nephrectomy and transplant nephrectomy. They are handled similarly by the laboratory with some notable exceptions as detailed below.

Initial procedure

- palpate and locate the tumour through the perinephric fat.
- if there seems to be a penetrating tumour, ink the surface prior to opening the perirenal fat/capsule. This helps to distinguish true tumour penetration of the perirenal fat and margins from the relatively common finding of elevation of the capsule by a protruding lobulated tumour margin. Ink also the parenchymal kidney resection margin in partial nephrectomy for renal tumours.
- the initial incision should pass through the midline of the kidney in the coronal plane.
- remove the perirenal fat (Gerota's fascia) with blunt dissection from the capsule and examine the surface for adenomas, adrenal rests and other subcapsular lesions.
- in tumours of adults, if parts of the capsule are adherent to the tumour, dissect around them leaving them in place so that they can be taken for histological examination.

- in paediatric tumours the renal capsule and perirenal fat should not be dissected from the kidney and tumour as the capsule retracts when the first cut is made and this may obscure the relationship of tumour, pseudocapsule, renal capsule and perirenal tissue.
- measurements:
    kidney – length (cm), breadth (cm), depth (cm) and weight (g).
    ureter – length (cm) and diameter (cm).
    tumour – length × width × depth (cm) or maximum dimension (cm), distances (mm) from perinephric fat, ureteric and parenchymal surgical margins.
- photograph the bisected kidney.
- next make a series of parallel slabs in the coronal plane at 1–2 cm intervals.
- use the first cut surface to collect tumour and kidney tissue for special purposes (EM, imprints, flow cytometry, cytogenetics, tissue culture, snap freezing, etc.).
- place the entire specimen in a large container of buffered formalin for fixation overnight (24–36 hours).

Description

- Tumour
    ball shaped, uni- or multinodular, uni- or multifocal.
    border: circumscribed, infiltrative, pseudocapsule.
    colour: yellow, grey–white, brown, tan–brown, beige.
    features of the tumour: homogeneous, solid, cystic, papillary, whorls.
    regression: necrosis, haemorrhage, scars (central), pseudocysts.
- surrounding kidney – nodules, other tumours, scars.
- extent of spread – consider the staging criteria (restricted to the kidney, infiltration of the perirenal adipose tissue or the hilar region (renal sinus), macroscopic invasion of hilar veins or pelvis).
- other – look for lymph nodes and dissect the adrenal gland.

Blocks for histology (Figure 28.3 – radical nephrectomy)

- separately label each block and clearly document the exact site of origin.
- sample margin blocks (perinephric fat, ureter, renal vein and artery). Ureteric and vessel blocks may be conveniently taken prior to dissection of the main specimen.
- sample to show relationships between tumour and the radial margin; tumour and adrenal gland (upper pole tumours); tumour and renal pelvis/sinus and surrounding renal parenchyma.
- sample one block from each tumour area that differs in colour.
- one block of tumour per 2 cm of tumour diameter is probably sufficient (minimum of four blocks).
- count and sample all lymph nodes.
- sample the adrenal gland when present (one block).
- sample the surrounding kidney and particularly if any nodules are seen (adenoma, adrenal rests or multifocal carcinoma).
- in transplant nephrectomies, blocks should be taken serially (from without in) of the hilar vessels to examine the nature of the renal vein and artery.
- in nephrectomies for benign disease, samples to be taken include any abnormal area and one random from otherwise normal parenchyma.

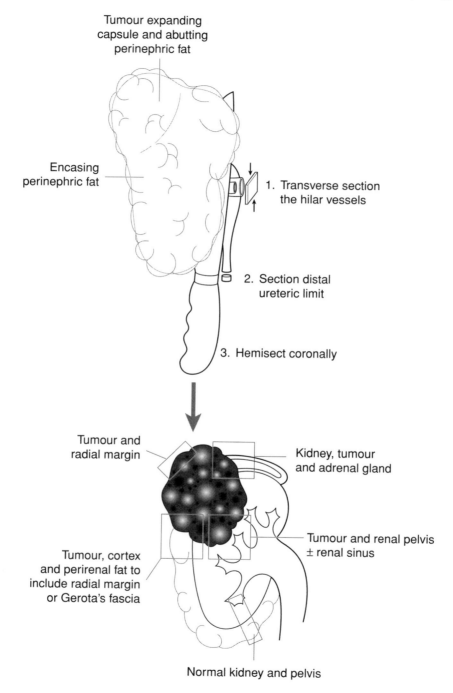

Figure 28.3.   Blocking of a nephrectomy specimen for upper pole renal carcinoma.

Blocks for histology (Figure 28.4 –nephroureterectomy/ureterectomy)

- separately label each block, and clearly document the exact site of origin.
- take one block from each tumour area that differs in colour.
- one block of tumour per 1 cm of tumour diameter is probably sufficient (minimum of four blocks).
- sample to show the relationships between tumour and renal pelvis; tumour, renal pelvic wall and peripelvic fat; tumour, cortex and perirenal fat.
- in renal pelvic tumours sample areas of unremarkable and abnormal mucosa away from the tumour in the renal pelvis and ureter.
- with ureteric tumours, serially section the tumour transversely at 3 mm intervals and sample a minimum of three blocks to assess the deepest point of invasion.
- if ureteric tumour is not seen grossly, sample and correspondingly label unremarkable and abnormal mucosal areas.
- transverse sections of the distal ureteric/bladder cuff margin.
- count and sample all lymph nodes.
- additional sections should include renal pelvis, renal artery, renal vein and ureter.

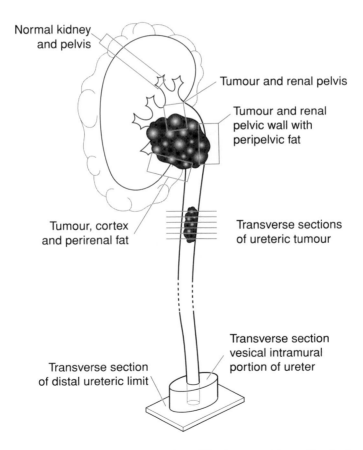

Figure 28.4.   Blocking of a nephroureterectomy for multifocal ureteropelvic transitional cell carcinoma.

- sample the adrenal gland if present (one block).
- sample the surrounding kidney.

Histopathology report

Renal tumours

- tumour type – clear cell/chromophil/chromophobe/collecting duct/unclassified/other.
- tumour differentiation/grade (Fuhrman) – sarcomatoid?

Fuhrman grade
  Grade 1: nuclei round, uniform, approximately 10 μm in diameter; nucleoli inconspicuous or
    absent.
  Grade 2: nuclei slightly irregular, approximately 15 μm in diameter; nucleoli evident.
  Grade 3: nuclei very irregular, approximately 20 μm in diameter; nucleoli large and prominent.
  Grade 4: nuclei bizarre and multilobated, 20 μm or greater in diameter, nucleoli prominent,
    chromatin clumped.

- tumour edge – infiltrative/pushing.
- extent of local tumour spread.
  - pT1 tumour ≤ 7 cm in greatest dimension, limited to the kidney.
  - pT1a ≤ 4 cm.
  - pT1b > 4 but ≤ 7 cm.
  - pT2 tumour > 7 cm in greatest dimension, limited to the kidney.
  - pT3 tumour invades:
    a. perinephric fat, adrenal gland.
    b. renal vein, IVC below diaphragm.
    c. IVC above diaphragm.
  - pT4 tumour invades neighbouring organs, abdominal wall, beyond Gerota's fascia.

- lymphovascular invasion – present/not present. Note perineural invasion.
- regional lymph nodes
  - pN0 no regional lymph node metastasis
  - pN1 metastasis in a single regional lymph node
  - pN2 metastasis in more than one regional lymph node.
- excision margins: perinephric fat, ureter, renal vein and in partial nephrectomy, the renal
  parenchymal margin of tumour clearance (mm).
- other pathology: multifocal papillary, synchronous tumours, amyloid in tumour, adrenal
  rests, adenomas, tumour regression, cystic disease.
- transplant nephrectomy: comment on hilar vessels, presence or absence of acute vascular
  and/or cellular rejection, donor related changes.

Histopathology report

Renal pelvis and ureter

- tumour type – transitional/squamous/adenocarcinoma/other.
- tumour differentiation – WHO grades I–III.

- pattern of growth:
  1. non-invasive (pure) – papillary/flat CIS/papillary and flat CIS.
  2. invasive (pure).
  3. mixed, non-invasive and invasive.
  4. indeterminate.
- extent of invasion:
  - pTa non-invasive papillary carcinoma.
  - pTis carcinoma in situ.
  - pT1 tumour invades subepithelial connective tissue.
  - pT2 tumour invades the muscularis.
  - pT3 (for renal pelvis only) tumour invades beyond muscularis into peripelvic fat or the renal parenchyma.
  - pT3 (for ureter only) tumour invades beyond muscularis into periureteric fat.
  - pT4 tumour invades adjacent organs, or through the kidney into the perinephric fat.
- lymphovascular invasion – present/not present. Note perineural invasion.
- regional lymph nodes – those within the true pelvis; all others are distant nodes.
  - pN0 no regional lymph node metastasis.
  - pN1 metastasis in a single lymph node, ≤ 2 cm in greatest dimension.
  - pN2 metastasis in a single lymph node, > 2 cm but ≤ 5 cm in greatest dimension, or multiple lymph nodes, none > 5 cm in greatest dimension.
  - pN3 metastasis in a lymph node > 5 cm in greatest dimension.
- margins: ureteral, bladder neck, Gerota's fascia (perinephric fat margin), hilar soft tissue, renal parenchyma (partial nephrectomy) tumour clearance (mm).
- additional pathologic findings, if present: carcinoma in situ (focal/multifocal), dysplasia, inflammation/regenerative changes, therapy related (BCG, mitomycin).
- other pathology: cystitis cystica glandularis, keratinising squamous metaplasia, intestinal metaplasia.

29 Bladder

1. Anatomy

The empty bladder is a pyramidal-shaped organ which lies entirely within the pelvic cavity. Upon filling (capacity approximately 500 ml) the bladder assumes a more ovoid shape, rises out of the pelvis and separates the peritoneum from the anterior abdominal wall. The bladder has an apex (anteriorly), a base (posteriorly), a superior surface (the dome) and two inferolateral surfaces. The apex is anchored to the anterior abdominal wall by the urachus, a fibrous embryological remnant which, during development, connects the bladder to the allantois. The superior bladder surface is covered by peritoneum, which reflects onto the anterior abdominal and lateral pelvic walls. The base is triangular in shape, limited superolaterally by the entrances of the ureters into the bladder and inferiorly by the urethral orifice. The area immediately adjacent to the urethral orifice is known as the bladder neck. The seminal vesicles and vasa deferentia lie immediately posterior to the bladder base (Figure 29.1).

The mucosal surface lining the bladder base is known as the trigone. It is distinct in that, because of firm adherence to the underlying muscle coat, its surface is always smooth, in contrast to the remainder of the mucosa which, when the bladder is empty, assumes an undulated appearance.

The bladder is lined by transitional epithelium or urothelium, usually six cell layers thick. This rests on a thick layer of fibroelastic connective tissue, allowing considerable distention. Below this is the ill-defined muscularis mucosae, composed of wispy irregular bundles of smooth muscle. The main muscular coat of the bladder, the muscularis propria or detrusor muscle, is composed of interlacing bundles of larger smooth muscle fibres loosely arranged into inner longitudinal, middle circular and outer longitudinal layers. At the bladder neck the circular layer is thickened, forming a preprostatic sphincter which is responsible for maintaining urinary continence. This muscle is richly ennervated by sympathetic nerve fibres.

Lymphovascular Supply

The blood supply to the bladder is from the superior and inferior vesical arteries and venous drainage is to the internal iliac veins via the vesical venous plexus. Most of the lymphatic drainage is to the external and internal iliac lymph nodes (Figure 29.2).

2. Clinical Presentation

Bladder tumours most commonly present with the painless passage of blood in the urine (haematuria), sometimes with amorphous clots. This is a serious symptom necessitating immediate urologic investigation, particularly in the adult. Haematuria occurring at the end of micturition

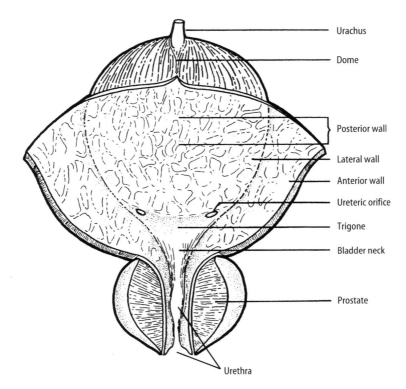

Urachus

Dome

Posterior wall

Lateral wall

Anterior wall

Ureteric orifice

Trigone

Bladder neck

Prostate

Urethra

Figure 29.1. Anatomy of the bladder. Reproduced from Hermanek P, Hutter RVP, Sobin LH, Wagner G, Wittekind Ch (eds.). TNM Atlas: illustrated guide to the TNM/pTNM classification of malignant tumours, 4th edition. Springer-Verlag: Berlin and Heidelberg, 1997.

(terminal haematuria) points specifically to pathology in the bladder neck region. There are usually no other symptoms unless there is secondary urinary obstruction and/or infection. Advanced bladder cancer may present with symptoms related to a pelvic mass, lower limb oedema due to lymphatic obstruction, or metastatic disease.

Acute urinary retention is more commonly due to prostatic enlargement than bladder disease. Overdistention causes a constant suprapubic pain relieved instantaneously by the passage of urine. Occasionally, with slowly progressive urinary obstruction and bladder distention, e.g., neurogenic (flaccid) bladder of diabetics, there is no associated pain.

Inflammatory conditions of the bladder, including bacterial infection and interstitial cystitis, often present with intermittent suprapubic discomfort or irritative symptoms of painful urination (dysuria), increased number of episodes of micturition daily (frequency) and a sensation of sudden, strong impulse to void (urgency). Diffuse carcinoma in situ of the bladder may also present in this way.

Bladder calculi may be asymptomatic or present with haematuria. There may be pain associated with intermittent bladder outlet obstruction or symptoms related to secondary infection.

Rarer conditions such as diverticula or urachal remnants are usually asymptomatic, although predisposing to stones and infection. Vesicocolic fistula due to colonic diverticulitis, Crohn's disease or malignancy can present with the unusual symptoms of passage of gas (pneumaturia)

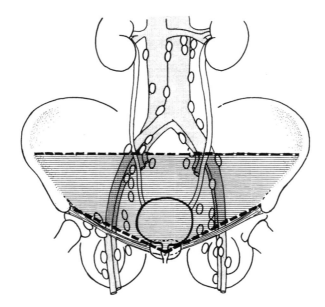

Figure 29.2.   Bladder – regional lymph nodes (pelvic nodes below the bifurcation of the common iliac arteries). Reproduced from Hermanek P, Hutter RVP, Sobin LH, Wagner G, Wittekind Ch (eds.). TNM Atlas: illustrated guide to the TNM/pTNM classification of malignant tumours, 4th edition. Springer-Verlag: Berlin and Heidelberg, 1997.

or faecal material (faecaluria) in the urine. Vesicovaginal fistula due to malignancy may result in the passage of urine vaginally.

3. Clinical Investigations

Urinalysis: a "dipstick" test will detect microscopic haematuria (not visible grossly) which can indicate bladder disease, or pick up other substances such as protein or sugar in the urine which may flag up bladder infection or an underlying medical condition such as diabetes mellitus.

Mid-Stream Sample of Urine culture (MSSU): will confirm the presence of bacterial infection.

Intravenous Urogram (IVU): of limited value in the diagnosis of bladder disease. Tumours may present as filling defects.

Cystoscopy and cytology/biopsy.

Cystography: occasionally indicated to demonstrate vesicocolic or vesicovaginal fistulae, to evaluate bladder diverticula or post-bladder surgery to look for an anastomotic leak.

Micturating Cystourethrography: assesses the pathophysiology of micturition as well as the lower urinary tract anatomy. In bladder disease, useful for evaluating neurogenic bladder, diverticula and vesicoureteral reflux.

Loopography: occasionally performed to examine reconstructed urinary reservoirs or conduits after resection of the native bladder, e.g., to look for obstruction in an ileal conduit.

USS: can be used to detect radiolucent bladder stones or diverticula or to confirm the presence of bladder tumour in suspicious filling defects on IVU. Endoluminal ultrasound (ELUS) is used to stage bladder cancer in some specialized centres.

CT/MRI: both modalities are used to stage bladder cancer, primarily in looking for metastatic disease in regional lymph nodes and other organs.

4. Pathological Conditions

Non-neoplastic Conditions

Bacterial cystitis: this, the most common cause of cystitis, is usually due to coliform organisms (e.g., *E. coli*) ascending the urethra. Underlying structural (diverticula, fistulae, malformations, stones) or medical (diabetes mellitus, chronic renal failure, immunosuppression) conditions predispose. Recurrent infections, especially in men, should trigger investigation for an underlying cause.

Malakoplakia: is caused by a defect in the host macrophage response to bacterial infection and can affect practically any organ in the genitourinary system or indeed elsewhere. It is seen primarily in middle-aged women and presents as multiple soft, yellow mucosal plaques on cystoscopy, sometimes mistaken for carcinoma. Biopsy reveals collections of granular histiocytes in the lamina propria, some with characteristic intracytoplasmic concentrically laminated inclusions (Michaelis–Gutmann bodies).

Polypoid/papillary cystitis: these closely related conditions describe localised non-specific inflammation and oedema of the bladder mucosa commonly seen in association with indwelling urinary catheters and less often with vesical fistulae. They may be difficult to differentiate endoscopically and microscopically from papillary urothelial carcinoma, which tends to have finer stromal papillary cores, more urothelial atypia and less associated inflammation.

Nephrogenic adenoma: often associated with previous surgery, stones or infection, these are small, usually polypoid lesions of metaplastic origin and, although most commonly found in the bladder (75%), can be seen anywhere in the urinary tract.

Interstitial cystitis: usually in middle-aged women, the aetiology is obscure and the diagnosis essentially one of exclusion. Symptoms may be extremely severe. On cystoscopy the typical appearances of diffuse punctate haemorrhage with or without ulceration can closely mimic carcinoma in situ. The histological appearances are non-specific, with lamina propria congestion, oedema and inflammation featuring lymphocytes, plasma cells and variable numbers of mast cells (best seen histologically if sample submitted in alcohol rather than formalin). Urine cytology to exclude malignancy and culture for infection are other important investigations. Treatment is initially medical for symptom relief (amitriptyline, antihistamines, analgesics) with intravesical therapy an alternative and eventually surgical intervention, in the form of urinary diversion with or without cystourethrectomy, as a last resort.

Bladder stones: most commonly seen in men with bladder outlet obstruction, and associated with renal or ureteric stones. Rarely result in surgical material.

Diverticula: most are seen in elderly males and attributed to increased luminal pressure secondary to prostatic enlargement causing outlet obstruction. Few cause symptoms or require surgical treatment. Most are located close to the ureteric orifices. Possible complications include ureteric obstruction, infection, stone formation and rarely malignancy (urothelial, adeno- or squamous cell carcinoma).

Urachal-related lesions: persistence of the urachus can result in a completely patent tract from bladder to umbilicus, a blind-ended sinus opening onto the bladder mucosa or umbilical skin, or an enclosed sinus blind at both ends. The lining epithelium may be of urothelial or columnar type. Presentation is usually in childhood. Stasis of urine and epithelial debris predispose to infection, abscesses and rarely stones. Cysts may occur at any point within the urachal remnant.

Neurogenic bladder: a wide range of neuromuscular conditions (e.g., cerebrovascular accident, multiple sclerosis, spinal cord trauma, diabetes mellitus) can cause voiding dysfunction by interfering with bladder wall compliance, detrusor muscle activity or sphincter function, resulting eventually in either a tightly contracted or flaccid bladder. These are usually treated by behavioural, pharmacological or electrophysiological means but occasionally surgical intervention may be indicated, e.g., augmentation cystoplasty to increase capacity in a contracted bladder, where a segment of stomach or intestine is isolated and anastomosed to the native bladder. Rarely, adenocarcinoma may supervene later in the augmented bladder.

Tumour-like Conditions

Postoperative necrobiotic granulomas: seen following transurethral surgery with diathermy. Microscopy reveals central necrosis with peripheral palisading of histiocyes and occasional giant cells.

Postoperative spindle cell nodule: nodular bladder masses seen up to several months following surgery. Histology shows interlacing fascicles of mitotically active bland spindle cells resembling leiomyosarcoma. Clinical history is most important. Behaviour is benign with spontaneous resolution in many cases. Follow-up with repeat cystoscopy and biopsy is indicated.

Pseudosarcomatous fibromyxoid tumour (inflammatory pseudotumour): another reactive proliferative condition seen in a younger age group without a history of surgery. Gross appearances vary from pedunculated lesions to mucosal ulcers. Histology shows a haphazard spindle cell proliferation in an inflammatory and myxoid background with prominent vascularity, resembling nodular fasciitis. Differentiation from sarcoma may be difficult. Behaviour is generally indolent although occasional infiltration into the muscularis propria has been reported.

Miscellaneous: other causes of cystitis include pelvic radiotherapy, intravesical BCG immunotherapy (granulomatous) or chemotherapy, oral drugs (cyclophosphamide), viral infection (CMV, HSV) and parasite infestation (schistosomiasis). Amyloidosis may present as a localised, nodular bladder mass ("amyloid tumour").

Neoplastic Conditions

Benign tumours: inverted urothelial papilloma, villous adenoma, paraganglioma, leiomyoma, haemangioma and granular cell tumour of the bladder are occasionally encountered. Benign urothelial papilloma is a rarely-made diagnosis.

Urothelial dysplasia/carcinoma: many carcinogenic agents are known to predispose to urothelial malignancy. These include cigarette smoke, industrial aniline dyes (aromatic amines), petrochemicals, cyclophosphamide and the analgesic phenacetin. Most invasive tumours are associated with urothelial dysplasia or flat carcinoma in situ.

Urothelial carcinoma in situ: occurs rarely in the absence of invasive tumour, when it can closely mimic interstitial cystitis both clinically and cystoscopically, presenting with irritative bladder symptoms and appearing as multifocal red, velvety patches. More often seen in association with prior or synchronous invasive malignancy which can be multifocal. Diagnosis is made by urine cytology and bladder biopsy, which shows severe (often, but not necessarily, full-thickness) dysplasia of the surface urothelium. Papillary architecture is lacking. Lesser grades of atypia may merit the term urothelial dysplasia. Careful distinction should be made from "superficial carcinoma", which is used by urologists to describe tumours that have not invaded into the muscularis propria, regardless of histological type and grade. Carcinoma in situ is usually treated with intravesical chemotherapy (e.g., mitomycin) or immunotherapy (BCG vaccine), although localised disease may be controlled by transurethral resection (TURB). Radical surgery is indicated for widespread field change in the urothelium, which may involve the bladder, ureters, urethra, prostatic ducts and seminal vesicles. Careful follow-up with urine cytology and biopsy is advocated following conservative management to monitor recurrence or progression (up to 80% at five years). Particularly on cytological material, recurrent disease may be difficult to distinguish from reactive atypia due to treatment.

Urothelial carcinoma: urothelial (or transitional cell) carcinoma (TCC) accounts for over 90% of primary bladder tumours, most commonly presenting in elderly males as a cystoscopic mass showing an exophytic or endophytic growth pattern. Diagnosis is confirmed by biopsy which commonly shows a papillary or solid growth pattern. Urine cytology is of limited value in the initial evaluation of bladder tumours and is more useful in industrial screening and follow-up after treatment. Note that non-invasive papillary TCC (> 7 cell layers thick, stage pTa) is also classified as carcinoma to avoid confusion with flat carcinoma in situ (stage pTis). Pathological staging is extremely important for prognostic and treatment purposes and is determined by the extent of local tumour spread. Assessment of small bladder biopsies is crucial and they must be carefully examined. Specifically, the ill-defined muscularis mucosae must be distinguished from the muscularis propria, infiltration of which defines true deep or muscle-invasive urothelial carcinoma (stage pT2). In bladder biopsy material, distinction is not made between invasion of the inner (superficial, pT2a) and outer (deep, pT2b) muscularis propria due to problems of orientation (reported as "at least" stage pT2a). Biopsies should also be examined closely for coexistent carcinoma in situ. Separate biopsies may be submitted to assess prostatic involvement. There is a correlation between tumour stage and grade, based on the degree of nuclear atypia, in that more poorly differentiated tumours (WHO grade III) show a much higher rate of concurrent or subsequent muscle invasion. High-grade tumours commonly show focal squamous or glandular differentiation.

Non-muscle invasive papillary urothelial carcinoma (stages pTa and pT1) is treated primarily by transurethral resection, with adjuvant intravesical therapy for higher-risk or recurrent disease. Muscle-invasive tumours (and sometimes grade III, pT1 tumours) are treated surgically, usually by total cystectomy or cystoprostatectomy and pelvic lymphadenectomy, with or without adjuvant chemotherapy depending on pathological assessment of the resection specimen. Partial cystectomy is reserved for solitary tumours with no previous history of bladder tumours and no carcinoma in situ, bladder neck or trigone involvement. Radiotherapy as a treatment modality alone is not as effective as surgery and is more commonly administered in a palliative setting, with or without chemotherapy, in advanced, unresectable bladder cancer.

Prognosis: multifocality, tumour size, histological grade, depth of invasion, coexistent urothelial dysplasia/carcinoma in situ and cystoscopic appearance at three-month follow-up are the best predictors of recurrence or progression. Involvement of the prostatic stroma is an adverse prognostic sign. Prostatic urethra involvement is associated with a high rate of urethral recurrence. Overall prognosis depends largely on stage, with a 70% five-year survival rate for stages pTa and pT1 and 50% for pT2b. Within the pT1 group, grade III decreases the five-year survival to 60%.

Variants of urothelial carcinoma are: nested (mimics benign von Brunn's nests – look for deep invasion and cytological atypia); microcystic (cysts or tubules containing proteinaceous debris); inverted (architecturally like inverted papilloma but with marked atypia); also giant cell, clear cell, lymphoepithelioma-like and micropapillary variants.

Squamous cell carcinoma: accounts for less than 5% of bladder tumours in the UK. Chronic irritation from stones, long-term indwelling catheters, diverticula, chronic urinary infections and, in particular schistosomiasis predispose, hence a much higher incidence of bladder squamous cell carcinoma in countries where the latter is endemic e.g., Egypt. High-grade urothelial carcinoma showing squamous differentiation (look for urothelial carcinoma in situ) and secondary involvement by primary cervical carcinoma should be excluded. Disease is often of advanced stage at presentation and prognosis therefore poor (overall five-year survival 15%).

Adenocarcinoma: constitutes 2% of bladder malignancies; may arise from metaplastic epithelium (cystitis glandularis) following chronic inflammation (60%) or in bladders with exstrophy, diverticula or urachal remnants (occur at the dome and usually lack a bladder mucosal component). Mucinous, clear cell, enteric and signet ring cell types exist. Overall five-year survival is poor (30%).

Other cancers: spindle cell carcinoma, small cell carcinoma, malignant melanoma, leukaemia/ malignant lymphoma, leiomyosarcoma, rhabdomyosarcoma, choriocarcinoma, yolk sac tumour and metastases (direct spread – prostate, cervix, uterus, rectum; distant spread – breast, malignant melanoma, lung, stomach).

5. Surgical Pathology Specimens – Clinical Aspects

Biopsy Specimens

Rigid or flexible cystoscopy allows direct visualisation of macroscopic bladder pathology for evaluation and biopsy of small lesions using either "cold" cup forceps or a small diathermy loop. The latter may cause significant heat artefact, reducing the value of histologic assessment. Rigid cystoscopy employs a larger lumen allowing superior visualisation (better optics and water flow), greater versatility in the passage of accessory instruments and easier manipulation. It also provides suitable access for transurethral resection of superficial bladder tumours with diathermy (TURB). Flexible cystoscopy is more comfortable for the patient, may be easier to pass and allows a range of angles of visualisation within the bladder. Cystoscopy should be avoided during active urinary tract infection as instrumentation can exacerbate the condition. Carcinoma in situ may be invisible to the endoscopist and necessitate random biopsies to make the diagnosis. Distinction from interstitial cystitis may require multiple biopsies as the surface can be extensively denuded. In the presence of an overt tumour it is important to sample abnormal mucosa (red, velvety) distant from the lesion to look for in situ malignancy. Sampling normal-looking mucosa adjacent to tumour is not advised due to the potential risk of tumour re-implantation. Deep biopsies (including muscularis propria) are essential to provide important staging information in invasive tumours.

Resection Specimens

Obviously there are important surgical differences between the sexes. Radical surgery for bladder cancer in the male comprises cystoprostatectomy, with urethrectomy if there is prostatic urethra involvement, and in the female an anterior exenteration (bladder, uterus and adnexae – see Chapter 34). With surgical and anaesthetic advances, operative mortality from radical cystectomy has fallen from 20% to < 1%.

In the male, the bladder is approached through a midline lower abdominal incision. The urachus and vasa deferentia are identified and ligated. A pelvic lymphadenectomy is performed and the ureters identified and divided close to the bladder. Ureteric margins are ideally submitted separately from the main resection specimen for pathological assessment. The bladder, prostate and seminal vesicles are separated from the rectum and the puboprostatic ligaments divided. The urethral sphincter is then divided unless a urethrectomy is being considered.

Simple cystectomy is quite a rare operation, typically performed for benign conditions such as interstitial cystitis or neurogenic bladder complicated by chronic infection. It involves bladder removal with maintenance of the urethra in women or the prostate and seminal vesicles in men.

The need for an alternative urinary drainage system following cystectomy has raised difficulties of acceptance for many patients. However, new developments in surgical techniques mean several options are now available:

1. urinary diversion and intestinal conduit formation; an isolated segment of small or large intestine (usually ileum) is anastomosed to both ureters and a stoma formed on the anterior abdominal wall. Drainage is continuous into a worn device.
2. continent cutaneous diversion (e.g., Indiana pouch, which uses the ileocaecal valve as a continence mechanism); requires intermittent self-catheterisation.
3. continent orthotopic reservoir; a "neobladder" is formed from an ileal or ileocolonic segment and sutured directly onto the urethra; usually confined to men but also possible in women with an intact urethra.
4. ureterosigmoidostomy (sigma rectum pouch); the ureters are anastomosed directly onto a detubularised segment of sigmoid colon still in continuity, i.e., remains in contact with faeces. This avoids the need for a stoma or self-catheterisation but results in the frequent passage of liquid faeces.
5. rarely, cutaneous ureterostomy.

Long-term complications following these procedures include stenosis, adenomatous polyps and tumour formation (usually adenocarcinoma). These may necessitate subsequent resection.

Partial cystectomy is infrequently performed, but may be indicated for a solitary urothelial carcinoma at the bladder dome or for tumour arising in a urachal remnant or diverticulum. Excision of a benign bladder diverticulum may be performed intravesically, extravesically or, if small, transurethrally.

6. Surgical Pathology Specimens – Laboratory Protocols

Biopsy Specimens

Tiny pieces of tissue (several mm) retrieved using either "cold" cup forceps or a small diathermy loop are counted, measured, processed intact and examined histologically through three levels. TURB specimens contain larger fragments possibly recognisable as papillary tumour grossly. These are weighed collectively and all tissue embedded if possible. If sampling is required, at least six blocks are processed, concentrating on more solid tissue and fragments containing identifiable muscle. It will not normally be feasible to orientate such fragments. Tissue from the tumour base may be submitted separately.

Resection Specimens

Specimen

- most bladder resections are for biopsy-proven malignant tumours: cystourethrectomy, cystoprostatectomy (including seminal vesicles), cystoprostatourethrectomy, anterior exenteration (including uterus and adnexae), simple cystectomy, partial cystectomy.

Initial procedure (Figure 29.3)

- orientate the specimen with the help, if present, of attached pelvic organs (uterus and seminal vesicles are posterior to the bladder) or the peritoneal reflection, which descends further on the posterior bladder wall than anteriorly.

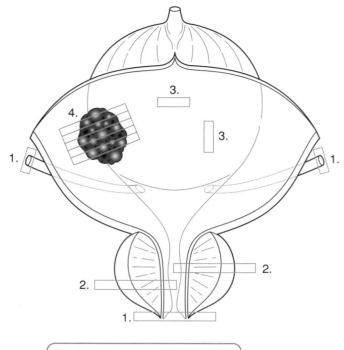

Blocks
1. Urethral and ureteric limits
2. Prostate
3. Bladder away from tumour
4. Tumour with adjacent mucosa, underlying wall and perivesical fat

Figure 29.3. Blocking a cystoprostatectomy specimen for bladder cancer. Based on Hermanek P, Hutter RVP, Sobin LH, Wagner G, Wittekind Ch (eds.). TNM Atlas: illustrated guide to the TNM/pTNM classification of malignant tumours, 4th edition. Springer-Verlag: Berlin and Heidelberg, 1997.

- locate both ureters in the lateral perivesical fat (may be marked with sutures).
- place a probe in the bladder via the urethra and open the specimen anteriorly (through the prostate if present) with a sagittal cut using a knife or scissors, trying if possible to avoid cutting into any localised tumour. Keep the posterior aspect of the specimen intact to maintain orientation. Some pathologists prefer to inflate the bladder with 10% formalin and allow fixation prior to opening. Others like to divide the specimen into anterior and posterior halves.
- if there is an obvious tumour, paint the nearest deep perivesical soft tissue margin; if no tumour is grossly obvious (e.g., following preoperative treatment), paint all peripheral soft tissue margins, using different coloured inks for orientation. Paint the prostate, if present.

- measurements:
    - dimensions (cm) of bladder and, if present, prostate, seminal vesicles, female pelvic organs.
    - lengths(cm) of ureters (limits may be submitted separately) and urethra, if attached.
    - tumour: dimensions (cm).
                 distances to urethral and ureteric margins (cm).
- photograph.
- fix by immersion in 10% formalin for at least 24–36 hours preferably pinned out or using a wick to fully expose the mucosal surface.
- locate the ureteric orifices at the trigone and open the ureters along their full length with small scissors.
- make 3–5 mm parallel, transverse sections through the tumour to demonstrate its deepest point of invasion and its relationship to the ureters, prostate or any other adjacent structures.
- look for and measure lymph nodes in perivesical fat (usually none found).
- if not involved by the bladder tumour, serially section the prostate perpendicular to the urethra looking for occult primary tumour.
- if not involved by the bladder tumour, process female pelvic organs.
- photograph suitable slices.
- partial cystectomies are processed in a similar manner, although orientation may be more difficult (or impossible). The mucosal edges should be treated as surgical margins, i.e., inked and measurements given from tumour (cm).
- if a tumour is identified as arising from the urachal tract (usually in a partial cystectomy specimen comprising dome of bladder, urachal tract and umbilicus), the bladder portion is processed as before, soft tissue margins surrounding the urachal tract are painted and the tract serially sectioned transversely up to the umbilicus.
- conduits, augmentation cystoplasty and neobladder specimens containing tumours are processed as before, opening along the urethra and ureters if possible, painting the nearest deep soft tissue margin and noting the relationship of the tumour to the enteric, bladder or ureteric mucosa. It may be best to serially section the tumour perpendicular to lines of anastomoses.

Description

- tumour: site (trigone, lateral walls, dome, neck, ureteric orifices).
             single/multifocal.
             appearance (papillary/sessile/ulcerated/mucoid/keratotic).
             edge (circumscribed/irregular).
- mucosa: red, velvety carcinoma in situ away from tumour.
- wall: tumour confined to mucosa, into muscle wall or through wall into perivesical fat.
- other: fistula, diverticulum, stones, urachal remnant.

Blocks for histology (Figure 29.3)

- transverse section the urethral and ureteric limits.
- if bilateral ureteric limits are submitted separately, measure the two lengths and sample the proximal surgical margin of each (if orientated by the surgeon), then serially section the remainder and process separately.
- sample at least four blocks of tumour to demonstrate depth of invasion, distance to perivesical soft tissue margins and relationship to adjacent mucosa, ureters, prostate or other organs.
- sample any suspicious background mucosa or take at least two random mucosal sections.

- if tumour is not seen grossly, sample and carefully label all bladder mucosal surfaces including the trigone, dome, lateral, anterior and posterior walls.
- sample any suspicious ureteric mucosa or submit random ureteric transverse sections.
- if not suspicious of harbouring malignancy on serial sectioning, sample each lobe of the prostate and the prostatic urethra. If suspicious, multiple site-orientated blocks are taken to include the prostatic capsule and relevant surgical margins.
- sample the seminal vesicles and vasa deferentia.
- sample any attached female pelvic organs.
- count and sample all lymph nodes identified.
- in a partial cystectomy, it is important to take perpendicular blocks of tumour which include the nearest lateral mucosal margins.
- a tumour arising in the urachus should be sampled as before, but also to include blocks of the soft tissue margins surrounding the urachus and the skin margin surrounding the umbilicus.
- conduits, augmentation cystoplasty and neobladder specimens containing tumour should be sampled as before, also taking tumour blocks to demonstrate the relationship with enteric/urothelial mucosa and anastomotic lines.

Histopathology report

- tumour type – urothelial/squamous/adenocarcinoma/other.
- tumour growth pattern – papillary/invasive/flat in situ.
- tumour differentiation – use WHO grades I–III (based on cytological atypia).
- tumour edge – pushing/infiltrative.
- extent of local tumour spread.
    - pTis   flat carcinoma in situ.
    - pTa   papillary non-invasive.
    - pT1   invasion of subepithelial connective tissue.
    - pT2a   invasion of superficial muscle (inner half).
    - pT2b   invasion of deep muscle (outer half).
    - pT3   invasion of perivesical fat.
            a.   microscopically.
            b.   macroscopically.
    - pT4   invasion of:
            a.   prostate, uterus, vagina.
            b.   pelvic wall, abdominal wall.
- lymphovascular invasion – present/not present.
- regional lymph nodes.
    - pelvic nodes below the bifurcation of the common iliac arteries.
    - pN0   no regional lymph node metastasis.
    - pN1   metastasis in a single regional node ≤ 2cm.
    - pN2   metastasis in a single regional node > 2cm but ≤ 5cm or multiple regional nodes each ≤ 5cm.
    - pN3   metastasis in a regional node > 5cm.
- excision margins:
    - distances (mm) to the ureteric, urethral and nearest perivesical soft tissue margins.
    - presence/absence of dysplasia/carcinoma in situ at ureteric/urethral limits.
- other pathology:
    - urothelial carcinoma in situ, diverticulum, inflammation, squamous/glandular metaplasia, urachus, prostate pathology.

30 Prostate

1. Anatomy

The normal prostate weighs 20 g by early adulthood and is best thought of as having an inverted pyramid shape, with anterior, posterior and lateral surfaces, a narrow apex anteroinferiorly and a broad base superiorly which lies against the bladder neck. It is related anteriorly to the symphysis pubis, laterally to the anterior fibres of the levator ani muscle and posteriorly to the seminal vesicles and rectum, separated from the latter by Denonvilliers' fascia. The prostate is surrounded by an ill-defined fibrous capsule which blends with the pelvic fascia. Numerous neurovascular bundles are found within this connective tissue. At the apex, skeletal muscle fibres of the urethral sphincter are admixed with occasional benign prostatic glands and, at the base, fibres from the bladder detrusor muscle blend imperceptibly with the prostate capsule. At these points the boundaries of the organ are particularly obscure, rendering difficult in resection specimens the interpretation of capsular penetration by carcinoma and capsular incision during surgery. Adipose tissue is occasionally found just inside the prostatic capsule.

The prostate is composed of branching tubuloalveolar glands lined by cuboidal or columnar epithelium and invested and surrounded by fibromuscular stroma which is continuous with the prostatic capsule. The urethra transverses the full diameter of the prostate in a curved fashion, entering at the centre of the prostate base and exiting just anterior to the apex. Prostatic ducts empty into the prostatic urethra. The ejaculatory ducts, formed at the juncture of the vasa deferentia and seminal vesicle, also secrete into the prostatic urethra.

The glandular prostatic tissue has been divided into four distinct zones, characterised by differing embryological origin, location and pathologies (Figure 30.1a). The anterior fibromuscular stroma, composed mainly of fibromuscular tissue with very few glands, merges with the bladder neck superiorly and the external sphincter at the apex inferiorly. The preprostatic zone surrounds the urethra proximal to the ejaculatory ducts and comprises the periurethral ducts and the larger transition zone. This region commonly gives rise to benign prostatic hypertrophy and approximately 25% of adenocarcinomas. The central zone, surrounding the ejaculatory ducts, is felt to differ embryologically from the remainder of the gland and is least commonly affected by pathological abnormality. Glands in the central zone may show complex papillary infoldings and a cribriform architecture on histology. Lack of cytological atypia distinguishes them from prostatic intraepithelial neoplasia (PIN). The peripheral zone occupies approximately 70% of the normal prostate in a horseshoe shape around the posterior and lateral aspects of the organ. Glands are normally small and simple but this zone is the main site of origin for prostatic adenocarcinomas (70%).

To simplify the concept of zones, the prostate may be considered to have significantly differing inner (transition zone) and outer (peripheral and central zones) regions.

Clinically, the prostate gland is often described as having right and left lateral lobes, a central sulcus and a middle lobe. These do not equate to any anatomically defined structures but rather

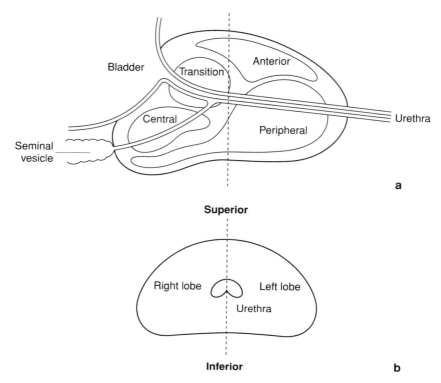

Figure 30.1.   (**a**) Prostatic zones (lateral view). (**b**) Prostatic lobes (anterior view).

relate to palpable masses on rectal examination, usually enlargement of the transitional zone later-ally and periurethral glands centrally.

For the purposes of TNM staging the prostate gland is simply divided into right and left lobes (Figure 30.1b).

Lymphatic Drainage

Lymphatic drainage from the prostate is to the obturator, hypogastric and external iliac nodes (Figure 29.2).

The seminal vesicles are paired, convoluted glands measuring approximately 5 cm in length and lying on the posterior wall of the prostate. Their function is to add a significant volume of alkaline secretion to the ejaculate, which promotes sperm motility and survival. Cowper's (bulbourethral) glands are paired, pea-sized, tubular glands found periurethrally immediately distal to the prostate.

2. Clinical Presentation

Benign prostatic enlargement, usually affecting the periurethral glands, causes urinary tract obstructive symptoms of delayed start to micturition (hesitancy), decreased force of urination, intermittency of the urinary stream and post-micturitional dribbling. Secondary changes in bladder compliance later lead to irritative symptoms of frequency (increase in daily episodes of micturition), urgency (sudden, strong desire to micturate) and nocturia (nocturnal frequency), the latter being the most common presenting complaint. Patients may also present in acute urinary retention. Digital rectal examination (DRE) usually reveals a rubbery, smoothly-enlarged prostate, although there is poor correlation between symptoms and gland size. Alternatively, an enlarged asymptomatic benign prostate gland may be detected incidentally on performing DRE to investigate lower gastrointestinal symptoms or on screening for prostate cancer. This is a very common finding in men over age 50 and per se is not a reason to precipitate further urologic investigation.

In contrast, carcinoma of the prostate, usually involving the periphery of the gland, rarely causes urinary symptoms and is often clinically silent. Indeed, presentation with obstructive urinary symptoms implies advanced disease. Patients present most commonly with advanced metastatic disease in lymph nodes or bone. Early cancer may be picked up by DRE, which frequently reveals a firm, indurated mass. This may be performed as part of a routine physical examination, to investigate urinary, gastrointestinal or generalised symptoms or as part of a screening procedure along with serum prostatic specific antigen (PSA) (see Clinical Investigations). DRE alone is of limited accuracy and cannot reliably differentiate malignancy from prostatic stones and granulomas. Early-stage, commonly low-grade prostatic carcinoma may be detected incidentally in transurethral resection specimens from men with concomitant benign hyperplasia.

Acute or chronic inflammation of the prostate (prostatitis) usually associated with bacterial infection may cause perineal pain which can be referred to the back, inguinal region or testes. It is frequently associated with irritative urinary symptoms of frequency and dysuria. DRE may reveal a tender, fluctuant or boggy prostate but is often extremely uncomfortable for the patient.

3. Clinical Investigations

Serum prostate specific antigen (PSA) – a highly organ-specific biochemical marker used as a diagnostic tool in those suspected as having prostatic cancer clinically and to screen for prostatic cancer in asymptomatic men. Normal value is < 4.0 ng/ml although this rises slightly with age. PSA is mildly elevated in benign hyperplasia, infection and post-biopsy but not in PIN. The risk of cancer is directly related to the PSA level (e.g., 25% of men with PSA 5–10 ng/ml, 66% of men with PSA 11–20 ng/ml have prostate cancer). Free:total PSA ratio < 15% increases the cancer risk. Increasing PSA value correlates with tumour volume and organ-escape (e.g., 50% of men with PSA > 10 ng/ml already have capsular penetration; PSA > 50 ng/ml is associated with bone metastases). However, 25% of prostate cancer cases have no PSA elevation. Following prostatectomy, PSA should fall to undetectable levels. Persistent or subsequent elevation provides a sensitive indicator of residual or recurrent disease.

Transrectal ultrasound (TRUS) and biopsy – US is more sensitive and accurate than DRE and may detect prostate cancer as peripheral hypoechoic regions. However, many prostate cancers are not detected on US appearances and most hypoechoic lesions are not cancer (may represent PIN, benign hyperplasia, atrophy, infarction or infection). TRUS is therefore mainly used to guide needle biopsy sampling for definitive diagnosis after an abnormal DRE or elevated serum PSA. As regards staging, locally extensive disease will be easily detected but not unexpectedly US will understage microscopic capsular penetration. TRUS biopies can be taken to monitor progression following non-surgical treatment.

CT/MRI – to determine pretreatment tumour stage by assessing capsular penetration and regional lymph node metastases (by size), although both are of limited sensitivity and specificity.

Radiolabelled isotope bone scan – investigation of choice to detect distant skeletal metastases.

4. Pathological Conditions

Non-neoplastic Conditions

Benign nodular hyperplasia (BNH): an extremely common androgen-dependent disorder (castration is protective) caused by hormonal imbalance affecting the stromal–epithelial relationship. No other clear risk factors apart from ageing have been identified. Benign prostatic hypertrophy (BPH) is variably defined by the presence of urinary obstructive symptoms, macroscopic prostate enlargement or histological hyperplasia. The average weight of the prostate with histologically confirmed BPH is 33 g but weights of over 800 g have been recorded. Incidence increases with age (approximately 50% in the fifth decade and 75% in the eighth decade). BPH first develops in the transition and periurethral (preprostatic) zones, giving rise to enlargement of the clinical lateral and middle lobes respectively. Grossly, the apearances are those of multiple, variably sized, grey to yellow central nodules, compressing the urethra and the peripheral zone. Histology shows hyperplasia of both prostatic glandular and stromal elements (benign prostatic *hypertrophy* is pathologically incorrect). This can adopt various forms, some reminiscent of benign breast disease such as fibroadenoma-like hyperplasia or sclerosing adenosis. Pure stromal nodules composed almost entirely of smooth muscle may also be seen. Treatment may be initially medical in the form of alpha₁-adrenergic blockers, which ease obstruction by relaxing prostatic smooth muscle, or androgen suppression. Aromatase inhibitors are a newer approach. Patients suffering serious complications of BPH such as recurrent urinary retention or infections, renal insufficiency or bladder stones are not suitable for medical therapy and should be offered surgery. Similarly, patients whose quality of life is significantly affected by their urinary symptoms are appropriate surgical candidates. Transurethral resection of prostate (TURP) has been the gold standard for surgical treatment of BPH for many years against which new treatments are compared. High-volume disease is best treated by enucleation of the entire gland using a retropubic or suprapubic approach (open prostatectomy). Newer, less invasive and less morbid alternatives to TURP include the following:

- transurethral incision of the prostate,
- transurethral balloon dilatation of the prostate,
- intraurethral stenting,
- hyperthermia and thermotherapy,
- high-intensity focussed ultrasound (HIFU),
- laser therapy,
- transurethral electrovaporisation of the prostate,
- transurethral needle ablation of the prostate.

Prostatitis: Acute bacterial prostatitis is associated with urinary tract infection (UTI) and responds to the same antimicrobial therapy so is rarely seen in surgical pathology practice. Chronic bacterial prostatitis is characterised by recurrent UTIs caused by the same pathogen and is less responsive to medical treatment. Large infected prostatic stones predispose and resection by TURP may be attempted, providing surgical material. On histological examination, reactive glandular atypia may mimic carcinoma. The presence of inflammatory cells and glandular atrophy, obvious on low power, should prevent misdiagnosis. Often in prostatic tissue showing chronic inflammation no organisms are cultured (non-bacterial prostatitis), hence it is better to report the histology as chronic inflammation rather than chronic prostatitis.

Abscess: Most commonly seen with bladder outlet obstruction as a complication of urinary tract infection or, less often, following biopsy. DRE and TRUS are diagnostic. Treatment is transurethral drainage and antimicrobial therapy.

Infarction: often found in prostates with significant BNH. Histology shows coagulative necrosis of glands and stroma often with prominent surrounding squamous metaplasia, not to be confused with squamous cell carcinoma (exceptionally rare in prostate).

Granulomatous prostatitis: seen following BCG therapy for bladder cancer (look for suburethral distribution of granulomas), with prostatic involvement in systemic mycobacterial or fungal infection (in an immunocompromised host), and in association with eosinophilia and possibly systemic vasculitis (allergic granulomatous prostatitis). Non-specific granulomatous prostatitis, due to an immune response to extravasated prostatic secretions, is the most commonly diagnosed non-infectious granulomatous prostatitis and clinically can closely mimic prostate cancer.

Postoperative necrobiotic granuloma: may be identified years following TURP and has a characteristic histological appearance of central fibrinoid necrosis with palisading histiocytes.

Miscellaneous: malakoplakia, stones, pseudosarcomatous fibromyxoid tumour (inflammatory pseudotumour), postoperative spindle cell nodule (following TURP), although all more commonly seen in the bladder, may be found in the prostate.

Neoplastic Conditions

Benign tumours

E.g., leiomyoma, cystadenoma, extremely rare.

Malignant tumours

Prostate cancer is the second leading cause of cancer-related death in men after lung cancer. It is androgen-dependent and risk factors include ageing, positive family history, black race and probably high dietary fat. Prostatic intraepithelial neoplasia (PIN) represents a precancerous condition confined to prostatic ducts and acini.

Prostatic intraepithelial neoplasia (PIN): PIN features cytologically atypical epithelial cells lining architecturally benign ducts or acini. It is subdivided into high-grade and low-grade types based on the degree of atypia. High-grade PIN, of which there are four architectural types (tufting, micropapillary, cribriform and flat) is recognised by significant nuclear atypia, crowding and stratification, prominent nucleoli and focal disruption of the basal cell layer. It is most commonly found in the peripheral zone and is a precursor to many intermediate-to-high-grade prostatic adenocarcinomas. Low-grade carcinomas do not have the same association. High-grade PIN may be confused histologically with several benign entities (e.g., lobular atrophy, atypical basal layer hyperplasia) as well as cribriform type acinar/ductal adenocarcinoma. The finding of high-grade PIN on a needle biopsy (and to a lesser extent on TURP chippings) is highly significant. There is a 30–50% chance of finding carcinoma on subsequent biopsies. DRE and TRUS are not helpful in deciding if carcinoma is already present. However, it is important to note that PIN alone does not cause an elevated serum PSA. The management of high-grade PIN is immediate clinical reassessment and rebiopsy. Its detection in chippings necessitates the processing of more tissue.

Prostatic adenocarcinoma: of acinar/proximal duct origin, accounts for over 95% of primary prostate cancers. Seventy per cent arise in the peripheral zone and most cause few symptoms initially, often presenting insidiously in elderly men. DRE or serum PSA may raise suspicion and diagnosis is usually confirmed on TRUS-guided needle biopsy. Alternatively, cancer may be an incidental finding in prostatic chippings following TURP. This may either have arisen in the transition zone (20% of cancers – often low volume and grade) or represent spread from a larger, often high-grade peripheral tumour. Prostatic carcinoma can be difficult to identify grossly, even on radical resection specimens. It may be visible as solid, firm, pale yellow foci found peripherally in the gland.

Histology shows small acini arranged in a variety of architectural patterns (acinar, papillary, cribriform, comedo, solid) with cytological atypia, at least focal nucleolar prominence and absence of surrounding basal cell layer on high power (confirmed with immunohistochemical staining for the high-molecular-weight cytokeratin marker 34ßE12 or cytokeratin 5/6). Ancillary features which may be seen in carcinoma include perineural invasion and intraluminal wispy secretions or crystalloids. These features should help distinguish carcinoma from PIN and from the many benign small acinar proliferations which, especially on needle biopsy, may cause misdiagnosis (e.g., atypical adenomatous hyperplasia, basal cell hyperplasia, post-atrophic hyperplasia, sclerosing adenosis). Insufficient diagnostic criteria for malignancy present in a limited focus of acinar proliferation on needle core biopsy may lead to a report of "suspicious but not diagnostic of malignancy", usually prompting rebiopsy.

The relative proportions of the various architectural patterns present are the basis of the Gleason grading system, which, because of limited tumour volume, may be difficult to apply accurately to needle core specimens and often tends to undergrading. Following a diagnosis of carcinoma on needle biopsy or TURP chippings, the Gleason score, clinicopathological stage (any evidence of extracapsular spread) and tumour volume (or length/proportion of needle core/tissue involved), together with the patient's age, serum PSA, general health and personal preferences, will direct treatment. It should be noted that the presence of a few prostatic glands in skeletal muscle or adipose tissue does not necessarily imply capsular penetration, as these features may be entirely innocent (look for cytological atypia). The best indicator of capsular penetration on TRUS biopsy is perineural spread. Seminal vesicle involvement may be another highly significant finding on TRUS biopsy.

At present there are four main treatment options available for prostate cancer:

- active surveillance (watchful waiting),
- radical prostatectomy,
- radiotherapy,
- androgen-deprivation therapy.

The most appropriate treatment for prostate cancer is highly controversial and truly valid analytical comparisons between options are lacking. In elderly men or those with serious comorbid disease, a low-grade, low-volume tumour (often picked up incidentally on TURP chippings) is unlikely to pose a serious threat to health or life expectancy. These individuals are highly appropriate candidates for conservative therapy in the form of watchful waiting. Radical prostatectomy should be reserved for men with curable disease (i.e., organ-confined) who will live long enough to benefit from the cure (at least 10 years). Clinicopathological index of suspicion of extracapsular extension is the main determinant in a man of suitable age and health contraindicating this major operation.

Radical radiotherapy is an alternative curative option in men unsuitable for surgery. It can have a similar success rate with a slightly lower rate of complications compared to radical prostatectomy. Radiotherapy may be given following androgen-deprivation therapy to downsize the tumour or with chemotherapy to sensitise the tumour cells. Another option is to implant the prostate with radioactive seeds (brachytherapy). Positive surgical margins following radical prostatectomy, although not shown to decrease long-term disease control or survival, are usually treated with pelvic radiotherapy, as is extracapsular extension (stage pT3) in the resection. Palliative radiotherapy may also be appropriate in metastatic disease, to treat bone pain.

Disease which is locally advanced or metastatic at diagnosis is best treated with androgen-deprivation therapy, which blocks the hormonal drive that sustains tumour cells. This was achieved previously with surgical castration (bilateral orchidectomy) but now much more commonly with "medical castration" using luteinising hormone-releasing hormone (LHRH) agonists or oestrogens. Anti-androgens are an alternative endocrine therapeutic option and can be administered with a LHRH agonist (maximal androgen blockade). Cytotoxic chemotherapy is reserved for androgen-resistant prostate cancer, i.e., when symptoms recur following endocrine therapy.

Prognosis: grade (Gleason score), pathological stage (notably extracapsular extension) and tumour volume are the most important prognostic indicators. Other factors are positive surgical margins following radical prostatectomy, perineural and lymphovascular invasion and serum PSA level, which is an indirect measure of tumour volume and spread. Overall ten-year survival is approximately 50%, with a 90% ten-year survival in organ-confined (pT1/pT2) disease, 60% in pT3/pT4 disease and only 10% in disease with bone metastases.

Variants of prostatic adenocarcinoma are: mucinous adenocarcinoma (exclude colorectal or bladder primary), signet ring cell adenocarcinoma (exclude gastric, bladder or colorectal primary), periurethral duct adenocarcinoma (syn. endometrioid carcinoma), adenoid basal carcinoma and clear cell adenocarcinoma.

Other carcinomas: rarely, urothelial carcinoma arises in periurethral prostatic ducts; small cell carcinoma; squamous/adenosquamous carcinoma; sarcomatoid carcinoma.

Other cancers: prostate is a common site for rhabdomyosarcoma (usually embryonal) in children; leiomyosarcoma is the commonest prostatic sarcoma in adults; leukaemia/malignant lymphoma (especially secondary involvement by chronic lymphocytic leukaemia); metastases (direct spread – bladder, colorectum; distant spread – lung, malignant melanoma).

5. Surgical Pathology Specimens – Clinical Aspects

Biopsy Specimens

Transrectal Ultrasound (TRUS) Biopsy

The peripheral location of most prostate cancers is ideal for transrectal sampling. This may be guided by suspicious US appearances (peripheral hypoechoic areas) or represent random, multiple biopsies. Ten biopsies (five from each lobe) provides a high diagnostic yield. Any patient with a suspicious DRE or serum PSA level should be biopsied even if TRUS appearances are normal. If random, the biopsies should be carefully labelled to direct further biopsies in the event of a non-diagnostic histology report. Biopsies are obtained in such a way as to maximise sampling of the peripheral zone in each sector sampled.

Transurethral Resection of the Prostate (TURP)

This procedure is performed via a cystoscope using a diathermy loop for resection (resectoscope) and bladder irrigation to wash out the resected chippings. Haemostasis is controlled using electrocoagulation. The bladder neck may be incised following resection. Rarely, dilutional hyponatraemia due to absorption of bladder irrigation fluid causes confusion, nausea and vomiting postoperatively (transurethral resection syndrome).

Resection Specimens

Open (Simple) Prostatectomy

This operation is reserved for BPH where the prostate weighs over 50–75 g. It is also appropriate where there is concomitant benign bladder disease requiring treatment such as a symptomatic diverticulum or a large stone. Potential risks are urinary incontinence, erectile dysfunction, retrograde ejaculation and urinary tract infection. The advantages over TURP are complete removal of the gland (therefore no recurrence) and no risk of dilutional hyponatraemia. However, there is an increased risk of intraoperative haemorrhage and a longer hospital stay. Previous prostatectomy, prior pelvic surgery and prostate cancer are contraindications to the operation.

There are two possible approaches to enucleation of the prostate gland via open prostatectomy:

- retropubic – through a direct incision of the anterior prostatic capsule,
- suprapubic – through an extraperitoneal incision of the lower anterior bladder wall.

The retropubic approach allows excellent exposure and visualisation of the prostate and prostatic fossa during enucleation, ensuring complete removal and control of bleeding sites. There is minimal trauma to the bladder and precise transection of the urethra distally to preserve urinary continence. The suprapubic approach allows direct access to the bladder and bladder neck and is suited to patients with bladder pathology (diverticulum, stone) or a large "middle" lobe of prostate protruding into the bladder.

Radical Prostatectomy

The three aims of this operation are cancer control, preservation of urinary continence and of sexual function. Two approaches are available: the perineal approach was pioneered first and has the advantages of usually less blood loss and greater exposure of and access to the apex of the prostate, thus optimising removal of tumour from this critical margin and allowing precise transection of the urethra. However, its main disadvantage is that it does not allow access to perform a pelvic lymphadenectomy. Furthermore, a greater understanding of periprostatic anatomy and developments in surgical technique over the years have reduced blood loss and improved tumour clearance using the retropubic approach, to the extent that currently the perineal procedure is seldom performed. It may be indicated for small, low-grade tumours when pelvic lymphadenectomy can be safely omitted.

Surgery should be deferred for at least six weeks following needle biopsy and twelve weeks following TURP to allow any inflammatory adhesions or haematoma to resolve. In retropubic prostatectomy, a midline extraperitoneal lower abdominal incision is made from pubis to umbilicus and, after appropriate dissection, a bilateral pelvic lymphadenectomy is performed. This is a staging rather than a curative procedure and, in some centres, the surgeon may ask for a frozen section lymph node analysis, halting the operation should tumour be detected in the node. Prostatectomy proceeds with dissection of the periprostatic fascia, division of the pubo-prostatic ligaments, dorsal vein complex, urethra and bladder neck and excision of the seminal vesicles. Newer nerve-sparing surgical techniques are possible, with the aim of maintaining erectile function postoperatively. These involve preserving the neurovascular bundles, which run between two layers of periprostatic fascia (prostatic and levator). This is most successful in young patients with organ-confined disease but involves a higher risk of positive surgical margins. An option is to remove one neurovascular bundle, on the side of the palpable lesion or positive biopsy, leaving the other intact. Alternatively, if there is a high probability of capsular extension on preoperative assessment, or if the patient is impotent, the bundles should be widely excised.

This major operation has surprisingly low postoperative mortality (0.2%) or serious morbidity. Urinary incontinence, possibly due to distal urethral sphincter dysfunction or bladder neck contracture, is often the most troublesome side effect. Loss of erectile function is now less of a problem thanks to modern surgical alternatives.

6. Surgical Pathology Specimens – Laboratory Protocols

Biopsy Specimens

TRUS needle biopsy: the wide-bore needle cores (18 gauge) are counted and measured (in mm), submitted separately if labelled accordingly and processed for initial histological examination through three levels. Careful handling is necessary to avoid crush artefact. Cores may be painted with alcian blue so that they are easily visible on facing the paraffin block. When sectioning, intervening ribbons of unstained sections are usefully kept for ancillary immunohistochemical studies if required.

TURP chippings: are weighed and sampled according to laboratory protocol. Fourteen per cent of specimens will reveal an unexpected carcinoma (stage pT1) and the more tissue processed the higher the detection rate. The availability of serum PSA now means that the chances of missing a clinically significant carcinoma are reduced. The potential management of such a detected cancer should ideally be known to avoid a substantial waste of resource. If aggressive treatment (radical prostatectomy) might be considered, for example in a younger patient, all tissue is embedded and examined histologically, as is also the case if there is any clinical suspicion of malignancy.

Otherwise, initial sampling of TURP specimens is recommended along the following Royal College of Pathologists guidelines:

For 12 g or less of tissue, all is processed; for over 12 g, 12 g plus an extra 2 g for every 5 g of tissue in excess of 12 g should be processed. This will normally equate to approximately six to eight cassettes for the average case. The suggestion of scrutinising chippings for suspicious (yellow or indurated) areas is felt to be impractical. One level is examined from each block. If carcinoma (or high-grade PIN) is found, all tissue should be processed to give an accurate stage (pT1a tumour in $\leq$ 5% of tissue resected; pT1b tumour in > 5% of tissue resected).

If there is a previous diagnosis of carcinoma of the prostate, only a small amount of tissue, say 6 g or four cassettes, need be embedded.

Resection Specimens

Specimen

- most prostate resections are retropubic radical prostatectomy specimens (including seminal vesicles) for biopsy-proven adenocarcinoma.
- occasionally, simple (retropubic/suprapubic) prostatectomy is performed for BPH. This is an enucleation procedure and usually produces an intact nodule with a wedge-shaped cut in one side. Orientation is not usually possible, although two distinct lobes should be identifiable. The specimen is weighed and measured (three dimensions, mm), then serially sectioned at 3–4 mm intervals. These sections are carefully examined for areas suspicious of carcinoma (yellow, firm) and six to eight cassettes of tissue processed, labelling the two lobes separately.

Radical Prostatectomy

Initial procedure

- orientate the specimen using the seminal vesicles (situated on the posterior aspect) and by placing a probe (sometimes a catheter is in situ) into the prostatic urethra. This will allow identification of the flat base superiorly (proximal, bladder, base margin) and the more conical apex anteroinferiorly (distal, urethral, apical margin).
- weigh the entire specimen, measure the prostate in three dimensions (mm) and give the lengths (cm) of the attached seminal vesicles and vasa deferentia.
- paint the right, left, anterior, posterior, superior and inferior surfaces of the prostate using six different-coloured inks, including the soft tissue around the base of the seminal vesicles but not the seminal vesicles themselves. Make a note of any areas where the prostatic tissue has been disrupted by the surgical knife, as this may lead to a false positive surgical margin.
- fix the specimen by immersion in 10% formalin for at least 24–36 hours .

- dissect off the seminal vesicles and vasa deferentia and serially section these.
- the proximal and distal margins are then removed. One option is to perform a very thin (1 mm) shave and submit these intact, ensuring they are embedded such that the true margin is sectioned. Note that in respect of the distal margin, one is interested in the prostatic tissue surrounding the distal urethral limit, rather than the urethra itself, which often seems to retract into the fixed specimen.

An alternative method involves amputating the proximal and distal 5 mm of the prostate (corresponding to the bladder and urethral margins respectively) and serially sectioning these at 3 mm intervals perpendicular to the amputating cut (i.e., parallel to the urethra – Figure 30.2). This technique allows a more accurate assessment of how close the tumour extends to these margins but, as only one section is examined for each 3 mm slice, the entire margin will not have been sampled.

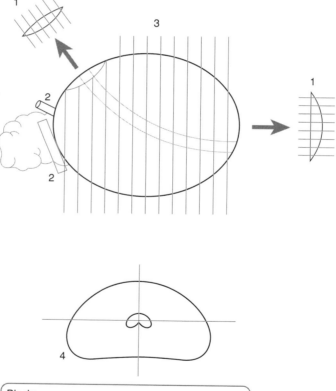

Blocks
1. Proximal (base) and distal (apex) margins
2. Base of seminal vesicles and vas limits
3. Prostate serial sections
4. Slices are bisected/quadranted to fit cassettes (or whole mounted)

Figure 30.2. Blocking a radical prostatectomy specimen.

• after removal of the margins, the prostate is serially sectioned at 3–4 mm intervals in the coronal plane from anterior to posterior. Some pathologists prefer to section the prostate in a horizontal plane. The slices are laid out sequentially and carefully examined, maintaining orientation with the help of the coloured inks. Malignancy is often not obvious macroscopically, but may appear as multifocal, peripheral, usually posterior, solid, grey-to-yellow nodules, contrasting with the central, spongy, non-neoplastic tissue. Asymmetry between lobes may be another clue.

Description

• tumour: site (right/left, peripheral/central, anterior/posterior).
              size (mm).
              multifocality.
              appearance (soft/firm, pale/yellow/granular).
              edge (circumscribed/irregular).
              extension beyond capsule/into seminal vesicles.
• non-neoplastic tissue: appearance (colour, consistency, nodularity).

Blocks for histology (Figure 30.2)

• sample proximal (base) and distal (apical) margins as described.
• sample the seminal vesicles at their bases (junction with the prostate) and the vasa deferentia at their limits.
• each serial section is bisected into right and left halves (and if necessary into superior and inferior quadrants) to fit into routine cassettes and the entire gland processed for histological examination, labelling each block carefully to aid microscopic interpretation.
• alternatively, some pathologists prefer to partially sample the prostate initially, concentrating on suspicious areas and random sections from the circumferential margin.
• whole mount sectioning may be available in some centres, greatly facilitating histological interpretation, but is usually reserved for teaching and research purposes.
• all pelvic lymph nodes (usually submitted separately) should be counted and sampled.

Histopathology report

• tumour type: acinar (proximal duct) adenocarcinoma/other.
• tumour differentiation: use the Gleason grading system. Each tumour is assigned two grades, based on the most predominant of five different architectural patterns present, ranging from grade 1 (well-differentiated) to grade 5 (undifferentiated). The two grades are summed to give the Gleason score (maximum 10). If only one grade is present, the grade is doubled to give the score, e.g., 3 + 3 = 6.
• tumour volume: the tumour is outlined microscopically on each glass slide and the area involved measured (mm^2). The areas for all sections are summed and the overall tumour volume (mm^3) is derived from multiplying by the average slice thickness (3–4 mm). This may be expressed as a proportion of the total volume of the prostate, to give the percentage gland involvement.
• tumour edge: pushing/infiltrative.
• extent of local tumour spread
    –   pT1   clinically inapparent tumour not palpable or visible by imaging.
               T1a   incidental finding in ≤ 5% of tissue resected.

> T1b incidental finding in > 5% of tissue resected.
> T1c identified by needle biopsy.
> - pT2 tumour confined within the prostate.
>   T2a involves ≤ one half of one lobe .
>   T2b involves > one half of one lobe but not both lobes.
>   T2c involves both lobes.
> - pT3 tumour extends through the prostatic capsule.
>   T3a extracapsular extension (unilateral or bilateral).
>   T3b invades seminal vesicle(s).
> - pT4 tumour is fixed or invades neighbouring structures other than seminal vesicles: bladder neck, external sphincter, rectum, levator muscles, and/or pelvic wall.
>   Note a positive surgical resection margin at a point lacking extraprostatic tissue can be reported as pT2+, i.e., extracapsular extension cannot be accurately assessed.

- lymphovascular invasion – perineural and lymphovascular space.
  - present/not present.
  - inside/outside capsule.
- regional lymph nodes.
  - pelvic nodes below the bifurcation of the common iliac arteries.
  - pN0 no regional lymph node metastasis.
  - pN1 metastasis in regional lymph node(s).
- excision margins
  - proximal (base), distal (apical), circumferential margins involved/uninvolved.
  - distances (in mm) to nearest margins.
- other pathology
  - high-grade PIN, effects of radiotherapy or androgen-deprivation therapy (glandular atrophy, apoptosis, vacuolation, stromal fibrosis).

31

Urethra

1. Anatomy

The urethra extends from the internal urethral orifice at the bladder neck to the external meatus. In the male it is approximately 15–20 cm long and is divided into three sections (Figure 31.1).

The prostatic urethra is 3–4 cm long, traversing the prostate in a curved manner. Throughout its length, a midline ridge on the posterior wall known as the urethral crest projects into the lumen causing it to appear crescentic on transverse section. The most prominent part of this ridge, close to the midpoint, is called the verumontanum. Here lies the orifice of the prostatic utricle, a short, blind-ending vestigial sac. The openings of the ejaculatory ducts lie on either side of the verumontanum. Prostatic ducts empty into the urethral sinuses, gutters flanking the urethral crest.

The membranous urethra extends from the prostatic apex to the bulb of the penis and measures 1 cm approximately. Small bulbourethral or Cowper's glands lie on either side and secrete into it.

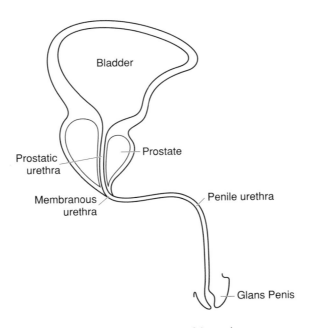

Figure 31.1.   Anatomy of the urethra.

The penile urethra measures 10–15 cm and is surrounded by the corpus spongiosum throughout most of its length. It includes the bulbous urethra proximally and the pendulous urethra distally. Scattered mucus-secreting (Littre's) glands are present periurethrally. The distal portion within the glans penis is dilated to form the fossa terminalis, before narrowing at the external meatus.

The female urethra is approximately 4 cm long and extends from the bladder neck to the external urethral meatus, embedded throughout its length in the adventitial coat of the anterior vaginal wall. Like the male counterpart it has a posterior midline ridge, the urethral crest, which gives a crescentic shape on sectioning, and periurethral mucus-secreting (Skene's) glands.

The urethra is lined proximally by urothelium and distally by non-keratinising stratified squamous epithelium and, in males, the intervening membranous urethra (and part of the penile urethra) by pseudostratified columnar epithelium. However, it should be noted that most urethral tissue submitted for pathological examination is diseased or altered by instrumentation and hence highly susceptible to metaplastic change.

Lymphovascular Drainage

The lymphatics of the proximal urethra drain to the external iliac, obturator and hypogastric nodes (Figure 29.2), while the distal urethra drains to the superficial and then deep inguinal nodes.

2. Clinical Presentation

Urethral lesions may be asymptomatic or, if causing obstruction, can present with haematuria, urinary retention or symptoms of infection. Urethral stricture can mimic benign prostatic enlargement, presenting with obstructive symptoms in the absence of haematuria. Primary urethral malignancy usually presents at a late stage when arising in the proximal urethra. Urethral diverticula may cause irritative symptoms or dribbling.

3. Clinical Investigations

Urethroscopy and biopsy.
Urethrography (micturating and retrograde) – the best methods for the evaluation of urethral strictures, diverticula and, less often, neoplasms.
CT/MRI – to determine tumour stage.

4. Pathological Conditions

Non-neoplastic Conditions

Urethritis: usually a sexually transmitted infection due to *Chlamydia trachomatis*, *Neisseria gonorrhoea* or *Gardnerella vaginalis*. Usually symptomatic in females but not in males, with urethral smear diagnostic. Occasionally seen in young males as part of Reiter's syndrome (urethritis, arthritis and conjunctivitis). Rarely provides surgical biopsy material.

Polypoid urethritis: the urethral equivalent of polypoid cystitis, this is an oedematous, inflammatory growth which may be confused with a papillary neoplasm. It is most commonly seen in the prostatic urethra, near the verumontanum. An association with indwelling catheters has not been shown.

Caruncle: a polypoid, fleshy and friable lesion seen near the meatus exclusively in women. Irritative urinary symptoms are common. Histology reveals a hyperplastic urothelial lining with prominent stromal inflammation and vascularity. Scattered bizarre stromal cells may cause diagnostic confusion with sarcoma.

Benign stricture: may result from previous inflammation or trauma, e.g., catheterisation, and can closely mimic malignancy, resulting in biopsy.

Diverticula: usually seen in women and may be palpated through the vagina. Most are acquired, following infection, obstruction and dilatation of a periurethral gland. Histology often fails to reveal an epithelial lining. An infected diverticulum may be the source of recurrent urinary tract infections. Other possible complications include stones, bladder outlet obstruction and, rarely, malignancy (most commonly adenocarcinoma). Diverticulectomy is the recommended treatment.

Urethral valves: are folds of mucosa that project into the urethral lumen. They are rarely seen in surgical pathology material unless they cause obstruction, when they may be associated with bladder neck hypertrophy.

Urethral polyps: prostatic urethral polyps are small, papillary growths seen in the prostatic urethra of adult males. They are usually asymptomatic but may cause haematuria. Histology shows a lining of benign prostatic acinar epithelium. These polyps are often seen incidentally at cystourethroscopy and sometimes biopsied. Congenital urethral polyps, seen in young males most commonly in the prostatic urethra, are rare growths lined by urothelium which can occasionally cause obstructive symptoms.

Miscellaneous: inverted urothelial papilloma, villous adenoma, nephrogenic adenoma, malako-plakia, amyloidosis and condylomata acuminata are infrequently encountered within the urethra.

Neoplastic Conditions

Benign tumours

The benign urothelial neoplasms of papilloma and inverted papilloma share the same morphological features as their bladder counterparts and rarely arise primarily in the urethra. Haematuria is the commonest symptom. Both should be managed by transurethral resection alone. Leiomyomas and haemangiomas are seen only rarely.

Malignant tumours

The urethra is much more commonly involved secondarily by urothelial carcinoma of the bladder than by primary carcinoma. As with bladder cancer, secondary urethral involvement is more common in males, with a reported incidence of approximately 10–20%. This may take the form of papillary carcinoma, flat carcinoma in situ (which may extend into periurethral ducts) or prostatic stromal invasion. Distinction is important as the latter has a worse prognosis. The same diagnostic histological criteria apply as in the bladder. In females, total urethrectomy is usually performed as part of the cystectomy procedure but, in males, urethrectomy is only performed when separate biopsies show prostatic urethra involvement. Recurrence of urothelial carcinoma in the urethral stump following a urethra-sparing cystectomy may be treated by instillation of BCG immunotherapy or, if there is stromal invasion, transurethral resection or urethrectomy.

Primary urethral carcinoma is more common in females than males and affects mainly those over 50 years of age. Aetiological factors have not been clearly elucidated, although chronic inflammation may play a role. Most tumours arising proximally in the urethra are urothelial in type whereas distal lesions are more often squamous, reflecting the normal epithelial linings at these sites. Adenocarcinoma is seen in association with diverticula, prostatic adenocarcinoma or, in women, arising in periurethral glands. The clear cell variant should be distinguished from nephrogenic adenoma and spread of malignancy from the female genital tract or kidney. In males, primary urothelial carcinoma is usually treated by surgical excision, the extent of which depends on the location and stage of the tumour. Radiotherapy has the advantage of preserving the penis but has a higher rate of tumour recurrence and may result in urethral stricture. Primary urethral carcinoma in the female usually involves the proximal urethra and is locally advanced at presentation. Aggressive surgery, radiotherapy or a combination of both is often required for local control or palliation. Brachytherapy or adjuvant radiosensitising chemotherapy are other treatment options. Local excision is often adequate for distal urethral carcinoma in the female.

Prognosis: prognosis relates to anatomical location and pathological stage. Distal carcinomas have a better prognosis as they are often well-differentiated squamous cell or verrucous types and present earlier. Proximal tumours are more frequently high-grade and present at a later stage, hence prognosis is worse. In men, overall five-year survival rates are 60–70% for penile urethral carcinomas and only 20% for membranous/prostatic urethral lesions.

Other cancers: rare but include adenosquamous carcinoma, small cell carcinoma, malignant melanoma, lymphoma/leukaemia, embryonal rhabdomyosarcoma (in children), aggressive angiomyxoma (in women) and metastatic carcinoma.

5. Surgical Pathology Specimens – Clinical Aspects

Biopsy Specimens

Urethroscopy may be undertaken in isolation or, more commonly, in tandem with cystoscopy. Small urethral lesions are snared using "cold" cup forceps or resected with a small diathermy loop. Staging biopsies of the prostatic urethra are frequently undertaken at the time of cystourethroscopy for evaluation of bladder cancer. Follow-up after cystectomy may require biopsy from the urethral stump, in the event of positive urethral washings.

Resection Specimens

Urethrectomy is performed in one of three situations:

- for bladder cancer in continuity with cystoprostatectomy.
- for recurrence of bladder cancer in the urethral stump (secondary urethrectomy).
- for primary urethral carcinoma.

In women, up until recently the urethra was routinely resected as part of a radical cystectomy procedure for bladder cancer. However, with careful preoperative evaluation it is now sometimes possible to preserve the urethra for orthotopic functional reconstruction of the urinary tract using a neobladder.

In men with bladder cancer, the standard surgical procedure is a radical cystoprostatectomy. Carcinomatous involvement of the urethra (usually prostatic) assessed on preoperative biopsies, is an indication for concomitant urethrectomy.

This is performed in two stages. Prior to the cystoprostatectomy the membranous urethra is dissected from the urogenital diaphragm and transected. This facilitates the subsequent perineal dissection and preservation of the neurovascular bundle. Cystoprostatectomy is completed and then the remainder of the urethra is resected from a perineal approach, dividing it distally and dissecting the bulbar urethra up to the urogenital diaphragm.

Secondary urethrectomy is indicated if urethral washings or biopsy following previous cystoprostatectomy for bladder cancer reveal recurrent tumour. This involves perineal dissection as described for primary urethrectomy but, because of scarring and proximity of small bowel to the urogenital diaphragm, is a much more difficult operation. Complete excision of the membranous urethra proximally is less certain, but frozen section may offer reassurance that a negative margin has been attained.

The best treatment of primary urethral carcinoma in the male is surgical excision. Distal tumours may be treated by transurethral resection, local excision, partial or radical penectomy depending on the extent of tumour infiltration. Carcinoma of the bulbomembranous urethra usually requires radical cystoprostatectomy, pelvic lymphadenectomy and total penectomy. This procedure may be extended to include in-continuity resection of the pubic rami and adjacent urogenital diaphragm to improve the margin of resection. Primary prostatic urethral carcinoma may be treated by transurethral resection if superficial but otherwise requires cystoprostatectomy and total urethrectomy.

6. Surgical Pathology Specimens – Laboratory Protocols

Biopsy Specimens

Tiny pieces of tissue (several mm) retrieved using either "cold" cup forceps or a small diathermy loop are counted, measured, processed intact and examined histologically through three levels. Transurethral specimens should be weighed collectively, the number of fragments counted and all tissue embedded if possible.

Resection Specimens

Specimen

- most urethrectomy resection specimens are for neoplasia as part of a cysto (prostato) urethrectomy. Occasionally, isolated urethrectomy is performed.

Initial procedure

- the specimen may be in several tubular fragments labelled separately or with attached sutures to aid orientation; in the absence of such markers, definitive orientation may not be possible, although the distally resected urethra may be identifiable, having a smaller diameter.
- weigh (g) and measure (cm) each fragment; record the number of fragments.
- paint the external CRM comprising adventitial connective tissue.
- fix the specimen by immersion in 10% formalin for at least 24–36 hours .

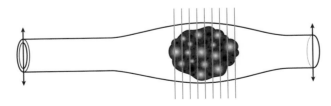

Figure 31.2.   Blocking a urethrectomy specimen. Transverse section the limits and the tumour at 3 mm intervals.

- remove the proximal and distal surgical resection limits (Figure 31.2) by taking circumferential transverse sections (rings) from the ends of the appropriate fragments; if separate fragments are not labelled, take sections from both ends of all fragments, for later possible correlation with clinical information.
- after removal of the limits, the remaining urethra is serially sectioned transversely throughout its length at 3 mm intervals, and the sections laid out sequentially for examination and photography, if desired. Alternatively, if a grossly obvious tumour is identifiable on one luminal surface of the urethra, the specimen is opened longitudinally with small scissors along the opposite surface, taking care not to disturb the tumour. A combination of both approaches often provides the best histological material.

Description

- tumour: site (prostatic/membranous/bulbar/pendulous urethra; meatus).
              length × width × depth (mm).
              multifocality.
              appearance (papillary/polypoid/verrucous/sessile/ulcerated/colour).
              edge (circumscribed/irregular).
- mucosa: carcinoma in-situ away from tumour may appear red and velvety.
- wall: tumour confined to mucosa or infiltrative.
- other: stricture, dilatation, diverticulum.

Blocks for histology (Figure 31.2)

- sample the proximal and distal limits of surgical resection as complete circumferential rings; more than one fragment may need to be sampled.
- sample at least three blocks of tumour, in the form of transverse or longitudinal sections or both, to show the deepest point of circumferential invasion and the relationship to the painted circumferential margin and the adjacent mucosa.
- sample at least one random block of background mucosa to look for carcinoma in situ.
- count and sample all lymph nodes (usually submitted separately).

Histopathology report

- tumour type – squamous/urothelial/adenocarcinoma/other.
- tumour growth pattern – papillary/invasive/flat in situ.
- tumour differentiation – use WHO grades I–III (based on cytological atypia).
- tumour edge – pushing/infiltrative.
- extent of local tumour spread

Urethra (male and female)

- pTa   non-invasive papillary, polypoid or verrucous carcinoma.
- pTis   carcinoma in situ.
- pT1   invasion of subepithelial connective tissue.
- pT2   invasion of any of: corpus spongiosum, prostate, periurethral muscle.
- pT3   invasion of any of: corpus cavernosum, beyond prostatic capsule, anterior vagina, bladder neck.
- pT4   invasion into other adjacent organs.

Urothelial carcinoma of prostatic urethra

-     –   pTis pu   carcinoma in situ, involvement of prostatic urethra.
-     –   pTis pd   carcinoma in situ, involvement of prostatic ducts.
-     –   pT1   invasion of subepithelial connective tissue.
-     –   pT2   invasion of any of: prostatic stroma, corpus spongiosum, periurethral muscle.
-     –   pT3   invasion of any of: corpus cavernosum, beyond prostatic capsule, bladder neck (extraprostatic extension).
-     –   pT4   invasion into other adjacent organs (invasion of the bladder).

- lymphovascular invasion – present/not present.
- regional lymph nodes
  - inguinal/pelvic
  - pN0   no regional lymph node metastasis.
  - pN1   metastasis in a single regional node $\leq$ 2cm.
  - pN2   metastasis in a single regional node > 2cm or multiple regional nodes
- excision margins
  - distances (in mm) to the nearest longitudinal and circumferential periurethral resection limits.
  - presence/absence of carcinoma in situ at longitudinal limits.
- other pathology
  - urothelial carcinoma in situ, diverticulum.

32
Testis, Epididymis and Vas

1. Anatomy

The testes are suspended in the scrotum by the spermatic cords, the left testis hanging somewhat lower (Figure 32.1). The average size is 4–5 cm in length, 2.5 cm in breadth, and 3 cm in the antero-posterior diameter. Weight varies from 10.5 to 14 g. Within the scrotum the testis is covered on its anterior, medial and lateral surfaces by tunica vaginalis, the remnant of a developmental connection with the peritoneal cavity. Each testis is covered by a tough fibrous coat, the tunica albuginea. The substance of the testis is subdivided by septa which run inwards from the tunica albuginea. The glandular structure consists of numerous lobules (~ 400) contained in one of the intervals between the fibrous septa. They consist of from one to four seminiferous tubules, between which lie the interstitial or Leydig cells, responsible for the production of testosterone. In the apices of the lobules, the tubules become less convoluted and unite together

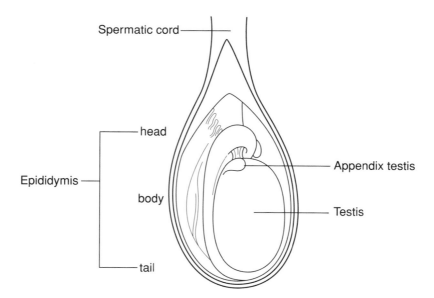

Figure 32.1. Anatomy of the testis, epididymis and spermatic cord. Reproduced from Hermanek P, Hutter RVP, Sobin LH, Wagner G, Wittekind Ch (eds.). TNM Atlas: illustrated guide to the TNM/pTNM classification of malignant tumours, 4th edition. Springer-Verlag: Berlin and Heidelberg, 1997.

to form twenty to thirty larger ducts (tubuli recti). The tubuli recti enter the fibrous tissue of the mediastinum forming a close network of anastomosing tubes (rete testis). The rete testis perforate the tunica albuginea, and carry the seminal fluid from the testis to the epididymis.

The epididymis lies on the posterior surface of the testis. It consists of a central portion or body, an upper enlarged extremity (the head), and a lower pointed end (the tail), which is continuous with the ductus (vas) deferens. The head is intimately connected with the upper end of the testis by means of the efferent ductules of the gland; the tail is connected with the lower end by cellular tissue, and a reflection of the tunica vaginalis. The epididymis is connected to the back of the testis by a fold of the serous membrane. On the upper extremity of the testis, just beneath the head of the epididymis, is a minute oval, sessile body, the appendix of the testis (hydatid of Morgagni). It is the remnant of the upper end of the Mullerian duct. On the head of the epididymis is a second small stalked appendage (appendix epididymis) usually regarded as a detached efferent duct.

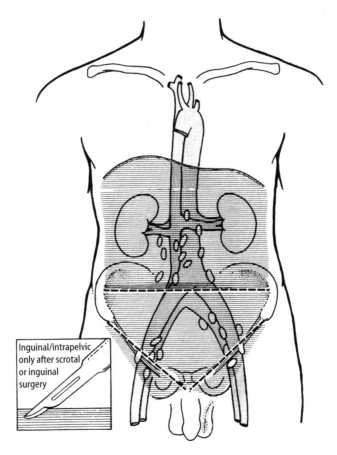

Inguinal/intrapelvic only after scrotal or inguinal surgery

Figure 32.2.   Testis – regional lymph nodes. The regional lymph nodes are the abdominal para-aortic (periaortic), preaortic, interaortocaval, precaval, paracaval, retrocaval and retroaortic nodes. Nodes along the spermatic vein should be considered regional. Laterality does not affect the N classification. The intrapelvic nodes and the inguinal nodes are considered regional after scrotal or ingiuinal surgery. Reproduced from Hermanek P, Hutter RVP, Sobin LH, Wagner G, Wittekind Ch (eds.). TNM Atlas: illustrated guide to the TNM/pTNM classification of malignant tumours, 4th edition. Springer-Verlag: Berlin and Heidelberg, 1997.

The vas deferens consists of a muscular tube, formed of three layers, which connects the tail of the epididymis to the ejaculatory duct at the prostate. The vas passes up in the spermatic cord through the superficial inguinal ring, inguinal canal and deep ring to reach the posterior surface of the bladder. At the ejaculatory duct it is joined by the duct from the seminal vesicles. The vas is lined by a tall columnar epithelium.

Lymphovascular Drainage

The lymphatic vessels of the testes form from four to eight collecting trunks which ascend with the spermatic veins in the spermatic cord. The testicular lymphatics drain to the periaortic and pericaval abdominal nodes. Intrapelvic (common and external iliacs) and inguinal nodes are considered regional after scrotal or inguinal surgery (Figure 32.2).

2. Clinical Presentation

A painless testicular mass is pathognomonic of a primary testicular tumour, occurring in only a minority of patients. The majority presents with diffuse testicular pain, swelling, hardness, or some combination of these findings. Since infectious epididymitis or orchitis is more common than tumour, a trial of antibiotic therapy is often undertaken. If testicular discomfort does not abate or findings do not revert to normal within two to four weeks, a testicular ultrasound examination is indicated. Delays in patients seeking definitive treatment after recognition of the initial lesion are frequent (3–6 months) and correlate with development of metastases. Trauma to the testis can sometimes lead to confusion in diagnosis. Endocrine manifestations such as gynaecomastia (2–4% of patients) are sometimes seen in association with sex cord-stromal tumours. In 5–10% of patients symptoms result from metastasis, e.g., back pain.

Undescended testicular tumours present with a suprapubic lump, urinary or bowel complaints. Development of torsion in an undescended testicle can sometimes be the warning sign of testicular tumour. Rarely, testicular tumours may present with metastases and symptoms of abdominal lump, chronic cough or as a "neck node with unknown primary".

3. Clinical Investigations

Radiological Evaluation

- Scrotal ultrasound – an important non-invasive diagnostic tool. Testicular tumours appear as a hypoechoic lesion.
- Chest X-ray – preliminary evaluation of pulmonary involvement.
- CT scan – imaging of the abdomen and pelvis is required. CT or MRI of the brain is performed in patients with neurologic signs or symptoms.
- FNAC of testicular tumours is generally not recommended as it is useful only if it is positive, and there is a theoretical risk of needle tract recurrence. FNAC is valuable in the investigation of possible metastatic lesions (seminoma versus non-seminomatous).

Serum Tumour Markers

Serum tumour marker concentrations are determined before, during, and after treatment and throughout long-term follow-up. Increased or rising concentrations of alpha-fetoprotein (AFP), human chorionic gonadotrophin (HCG), or both, without radiographic or clinical findings, imply active disease and are sufficient reason to initiate treatment if likely causes of false positive results have been ruled out.

Alpha-fetoprotein: production is restricted to non-seminomatous germ cell tumours, specifically embryonal carcinoma and yolk sac tumours.

HCG: may be observed in both seminomas and non-seminomatous tumours.

Lactate dehydrogenase (LDH): is less specific but has independent prognostic value in patients with advanced germ-cell tumours.

4. Pathological Conditions

Testis

Non-neoplastic Conditions

Pyogenic epididymo-orchitis: usually due to E. coli and presents as a painful mass often clinically confused with testicular cancer. Generally differentiated by ultrasound scanning. Histology resembles a granulomatous orchitis. This can be complicated by venous thrombosis and septic testicular infarct.

Granulomatous orchitis: aetiology and pathogenesis unknown but there is speculation that the disease may have an autoimmune basis. It presents in middle-aged males with painful unilateral testicular mass and associated fever. Some cases are associated with urinary tract infections, history of prostatectomy, inguinal hernia repair and trauma. Grossly, the testis is enlarged and the cut surface is vaguely nodular, yellowish, and hard. Testicular involvement may be total or partial. Histologically, there is a mixed chronic inflammatory infiltrate, fibroblasts and scattered multinucleated giant cells.

Other infections: syphilis, tuberculosis, mumps.

Cysts: epidermoid cysts (below), cysts of tunica albuginea, rete testis, efferent ducts or testicular parenchyma have been described. Cystic dysplasia is a rare congenital disorder with numerous irregular cystic spaces in the mediastinum testis.

Epidermoid cyst: may represent monodermal teratoma, but not potentially metastatic if no adnexal structures or other tissue types are found after thorough sampling. It usually affects ages 10–39 and grossly consists of an intraparenchymal lesion containing white grumous keratin debris, with a keratinised squamous epithelial lining. There is no intratubular germ cell neoplasia.

Hydrocele: accumulation of clear serous fluid between the visceral and parietal layers of the tunica vaginalis, associated with trauma and epididymitis. Histology shows loose to fibrotic connective tissue with a mesothelial lining.

Rare lesions: include malakoplakia, inflammatory pseudotumour.

Neoplastic Conditions

Testicular neoplasms represent less than 1% of all malignancies in males although their incidence is rising. They are highly curable even if advanced; 95% are germ cell tumours and 5% sex cord-stromal tumours. The rest are rare but include mixed tumours not specific to the testis and metastases. Predisposing factors include cryptorchidism, genetic, testicular dysgenesis, Li–Fraumeni syndrome, prior testicular germ cell tumour or intratubular germ cell neoplasia.

Germ cell tumours: the British and American histological classifications of teratoma differ but the terminology can be correlated (Table 32.1). For management and prognostic purposes the most important distinction is between seminomatous and non-seminomatous tumours. Pathological staging has minor clinical significance as therapy is largely dependent on clinical

Table 32.1.   Malignant teratoma classification

British (BTTP)	American/WHO
Teratoma Differentiated (TD)	Mature Teratoma
	Immature Teratoma
Malignant Teratoma Intermediate (MTI)	Teratoma with embryonal carcinoma and/or yolk sac tumour
Malignant Teratoma Undifferentiated (MTU)	Embryonal carcinoma
Malignant Teratoma Trophoblastic (MTT)	Choriocarcinoma (only element)

staging (TNM and the modified Royal Marsden systems) based on imaging techniques (for abdominal/pulmonary/cerebral metastases) and levels of serum tumour markers.

Intratubular germ cell neoplasia (ITGCN): in situ stage of germ cell neoplasia seen in 90–100% of testes adjacent to germ cell tumours. There is an association with infertility (0.4–1.0%), cryptorchidism (2–8% of patients) and in the contralateral testis in patients with prior testicular tumour (5%). Fifty per cent progress to germ cell tumour in five years. Histology shows large seminoma-like cells present along a thickened/hyalinised tubular basement membrane. Spermatogenesis is usually absent. There is positive staining with PLAP (97% of cases) and PAS without diastase (glycogen). It can be treated with low-dose radiation but watchful waiting (clinical, ultrasound examination and serum markers) is advocated by some.

Seminoma: represents 30–50% of testicular germ cell tumours with a mean age at diagnosis of 40 years. Forty per cent have increased serum PLAP and 70% of patients have stage I disease. Metastases are to lymph nodes or bone. The presence of elevated serum HCG does not change the classification and has no clinical significance. However, elevated AFP indicates a non-seminomatous germ cell component (or liver disease), even if not seen histologically. The gross appearance is that of a bulky, homogeneous, pale tumour with lobulated and bulging cut surface. Histology consists of sheets of relatively uniform large, polyhedral, glycogenated tumour cells and delicate fibrous septa with T lymphocytes and plasma cells. Granulomatous inflammation, trophoblastic giant cells and Pagetoid spread to the rete are seen in a minority of cases. There is positive staining with PLAP (almost all), PAS and vimentin. Cytokeratins may be weak/focal and the tumour cells are negative for AFP, HCG (syncytiotrophoblastic giant cells are positive), CD30 and EMA.

Treatment consists of orchidectomy and or radiotherapy (very radiosensitive). Cis-platinum-based chemotherapy is used for bulky retroperitoneal disease or supradiaphragmatic involvement. Prognosis is excellent with a 95% cure rate for stage I (testis confined) or II (infradiaphragmatic nodes) disease. Adverse prognostic factors include tumour > 6 cm, age > 35 years and lymphovascular invasion.

Spermatocytic seminoma: One to two per cent of germ cell tumours with a mean age of 55 years. Regarded as benign but occasionally associated with sarcoma (rhabdomyosarcoma), they are pale with a soft, friable cut surface and 10% are bilateral. Microscopy reveals three types of cells; small (lymphocyte size), medium cells and large (giant) cells and mitoses. They are distinguished from seminoma by the absence of stroma, lymphocytes, glycogen, granulomas and ITGCN. They are positive for CAM5.2 (40%) and negative for PLAP, HCG, AFP and EMA.

Non-seminomatous germ cell tumours (NSGCT): in general more aggressive and metastasise earlier than seminomas. The metastases may not resemble the primary tumour and are radioresistant. Eighty per cent have elevated AFP or HCG at diagnosis. The prognosis is good with 95% cure rate if there is no lymph node or metastatic involvement but ranges from 40 to 95% with metastases. There is a poor prognosis if extensive pulmonary disease is present. Traditionally, the treatment for stage I non-seminomatous germ cell tumours has been orchidectomy followed by retroperitoneal lymph node dissection to eradicate the disease while confined to the local lymph nodes. It is now believed, however, that most patients with such tumours do not benefit from this dissection, a procedure which is not without complications. More recently, stage I non-seminomatous germ cell tumours have been managed by surveillance (regular serum tumour markers and CT scanning). Stage I tumour with lymphovascular invasion and more advanced disease are best treated with chemotherapy. If the concentrations of tumour markers fall after chemotherapy and residual retroperitoneal masses are seen on CT then lymph node dissection is appropriate as 20% of such nodes will harbour residual tumour. When the tumour markers do not fall to normal concentrations after chemotherapy, opinion on treatment is divided between lymph node dissection and further chemotherapy.

Teratoma: represent five per cent of germ cell tumours and contain cellular components derived from two or three germ layers. It is the second most common testicular tumour after yolk sac in children (age < 3), is not associated with intratubular germ cell neoplasia and almost never metastasises. In adults there is a presumption of malignant behaviour regardless of tumour differentiation. Grossly large (5–10 cm), multinodular and heterogeneous (solid, cartilaginous, cystic). Histologically mature teratomas contain differentiated tissues including cartilage, nerve and various epithelia, whereas immature teratomas have foci resembling embryonic or fetal structures including primitive neuroectoderm, poorly formed cartilage, neuroblasts, loose mesenchyme and primitive glandular structures (amount important). Occasional cases undergo malignant transformation with focal malignancy such as squamous cell carcinoma, adenocarcinoma or sarcoma (adults).

Mixed germ cell tumours: mixed forms are common, accounting for one third of germ cell tumours and 70% of non-seminomatous tumours of the testes. Common combinations include embryonal and teratoma; embryonal and seminoma; embryonal, yolk sac tumour and teratoma. Clinical presentation and management are the same as non-seminomatous germ cell tumour and the prognosis is usually that of the worst component.

Embryonal carcinoma: pure tumours represent 2% of germ cell tumours, but 85% of NSGCTs have an embryonal carcinoma component. Histologically solid, alveolar, tubular or papillary patterns of large, epithelioid, anaplastic cells. There is positive staining with HCG or AFP in mixed tumours, cytokeratin, CD30, PLAP and negative staining with EMA.

Yolk sac tumour: considered a unilaterally developed teratoma mimicking embryonal yolk sac tissue. It is the most common testicular tumour age three or less and often pure with a good prognosis (80%+ are stage I). In adults it is usually part of a mixed tumour and has the prognosis of embryonal carcinoma. Most patients have elevated serum AFP. Microscopy varies greatly but includes papillary Schiller Duval bodies, PAS-positive hyaline globules, solid and microcystic patterns.

Choriocarcinoma: Between 0.3% and 1% of germ cell tumours are pure choriocarcinoma, but mixed tumours are more common. It may present initially with early haematogenous metastases (liver, lung, mediastinum, retroperitoneum) and a normal testis or small tumour, but with increased serum HCG. It is usually fatal if pure. Histologically there is haemorrhage and necrosis with a biphasic arrangement of cytotrophoblast and syncytiotrophoblast cells. There is positive staining with HCG, HPL and EMA (syncytiotrophoblast, not cytotrophoblast), cytokeratin, PLAP (50%) and CEA (25%).

Sex cord-stromal tumours: Four per cent of testicular neoplasms and containing epithelial elements of sex cord origin (Sertoli and granulosa cells) admixed with mesenchymal components (Leydig and theca-lutein cells) in varying combinations and degrees of differentiation. Almost all are immunoreactive for inhibin.

Leydig (interstitial) cell tumours: Between 1 and 3% of testicular tumours (age 20–60) with 3% bilateral. They secrete sex hormones and symptoms include gynaecomastia with virilism, precocious puberty and a testicular mass. In adults 10% have malignant behaviour with metastases to lymph nodes, lung and liver. Features suggesting malignancy include large size (> 5 cm), necrosis, vascular invasion, nuclear atypia, numerous and atypical mitoses, infiltrative margins, older patients, aneuploidy and higher MIB-1 activity. Mean survival when malignant is four years. Grossly they are solid brown tumours and 10% have extratesticular extension. Histology reveals sheets of large, round/polygonal cells with eosinophilic cytoplasm and round central nuclei. Reinke crystals are present in 25% of cases. Treatment includes orchidectomy and/or lymph node dissection if malignant.

Granulosa cell tumour: resembles analogous ovarian tumour. The adult form is rare with an age range 20–53 years, usually non-functional and rarely associated with gynaecomastia. It is usually benign but metastases occur in 10% (associated with size > 7 cm, haemorrhage, necrosis, lymphovascular invasion). The juvenile form is the most common neonatal testicular tumour with an average age of onset less than one month or even congenital. There is an association with trisomy 12 and sex chromosome mosaicism if abnormal external genitalia. There is no association with endocrine manifestations. It has a benign behaviour following orchidectomy.

Sertoli cell tumours: one third present with gynaecomastia without virilism and 10% are malignant (to local lymph nodes), indicators being nuclear pleomorphism, size > 5 cm, mitoses, necrosis and lymphovascular invasion. Grossly firm, small, well-circumscribed yellow–white nodules. Histology shows trabeculae lined by Sertoli-like cells. They show positive staining for vimentin, cytokeratin AE1/AE3, and inhibin (variable) but are PLAP negative. Treatment is orchidectomy (radiation and chemotherapy have little effect).

Mixed germ cell-sex cord stromal tumours (gonadoblastoma)

Other tumours not specific to testis:

Leukaemia: testis may be first site of relapse, e.g., ALL in children.

Lymphoma: Fifty per cent of testicular neoplasms in men age 60+, 20% bilateral, often representing spread from systemic disease.

Granulocytic sarcoma: 20–35% patients involved.

Carcinoid: presumed to be a monodermal teratoma, although 20% have other teratomatous elements. It is rare and 10% have clinical carcinoid syndrome.

Metastases to testes: rarely the first clinical sign of disease. Lung, prostate and skin (Merkel cell tumours, melanoma) are the usual primary sites. Immunohistochemistry may help in distinguishing the primary site.

Epididymis

Non-neoplastic Conditions

Epididymitis: primary cause of epididymal obstruction and usually related to cystitis, prostatitis or urethritis that spreads through the vas deferens or lymphatics. It may cause testicular ischaemia and necrosis. Causes include chlamydia trachomatis, neisseria gonorrhoea, E-coli, pseudomonas, other urinary tract infection organisms and rarely tuberculosis and brucellosis.

Cysts of epididymal appendix and epididymal cysts: the former can twist, necrose and present with pain while the latter form an epididymal mass separate from the testis. Treatment is resection of the necrotic appendix and cyst aspiration, respectively, or if persistent epididymectomy.

Spermatic granuloma/epididymitis nodosa: inflammation or trauma damage to the epithelium or basement membrane, causing spillage of spermatozoa into the interstitium (similar to vasiitis nodosa). It consists of a nodule up to 3 cm in the head of the epididymis with histological features of non-caseating granulomas around spermatozoa.

Spermatocele: cystic dilation of efferent ducts lined by ciliated columnar cells with thin connective tissue wall; no smooth muscle. The cysts are usually translucent and contain spermatozoa and proteinaceous fluid.

Neoplastic Conditions

Adenomatoid tumour: most common tumour of the epididymis (age 20–39) and often painful. It is similar to the tumour in spermatic cord, fallopian tube and uterus. It has a mesothelial origin and may be a peculiar form of nodular mesothelial hyperplasia instead of a neoplasm. It is benign, even if it extends into testis. Grossly, a circumscribed white mass up to 5 cm. Histology shows cuboidal cells forming cords and channels with dilated lumina simulating vessels (cytokeratin positive). Resection is curative.

Papillary cystadenoma: familial, unilateral or bilateral (40%) with a mean age of 36 years. Associated with von Hippel–Lindau disease.

Carcinoma of epididymis: rare, with a poor prognosis. It usually presents as a scrotal mass, is large and often haemorrhagic or necrotic.

Rete Testis

Non-neoplastic Conditions

Adenomatous hyperplasia: solid/cystic mass in testicular hilus and usually an incidental microscopic finding.

Cystic dilation (transformation): due to obstruction of epididymis or intratesticular excretory ducts and also seen after haemodialysis.

Cystic dysplasia: presents as testicular mass in infants and children. Consists of cystic dilation of rete testis with compression/atrophy of seminiferous tubules. It is thought to be a developmental anomaly sometimes associated with ipsilateral renal agenesis.

Neoplastic Conditions

Rete testis adenocarcinoma: very rare and resembles mesothelioma of the tunica vaginalis. Wide age range with a poor prognosis.

Sertoliform cystadenoma of rete testis: extremely rare benign tumour (ages 34–62) usually presenting as a unilateral painless testicular mass.

Spermatic Cord and Paratesticular Region

Non-neoplastic Conditions

Torsion: may cause testicular infarct if not treated quickly. This usually occurs in the first year of life or also towards puberty due to trauma . It is associated with incomplete descent, absent scrotal ligaments, absent gubernaculum testis or testicular atrophy causing the testis to be abnormally mobile. Torsion must last at least 6–24 hours to cause an infarct. Treatment consists of untwisting and fixing the testis to dartos muscle or orchidectomy. The opposite testis should be fixed to dartos muscle as a preventive measure.

Vasiitis nodosa: condition of the vas deferens, which resembles spermatic granuloma of the epididymis. It is usually post vasectomy or herniorrhaphy and occasionally associated with recanalisation. Histology shows proliferating ductules and dilated tubules containing spermatozoa in the wall of the vas deferens with hyperplastic smooth muscle. May see perineural or vascular invasion by the proliferating ductules.

Varicocele: abnormal dilation and tortuosity of veins in the pampiniform plexus of the spermatic cord probably due to insufficiency of venous valves. It is often associated with infertility. Ninety per cent are on the left and 10% bilateral. Treatment consists of ligation or occlusion of the left spermatic vein and after treatment 40–55% are fertile.

Neoplastic Conditions

Benign tumours are usually lipomas. Fat collections around a hernia sac are not true lipomas. Non-neoplastic masses include mesothelial and dermoid cysts.

Aggressive angiomyxoma: more usual in the vulva with local recurrence common, but no metastases. Grossly mixed and non-encapsulated with bland spindle cells in myxoid stroma containing prominent thick-walled/hyalinized vessels.

Angiomyofibroblastoma: benign soft tissue tumour which is well circumscribed consisting of alternating hypocellular and hypercellular zones.

Embryonal rhabdomyosarcoma: most common childhood malignant tumour of the spermatic cord. The peak age is 9 years with an 80% overall survival. It is a fleshy white-to-tan tumour, 4–6 cm, and may be mucoid. Small cells, eosinophilic cells and spindle cells with variable cross striations. Immunopositive staining with desmin, muscle-specific actin and myoglobin.

Sarcomas: adults – most common tumours are liposarcoma, MFH, leiomyosarcoma and fibrosarcoma. Treatment is orchidectomy with high ligation of the cord and radiation therapy.

Liposarcoma: usually well differentiated or sclerosing types. There is a 20% recurrence rate following local removal.

Mesothelioma: cystic/solid/nodular masses lining a hernial sac. They have an aggressive behaviour.

Desmoplastic small round cell tumour: occurs in young men and is an aggressive primitive neuroectodermal tumour with a 3–4 cm grey–white firm mass, often near the epididymis. Comprises small cells in a desmoplastic stroma and the prognosis is very poor.

Lymphoma: rare to involve paratesticular regions without testicular involvement.

5. Surgical Pathology Specimens – Clinical Aspects

Biopsy Specimens

1. Inguinal exposure with testicular isolation and biopsy; Testicular biopsy is standard management in patients at high risk of ITGCN as it is thought to progress to invasive tumour in 50–100% of cases and therapy should be considered. It is also useful in the management of the contralateral testis in patients with germ cell tumours, approximately 5% of whom have ITGCN of the opposite testicle. A high incidence of ITGCN (35%) is found in young (< 30 years) patients where the contralateral testis is small (< 16 ml) and of poor quality (soft). These patients constitute a high risk group in whom it is appropriate to recommend biopsy at initial presentation. Biopsy should be 0.3–1.0 cm in maximum dimension and removed atraumatically without squeezing the tissue or handling it with forceps. Open biopsy is considered the normal procedure but needle biopsy may be adequate.
2. Transscrotal open or needle biopsy; rarely performed due to the presumed risk of wound seeding and lymphovascular spread to inguinal lymph nodes.

Resection Specimens

Radical inguinal orchidectomy is performed when a testis tumour is appreciated on examination and/or preoperative imaging studies. This is accomplished via an inguinal incision in order not to alter the lymphatic drainage pattern of the testicle (to the retroperitoneal lymph nodes) by violating the scrotal wall (drainage to the superficial inguinal lymph nodes). Radical orchidectomy also allows ligation of the vas deferens and testicular vessels at the internal inguinal ring, so that, should subsequent surgical removal of the spermatic cord and retroperitoneal lymph nodes be required (for therapy or staging), the inguinal canal need not be explored again.

6. Surgical Pathology Specimens – Laboratory Protocols

Biopsy Specimens

Testicular biopsy (0.3–1.0 cm): placed in Bouin's fixative for a minimum of 2 hours (smaller biopsies) and a maximum of 24 hours. Paraffin sections are cut through levels and stained routinely with haematoxylin and eosin. Comment should be made on the presence or absence of ITGCN, the degree of spermatogenesis, and evidence of atrophy of seminiferous tubules. Immunohistochemical assessment of PLAP (present in ITGCN cells) is helpful in a biopsy showing equivocal morphology.

Epididymectomy: weigh (g) and measure (cm), bisect or serially slice noting any focal lesions (abscess/adenomatoid tumour) and submit representative blocks. Cysts are submitted in total, or if large, blocks of the wall are sampled. Fluid contents can be examined microscopically for sperm to distinguish from a hernial sac.

Appendix epididymis (Hydatid of Morgagni): measure (mm), process intact.

Vasectomy: measure (cm) the segments of right and left vas and submit two complete transverse sections of each. Lengths vary from 0.5 cm to 5 cm – small specimens are often distorted by surgical clamping and care needs to be taken with blocking and embedding to obtain a representative cross-section. Levels or reembedding may be required.

Hydrocele wall: weigh (g), measure (cm) and submit representative blocks. Note any contents, e.g., blood/fibrin.

Resection Specimens

Specimen

- most radical orchidectomy specimens are for malignant tumours but the diagnosis usually cannot be definitively made preoperatively.

Initial procedure

- testes are often received having been incised prior to receipt and this may make assessment of invasion through the tunica albuginea difficult and accurate staging impossible. Urologists should be encouraged to send the intact testis to the laboratory rapidly to allow bisection by the pathologist.
- some tumours spread to involve the cord and this should be looked for and sampled prior to opening the testis to minimise the risk of contamination by tumour.
- the testis is incised in a plane that bisects the epididymis and rete testis such that invasion of these structures can be recognised (Figure 32.3).
- fix by immersion in 10% formalin for 24–36 hours.
- cuts parallel to the incised plane to examine the entire testis are then performed.
- photograph tumour and individual slices if appropriate.
- measurements:
  - dimensions (cm) of testis and length (cm) of spermatic cord.
  - weight of specimen in total (g).
  - tumour – length × width × breadth or maximum dimension (cm).
- identify different tumour appearances looking particularly for areas of haemorrhage and necrosis.
- all areas of different macroscopic appearances should be sampled in order to identify all the histological patterns present (seminomatous versus NSGCT).

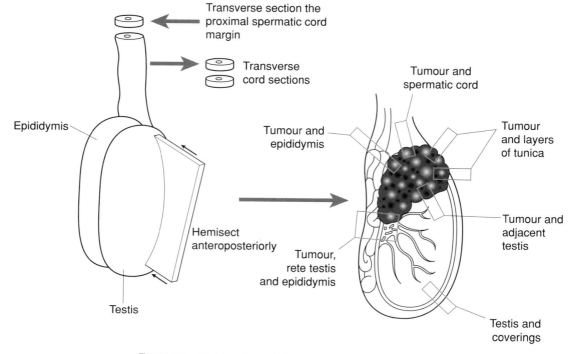

Figure 32.3. Blocking of an orchidectomy specimen for tumour.

- count and submit any lymph nodes with the main specimen.
- examine the cord and surrounding tissue for abnormality.

Description

- tumour: location (testis, rete, epididymis, tunica albuginea, spermatic cord).
  single/multifocal – mixed germ cell.
  colour (pale/uniform – seminoma or lymphoma).
  necrosis (embryonal – MTU).
  haemorrhage (choriocarcinoma).
  cysts/cartilage (teratoma – MTD).
- surrounding testis – normal, scar, calcification.
- other – epididymal cysts, scarring, cord or paratesticular involvement, other lesions.

Blocks for histology (Figure 32.3)

- all areas of different macroscopic appearances are sampled in order to identify all the histological patterns present.
- one block of tumour per centimetre diameter is taken.
- sample areas demonstrating the relationship of tumour, rete and epididymis and of any area where tumour appears to invade these structures or the tunica (Figure 32.3).
- sample, where possible, adjacent non-tumourous tissue to look for vascular invasion.

- sample the surrounding normal testis to look for ITGCN and status of the normal testis (i.e., scar, inflammation, regressional changes, other tumours, calcification).
- sample a transverse section of the cut end of the spermatic cord and ideally this should be done before opening the testis to minimise the risk of contamination by tumour.
- sample the cord in one or two other areas.
- samples for special studies (e.g., electron microscopy, cytogenetics, molecular biologic studies, flow cytometry, image analysis).

Histopathology report

- tumour location: testis/rete/epididymis/cord involvement.
- tumour type – seminomatous/non-seminomatous/sex cord-stromal tumour.
- tumour classification (BTTP or WHO).
- estimate percentage of each component for mixed tumours.
- intratubular, invasive, or both.
- extent of invasion:
  - invasion or penetration of tunica albuginea (specify).
  - involvement of paratesticular structures.
    pT0 no evidence of primary tumour (i.e., scar in testis).
    pTis intratubular germ cell neoplasia (carcinoma in situ).
    pT1 tumour involves testis and epididymis or tunica albuginea, no lymphovascular invasion.
    pT2 tumour involves testis and epididymis or tunica vaginalis with lymphovascular invasion.
    pT3 tumour invades spermatic cord ± lymphovascular invasion.
    pT4 tumour invades scrotum ± lymphovascular invasion.
- lymphatic/blood vessel invasion (specify if in testis or paratestis/spermatic cord).
- regional lymph nodes – usually not removed at surgery but retroperitoneal lymph node dissection occasionally performed – usually following orchidectomy and chemo/radio-therapy.
  - abdominal, periaortic and pericaval and those along the spermatic veins.
    pN0 no regional lymph node metastases.
    pN1 regional lymph node metastasis ≤ 2 cm but ≤ 5 positive nodes.
    pN2 regional lymph node metastasis > 2 cm but ≤ 5 cm, or > 5 positive nodes, or extra-nodal extension.
    pN3 regional lymph node metastasis > 5 cm.
- other tissue(s) – involved/uninvolved by tumour.
- results of special studies (immunohistochemistry – alpha-fetoprotein, HCG, PLAP, CAM 5.2, EMA (germ cell tumours), inhibin (sex cord stromal)).
  - comments – correlation with other specimens, as appropriate
  - correlation with clinical information, as appropriate
  - presence/absence of embryonal carcinoma, yolk sac tumour and lymphovascular invasion are prognostically significant.
- resection margin(s), including spermatic cord.
- additional pathologic findings; Leydig cell hyperplasia (correlated with HCG), scarring, the presence of haemosiderin-laden macrophages and intratubular calcification (tumour regression), testicular atrophy, and abnormal testicular development (e.g., dysgenesis).

33 Penis

1. Anatomy

The penis (Figure 33.1) comprises the body or shaft and the two ends, anterior and posterior (root). The anterior portion is composed of the glans, coronal sulcus and foreskin (prepuce). There is a vertical cleft, the meatus, in the apex 5 mm in length and this is attached to the foreskin by a triangular piece of mucosa, known as the frenulum. The base of the cone is represented by the corona, an elevated ridge surrounding the glans. The coronal sulcus below the corona separates the glans from the foreskin.

The glans is composed of the following layers: epithelium, lamina propria, corpus spongiosum, tunica albuginea and corpus cavernosum. The stratified epithelium is thin and non-keratinised in uncircumcised males but keratinised in circumcised males. The lamina propria is loose, 1–4 mm thick, and separates the epithelium from the corpus spongiosum. The corpus spongiosum is the main component of the glans and consists of specialised erectile tissues with numerous anastomosing venous sinuses. It is 8–10 mm in thickness. The tunica albuginea is a very dense, white, fibrous membrane which terminates in or near the glans separating the corpus spongiosum from the corpora cavernosa and constitutes an important barrier to the spread of cancer to the latter. The coronal sulcus is a narrow and circumferential "cul-de-sac" located just below the glans corona. It is a common site for recurrence of carcinoma or of a positive margin in cases of foreskin carcinoma. The foreskin is a double membrane which encases the glans and from which it is separated by a potential space.

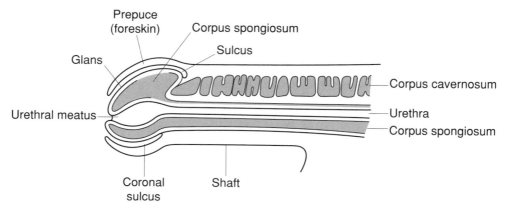

Figure 33.1. Anatomy of the penis. Reproduced from Hermanek P, Hutter RVP, Sobin LH, Wagner G, Wittekind Ch (eds.). TNM Atlas: illustrated guide to the TNM/pTNM classification of malignant tumours, 4th edition. Springer-Verlag: Berlin and Heidelberg, 1997.

The shaft comprises three cylindrical masses of cavernous erectile tissue bound together by the fibrous tunica albuginea and encased in Buck's fascia. These cylinders are the ventral corpus spongiosum with a centrally located urethra and two corpora cavernosa separated by a median raphe.

The posterior part (root) of the penis is deeply embedded in the perineum. It is fixed to the anterior wall of the pelvis by a ligamentous insertion of the corpora cavernosa to the ischium and pelvic bones.

Lymphovascular Drainage

A rich network of lymphatics in the glans and corpora cavernosa courses along the dorsal vein and drains into superficial and deep inguinal lymph nodes. The foreskin and shaft skin lymphatics drain also to the superficial inguinal lymph nodes. The sentinel group of the superficial inguinal nodes lymph nodes is the most common site for lymph node metastasis. Within the deep inguinal nodes, the node of Cloquet (highest) is significant as the next level of drainage is the iliac nodes.

2. Clinical Presentation

Infectious lesions present with an area of induration or erythema on the glans which is often painful and itchy. Biopsy or microbiological culture are usually confirmatory and treatment decided depending on the nature of the lesion.

Early symptoms of penile cancer include the appearance of a painless nodule, warty growth or ulcer, especially on the glans or foreskin, or swelling at the end of the penis. Any abnormality including warts, blisters, sores, ulcers, white patches, rash or bumps, should be evaluated. Most penile cancers do not cause pain, but can result in ulceration and bleeding in later stages. Circumcision as a preventive factor for penile cancer remains unproven. A number of benign conditions, such as genital warts or infections, can have similar symptoms.

3. Clinical Investigations

- Full blood picture (low Hb).
- Biochemistry – raised calcium in bone metastasis in 20%.
- Swab if suspected local infection – candida, etc.
- Chest X-ray.
- CT scan of abdomen and pelvis.
- Bone scan if indicated.

4. Pathological Conditions

Non-neoplastic Conditions

Paraphimosis: forceful retraction of phimotic foreskin over the glans may cause marked swelling which blocks replacement of the foreskin. This is often painful, and associated with constriction and urinary retention. Treatment consists of circumcision.

Phimosis: the foreskin orifice is too small to permit its retraction; usually due to scarring from repeated infection. Smegma (desquamated epithelial cells, sweat, debris) accumulates, causes secondary infections and possibly carcinoma.

Inflammatory Lesions

Balanitis circumscripta plasmacellularis (Zoon's balantitis): occurs in uncircumcised men with an unknown aetiology (possibly autoimmune). It consists grossly of well-defined brown/red plaques, solitary or multiple, and clinically resembles erythroplasia of Queyrat.

Balanitis xerotica obliterans (BXO): this is the male equivalent of lichen sclerosus et atrophicus of vulva. It may cause narrowing of the urethral meatus or phimosis. There is a weak association with carcinoma of the foreskin. The gross appearances are that of grey–white foci of atrophy in the foreskin or perimeatal glans.

Balanoposthitis: infection of the glans and foreskin, usually due to candida, anaerobes, gardnerella or pyogenic bacteria. It is common in uncircumcised newborns or uncircumcised men with poor hygiene and accumulation of smegma and due to the propensity of pathogenic bacteria to adhere to the mucosal surface of foreskin. It causes phimosis.

Fournier's gangrene: necrotizing fasciitis of the genitalia due to bacterial infection. Risk factors include trauma, burns, anorectal disease, diabetes, leukaemia and alcoholic cirrhosis.

Sexually transmitted disease: these include granuloma inguinale (calymmatobacterium granulomatis), herpes simplex virus, lymphogranuloma venereum (chlamydia trachomatis), candida, molluscum contagiosum, scabies and syphilis.

Neoplastic Conditions

Condyloma accuminatum: benign tumour caused by HPV 6 or 11 and related to verruca vulgaris (common wart). It is usually sexually transmitted and seen near the coronal sulcus and inner surface of the foreskin. It has a propensity for recurrence but does not evolve into invasive cancer. The gross features are of papillary, wart-like, often multiple lesions, 1 mm or larger. Treatment involves local preparations (podophyllin).

Giant condyloma accuminatum: very rare, benign, exophytic papillary growth of penis (Buschke–Löwenstein tumour). Grossly, usually involves the foreskin and coronal sulcus, 5–10 cm cauliflower like verruciform tumour. Histology resembles that of a condyloma.

Peyronie's disease: fibrous dermal and fascial thickening causing curvature towards the side of the lesion and restricting movement during erection. There is an association with Dupuytren's contracture and it is considered a form of fibromatosis. It may regress spontaneously, but responds to small amounts of irradiation, steroids and excision.

Carcinoma in situ (Penile intraepithelial neoplasia): known as Bowen's disease, Bowenoid papulosis and erythroplasia of Queyrat.

Bowen's disease (squamous cell carcinoma in situ): affects skin of the shaft and scrotum. Ten per cent progress to invasive squamous cell carcinoma and one third may have unrelated visceral malignancy (lung, GI, urinary tract). It is HPV positive and grossly consists of a sharply demarcated, grey–white plaque with shallow ulcer and crusting. Histology shows markedly dysplastic cells in all layers of the epithelium.

Bowenoid papulosis: sexually active young men (mean age 30), usually on skin of the shaft, glans or scrotum and associated with HPV 16 or 18. It almost never becomes invasive and may spontaneously regress. Grossly, may resemble condyloma accuminatum and histologically Bowen's disease.

Erythroplasia of Queyrat: one or more shiny red, velvety plaques, usually on the glans and prepuce, which is histologically similar to Bowen's disease but occurs at an older age. It is also HPV positive.

Squamous cell carcinoma of penis: this is relatively rare in the UK (< 1% of carcinomas in men vs. 10–20% in Asia, Africa, South America) affecting ages 40–70 years. It is particularly rare with early circumcision (at birth). There is an association with paraphimosis, phimosis, HPV 16, smoking, psoriasis and patients treated with UVB radiation. One third of non-HPV cases are associated with balanitis xerotica obliterans.

Most tumours arise from the glans or inner foreskin near the coronal sulcus as a slow-growing, irregular mass. Patients occasionally present with inguinal nodal metastases and occult penile cancer due to severe phimosis or a very small primary tumour. Metastases to inguinal lymph nodes, lung, liver or bone occur and are present in 15% of cases at diagnosis. Lymph nodes may be enlarged at clinical presentation due to infection alone.

The gross appearance is papillary or flat (ulcerated papule). The cut surface shows a white, solid, irregular tumour with superficial or deep penetration. The microscopy is classified according to growth patterns as superficial spreading, vertical growth, verruciform, multicentric or mixed. They are graded on differentiation as well, moderate or poor (G1, G2, G3) depending on the extent of keratinisation. Undifferentiated carcinomas are rare. Most cases have associated carcinoma in situ and/or squamous hyperplasia.

Prognosis: dependent on histologic grade, nodal status and depth of penetration into the various anatomical compartments. Poor prognostic factors are lymphovascular invasion, vertical growth pattern, basaloid, sarcomatoid, solid, anaplastic and pseudoglandular subtypes. The average five-year survival is 70–80%.

Basaloid carcinoma: an aggressive high-grade and deeply invasive tumour in which 50% have enlarged inguinal nodes (due to metastasis) at diagnosis. It is usually associated with human papillomavirus (HPV) and represents 5–10% of penile cancers.

Sarcomatoid carcinoma: is a rare, aggressive, large tumour with a predominance of anaplastic spindle cells. It usually involves the glans and there are frequent recurrences due to inadequate surgery.

Verrucous carcinoma: this is a slow-growing, extremely well-differentiated variant of squamous cell carcinoma (5–10%) with low malignant potential. It is locally invasive, one third recur (inadequate surgery or multifocal tumour) but rarely/never metastasises. It is associated with HPV 6 and 11. The tumour involves all penile compartments (glans most common) and penetrates through lamina propria with a broad base and pushing borders. It is prone to local recurrence if incompletely excised and may dedifferentiate with radiotherapy.

Malignant melanoma: is the most common tumour after squamous cell carcinoma, but is still rare (< 1%). It is similar to melanoma at other sites but shows propensity for lymph node spread (50%).

Sarcomas: extremely rare but include Kaposi's sarcoma, leiomyosarcoma, epithelioid sarcoma, rhabdomyosarcoma.

5. Surgical Pathology Specimens – Clinical Aspects

Biopsy Specimens

Macules, papules, nodules and ulcers from the glans are biopsied to exclude neoplasia or confirm the diagnosis particularly if these lesions have been long standing. Specimens are either punch biopsies (3–5 mm) or excision skin ellipses.

Circumcision specimens consisting of the foreskin are removed more often in the context of benign penile conditions (BXO, Zoon's, phimosis and paraphimosis). Occasionally a small cancer is removed in this fashion and margins in this case will be important. These are dealt with below.

For carcinoma in situ of the glans with or without adjacent skin involvement, therapeutic options include local applications of fluorouracil cream or microscopically controlled surgery. Wide local excision with circumcision may be adequate therapy for control of lesions limited to the foreskin.

Resection Specimens

The goal of treatment in invasive penile carcinoma is complete excision with adequate margins. For lesions involving the prepuce, this may be accomplished with simple circumcision. For infiltrating tumours of the glans, with or without involvement of the adjacent skin, the choice of therapy is dictated by tumour size, extent of infiltration, and degree of tumour destruction of normal tissue. The options include penile amputation (partial or total penectomy) and irradiation. Stage I and II penile cancer is most frequently managed by penile amputation for local control. Whether the amputation is partial, total, or radical will depend on the extent and location of the neoplasm. Radiation therapy with surgical salvage is an alternative approach. There is no standard treatment which is curative for stage IV penile cancer. Therapy is directed at palliation, which may be achieved either with surgery or radiation therapy.

Glansectomy

This procedure involves removing the foreskin and glans and although not commonly performed, is indicated for localised tumours and carcinoma in situ of the glans. There is a higher risk of incomplete removal and therefore tumour recurrence.

Partial Penectomy

Successful local control by partial penectomy depends on division of the penis 2 cm proximal to the gross tumour extent. During the operation the skin is incised circumferentially and the cavernous bodies are divided sharply to the urethra. The dorsal vessels are then ligated and the urethra is dissected proximally and distally to attain a 1 cm redundancy. After a dorsal urethrotomy a skin-to-urethra anastomosis is performed and the redundant skin approximated dorsally to complete the closure.

Modified Partial Penectomy

When the penile stump after partial penectomy is too short for directing urinary stream, releasing the corpora from the suspensory ligament, dividing the ischiocavernosus muscle, and partially separating the crura from the pubic rami can obtain further length. The scrotum is incised and skin flaps fashioned for penile coverage.

Total Penectomy

If the size/site precludes partial penectomy, then as part of penile amputation the proximal urethra is dissected and transposed to the perineum with an indwelling catheter placed for adequate urinary stream.

Radical Surgery

This is rarely performed but involves penectomy including removal of the scrotum, testes, spermatic cords and ilioinguinal lymph node dissection.

Ilioinguinal Lymph Node Dissection

Inguinal lymphadenopathy in patients with penile cancer is common but may be the result of infection rather than neoplasm. If palpable enlarged lymph nodes persist three or more weeks after removal of the infected primary lesion and a course of antibiotic therapy, lymphadenectomy should be considered.

In cases of proven regional inguinal lymph node metastasis (fine needle aspiration cytology or biopsy) without evidence of distant spread, bilateral ilioinguinal dissection is the treatment of choice. Radiation therapy may be an alternative in patients who are not surgical candidates. Postoperative irradiation can decrease incidence of inguinal recurrences. Because of the high incidence of microscopic node metastases, elective adjunctive inguinal dissection of clinically uninvolved (negative) lymph nodes in conjunction with amputation is often used for patients with poorly differentiated tumours. However, lymphadenectomy can carry substantial morbidity, such as infection, skin necrosis, wound breakdown, chronic oedema, and even a low, but finite, mortality rate. The impact of prophylactic lymphadenectomy on survival is not known. For these reasons, there are varying opinions on its use.

6. Surgical Pathology Specimens – Laboratory Protocols

Biopsy Specimens

Diagnostic punch and incisional biopsies: count, measure (mm), process intact and cut through three levels. PAS stain for fungi if suspected.

Elliptical excisions: measure (mm), ink the deep and lateral (circumferential) margins and cut into multiple transverse serial slices.

Foreskin: stretch and pin out to a rectangular shape and fix for 24–36 hours. Make serial vertical slices to include skin, mucocutaneous junction and margins of excision.

Resection Specimens

Specimen

Glansectomy, penectomy (partial or total).

Initial procedure

The various anatomical components of the penis should be examined as any of these may be the site of involvement.

- photograph.
- fix in 10% formalin for 24–36 hours.
- measurements:
  - dimensions (cm) of specimen and individual components (foreskin, shaft and glans).
  - tumour: length × width × depth (cm) or maximum dimension (cm).
    distances (cm) to the urethral and surgical resection margins.
- identify the shaft and glans.
- remove the foreskin, leaving a 2–3 mm redundant edge of skin around the sulcus. This permits better evaluation of the coronal sulcus. Proceed with foreskin as above.
- ideal sectioning is longitudinal, centred along the urethra, with additional parallel sections on both sides. With a probe as a guide the urethra is opened along the ventral aspect where it is closest to the surface and the cut is then continued to bisect the penis.
- involvement of the foreskin, frenulum, glans, meatus, corpora cavernosa, urethra and corpus spongiosum are recorded.
- a transverse section of the urethral margin should include the mucosal surface, surrounding lamina propria and corpus spongiosum. This is usually long in partial penectomy specimens because the surgical technique uses a long urethra stump for reconstruction.
- shaft margin: usually a large specimen. Divide it in two, from dorsal to ventral along the central septum and submit the cut surface entirely. Each half should be labelled left or right. If the specimen has a long shaft, cut two or three additional sections distal to the margin.

- examination of the cut surface of the glans represents the best approach for surgical pathology evaluation.
- glans (glansectomy): several longitudinal sections should be taken. Cut the specimen into two halves labelling them left and right, going from meatus to proximal urethra. Cut three to six serial sections, 2–3 mm in width from each half.
- photograph suitable individual slices.

Description

- tumour: site (urethral meatus/glans/prepuce/coronal sulcus/shaft – dorsal, ventral, lateral). single/multifocal.
             appearance (verrucous/warty/exophytic/sessile/ulcerated).
             edge (circumscribed/irregular).
- foreskin – ulcerated/thickened/papule/warty.
- glans – erythematous/ulcerated/macule/papule/warty.
- other – BXO, scars of previous surgery/biopsy.

Blocks for histology (Figure 33.2)

- shave section from shaft margin (including skin, erectile bodies and urethra).
- samples of foreskin to include associated conditions.
- sample four sections of tumour to demonstrate depth of invasion, relationships to the adjacent surface epithelium, corpora cavernosa, corpus spongiosum and urethra.
- sample two to three transverse sections through the shaft at different levels.

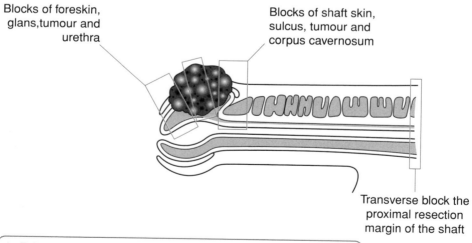

1. Paint and transverse block the shaft proximal resection margin
2. Multiple serial longitudinal blocks to represent tumour in relation to foreskin, sulcus, glans, corpora and urethra

Figure 33.2.   Blocking a penectomy specimen.

- sample longitudinal sections through the glans to include the urethra.
- in larger specimens it is important to submit two to three additional sections of the more distal urethral cylinder to ensure adequacy of the resection margin.
- count and sample all lymph nodes accompanying the specimen.

Histopathology report:

- tumour site (urethra, foreskin, glans, shaft).
- tumour size.
- patterns of growth and histological type.
- tumour grade (well, moderately, poorly differentiated, or verrucous).
- tumour extension: subepithelial connective tissue, tunica albuginea, corpus spongiosum, corpus cavernosum, urethra.
- in-situ component (present/absent/extent, multifocal).
      pTis carcinoma in situ.
      pTa noninvasive verrucous carcinoma.
      pT1 tumour invades subepithelial connective tissue.
      pT2 tumour invades corpus spongiosum or corpus cavernosum.
      pT3 tumour invades urethra or prostate.
      pT4 tumour invades other adjacent structures.
- lymphovascular space invasion (present/absent).
- regional lymph nodes: superficial and deep inguinal nodes
      pN0 no regional lymph node metastases.
      pN1 metastasis in a single superficial, inguinal lymph node.
      pN2 metastasis in multiple or bilateral superficial inguinal lymph nodes.
      pN3 metastasis in deep inguinal or pelvic lymph node(s) unilateral or bilateral.
- excision margins: urethra, corpora, skin – distances (mm).
- other pathology: status of non-neoplastic epithelium (condyloma, BXO, Zoon's, inflammatory process).

Pelvic and Retroperitoneal Specimens

Maurice B Loughrey, Damian T McManus

34 Pelvic Exenteration Specimens

1. Anatomy

The relevant anatomy is discussed in other sections pertaining to the various organs in which cancers originate. Specimens may be classified into one of three groups (Figure 34.1):

Anterior Pelvic Exenterations: bladder, lower ureters, reproductive organs, draining lymph nodes and pelvic peritoneum.

Posterior Pelvic Exenterations: rectum, distal colon, internal reproductive organs, draining lymph nodes and peritoneum. Such procedures are also known as composite resections.

Total Pelvic Exenteration: bladder, lower ureters, rectum, distal colon, reproductive organs, draining lymph nodes and peritoneum.

2. Clinical Presentation

Pelvic exenteration is performed for locally advanced or recurrent malignant tumours within the pelvis. Whilst locally advanced (stage IV) cervical carcinoma was formerly the commonest indication, this is now much rarer as a result of earlier detection of cervical cancer by screening programmes. Exenteration is now performed with increasing frequency for pelvic recurrence of rectal adenocarcinoma or anal carcinoma. Patients undergoing this procedure for these cancers will often have been treated by radiotherapy preoperatively.

More detailed discussion of the symptoms and clinical signs of the various malignant tumours that might result in a pelvic exenteration are found in the relevant chapters relating to gastrointestinal tract and gynaecological specimens. Locally advanced malignancies may produce fistulae between viscera such as the rectum and vagina. Specific symptoms and signs result, e.g., fistulae between the rectum and urinary bladder may result in pneumaturia (gas bubbles in the urine) and contamination of the urine by faeces (faecaluria).

3. Clinical Investigations

Exenterations are performed for advanced or recurrent pelvic malignancy in the absence of extra-pelvic metastatic spread. Patients will usually have been staged by one or more radiological techniques:

CT scanning: this is particularly useful in the evaluation of pelvic and retroperitoneal lymphadenopathy and metastatic disease outside the pelvis. Magnetic resonance imaging has largely replaced CT scanning in the evaluation of the T stage of cervical, endometrial and rectal tumours. Pelvic exenteration is a major surgical procedure and carries with it considerable morbidity and

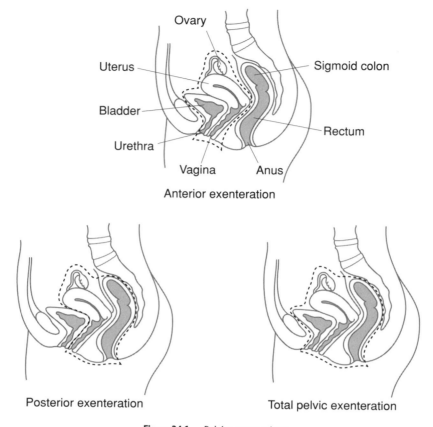

Figure 34.1. Pelvic exenterations.

mortality. Although occasionally it might be performed as a palliative procedure, it is contraindicated if there is evidence of widespread distant metastases.

Magnetic resonance imaging (MRI): this is used to clinically stage cervical, endometrial and rectal cancers preoperatively.

Positron Emission Tomography (PET scanning): PET scanning detects metabolic activity in malignant tumours and in combination with CT (CT–PET) is particularly useful in the identification and localisation of recurrent or metastatic disease.

4. Pathological Conditions

Pelvic exenteration may be performed for:

- advanced stage IV cervical carcinoma.
- locally advanced rectal adenocarcinoma.
- recurrent cervical, rectal or anal carcinoma with no evidence of distant metastasis.

- certain sarcomas, e.g., malignant fibrous histiocytoma or locally invasive tumours such as aggressive angiomyxoma. The pelvis is a common site for both types of tumour, which may be associated with advanced pelvic disease without distant metastasis elsewhere.
- pelvic exenteration may be used occasionally for advanced endometrial adenocarcinoma with involvement of the vagina but is generally not recommended in ovarian carcinoma as there is usually peritoneal disease outside the pelvis. Advanced vaginal or vulval squamous carcinoma with involvement of the rectum or urinary bladder may rarely be treated by pelvic exenteration but such locally advanced disease is frequently accompanied by pelvic side wall involvement or nodal metastasis.
- aggressive muscle-invasive transitional carcinoma can be treated by cystoprostatectomy or variants of pelvic exenteration. Prostatic carcinoma may be treated by radical prostatectomy in certain circumstances but pelvic exenteration has no role in the management of locally advanced prostatic carcinoma, as such disease is almost invariably accompanied by distant metastatic spread.

5. Surgical Pathology Specimens – Clinical Aspects

Advanced (stage IV) cervical carcinoma is usually treated preoperatively by radiotherapy or neo-adjuvant chemotherapy with radiotherapy. Locally advanced rectal cancer may be treated by long-course or short-course radiotherapy to downstage tumours prior to resection. Cervical carcinoma can show an excellent response to radical radiotherapy treatment and it is not uncommon to find no evidence of residual disease. There can be a similar downstaging of rectal carcinoma, in some instances obviating the need for composite resection, and macroscopically the tumour may only be represented by a small area of ulceration. Similarly, local lymph nodes hyalinise, becoming difficult to identify and harvest.

Contraindications to pelvic exenteration include significant co-morbidity or distant metastatic disease (except perhaps for isolated resectable liver metastasis from rectal carcinoma). Involvement of major pelvic vessels or nerves by carcinoma is generally felt to represent a contraindication to surgery for carcinomas, but not necessarily sarcomas. Involvement of pelvic side walls or sacral bone are also relative contraindications, although en-bloc resection of the sacrum can be used for locally advanced primary and recurrent rectal carcinoma.

6. Surgical Pathology Specimens – Laboratory Protocols

A general protocol is described. This can be modified according to the type of specimen received (anterior, posterior or total pelvic exenteration) and the primary site of the tumour.

Specimen

- anterior exenteration.
- posterior exenteration/composite resection.
- total pelvic exenteration.

Initial procedure

- identify and measure each organ that is present in the resection.
- identify and take a limit block from:
  - ureteric limits.
  - urethral limit.

-    –   vaginal limit.
-    –   proximal and distal bowel.
-    –   painted circumferential or radial fascial margins and serosal surface of rectum above peritoneal reflection if present. The quality of the mesorectal excision should also be assessed for advanced rectal tumours as discussed in Chapter 5.
- •   fixation can be problematic in such a large specimen. The bladder can be inflated with formalin from without. The bowel may be partially opened avoiding disruption of the serosa and radial margin in the vicinity of the tumour.
- •   after fixation the specimen can be bisected in a sagittal plane to give roughly equal left and right halves. This should allow visualisation of the anatomical relationship between cervical tumours and the rectum posteriorly, the vagina inferiorly and the urinary bladder anteriorly. Rectal tumours may spread anteriorly to involve the vagina and also the urinary bladder. Fistulae may be present and can be demonstrated by exploration with a probe.

Description

- •   list organs present and dimensions.
- •   presence or absence of tumour.
- •   site of tumour.
- •   size of tumour.
- •   extent of tumour; relationship of tumour to adjacent organs and resection margins.
- •   fistulous tracts involving tumour or perforation.
- •   describe anatomical location, size and number of harvested lymph nodes.
- •   list of any separately submitted lymph node groups.
- •   other pathology, e.g., dilatation of ureter.

Blocks for histology

- •   it may be helpful to use a diagram such as Figure 34.2 to identify the origin of blocks for histology.
- •   longitudinal limit blocks of colon, rectum, ureters, urethra and distal vagina.
- •   the remaining blocks taken for histology depend on the type and origin of the tumour, if a tumour can be identified:

Cervical carcinoma

- •   blocks of tumour and tumour in relation to:
-    –   anterior rectal wall.
-    –   posterior bladder wall.
-    –   vagina.
-    –   pericervical tissues with lateral circumferential margins.
-    –   ureters.
-    –   peritoneum.
-    –   if no cervical tumour is apparent post-radiotherapy, then the cervix must be blocked to identify residual disease histologically. It may be "clock-faced", submitting the entire cervix for histology or more pragmatically, four quadrants taken from the transformation zone.
- •   representative sections are also submitted from uninvolved tissues:
-    –   bladder wall.
-    –   urethra.

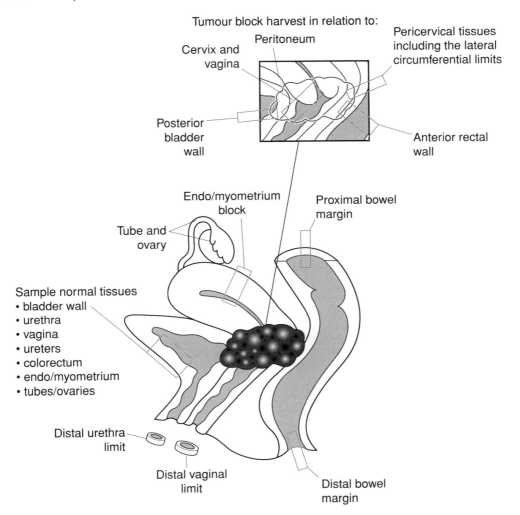

Figure 34.2. Blocking of total pelvic exenteration specimen for a pT4 cervical carcinoma.

- – ureters.
- – vagina.
- – endometrium/myometrium.
- – fallopian tubes and ovaries.
- – colorectum.
- • pelvic lymph node dissections will often be submitted separately and individually labelled and are described later.

Rectal Carcinoma

- blocks of tumour and tumour in relation to:
  - mucosa.
  - posterior vaginal wall.
  - dome of urinary bladder.
  - prostate and seminal vesicles (in males).
  - cirumferential margin of mesorectum.
  - peritoneum.
- the mesorectal fat must be dissected to identify lymph nodes.
- representative sections of uninvolved tissues are also submitted.

Histopathology report

- the specific features that should be included in pathology reports of cervical, rectal cancers and soft tissue tumours are detailed in other relevant chapters. The purpose of pelvic exenteration is one of complete local excision and in view of this the status of longitudinal and circumferential resection margins and peritoneum in relation to the tumour must be documented.

Sarcomas and tumour recurrence in soft tissues

- the dissection and precise blocking protocol must be adapted to suit the individual specimen.
- in general terms, blocks should be taken from tumour (one per centimetre), tumour and involved pelvic structures, tumour and resection margins and representative blocks of uninvolved structures.
- tumour stage; use the TNM system for soft tissue sarcomas where pelvis is a specific topographical site and pelvic tumours are classified as deep tumours.

35 Retroperitoneum

1. Anatomy

The retroperitoneal space may be defined as that part of the lumbo-iliac region which is bounded anteriorly by the parietal peritoneum, posteriorly by the posterior abdominal wall, superiorly by the twelfth rib and vertebra and inferiorly by the iliac crest and the base of the sacrum. The lateral borders are formed by the quadratus lumbora muscles.

This space contains the kidneys, adrenal glands, ureters, aorta and inferior vena cava and their tributaries and many lymph nodes. Numerous nerves, the lumbosacral nerve plexus and ganglia from both the sympathetic and parasympathetic autonomic nervous system are also present.

The retroperitoneal and pelvic lymph nodes are found around the aorta and its branches and may be divided into the following groups (Figure 35.1):

1. para-aortic.
2. inferior mesenteric.
3. common iliac.
4. internal iliac.
5. external iliac.
6. superficial and deep inguinal.
7. sacral.
8. pararectal.

The testes drain to the para-aortic lymph nodes and the prostate to the sacral and internal iliac nodes. The uterus drains to the external and common iliac nodes.

The genitourinary system is considered in detail in Chapters 21–33. This section will consider tumours of the retroperitoneum and retroperitoneal lymph node dissections. Diseases of the adrenal gland are discussed in Chapter 36.

2. Clinical Presentation

The retroperitoneum is rather inaccessible and because of its anatomical location tumours can grow to a large size before becoming clinically apparent. Symptoms and signs of a retroperitoneal tumour may be vague and only manifest late in the course of the disease because of obstruction/displacement of adjacent structures such as the ureter.

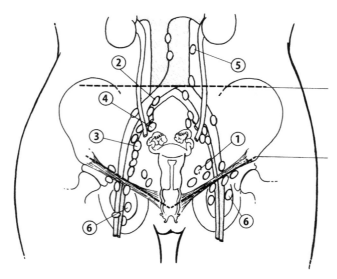

Figure 35.1. Retroperitoneal and pelvic lymph nodes. 1. Hypograstric (internal iliac). 2. Common iliac. 3. External iliac. 4. Lateral sacral. 5. para-aortic. 6. Inguinal. Reproduced from Hermanek P, Hutter RVP, Sobin LH, Wagner G, Wittekind Ch (eds.). TNM Atlas: illustrated guide to the TNM/pTNM classification of malignant tumours, 4th edition. Springer-Verlag: Berlin and Heidelberg, 1997.

3. Clinical Investigations

Plain abdominal X-ray, barium enema or an intravenous pyelogram may suggest the presence of a retroperitoneal tumour due to distortion of normal structures. However, the investigations of choice are ultrasonography, CT scanning or magnetic resonance imaging (MRI). Arteriography may also be useful, particularly if resection of a large tumour is contemplated. Historically, lymphangiograpy was the investigation of choice in the evaluation of lymphadenopathy in the retroperitoneum. Now CT scanning is more commmonly performed. Whilst CT is very good at detecting large nodal masses associated with malignant lymphoma, it is less effective in the assessment of metastatic disease to the pelvic and retroperitoneal nodes. The status of pelvic and retroperitoneal lymph nodes is particularly important in patients with stage 1 non-seminomatous malignant germ cell tumours of the testis for reasons discussed later and positron emission tomography (PET) scanning is currently being evaluated as an alternative imaging modality in the context of a clinical trial.

4. Pathological Conditions

A variety of tumours, both benign and malignant, may arise within the retroperitoneum. The commoner lesions are discussed here.

Liposarcoma: arising within the retroperitoneal fat, well-differentiated liposarcoma, particularly the sclerosing subtype, represents one of the commonest histological subtypes. There is a very low risk of metastasis with this type of lesion, which indeed has been described as an atypical lipoma at other sites. However, such lesions can be difficult to excise from the retroperitoneum and may prove lethal because of pressure effects on adjacent organs or local recurrence if incompletely excised. These tumours may also contain or develop a dedifferentiated spindle cell component, resembling a high-grade spindle cell sarcoma. Careful macroscopic examination and adequate sampling are important. Lipomas also arise at this site; careful evaluation is necessary to distinguish from well-differentiated liposarcoma as described above.

Other sarcomas: these include malignant fibrous histiocytoma and leiomyosarcoma. Careful consideration must be given before rendering a diagnosis of malignant fibrous histiocytoma as it is increasingly recognised that a proportion of such lesions represent anaplastic forms of other malignant tumours. At this site lesions such as sarcomatoid renal cell carcinoma should also be excluded. Both benign and malignant smooth muscle tumours may occur. Leiomyoma is reported as very rare and is to be distinguished from leiomyosarcoma and renal angiomyolipoma. Leiomyosarcoma may arise from the wall of the inferior vena cava or its tributaries.

Peripheral nerve tumours: relatively common at this site, although not as frequent as in the mediastinum. Schwannomas may be quite large and show cystic degeneration; neurofibromas and malignant peripheral nerve sheath tumours are also described. Rarer tumours include lesions such as paraganglioma (chemodectoma/aortic body tumour), ganglioneuroma, neuroblastoma and other small, round, blue cell tumours such as Ewing's sarcoma/PNET and intra-abdominal desmoplastic small cell tumour.

Solitary fibrous tumour, haemangiopericytoma and carcinoid tumours: although haemangiopericytoma-like areas may be seen in various soft tissue tumours, the retroperitoneum remains a typical site for true haemangiopericytomas in middle-aged female patients. The histogenesis of retroperitoneal carcinoid tumours is uncertain. Some may represent a form of germ cell tumour, which also occur at this site either as primary tumours or more commonly as lymph node metastases from a testicular or ovarian primary.

Malignant lymphoma and metastatic disease: lymphoma may involve the retroperitoneal lymph nodes and lead to massive enlargement. Diffuse large B cell lymphoma (and variants such as T-cell-rich B cell) and follicle centre cell lymphomas are among the commonest. Pelvic and retroperitoneal nodes are a common site for metastatic disease from malignant germ cell tumours of the testis, prostatic carcinoma or gynaecological malignancy.

Miscellaneous: abdominal aortic aneurysms are only rarely biopsied. Idiopathic retroperitoneal fibrosis is an uncommon reactive, inflammatory condition that may simulate a tumour at laparotomy – it strictures and distorts the ureters resulting in hydronephrosis. Most cases are of unknown aetiology, a minority being drug related or associated with inflammatory type aortic aneurysms.

5. Surgical Pathology Specimens – Clinical Aspects

Biopsy Specimens

Percutaneous CT guided needle core biopsy or fine needle aspiration may be performed for retroperitoneal tumours or if there is evidence of lymphadenopathy suggestive of lymphoma. It is not commonly used in the investigation of suspected metastatic disease at this site.

Resection Specimens

Retroperitoneal tumours: these may be very large and structures such as the kidney enveloped by the tumour. A smaller wedge biopsy, obtained at laparotomy, may also be submitted if it is not possible to excise the whole tumour or if a needle core biopsy has proven inconclusive.

Retroperitoneal and pelvic lymph node dissections: nodal dissections are frequently performed in association with cervical carcinomas unless these fall into the micro-invasive category and/or are being managed by a non-radical surgical approach. Nodal dissection is also indicated for late-stage and high-grade endometrial cancers, radical prostatectomy and cystectomy but the situation for testicular germ cell tumours is more complex.

Metastatic seminoma is generally treated by radio/chemotherapy. Retroperitoneal lymph node dissection (RPLND) may be performed as prophylaxis against abdominal recurrence in clinical stage 1 non-seminomatous germ cell tumours or in the context of a residual mass post-chemotherapy. Prophylactic RPLND is generally not performed in the United Kingdom for clinical stage 1 non-seminomatous germ cell tumours, in contrast to Europe or the United States, where such operations are more common.

Clinical stage 1 non-seminomatous testicular germ cell tumours may be managed conservatively by surveillance with CT scanning and serial serum tumour markers or by chemotherapy. The prognostic factors influencing the administration of chemotherapy are considered in more detail in Chapter 32. However, about 25% of patients managed by surveillance will relapse, with abdominal nodal disease being the most frequent site. Chemotherapy will then be administered and if a residual mass persists this will be excised. Such specimens frequently show widespread necrosis and fibrosis but there may be residual areas of viable tumour. This can range from differentiated, mature tissues that are insensitive to chemotherapy and form cystic masses that press on local structures (growing teratoma syndrome) to mixed solid/cystic lesions containing immature/undifferentiated teratoma (10–25% of cases). The factors influencing an increased risk of progression are the presence of MTU (embryonal carcinoma), yolk sac tumour or trophoblastic tumour and incomplete resection (as judged by the surgeon). These criteria will influence the decision to give further chemotherapy and this should be borne in mind when the pathologist is examining these specimens so that sufficient blocks are sampled and margins inked.

6. Surgical Pathology Specimens – Laboratory Protocols

Retroperitoneal Tumours

Needle Core Biopsy Specimens

These are counted, their length recorded (in mm) and embedded for histological examination through multiple levels. Fine cores may be painted with alcian blue to allow visualisation when facing the paraffin block at section cutting.

Excision Biopsy

These are weighed (g) and their dimensions (cm) recorded. The lesion is serially sectioned and either representative sections taken for histology or all the tissue is processed. If the biopsy is received unfixed and depending on the clinical differential diagnosis, material may be snap frozen or sent for cytogenetics, tumour imprints made and tissue fixed in glutaraldehyde for EM.

Resection Specimens

Initial procedure

- the specimen is weighed (g) and measured (cm). The relationship of tumour to any recognisable organs such as the kidney that are present in the resection is noted.
- the surface of the specimen is painted with ink.
- if the specimen is received unfixed then consideration should be given to the use of ancillary techniques as described above.

- the specimen is fixed in formalin for 24–36 hours. It may be advantageous to cleanly bisect large specimens after a few hours to allow adequate fixation in the centre.
- the specimen is serially sectioned at intervals of 1–2 cm.

Description

- weight (g), dimensions (cm) of specimen and constituents (fat, connective tissue, kidney, lymph nodes, etc.).
- tumour size (maximum diameter or three dimensions (cm)).
- edge of tumour (well circumscribed, encapsulate or infiltrative) and relationship to surrounding structures.
- appearance of cut surface of tumour (haemorrhage, necrosis, cystic degeneration, etc.).

Blocks for histology

- representative samples of tumour (approximately one block per centimetre to include any macroscopically different-looking areas).
- tumour and adjacent structures.
- tumour and inked circumferential margin of specimen.
- lymph nodes.
- uninvolved organs/tissues.

Histopathology report

- tumour type.
- maximum diameter of tumour.
- tumour grade (if applicable).
- tumour stage; use the TNM system for soft tissue sarcomas where retroperitoneum is a specific topographical site and retroperitoneal tumours are classified as deep tumours.

Retroperitoneal and pelvic lymph node dissections

- such specimens will often be submitted in multiple parts, each representing a specific anatomical nodal group and it is important that this information is preserved in the final histological report.
- weigh (g) each specimen and dissect out recognisable lymph nodes. The maximum dimension (cm) of the largest node should be recorded. Smaller lymph nodes may be submitted intact; larger nodes can be bisected or serially sectioned and then submitted in a separate tissue block. It is important to record on the final histology report the number of nodes identified. For example, in cervical carcinoma retrieval of 10 uninvolved lymph nodes is considered necessary for assignment to the pNO category.
- RPLNDs post-chemotherapy for testicular germ cell tumours present particular challenges. There may be a recognisable tumour mass present. The circumferential margin is inked to assess the adequacy of excision. Multiple representative sections are taken to ensure that any residual viable areas of embryonal carcinoma or yolk sac tumour are detected (Figure 35.2).

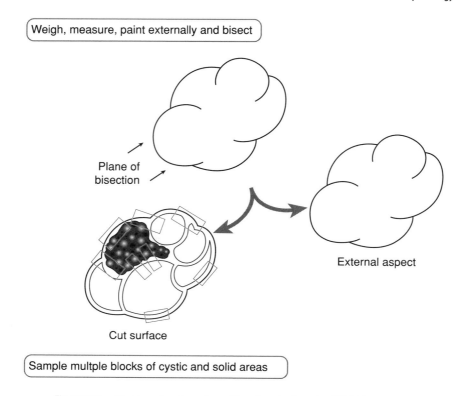

Weigh, measure, paint externally and bisect

Plane of
bisection

External aspect

Cut surface

Sample multple blocks of cystic and solid areas

Figure 35.2.   Blocking of a retroperitoneal lymph node dissection (RPLND) specimen.

Histopathology report

- anatomical location of lymph node groups.
- weight (g) of tissue. Number of nodes identified. Number of lymph nodes involved by metastatic disease. Maximum diameter of largest involved node. Presence or absence of extra-nodal spread.

RPLNDs for non-seminomatous germ cell tumours post chemotherapy.

- presence of fibrosis, tumour necrosis or other effects of chemotherapy.
- presence or absence of residual viable tumour. Mature cystic teratomatous components, immature elements, malignancies of somatic components, i.e., carcinoma or sarcoma.
- presence or absence of residual viable embryonal carcinoma, yolk sac tumour or choriocarcinoma.
- relationship to inked circumferential margin.

36 Adrenal Gland

1. Anatomy

The adrenal glands are paired, yellowish, retroperitoneal organs that lie close to the upper poles of the kidneys (Figure 28.1). They are surrounded by renal fascia but separated from the kidneys by perirenal fat. The left adrenal is almost crescentic in shape whereas the right is more pyramidal. In adults they average 5 cm in length and 5 g in weight, being proportionately larger at birth.

Each gland is divided into an outer cortex and inner medulla, the former being of mesodermal origin and the latter neuroectodermal. Both layers have important physiological roles in hormone secretion, which is the basis for the most common clinical presentations of adrenal pathological conditions. The cortex is divided into three zones (the glomerulosa, fasciculata and reticularis) and is under direct control from pituitary secretion of adrenocorticotrophic hormone (ACTH) via a negative feedback system. The adrenal cortex secretes the mineralocorticoid hormone aldosterone which is responsible for maintaining fluid and electrolyte balance (mainly under influence of the renin–angiotensin axis), the glucocorticoid hormone cortisol (important in control of metabolism), and small amounts of sex hormones. The outer cortex is lipid-laden and golden-yellow in colour whereas the inner cortex (zona reticularis) is brown due to high lipofuscin content. The grey–white medulla secretes the catecholamines noradrenaline and adrenaline.

Lymphovascular supply

Arterial blood supply is from adrenal branches of the aorta, renal and inferior phrenic arteries. The right adrenal vein drains directly into the inferior vena cava whereas the left drains into the left renal vein. Lymphatics pass to the lateral aortic nodes.

2. Clinical Presentation

Because of their location, adrenal tumours seldom present with symptoms due to mass effect. Rarely, a large adrenal carcinoma may cause abdominal pain, low-grade fever (due to tumour necrosis) and a palpable mass. Instead, presentation is more often as an incidental finding on CT scanning of the abdomen or as a result of symptoms related to hormones secreted by the adrenal tumour. These hormones give rise to characteristic constellations of symptoms and signs (clinical syndromes) and the initial diagnosis may be confirmed by appropriate biochemical investigation, after excluding an exogenous cause of hormone excess.

Hypercortisolism (Cushing's syndrome): central weight gain, "moon face", thin skin, striae, bruising, hirsutism, hypertension, osteoporosis, proximal myopathy.

Hyperaldosteronism (Conn's syndrome): urinary frequency, weakness, hypertension, hypokalaemia, hypernatraemia, metabolic alkalosis.

Hypoadrenalism/adrenal insufficiency (Addison's disease): anorexia, weight loss, fatigue, cutaneous pigmentation, orthostatic hypotension, hyponatraemia, hyperkalaemia, metabolic acidosis.

Virilising adrenal tumours: hirsutism and primary amenorrhoea.

Phaeochromocytoma: headaches, sweating, anxiety, chest pain, tachycardia, tremor, (paroxysmal) hypertension.

3. Clinical Investigations

Biochemical Assessment

Hypercortisolism
- morning and evening serum cortisols (diurnal variation is lost in hypercortisolism).
- 24-hour urinary cortisol.
- dexamethasone suppression test (cortisol normally suppressed).
- plasma ACTH (differentiates primary hypercortisolism (ACTH low) from pituitary-dependent hypercortisolism or ectopic ACTH production (ACTH high)).
- petrosal venous sinus sampling (to localise source of ACTH production).

Hyper/hypo-aldosteronism
- serum sodium, potassium, bicarbonate.
- serum aldosterone and plasma renin (primary/secondary hyperaldosteronism).
- erect and supine aldosterone:renin ratios (normally vary with posture).
- saline suppression tests (saline infusion normally suppresses aldosterone).
- adrenal vein sampling of aldosterone (for lateralisation of lesion in primary hyperaldosteronism).

Hypoadrenalism
- ACTH stimulation (Synacthen) test (low cortisol response indicates hypoadrenalism).
- adrenal auto-antibodies (+ve in autoimmune hypoadrenalism).

Virilising tumour
- serum adrenal androgen profile.

Phaeochromocytoma
- 24-hour urinary catecholamines.
- clonidine suppression test if above result ambiguous (normally suppresses catecholamine production).

Radiological Assessment

- CXR – to look for lung tumour as a possible ectopic source of ACTH in hypercortisolism.
- CT/MRI – to assess size, margins, multifocality, density, homogeneity and presence of necrosis or calcification in adrenal lesions; often poor, however, at distinguishing benign

from malignant apart from on size; in overt adrenal carcinoma used to assess staging and resectability preoperatively. Contralateral adrenal and pituitary assessment may be helpful in distinguishing adrenal hyperplasia from adenoma.

- Radioisotope metaiodobenzylguanidine (MIBG) scan – images medullary tissue and is particularly useful for detecting extra-adrenal phaeochromocytomas.
- Core biopsy and FNA.

4. Pathological Conditions

Cortex

Congenital adrenal hyperplasia: this autosomal recessive disorder is caused by an enzyme deficiency in the cortisol biosynthetic pathway, most commonly 21-hydroxylase. ACTH levels are elevated by negative feedback, causing adrenal enlargement. Symptoms are caused by diversion of cortisol precursors into androgenic steroid pathways, leading to virilisation. A spectrum of severity exists and the condition may go unrecognised in males. Affected females may present at birth with sexual ambiguity and adrenal failure, or later with hirsutism or primary amenorrhoea. Treatment consists of steroid replacement; surgical pathology specimens are seldom seen.

Addison's disease: chronic adrenal cortical insufficiency is most commonly of autoimmune aetiology but other causes include tuberculosis, malignant infiltration, fungal infection and sarcoidosis. Treatment is aimed at the underlying cause, in addition to steroid replacement. Surgical resection is seldom indicated.

Acquired hyperplasia: is usually due to overproduction of ACTH either by the pituitary gland (usually an adenoma) or an ectopic source, most commonly bronchogenic small cell carcinoma. Both cause bilateral (may be asymmetrical) adrenal enlargement, which may be diffuse or nodular. Histology shows thickening of and lipid depletion within the zona fasciculata of the adrenal cortex. Occasionally, pigmented cortical nodules are seen, possibly as part of Carney's syndrome. Pituitary-dependent adrenal cortical hyperplasia (Cushing's disease) accounts for 60–70% of adult cases of Cushing's syndrome. It is treated by transphenoidal pituitary surgery and irradiation if this fails. Bilateral adrenalectomy is now rarely performed. Ectopic ACTH production accounts for 15% of adult cases of Cushing's syndrome and treatment is aimed at the primary tumour. Conn's syndrome is due to bilateral adrenal hyperplasia in approximately 25% of cases. Treatment is primarily medical in the form of spironolactone, an aldosterone antagonist (may see spironolactone bodies on histology), but unilateral adrenalectomy is curative in some cases.

Adenoma: these may be incidental findings or present with hormone-related symptoms. They are usually solitary, sharply circumscribed and weigh less than 50 g.

Sectioning reveals a golden-yellow appearance, possibly with irregular mottling. Histology usually shows lipid-rich cells resembling those of the zona fasciculata, arranged in cords or nests. Focal, mild-to-moderate nuclear enlargement and pleomorphism is common and not an indication of malignancy. The best indication of hormone functionality is to look for cortical atrophy in the adjacent adrenal tissue (indicates Cushing's syndrome). Conn's syndrome caused by an aldosterone-secreting adenoma is significant as it represents a curable form of systemic hypertension. Regardless of functionality, most adrenal adenomas are surgically excised, although radiological monitoring (by CT or MRI) for size increase may be acceptable for small (< 5 cm), non-functioning masses.

Carcinoma: adrenal carcinoma is rare, affecting both sexes equally at an average age of 50. Because the hormone-producing capability is often deleted in tumour cells, clinical manifestations of hormone secretion usually only become apparent when the tumour has reached a large size. Symptoms are often mixed, e.g., Cushing's syndrome plus virilisation, and, together with patient age, give some indication as to the likelihood of underlying malignancy. Adrenal carcinoma rarely causes pure hyperaldosteronism. The tumours are usually large (almost all weigh over 100 g) with a variegated appearance showing focal haemorrhagic, necrotic or cystic change. A capsule may be seen, often with obvious tumour infiltration. Histology most characteristically shows a trabecular architectural arrangement of cells with small nuclei and eosinophilic cytoplasm but cytological atypia is highly variable. The best histological predictors of behaviour are mitotic index, a diffuse growth pattern, fibrous bands and vascular invasion. Distinction from metastatic renal cell carcinoma is important. Spread is via haematogenous and lymphatic routes to liver, lung and lymph nodes. In addition, there is often local invasion, into kidney and possibly inferior vena cava. Treatment is aimed at complete surgical removal of the tumour, if possible. Adjuvant mitotane (o,p'-DDD) therapy may control endocrine symptoms and tumour size. The overall five-year survival for these aggressive tumours is only 35%.

Medulla

Phaeochromocytoma: induces all its clinical manifestations through the production of catecholamines, which may be intermittent and life-threatening. Known as the 10% tumour (approximately 10% are bilateral, 10% are extra-adrenal, up to 10% are malignant), there is a strong association with multiple endocrine neoplasia (MEN) type 2A, von Hippel–Lindau disease and neurofibromatosis type 1. Extra-adrenal phaeochromocytomas, or paragangliomas, are morphologically identical and are most commonly found in the retroperitoneum, mediastinum, carotid body and urinary bladder. These have a higher incidence of malignant behaviour. Phaeochromocytomas average 3–5 cm in diameter and 75–150 g in weight and are therefore usually easily seen on radiographic imaging with CT or MRI. They are soft, pale-to-tan-coloured often with mottled areas of congestion, haemorrhage or necrosis, focal cystic degeneration and a fibrous pseudocapsule. Histology characteristically shows well-defined nests of cells ("Zellballen") separated by a delicate fibrovascular stroma. Nuclear enlargement and pleomorphism are common and are not an indication of malignancy, which is notoriously difficult to predict histologically. In fact, the presence of distant metastases is the only reliable criterion. Favoured metastatic sites include ribs and spine. Treatment is primarily surgical excision of the tumour, sometimes solely as a debulking procedure in the presence of advanced malignant disease. The overall five-year survival rate for phaeochromocytomas is under 50%. Background medullary hyperplasia is an indicator of familial disease.

Neuroblastoma: a paediatric tumour (80% occur < 4 years of age) of the sympathetic nervous system belonging to the family of "small, round, blue cell" tumours. Most present with an intra-abdominal mass. Forty per cent arise in the adrenal glands, most of the remainder being retroperitoneal or intrathoracic. Ganglioneuroblastoma and ganglioneuroma represent better-differentiated counterparts which are seen in an older age group and less commonly involve the adrenal gland. The clinical and laboratory aspects of these highly specialised paediatric tumours will not be discussed further.

Miscellaneous conditions: chronic adrenalitis is usually secondary to inflammation in adjacent organs, e.g., chronic pyelonephritis; adrenal haemorrhage (secondary to sepsis, shock, coagulopathy), cysts, myelolipoma (composed of fat and heamatopoietic tissue), lipoma, angioma, schwannoma and adenomatoid tumour (of mesothelial origin) are all occasionally encountered in surgical pathology practice.

Other malignant neoplasms: sarcomas (most commonly leiomyosarcoma) are very rare in the adrenal gland; malignant melanoma and malignant lymphoma/leukaemia usually secondarily involve the adrenals but may rarely be primary; metastatic carcinoma is the commonest pathological lesion and can closely mimic primary adrenal carcinoma (lung, breast and kidney most common primary sites).

5. Surgical Pathology Specimens – Clinical Aspects

Biopsy Specimens

Biopsies of adrenal masses, in the form of fine needle aspiration or needle core, are taken under CT guidance, most often to distinguish primary and secondary malignancy. Biochemical investigations often render biopsy of an adrenal mass unnecessary. Because of the potentially serious risk of hypertensive crisis, suspected phaeochromocytoma has been regarded as a contraindication to needle biopsy.

Resection Specimens

There are numerous surgical appoaches to the adrenal gland and the choice is determined by the underlying pathology, the size of the adrenal lesion, patient habitus and personal preference of the operating surgeon. Each case should be assessed individually.

A posterior (or modified posterior) approach is traditional for small, well-localised lesions. This approach was also used for bilateral adrenal exploration in primary hyperaldosteronism but as preoperative radiographic localisation is now mandatory the bilateral posterior approach is reserved for bilateral adrenalectomy.

A solitary large phaeochromocytoma or a large adrenal adenoma or carcinoma may be best approached through a thoracoabdominal (ninth or tenth rib) incision. Multiple phaeochromocytomas necessitate an abdominal approach to allow careful exploration for metastases. Children and those with MEN or a positive family history of phaeochromocytoma are considered at high risk for multiple lesions.

Surgical manipulation of a phaeochromocytoma causes extreme cardiovascular instability due to fluctuation in catecholamine release. Careful pre- and perioperative medical control of blood pressure with adrenergic blockade is essential, and requires expert anaesthetic technique.

Partial adrenalectomy may be occasionally performed, usually in cases of bilateral neoplasms to leave some functional cortical tissue, or in rare patients with a solitary adrenal gland.

Advances in laparoscopic surgery now mean laparoscopic adrenalectomy is commonly offered as an alternative to open adrenalectomy, especially for the excision of small, possibly incidentally found, adrenal tumours.

6. Surgical Pathology Specimens – Laboratory Protocols

Biopsy Specimens

Wide-bore needle cores are counted, measured (in mm) and embedded in entirety for histological examination through multiple levels. Careful handling is necessary to avoid crush artefact.

Resection Specimens

Specimen

- adrenalectomy specimens are usually complete gland resections to remove an adrenal tumour, or part of an en-bloc radical nephrectomy. Partial and bilateral adrenalectomy specimens are rare. Laparoscopic resection may result in a fragmented specimen. Extra-adrenal phaeochromocytomas (paragangliomas) are handled in a similar manner to their intra-adrenal counterparts, obviously with some variation depending on their location.

Initial procedure

- weigh the specimen (g) and measure in three dimensions (mm). If the gland appears grossly normal, attached soft tissue may be dissected off and the naked gland reweighed.
- identify and measure (cm) any adjacent organs or structures such as the adrenal vein, if attached.
- if the specimen is infiltrated by obvious tumour, paint the entire surrounding connective tissue; if there is a localised mass, paint its outer surface.
- fix the specimen by immersion in 10% formalin for at least 24 hours.
- serially section the entire specimen at 3 mm intervals perpendicular to the longest axis of any localised mass (Figure 36.1) and lay the sections out sequentially for examination and photography.
- look for lymph nodes in any attached soft tissue.

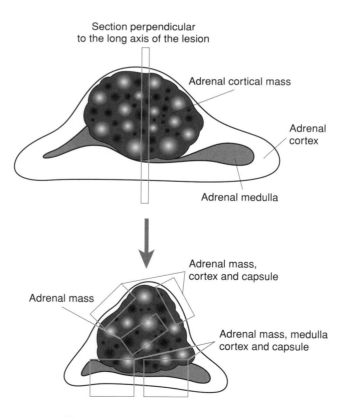

Figure 36.1. Sectioning an adrenal gland mass.

Description

- tumour: size in three dimensions (mm).
             colour (yellow, pale, white, tan, red–brown, mottled).
             site (relationship to cortex/medulla).
             appearance (haemorrhagic/necrotic/cystic/calcified areas).
             edge (capsule/circumscribed/irregular/invasion into soft tissue).
- non-neoplastic tissue: nodularity, colour, atrophy.
- other: cysts, haemorrhage.

Blocks for histology

- sample tumour according to size (at least two blocks plus one for each 5 cm tumour diameter) taking blocks to show all grossly different areas, capsule and the relationship to adjacent adrenal tissue, other structures if attached (e.g., the adrenal vein) and the painted circumferential soft tissue margin.
- one representative section should be submitted from grossly normal adrenal tissue.
- count and sample any lymph nodes identified.

Histopathology report

- tumour type – cortical adenoma/cortical carcinoma/phaeochromocytoma/other.
- features of malignancy – extremely difficult to predict using histological criteria alone but the following may be important and are usually reported:
  - nuclear pleomorphism, mitotic index, atypical mitotic figures, architecture, presence of necrosis, capsular penetration, broad fibrous bands.
- tumour edge – circumscribed/irregular/capsule/pseudocapsule.
- extent of local tumour spread – no AJCC/UICC TNM staging system currently exists for adrenal tumours. The following system for adrenal cortical carcinoma has been incorporated into the Royal College of Pathologists Minimum Dataset.
  - pT1 ≤ 5 cm, no invasion.
  - pT2 > 5 cm, no invasion.
  - pT3 any size, locally invasive but not involving adjacent organs.
  - pT4 any size with invasion of adjacent organs.
- lymphovascular invasion – present/not present.
- regional lymph nodes.
  - pN0 no regional lymph node metastasis.
  - pN1 regional lymph nodes involved.
  - pNX cannot assess regional nodes.
- excision margins: distances (in mm) to the nearest circumferential soft tissue limit.
- other pathology: nodularity, atrophy, spironolactone bodies, medullary hyperplasia.

Skin Specimens

Maureen Y Walsh

---

37 Skin Specimens

1. Anatomy

The skin is the largest organ in the body. There are regional variations in the structure and function of skin between different sites in the body, and this is reflected in the microscopic appearance of the skin. The skin at all sites consists of three layers: (a) epidermis, which provides a protective waterproof covering; (b) dermis, which gives structural support and contains skin appendages and (c) subcutaneous fat.

Epidermis: the epidermis is a keratinising stratified squamous epithelial layer. The cells arise from the basal layer and divide to form the spinous cell layer. At the granular layer cell death occurs and the dead cells form the keratin (horny) layer which is shed from the body. The epidermis also contains two other cell types: (a) melanocytes, which produce melanin pigment. These cells are scattered individually along the basal layer of the epidermis and (b) Langerhans cells which have a role in the immunoresponse of the body.

Dermis: the dermis is the layer of connective tissue and elastic tissue containing blood and lymphatic vessels, nerves and nerve endings with skin appendage structures. The dermis is divided into the papillary dermis, which is the superficial structure that folds between the rete pegs of the epidermis and the reticular dermis (deeper dermis).

Skin appendages: the skin appendage structure is derived from the epidermal cells which flow down into the dermis. These may form hair follicles and sebaceous glands which are closely associated with each other, forming a pilosebaceous unit. There are also eccrine and apocrine sweat glands. The skin appendage structures often extend into the subcutaneous fat.

Subcutaneous fat: beneath the dermis is a layer of adipose tissue with an associated fibrovascular stroma. Hair follicles and sweat gland structures extend into it.

Hair and nails: the hair and nails are specialised structures formed from keratin. They are located at specific specialised sites in the body.

Lymphovascular drainage:

Is to the locoregional lymph nodes of the body site at which the skin lesion occurs.

2. Clinical Presentation

Clinical dermatology can be divided into two broad categories: (a) skin rashes and (b) tumours/tumour-like lesions.

Skin rashes: skin rashes present with a wide range of clinical appearances and include blistering disorders, skin manifestations of systemic disease, congenital and genetic syndromes. The dermatologist usually makes a diagnosis based on the history and clinical appearance including the distribution of the rash. Pathologists dealing with specimens from these lesions need to have good clinico-pathological correlation and a knowledge of clinical dermatology to ensure that the appropriate and best diagnosis is arrived at for the patient.

Tumours/tumour-like lesions: the second category of dermatology involves removal of a vast array of "lumps and bumps" by the clinician. These can range from benign cysts and tumours through to malignant skin tumours. Once again, the clinical background appearance, site and distribution of the lesion may aid in the diagnosis.

3. Clinical Investigations

In skin disease the clinical history and examination of the patient will usually assist the dermatologist or plastic surgeon in making the correct diagnosis. Diagnostic biopsy for histological examination is often the next stage in the management process. Particularly in inflammatory disorders, the skin may be involved in systemic disease and full clinical examination and investigation of the patient are required. Similarly, patients with congenital anomalies often have multiple abnormalities, emphasising the need for full clinical assessment.

4. Pathological Conditions

Inflammatory disease biopsies require histology and close correlation with clinical details as do tumourous lesions which can arise from all the structures in the three skin layers resulting in a range of benign and malignant conditions.

Cysts: there is a variety of benign epithelial cysts that usually occur in the dermis and present as a dermal swelling. The type of cyst is determined by microscopic examination of the cell lining. Common examples are pilar and epidermal inclusion cysts – clinically termed sebaceous cysts.

Melanocytic naevi (moles): most Caucasians have several benign moles or naevi on their body, the number relating to sun exposure and to the age of the patient. Naevi vary both in size and colour. They may be the patient's skin tone, white or red through to shades of brown to blue/black in colour. Melanocytic naevi are removed for various reasons. They may have changed in appearance or develop symptoms suspicious clinically of malignant change requiring excision for histological examination. Naevi are also removed for cosmetic reasons, because they are being traumatised, occur at a hidden site on the body or constitute a newly formed naevus in an adult. There is a variety of histological types of benign naevi that are dependent on microscopic examination for correct diagnosis.

Malignant melanomas: malignant melanomas, like benign naevi, are derived from melanocytes. They may arise de novo or from within an existing melanocytic naevus. Changes in a pre-existing mole that cause concern include (a) asymmetry; (b) irregular borders; (c) change or variation in colour; (d) size > 6 mm; (e) elevation and also itching, bleeding or symptoms associated with a naevus. When the clinician is suspicious of a diagnosis of malignant melanoma the lesion is removed in total, usually with an ellipse of normal skin around it. Depending on the degree of certainty of the clinical diagnosis, a wide excision may or may not be done at that time. Melanomas are the third most common malignant skin tumour. Their incidence is rising and they are the primary skin tumour most likely to metastasise and cause death. Malignant melanomas typically occur after puberty and their incidence increases with advancing age.

Actinic keratosis, Bowen's disease, basal cell carcinoma, squamous cell carcinoma: most skin cancers and pre-cancerous lesions of the skin are related to chronic sun exposure in white skin and their incidence is increasing. Other aetiological factors include a genetic predisposition and immunosuppression. Patients who have had organ transplants are at greater risk of developing skin neoplasia.

Actinic (solar) keratosis: actinic keratoses present usually as multiple red scaly lesions on sites of chronic sun exposure, particularly the head and neck, back of hands and forearms. The lesions are usually removed and submitted for pathology when the clinician is concerned that there may be malignant change, and particularly invasive malignancy. Often, patients with actinic (solar) keratosis have multiple lesions which are treated by a variety of topical agents and are not submitted for histological examination. Various biopsy techniques may be used to remove actinic keratoses including curettage, shave, punch and excision biopsies.

Bowen's disease (carcinoma in situ): Bowen's disease is a pre-invasive or in situ malignancy of the skin usually presenting as a red scaly patch. Most of these lesions present in a background of solar damage although it can occur in areas of non-sun-damaged skin where it may be associated with a higher incidence of internal malignancy. Bowen's disease is often treated by dermatologists with topical agents and may be biopsied to confirm the diagnosis and to exclude invasive malignancy. Occasionally there will be a biopsy to remove the lesion. Depending on whether the biopsy is excisional or diagnostic in intent the laboratory will receive either a curettage, shave, punch or elliptical specimen.

Basal cell carcinoma: basal cell carcinoma is the commonest malignant tumour of the skin, and overall in humans. The vast majority is associated with chronic sun exposure and occur in the head and neck area of fair-skinned people. A few occur at sites of scarring in the skin and a small number of patients with a genetic predisposition develop multiple basal cell carcinomas. These patients often present at an early age. Basal cell carcinomas have a variety of clinical appearances from a nodular lesion to an ulcer or scarred areas and they may also be multifocal. The colour of the tumours can vary. The cell of origin of basal cell carcinoma is thought to be either the basal cell layer of the epidermis or hair follicle. Basal cell carcinomas are locally aggressive tumours, often infiltrating and destroying adjacent tissue. They do not, however, metastasise to other sites. The treatment of choice is surgical removal. The clinician may submit a variety of specimen types to the laboratory depending on the surgical technique used. These may be curettage, shave, punch or excision. Based on clinical need, Mohs' micrographic surgery is used in the treatment of a small number of cases. Occasionally, basal cell carcinomas may be treated by radiotherapy following a confirmatory diagnostic biopsy.

Squamous cell carcinoma: squamous cell carcinoma is the second most common malignant tumour of the skin typically at sun-exposed sites in patients with fair skin. A small number of squamous cell carcinomas occur in patients with predisposing genetic disorders, or at sites of chronic scarring. These tumours arise from the surface epithelium. They have a variety of clinical appearances including nodules and ulcers and they also can vary in colour. These tumours do have the potential to metastasise although the vast majority are cured by adequate local treatment. The treatment of choice is surgical and the clinician will submit various specimens including curettage, shave, punch and excision biopsies. Mohs' micrographic surgery may be used in selected cases. Some cases are treated with radiotherapy following a pathological diagnosis.

Other Skin Tumours

Merkel cell tumours: of neuroendocrine origin that occur in elderly patients, usually presenting as a rapidly growing nodule often in the head and neck area. They may present with skin involvement and lymph node spread. Prognosis in these tumours is poor. Secondary spread from small cell carcinoma of lung must be excluded.

Paget's disease of nipple: presents as an eczematous area on the nipple or areola. It is associated with underlying malignancy in the breast.

Extramammary Paget's disease: occurs at the vulva, perineum, scrotum, penis, anus and axilla. It presents as a red velvety area and on histological examination is an in situ carcinoma. It may or may not be associated with underlying carcinoma in the sweat glands of the skin or visceral malignancy in the gastrointestinal, urinary or gynaecological tracts.

Skin appendage tumours (benign and malignant): the hair follicle and sweat gland structures are capable of giving rise to a wide variety of skin appendage tumours. If multiple, they may be associated with clinical syndromes. Most of these lesions present as nodules in the skin and correct diagnosis is dependent on histological examination. The majority of lesions are benign, although a small number are malignant and may metastasise and cause death in the patient.

Benign epithelial tumours and tumour-like lesions: seborrhoeic keratosis is a benign epithelial tumour arising in the skin of middle-aged and elderly patients, presenting usually as a stuck-on, warty type of lesion. They are often pigmented and may be mistaken by the patient and clinician for a melanoma.

Viral warts: most viral warts are treated with topical agents and are not submitted for histological diagnosis, unless the diagnosis is unclear.

Benign mesenchymal tumours: the mesenchymal tissue in the dermis and subcutis can give rise to various tumours. Most present as nodules in the skin and may be biopsied or excised by the clinician using curettage, shave, punch and elliptical excision.

Malignant mesenchymal tumours (sarcomas): rare. These lesions are often large and may have a history of growth or change. They may be biopsied to establish the diagnosis or have a wide surgical excision to remove the lesion.

Leukaemia and lymphoma: leukaemias and lymphomas may affect the skin in two main ways: (a) as an inflammatory skin rash as a consequence of the underlying malignancy and (b) as a lymphoma/leukaemia involving the skin, either as a primary skin lesion or spread to the skin as part of systemic disease. Lymphoma and leukaemia involvement of the skin may present as a skin rash, plaques or nodules of tumour. Usually, a small diagnostic biopsy is taken in such cases, either as a punch or an ellipse.

Secondary tumours: secondary tumours may involve the skin, either as directly from an underlying tumour or as metastatic spread. A small biopsy is usually used for diagnostic purposes. FNA also has a role to play (see below).

5. Surgical Pathology Specimens – Clinical Aspects

Biopsy and Excision Specimens

A variety of biopsies are submitted depending on the clinical diagnosis and the type of information the clinician wants.

Curettage: a curetted specimen is used to remove or sample small warty-type lesions which are usually benign or small basal or squamous cell carcinomas. This can be associated with cautery to the lesion base (C+C). Occasionally, a basal cell carcinoma, actinic keratosis or squamous cell carcinoma may be removed by curettage and then formal surgical excision is carried out of the curetted area. The laboratory in this case will receive two specimens from the one patient: a curettage and the excision biopsy. This combined technique is used to give a good cosmetic result. The curettage removes the bulk of the tumour and the excision results in a neat scar.

Shave biopsy: shave biopsies are used to remove polypoid or raised lesions on the skin. Usually the clinician thinks the lesion is benign and a shave will give a good cosmetic result.

Diagnostic punch biopsy: a diagnostic punch biopsy is usually done to assist in the diagnosis of inflammatory diseases, or to establish the diagnosis of a tumour before formal wider excision is carried out.

Punch excision: a punch excision biopsy is used to remove completely a lesion on the skin such as a small mole or naevus. The lesion is removed with a rim of normal tissue surrounding it.

Diagnostic elliptical biopsy: an ellipse of skin may be removed to establish the diagnosis in skin rashes. This may involve lesional skin and surrounding normal skin, or only lesional skin. Where the biopsy is taken depends on the clinical diagnosis, and where the most likely diagnostic pathology is to be found. The dermatologist on the advice of the dermatopathologist must take the most appropriate site for diagnosis. Diagnostic elliptical biopsies are also done for skin tumours before, if necessary, formal excisions are carried out. They are not recommended for lesions where malignant melanoma is a suspected diagnosis clinically.

Elliptical excisions: elliptical excisions are carried out to remove skin tumours, both benign and malignant. The dermatological surgeon will usually remove the lesion with a surrounding rim of normal skin.

Pigmented lesions: where the clinician suspects that he is dealing with a possible malignant melanoma the biopsy should be an excision biopsy with a rim of normal surrounding skin. Only in exceptional circumstances should a diagnostic biopsy of a suspected melanoma be carried out, e.g., a pigmented lesion on a digit where full excision would result in an amputation.

Fine needle aspiration biopsies (FNA): FNAs are used to diagnose subcutaneous lumps in the skin and to establish the diagnosis in secondary carcinoma. The role of FNA in primary tumours of the skin is limited because the diagnostic biopsy often comprises surgical removal of the lesion.

6. Surgical Pathology Specimens – Laboratory Protocols

A variety of biopsies are submitted and received.

Curettage: a curetted specimen is usually received in multiple fragments which are all submitted for histological diagnosis. The pathologist, based on the curette, makes a diagnosis of the lesion but cannot comment on adequacy of excision. Deeper levels are employed as appropriate.

Shave: shave biopsies are measured, i.e., the length, breadth and depth, in millimetres. If a lesion is noted grossly, this is also measured in millimetres. Depending on the size of the shave, it is submitted in total (Figure 37.1) but if greater than 6 mm it is first bisected (Figure 37.2). Shave biopsies are not excisional biopsies and the lesion often extends to the deep margin. Excision margins are not commented on in benign lesions in a shave biopsy.

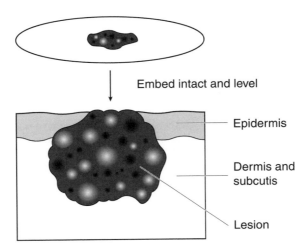

Figure 37.1.   Punch, ellipse or shave biopsy embedded intact.

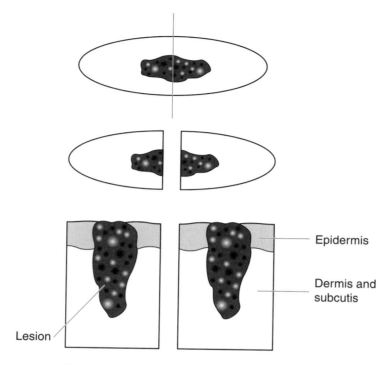

Figure 37.2.   Punch, shave or ellipse bisected and embedded.

Diagnostic punch biopsy: diagnostic punch biopsies come in a variety of sizes ranging from 2 mm to 8 mm. The smaller-sized punch biopsies are usually for diagnostic purposes. The size of the punch is recorded and a description of any lesion seen. Small punches less than 4 mm are submitted in total and will require examination of multiple levels (Figure 37.1). Punch biopsies 4 mm and above are bisected and then submitted in total. Bisecting the specimen through the centre of the lesion results in its representation in the initial levels.

Punch biopsy for alopecia: punch biopsies are taken to establish the cause of alopecia and are embedded in the usual manner. In some centres, depending on the experience of the dermatopathologist, the punch biopsy may be bisected, with one half embedded and sectioned in the usual vertical fashion and the other half sectioned transversely. This is thought to give a better view of the hair follicle structures and assist in the diagnosis of alopecia (Figure 37.3).

Punch excision: punch excisions, like diagnostic punch biopsies, come in a variety of sizes, usually 4 mm and greater. The size of the punch is measured and the edges inked. Depending on the size the punch may be embedded intact and adequate sections cut to see the full face of the lesion (Figure 37.1). Larger punch biopsies are bisected (Figure 37.2) or sliced through to examine the lesion (Figure 37.4). All punch excision biopsies and lesions present are described and measured in millimetres.

Elliptical biopsy: small ellipses of skin may be removed for diagnosis. They are usually processed intact or bisected longitudinally and examined through multiple levels (Figures 37.1 and 37.2). Biopsies are measured in millimetres and any lesion seen described and measured. They may have their edges inked.

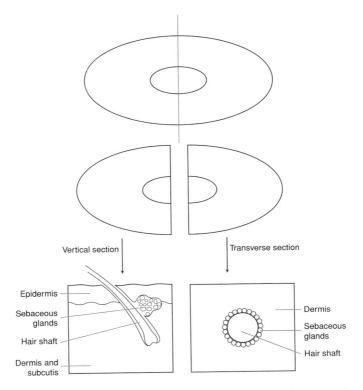

Figure 37.3. Vertical and horizontal sections of a punch biopsy for the diagnosis of alopecia.

Elliptical excision: skin ellipses are used to remove tumour with a rim of normal tissue around the lesion. The pathologist needs to see the full face of the lesion and examine for adequacy of excision. All skin ellipses are measured and described. Any sutures and pins, etc., placed by the clinician for orientation are noted and if any specific questions are asked on the request form regarding the excision, these are considered when sectioning the skin ellipse. Most elliptical skin excisions are not photographed unless the gross appearance is unusual when often it will have been photographed by the clinician before surgical removal. Photography or a photocopy of the lesion surface may be useful if sampling of the lesion is complex to indicate where blocks have been taken, but usually a diagram is adequate. The edges of the ellipse are inked to indicate the true surgical margins.

Elliptical excisions are dealt with in the laboratory in a variety of ways:

1. If small (< 6 mm), they can be processed intact and cut along the long axis. Multiple levels need to be examined to see the full face of the lesion (Figure 37.1).
2. Small ellipses may be bisected across the short axis and embedded to show the centre of the lesion. This provides information on the deep limit and nearest peripheral margins at the short axis but not the long axis (Figure 37.2).
3. Quadrant blocks of the lesion. A block is taken through the centre of the lesion across the short axis and two lateral blocks are taken across the long axis. This gives the full face of the lesion and margins on four quadrants (Figure 37.5).

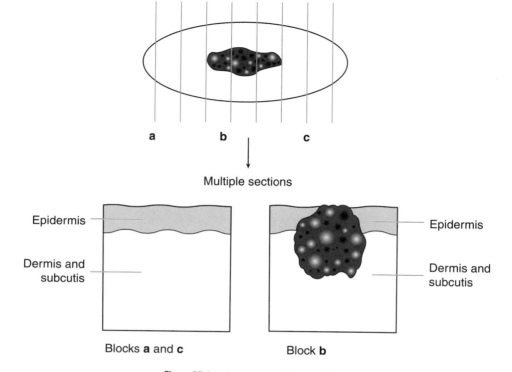

Figure 37.4. Serial section of a skin ellipse.

4. Skin ellipses may be serially sectioned or sliced like a loaf of bread through the lesion at 2–3 mm intervals. This ensures that the whole of the lesion is examined and is useful in melanocytic lesions of the skin (Figure 37.4).

Wedge excisions: wedge excisions are used to remove skin from the eyelid, lip, ear and vulval areas. These and any gross lesions are described and measured. The surgical limits are the outer margins of the wedge and these are sampled for histology. A section is then taken through the centre of the tumour (Figure 37.6).

7. Special Techniques and Considerations

Immunofluorescence: immunofluorescent examinations are required for the diagnosis of chronic blistering diseases and are useful in connective tissue diseases. The site of biopsy is important for immunofluorescence, particularly in the blistering disorders. In dermatitis herpetiformis a biopsy for immunofluorescence should be taken from clinically normal skin away from the area of blistering. In the other blistering disorders, perilesional skin is submitted. The skin should have an intact epidermal/dermal junction. In most of the connective tissue disorders lesional skin is submitted for immunofluorescence except for the lupus band test, where normal non-sun-exposed skin is used. Most patients having skin submitted for immunofluorescence should

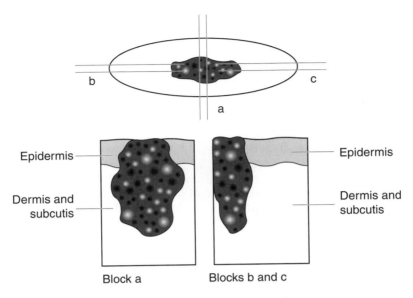

Figure 37.5. Quadrant blocks of a skin ellipse.

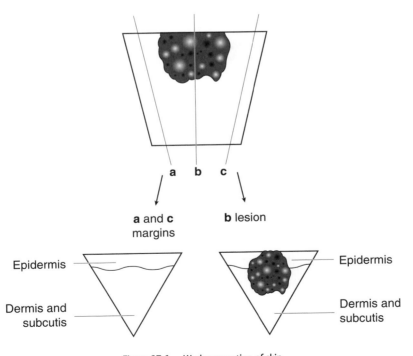

Figure 37.6. Wedge resection of skin.

also have a serum sample sent to the laboratory for examination for autoantibodies related to the disease process. Skin biopsy specimens for immunofluorescence are either snap frozen in liquid nitrogen or sent in the correct transport medium to the laboratory. Most laboratories doing immunofluorescence will supply the clinical area with the appropriate transport medium. Formalin fixation is inappropriate for immunofluorescence and will render the specimen unsuitable for examination. Specimens for immunofluorescence are either punch or elliptical biopsies.

Mohs' micrographic surgery: for the surgical removal of the tumour under microscopic control. The aim of the technique is to remove all the tumour with the minimum of surrounding normal tissue. This is a time-consuming and slow procedure for the patient, dermatological surgeon and laboratory staff but it is useful in a small number of cases. Mohs' micrographic surgery is used primarily for the treatment of basal cell carcinoma, but may be used for squamous cell carcinoma, some sarcomas of the skin especially dermatofibrosarcoma protuberans and, rarely, some types of desmoplastic melanoma and other malignant skin appendage tumours. It is especially useful for tumours occurring on the face around the eyelids, nose and mouth where a good cosmetic result is required. The technique involves examination of frozen sections of surgical margins with the patient and the surgeon awaiting the results. If limits are involved a further excision of this area is carried out and examined by frozen section. This is repeated until the margins are clear. The defect is then repaired by the surgeon on the same day. In some units the tissue is fixed, processed to paraffin, and margin sections examined the next day. If the margins are involved further tissue is removed, processed to paraffin and sections examined. Only when the margins are clear is repair carried out. This is a slower procedure over a period of days in which the patient has a defect which has to wait for confirmation of clearance before repair can take place. This technique is useful for rarer types of tumour where there may be an infiltrate of single spindle cells such as a desmoplastic malignant melanoma, or where immunocytochemistry is required to identify tumour cells.

Mohs' laboratory procedure: it is essential that there is clear communication between the surgeon and the pathologist examining the specimen by Mohs' micrographic surgery. The specimen should be laid out flat on a dish or board and the margins indicated either by sutures or pins of different colours. It is useful if the surgeon also draws a diagram of the lesion and its location on the patient with appropriate landmarks. The pathologist ensures that the complete surgical margins are examined. It is often necessary to divide the specimen into smaller blocks to be examined microscopically. They may need to be marked so that the area involved by tumour can be clearly pinpointed. On an ellipse skin margins can be marked in relation to the clockface or to compass points. The surgical margins are marked with different-coloured inks, to aid locating the correct area with tumour involvement (Figure 37.7).

Surgical margins: on excision biopsies the pathologist should comment on the adequacy of excision and, in line with protocols, measure the tumour distance from the margins. In punch biopsies the specimen is either embedded intact or bisected and embedded. The pathologist can comment on two lateral and deep margins. The edge of the punch biopsy can be inked to indicate microscopically the true excision margins, which are also often associated with red blood cells.

Similarly, in an elliptical biopsy the margin status is documented by the pathologist. Quadrant blocks result in four lateral margins and a deep margin being examined. Bread-loaf slicing through the ellipse results in all the margins being seen microscopically but this is only suitable for relatively small ellipses. The margins can be inked to assist microscopic identification, although usually red blood cells are present. To examine all the surgical margins in a large skin biopsy the best approach is a modified Mohs' technique. The pathologist sections the margins and these are marked with different-coloured inks to aid identification.

Sutures and markers: the surgeon will often mark margins with sutures to help orientate the specimen and an accompanying diagram is also useful. Techniques of margin sampling in large excisions may need to be modified in the light of attached sutures or clinical request form information.

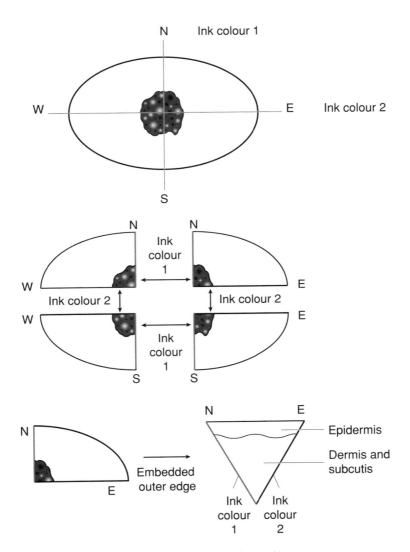

Figure 37.7. Sections for Moh's micrographic surgery.

Grafts: tumours may recur under and around an area of skin grafting. These specimens are dealt with in the usual manner for a skin ellipse.

Re-excisions: The most common cause for re-excision is when a malignant tumour is incompletely excised, or in the case of a malignant melanoma, despite complete primary excision, the margins are not wide enough to follow standard guidelines. Re-excision biopsies are sampled as for primary excisions. Tumour, if present, is usually at the edge of the previous biopsy scar. Again, margins of excision are commented on.

Diagrams: diagrams are also useful in orientating specimens.

Transmission Electron Microscopy (TEM): As in other branches of pathology, the role of diagnostic TEM is declining. Immunocytochemistry has reduced the need for it in diagnosing undifferentiated tumours and viral infections, although it is still useful for inborn errors of metabolism. All such samples of skin should be placed in a glutaraldehyde fixative. Other indications for TEM are in the diagnosis and subclassification of: (1) congenital anomalies, e.g., icthyosis, (2) blistering diseases as in the epidermolysis bullosa group (it may be necessary to obtain a fresh blister by rubbing up with an eraser) and (3) acquired blistering disorders (in conjunction with immunohistochemistry).

Scanning Electron Microscopy: Scanning electron microscopy is useful in the diagnosis of hair shaft anomalies. The hair sample should be sent unfixed to the laboratory.

Microprobe Analysis: A microprobe attached to the scanning electron microscope can be useful to detect small amounts of elements present in the skin that may be causing increased abnormal pigmentation.

Skin scrapings: scrapings from the skin surface can be examined for fungal particles or scabies mites. This may be a wet preparation by putting the scrapings in potassium hydroxide or fixing the tissue and processing it. This is a useful way to make a diagnosis without a full surgical biopsy.

Fixation: the usual fixation for skin biopsies for histology is 10% formalin. Mast cells are easier to demonstrate if the skin biopsy has been fixed in alcohol. Where a mast cell lesion is suspected the biopsy should be divided and halves placed in formalin and alcohol. However, if mast cells are present in large numbers they can still be seen in formalin-fixed tissue. Similarly, the ureate crystals in gout dissolve in formalin. It is still possible to diagnose gout on formalin-fixed tissue but it is easier to demonstrate the crystals if the tissue has been placed in alcohol fixative.

Special Sites

Hair: hair samples should be plucked, not cut, from the patient and sent unfixed to the laboratory. The hair is mounted unfixed on glass slides and examined for hair shaft anomalies, or to look at the hair roots and count the telogen:anagen ratio – this requires a minimum of 50 hairs. Scanning electron microscopy provides more information in patients with hair shaft anomalies and picks up more subtle changes than those seen at light microscopy.

Nails: fragments of nails may be submitted for examination, either to detect fungi or the cause of nail pigmentation. The fragments are softened in phenol and then processed in the usual way for histology. For pigmented lesions or growths beneath the nail, the nail must be removed by the surgeon before skin biopsy of the nail bed is taken. Nails may be involved in several skin diseases, but usually a biopsy of skin involved elsewhere is taken to confirm the diagnosis.

Digits: pigmented lesions beneath nails often cause diagnostic problems in distinguishing between benign lesions, trauma and malignant melanoma. Trauma to the nail which bleeds grows outwards as the nail grows whereas naevi and melanomas do not. If melanoma is suspected the clinician must first remove the nail and biopsy the lesion on the nail bed. Excision biopsy is ideal but if this is not possible then a diagnostic biopsy is permitted. This is allowed in the nail bed as treatment for melanoma is amputation of the digit. Because of this the pathologist should only diagnose melanoma when there is a high degree of certainty, otherwise another biopsy is requested. Digits are measured and described in the usual manner, including which joints have been disarticulated. The tumour is measured and described. The surgical margin of excision is blocked and the tumour sampled through its deepest area.

Eyelid: the eyelid margins can be involved in a variety of benign and malignant tumours. Benign tumours are dealt with in the usual manner. In malignant tumours, especially basal cell carcinomas, squamous cell carcinomas and melanomas, the surgeon's aim is to remove all the tumour with as little normal tissue as possible. The surgeon may use a modified Mohs' technique to do this or orientate the specimen with pins and sutures. This will then be treated in the laboratory as a wedge excision and the margins carefully marked.

Ear: the ear may be involved in skin rashes, benign and malignant tumours. Skin rashes rarely only involve the ear and skin from elsewhere should be sampled. Benign lesions will have a variety of biopsy samples which are dealt with in the usual way. Tumours are often removed as a wedge and dealt with accordingly (Figure 37.6).

Lip: lip biopsies from benign lesions are treated as other biopsies but malignant tumours are removed as a wedge and dealt with accordingly (Figure 37.6).

Pilonidal sinus: occurs in the natal cleft of young-to-middle-aged males due to insinuation of hair shafts into the dermis and subcutis forming a tract variably lined by epidermis and/or granulation tissue. It is associated with serous discharge and, potentially, infection with pain and abscess formation. There may be several tracts present and communication points with the surface epidermis. Treatment involves wide elliptical excision of the skin and subcutis down to the level of the sacral fascia. The specimen is measured and the presence of opening(s)/tract(s) noted. A horizontal transverse block of the deep limit allows microscopic assessment of tract extension to the deep margin. The tract is demonstrated by serial vertical slices (Figure 37.8).

Histopathology Reports

Inflammatory disease:

- specimen site, type and size (mm).
- description of histological findings.
- diagnosis or differential diagnosis with most likely diagnosis.

Benign tumours:

- specimen site, type and size (mm).
- tumour type and brief description of lesion.
- if excision biopsy, is the lesion excised?

Malignant tumours:

Basal Cell Carcinoma

- specimen site.
- specimen type.
- specimen size: length (mm).
  - breadth (mm).
  - depth (mm).
- size of lesion: length (mm).
  - breadth (mm).
  - depth (mm).
- growth pattern: nodular/superficial/infiltrative (morphoeic)/micronodular/other.
- differentiation: severely atypical or malignant squamous component present – yes/no.
- invasion:
  - lymphatic/vascular invasion: yes/no/uncertain.
  - perineural invasion: yes/no/uncertain.

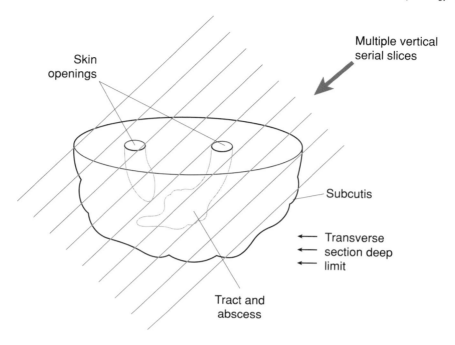

Figure 37.8.   Blocking a pilonidal sinus specimen.

- excision margins:
  - nearest peripheral: not involved (mm)/involved.
  - nearest deep: not involved (mm)/involved.
- extent of local tumour spread (see squamous cell carcinoma).

Squamous Cell Carcinoma

- specimen site.
- specimen type.
- specimen size: length (mm).
  - breadth (mm).
  - depth (mm).
- maximum diameter of lesion (mm).
- histology suptype: classical/spindle cell/acantholytic/verrucous/desmoplastic/other.
- differentiation: grade I (over 75% differentiated).
  - grade II (between 25 and 75% differentiated).
  - grade III (under 75% differentiated).
  - grade IV (no differentiation).
- tumour thickness (mm).
- *Clarke level: I/II/III/IV/V.
- invasion:
  - lymphatic/vascular invasion: yes/no/uncertain.
  - perineural invasion: yes/no/uncertain.

- excision margins:
  - nearest peripheral: clear (mm)/involved (in situ/invasive).
  - nearest deep: clear (mm)/involved (in situ/invasive).
- extent of local tumour spread:
  - pTis carcinoma in situ.
  - pT1 tumour ≤ 20 mm in greatest dimension.
  - pT2 tumour > 20 mm and ≤ 50 mm.
  - pT3 tumour > 50 mm in greatest dimension.
  - pT4 tumour invades extradermal structures (cartilage, skeletal muscle, bone).
  - pN0 no regional lymph node metastasis.
  - pN1 regional lymph node metastasis.

* Clarke levels – I (intraepidermal), II (papillary dermis), III (papillary-reticular interface), IV (reticular dermis), V (subcutaneous fat)

Malignant Melanoma

- specimen site.
- specimen type.
- specimen size: length (mm).
  - breadth (mm).
  - depth (mm).
- lesion size: length (mm).
  - breadth (mm).
  - depth (mm).
- lesion margins: regular/irregular.
- histogenic type: lentigo maligna/superficial spreading/nodular/acral lentiginous/desmo-plastic/neurotropic.
- Clarke level: I/II/III/IV/V.
- Breslow's depth: (mm).
- mitoses/mm^2.
- growth phase: radial/vertical.
- cross-sectional profile.
- ulceration: yes – diameter (mm)/no.
- pigmentation.
- cell type.
- lymphoid response at base.
- signs of regression.
- associated melanocytic naevus.
- vascular invasion.
- perineural invasion.
- desmoplasia.
- neurotropism.
- microscopic satellitosis.
- excision margins
  - nearest peripheral: clear (mm)/involved (in situ/invasive).
  - nearest deep: clear (mm)/involved (in situ/invasive).
- extent of local tumour spread.
  - pTis melanoma in situ.
  - pT1 tumour ≤ 1.0 mm.
    a. without ulceration and level II/III.
    b. with ulceration and level IV/V.

- pT2* tumour 1.01–2.0 mm.
- pT3* tumour 2.01–4.0 mm.
- pT4* tumour > 4.0 mm.
  * a. without ulceration.
    b. with ulceration.
- pN1* 1 lymph node involved.
- pN2* 2–3 lymph nodes involved.
- pN3*+ ≥ 4 lymph nodes involved.
  * a. micrometastasis.
    b. macrometastasis.
  + c. in-transit metastasis/satellites without metastatic lymph nodes.
- pM1a distant skin or nodal metastasis.
- pM1b lung metastasis.
- pM1c all other visceral metasases, any distant metastases with elevated serum LDH.

Lymph nodes: lymph nodes may be removed where there is tumour involvement in patients with squamous cell carcinoma or malignant melanoma. If the lymph node is subcutaneous a fine needle aspiration will be carried out to confirm the diagnosis prior to surgical removal. The node(s) should be weighed, measured, counted and submitted for histological examination

Sentinel node biopsy: sentinel node biopsy is used in some centres in patients with biopsy-proven malignant melanoma of the skin. The sentinel node is the first drainage node at the site of the excised malignant melanoma. This is removed and examined in the laboratory for microscopic tumour using multiple step sections through the node and using both haematoxylin and eosin and immunocytochemistry markers including S100, Melan-A and HMB45 to confirm small microscopic deposits of malignant melanoma.

Cardiothoracic Specimens and Vessels

Kathleen M Mulholland

38 Lung

1. Anatomy

The combined weight of both lungs is approximately 850 g in the male, 750 g in the female. The apex of each lung is situated in the root of the neck, the base of the lung on the diaphragm. The mediastinum is medial to the lungs and ribs are present laterally. The hilum of each lung contains a main bronchus, pulmonary artery, two pulmonary veins, pulmonary nerve plexus and lymph nodes.

The lungs are separated into lobes by invaginations of pleura along fissures (Figure 38.1). The right lung is divided into three lobes by the oblique and horizontal fissures, the left into two lobes by the oblique fissure. The inferior part of the left upper lobe (the lingula) is the homologue of the right middle lobe.

The trachea branches at the level of T4 and T5 into two main bronchi. The right bronchus enters the lung behind the right pulmonary artery, the left bronchus crosses behind the left pulmonary artery and enters the lung below it. The main bronchi divide to give five lobar bronchi. These then divide into segmental bronchi supplying the 19 bronchopulmonary segments. Segments are roughly wedge shaped with their base at the pleural surface. Each segment is supplied by a segmental artery and bronchus. Veins draining segments often anastomose with

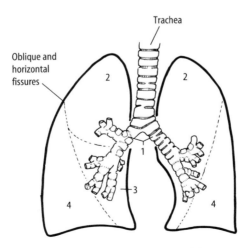

Figure 38.1. Anatomy of the lungs. 1. Main bronchus. 2. Upper lobe. 3. Middle lobe. 4. Lower lobe. Reproduced from Hermanek P, Hutter RVP, Sobin LH, Wagner G, Wittekind Ch (eds.). TNM Atlas: illustrated guide to the TNM/pTNM classification of malignant tumours, 4th edition. Springer-Verlag: Berlin and Heidelberg, 1997.

those from adjacent segments. Bronchopulmonary segments can be resected with little haemorrhage or leakage of air from adjacent raw surfaces. Further divisions of the bronchi produce bronchioles. Glands and cartilage are present in the walls of bronchi but not in bronchioles.

Bronchioles have a diameter of less than 1 mm. Terminal bronchioles lead to respiratory bronchioles which branch to produce alveolar ducts, alveolar sacs and then alveoli. The lung may be divided into lobules, areas that measure 1–2 cm across and are poorly demarcated by incomplete fibrous septa. Each lobule is made up of three to ten acini. An acinus or terminal respiratory unit is that portion of the lung supplied by one terminal bronchiole. Pulmonary arteries are found at the centres of each acinus alongside bronchioles, whereas pulmonary veins run in the interlobular septa. Flattened type 1 pneumocytes and occasional rounded type 2 pneumocytes line the alveoli.

Lymphovascular supply

Lymphatic drainage is by a superficial subpleural lymph plexus and a deep plexus of vessels accompanying the bronchi. Both groups drain through hilar (bronchopulmonary) lymph nodes into tracheobronchial nodes around the bifurcation of the trachea and from there into mediastinal lymph trunks.

Blood supply to the lungs is by a dual arterial supply – the pulmonary arteries and the bronchial arteries. Blood returns to the heart via the pulmonary veins or travels in the bronchial veins to the azygos or accessory hemiazygos veins.

2. Clinical Presentation

Respiratory symptoms include cough, sputum production, dyspnoea (undue respiratory effort), orthopnoea (breathlessness on lying down), wheeze due to airway obstruction, haemoptysis (coughing up blood) and chest pain. The commonest cause of haemoptysis is acute infection. Other causes include tuberculosis and pulmonary infarction. Tumour, e.g., carcinoid or bronchial carcinoma, may cause haemoptysis due either to ulceration of the expanding tumour or secondary infection caused by obstruction. Chest pain can be localised and pleuritic, due to infection or infarction or constant, severe and dull due to chest wall invasion by carcinoma. Lung cancer can produce secondary pneumonia, bronchiectasis, pleural effusions, hoarseness (laryngeal nerve involvement) and paralysis of the diaphragm (phrenic nerve involvement). Tumours in the apical part of the upper lobe (Pancoast's tumours) may result in unilateral Horner's syndrome due to involvement of sympathetic ganglia. Pancoast's tumours may also produce pain and weakness in the shoulder and arm due to invasion of the brachial plexus. Mediastinal disease may lead to superior vena cava syndrome with congestion and oedema of the face, neck and chest associated with dyspnoea.

Paraneoplastic syndromes are systemic effects of tumours not mediated by tumour spread. They include Cushing's syndrome, inappropriate antidiuretic hormone secretion and acromegaly. Weight loss may occur in chronic inflammatory diseases such as TB or secondary to tumours.

3. Clinical Investigations

Chest X-ray – primary technique for imaging the thorax.

CT scan – the only cross-sectional imaging technique that adequately evaluates the lung parenchyma and is equivalent to MRI in the evaluation of mediastinum, pleura and chest wall. CT has a sensitivity of 80–94% compared with results obtained by mediastinoscopy and lymph node sampling. CT scans are used to stage carcinoma of bronchus and may be extended to include liver, adrenal glands and brain.

High Resolution (thin section) CT scan (HRCT) – slices are 1–3 mm thick. HRCT is of value for the investigation of sarcoidosis, lymphoma, cryptogenic and extrinsic alveolitis, occupational lung disease, bronchiectasis and lymphangitis carcinomatosa. It is also used to distinguish emphysema from interstitial lung disease or pulmonary vascular disease.

Spiral CT scan and Ventilation/Perfusion (V/Q) scan – used in detection of pulmonary emboli.

MRI – less useful than CT because of poorer imaging of lung parenchyma. MRI may be used in assessing disease near the lung apex, the spine, the thoracoabdominal regions and the mediastinum. It can detect invasion into spinal cord, vertebral bodies, brachial plexus and chest.

PET scan – used to distinguish between benign and malignant conditions. If the lesion does not demonstrate high radiation activity, it is interpreted as having a low metabolic rate and is likely to be benign.

Respiratory function tests – include peak expiratory flow rate (PEFR), forced expiratory volume in one second (FEV1), vital capacity (VC), forced expiratory ratio (FEV/VC) and carbon monoxide transfer (Tco). These tests are helpful in differentiating between lung disease due to airways obstruction, restrictive conditions or respiratory muscle weakness.

Measurement of blood gases – important in the diagnosis of respiratory failure.

Full blood picture (FBP): haemoglobin – anaemia, PCV – secondary polycythaemia.

Biochemistry – alpha-1-antitrypsin levels, autoantibodies, aspergillus antibodies, IgE to specific allergens. Hypercalcaemia occurs in 1 in 5 patients with sarcoidosis, as a paraneoplastic syndrome notably in association with squamous cell carcinoma and secondary to bony metastases. Hyponatraemia is seen in association with small cell carcinoma.

Sputum – cytological examination of sputum can detect between 60 and 90% of malignancies if multiple specimens are examined. Gram stain and culture are of value in pneumonia, TB and aspergillus.

Transthoracic needle aspiration and biopsy (TTNA and TTNB)/percutaneous needle aspiration and biopsy – are performed under fluoroscopic or CT guidance. They successfully diagnose lung cancer with at least 85–90% accuracy. The most common indication for aspiration is to evaluate a solitary peripheral lung nodule suspicious of carcinoma. Biopsy is more appropriate when lymphoma or sarcoidosis is suspected. Needle core biopsies may be obtained from lesions close to the chest wall, while more central lesions require fine needle aspiration.

Bronchial brushings and washings – fibre optic bronchoscopy (FOB) can reach and sample up to 90% of malignancies.

Transbronchial fine needle aspiration – at the time of FOB makes submucosal and paratracheal lesions accessible.

Endobronchial and transbronchial biopsy – lead to a histological diagnosis in 95% of central lung carcinomas, but in only 50–75% of peripheral lesions. Transbronchial biopsy is of particular use in the diagnosis of sarcoidosis and lymphangitis carcinomatosa.

Bronchoalveolar lavage (BAL) – using a flexible fibre optic bronchoscope, small-volume lavages (up to 300 ml) are performed. BAL may be used to monitor progression of interstitial lung disease. It is useful in eosinophilic pneumonia, eosinophilic granuloma, pulmonary alveolar proteinosis and in the diagnosis of opportunistic infections, e.g., in the immunosuppressed.

Mediastinoscopy – allows access to, and biopsy of, lymph nodes. Cervical mediastinoscopy accesses paratracheal and subcarinal mediastinal nodes for diagnostic and staging purposes. Anterior mediastinoscopy is used primarily to sample enlarged nodes or tumour in the left aortopulmonary window region.

Frozen sections – sent intra-operatively to distinguish between inflammatory and neoplastic parenchymal lesions, as a prequel to a cancer resection operation or a lung-sparing wedge resection. These specimens should be handled with care in a microbiological safety cabinet. If there is any suspicion of tuberculosis, frozen sections are inappropriate and should not be performed. Such tissue needs thorough formalin fixation.

Open/closed lung biopsy – used to evaluate pleural/peripheral lesions and interstitial lung disorders.

4. Pathological Conditions

Non-neoplastic Conditions

Bacterial pneumonia: lobar pneumonia can be of rapid onset in otherwise healthy patients and entire lobes are involved by neutrophilic infiltrates. Bronchopneumonia affects older debilitated patients and is characterized by more circumscribed infiltrates.

Lung abscess: an area of infection with parenchymal necrosis. Primary lung abscess occurs more often on the right side as the right main bronchus leads more directly off the trachea and aspiration can occur more easily. Secondary abscesses occur when there are predisposing factors such as carcinoma, foreign body or bronchiectasis.

Viral infection: may occur in the lungs due to respiratory viruses such as influenza or in the immunocompromised patient (cytomegalovirus, respiratory syncytial virus, *Varicella zoster* or *Herpes simplex*). Histological examination shows alveolar cell injury with a mononuclear cell interstitial infiltrate.

Tuberculosis: the characteristic histological lesion is the caseating granuloma. Primary TB presents with a solitary parenchymal nodule and hilar lymph node involvement. Secondary TB may present as miliary TB, tuberculous pneumonia or cavitary TB.

Mycotic infections: tangled masses of fungal hyphae and debris may be found in lung cavities and are known as fungal balls. These are usually non-invasive unless the patient is immuno-compromised. *Aspergillus fumigatus* is the most common cause, the fungal balls being called aspergillomas. Surgery may be needed for diagnosis and treatment of disease resistant to medical treatment.

Pneumocystis carinii: a fungal organism, which occurs in immunocompromised patients. There is an acellular intra-alveolar exudate. Silver stains or antibody techniques demonstrate the organism.

Chronic bronchitis and *emphysema:* often occur together. Emphysema is characterized by an increase in the size of airspaces distal to the terminal bronchioles. It is classified into three types depending on the part of the lung involved by the process – centrilobular, panlobular (panacinar) and paraseptal. Chronic bronchitis results from hypersecretion from bronchial mucous glands.

Bronchiectasis: permanent abnormal dilatation of the bronchi with infection of the bronchial wall and obliteration of distal airways. Cystic fibrosis is the most common predisposing factor.

Endogenous lipoid pneumonia: may occur distal to a lung tumour and is secondary to break-down of lung parenchyma. The alveoli contain lipid-laden macrophages.

Pneumoconiosis: defined as permanent alteration of lung structure due to the inhalation of mineral dusts and the tissue reactions which follow this. Included in this group are *silicosis, asbestosis, coal worker's pneumoniosis, hard metal disease* and *berylliosis. Asbestosis* is a form of interstitial fibrotic lung disease secondary to asbestos exposure. Fibrosis is characteristically found in the lower lobes especially in the subpleural areas. Asbestos bodies are present in the lung parenchyma. Asbestosis may be graded depending on the amount of lung substance involved and the severity of the fibrosis. Other asbestos-related conditions include benign pleural plaques, diffuse pleural thickening and malignant mesothelioma. The incidence of carcinoma of the lung is increased in those with a history of asbestos exposure.

Interstitial pneumonia/cryptogenic fibrosing alveolitis/pulmonary fibrosis: chronic inflammatory disease, which shows thickening of the alveolar walls, initially by lymphocytes and plasma cells, later by fibroblastic proliferation. Eventually "honeycomb lung" is produced with scarring and multiple air-filled spaces. The need to assess both spatial and temporal distribution of the pathology means that open or thoracoscopic lung biopsies from different zones are usually required. Of clinical value is the sub-classification of interstitial pneumonia as prognosis and response to treatment varies between subgroups. These include *usual interstitial pneumonia (UIP), desquamative interstitial pneumonia (DIP), respiratory bronchiolitis-associated interstitial lung disease (RBILD)* and *non-specific interstitial pneumonia (NSIP)*. Prognosis and response to treatment are worse for UIP than other subgroups (five-year survival 55%).

Immune-mediated lung diseases: extrinsic allergic alveolitis is a chronic granulomatous disease of the lungs due to inhalation of organic dusts, e.g., farmer's lung, bird-fancier's lung, mushroom worker's lung. Upper lobes are more severely affected than basal portions with fibrotic changes occurring in advanced disease.

Wegener's granulomatosis: in the lungs is characterized by vasculitis and granulomas.

Sarcoidosis: occurs most often in the lungs although lymph nodes, skin, eyes, liver and spleen may also be affected. Characteristically, sharply circumscribed non-caseating epithelioid granulomas are present and 25% of cases show marked interstitial fibrosis.

Rare conditions include *Langerhans cell histiocytosis, lymphomatoid granulomatosis* and *pulmonary lymphangioleiomyomatosis.*

Pulmonary vascular disease: emboli that lodge in peripheral arteries cause pulmonary infarcts in patients whose pulmonary circulation is already compromised.

Pulmonary hypertension: primary or secondary. Changes in the arteries may be graded according to the Heath–Edward's classification.

Lung transplantation: the most common indication for lung transplantation is emphysema, e.g., secondary to alpha-1-antitrypsin deficiency. Other indications include chronic obstructive pulmonary disease, septic disease such as cystic fibrosis, fibrotic lung disease and primary pulmonary hypertension. Surveillance involves transbronchial biopsy to look for rejection, which is graded according to the 1995 working classification.

Neoplastic Conditions

Benign Tumours

Most benign tumours are identified incidentally on chest X-ray as solitary lung nodules. Recent advances in minimally invasive surgery, such as video-assisted thoracic surgery, have lowered the threshold for early referral and surgical excision.

Chondroid hamartoma: the most common benign lung tumour, it consists of a mass of cartilage with entrapped epithelial structures. Other connective tissue elements such as bone, adipose tissue, and fibrous tissue may be present.

Other benign tumours include *lipoma, sclerosing haemangioma* and *haemangiopericytoma.*

Malignant Tumours

Lung cancer causes approximately 40,000 deaths annually in the UK and has a strong association with cigarette smoking. Two thirds of lung cancers are inoperable at the time of diagnosis. The ability to classify lung cancer into either small cell carcinoma (SCLC) or non-small cell carcinoma (NSCLC) is important, as behaviour and treatment of the two groups differs. In general, SCLC is treated by chemotherapy, whereas NSCLC, after appropriate clinical staging, is either resected (stage pT2 N1 disease or less) or treated with radiotherapy or chemotherapy. Few patients with SCLC survive longer than 12–18 months. Patients with NSCLC have an average five-year survival of 10–15%.

Squamous cell carcinoma: the commonest carcinoma of the lung (30–45%). It is a malignant epithelial neoplasm showing at least one of the following: keratin, nuclear stratification or intercellular bridges. Squamous cell carcinomas mainly occur centrally in a main or lobar bronchus and can reach a considerable size with central necrosis. Histological variants include *papillary, clear cell, small cell* and the aggressive *basaloid carcinoma.*

Adenocarcinoma: a malignant epithelial neoplasm showing glandular differentiation. It is the lung malignancy which occurs most frequently in non-smokers, women and in the young. It often involves the upper lobes and may present peripherally as a subpleural mass or nodule, with retraction of the pleura. Central scarring in the tumour is quite common.

Secondary adenocarcinomas may come from pancreas, colon, ovary or kidney and show various patterns. If there is involvement of the hilar nodes and significant scarring, then the tumour is more likely to be a primary, if multiple tumours are present it is more likely to be secondary. Lung adenocarcinoma is classified into five subtypes. *Bronchioloalveolar carcinoma (BAC)* is a histological variant of adenocarcinoma, which has low-grade malignant behaviour. It is composed of tall, mucin-secreting cells or non-mucinous cells with distinctive hobnail appearances, which grow along the alveolar septa in a lepidic pattern. There is no stromal reaction or infiltration into the interstitium. BAC may be multifocal or diffuse, when it can mimic pneumonia. Other variants of adenocarcinoma include *papillary carcinoma, acinar adenocarcinoma, solid carcinoma with mucus formation* and *mixed adenocarcinoma. Adenosquamous carcinoma* shows areas of both squamous cell and adenocarcinomatous differentiation, with the minor component accounting for at least 10%. Prognosis is worse than for pure squamous cell carcinoma or adenocarcinoma.

Large cell carcinoma: accounts for 5–10% of all lung malignancies and early metastasis is common. Histological examination shows sheets of large tumour cells with no glands or keratinisation. Variants include *large cell neuroendocrine carcinoma, lymphoepithelioma-like carcinoma,* and *clear cell carcinoma.*

Typical carcinoid tumours: account for 90% of bronchial carcinoids. The vast majority are cured by complete excision with more than 90% ten-year survival. They are of low malignant potential – only 10–15% spread to local lymph nodes and distant metastases are rare. Typical carcinoids may occur either centrally or peripherally. Grossly they are yellowish or pale tan and may be "dumbbell"-like, as they extend into the lumen of the bronchus and the lung parenchyma. They are composed of a uniform cell population arranged in ribbons, cords or islands. In peripheral carcinoids the cells are often spindle shaped. Mitoses are infrequent. It is recommended that resection margins should be to within 5 mm of the tumour.

Atypical carcinoids: metastasise in 50–70% of cases with a five-year survival of 60%. Necrosis, which is usually focal, and increased mitotic activity (> 2/10 high power field), are the most reliable indicators of malignant behaviour.

Small cell carcinoma (SCLC): accounts for 20% of all lung cancers. SCLC is most often located centrally and tends to metastasise early. It is the lung carcinoma most frequently associated with paraneoplastic syndromes. It is primarily treated with chemotherapy, the role of surgery usually being limited to obtaining a definitive tissue diagnosis and for staging. Histological examination shows small- or medium-sized cells with scanty cytoplasm, arranged in nests, ribbons or strands but often showing a lack of an architectural pattern. A variant of small cell carcinoma is a combined tumour where other tumour elements such as squamous or adenocarcinoma are present.

Salivary gland tumours: adenoid cystic carcinoma is most commonly located in the trachea and major bronchi. The tumour shows a cribriform pattern with tubular and solid areas. Perineural infiltration is common. It is generally slow growing.

Mucoepidermoid carcinoma arises from minor salivary glands lining the tracheobronchial tree.

Other cancers: pleomorphic carcinoma, spindle cell carcinoma and *giant cell carcinoma* contain spindle cells and/or giant cells. *Carcinosarcomas* contain both malignant epithelial and sarcomatous elements. *Blastomas* have a biphasic pattern consisting of epithelial tubules or cords in an undifferentiated stroma.

MALT lymphoma is the commonest primary lung lymphoma. It may be solitary or multifocal. Histological examination shows a monomorphic population of centrocyte-like cells. Most MALT lymphomas are low-grade but can transform to high-grade. Lymphoma may also present in the lung secondary to nodal or systemic disease.

Hodgkin's disease is usually secondary to spread from mediastinal disease. *Malignant melanoma* is usually due to metastasis from another site.

Tracheal tumours: primary tracheal tumours are rare, secondary tumours being more common. In adults most primary tracheal tumours are malignant and include *squamous cell carcinoma*, which is usually locally advanced at the time of presentation, and *adenoid cystic carcinoma*.

Chest wall tumours: *malignant small cell tumour of the thoracopulmonary region (Askin Tumour)* occurs in the first two decades of life. It is composed of sheets of undifferentiated, small, hyperchromatic cells, which may form rosettes round a central tangle of fibrillary cytoplasmic processes. Other chest wall tumours include *extra-abdominal desmoid tumours*, *elastofibroma dorsi*, and primary tumours of muscle, fat, blood vessels, nerve sheath or bone.

5. Surgical Pathology Specimens – Clinical Aspects

Biopsy Specimens

Percutaneous/transthoracic needle biopsy: performed under X-ray guidance, an 18-gauge needle is inserted with the aid of a spring-loaded firing device. The biopsy is rinsed directly into fixative. Occasional cases require fresh tissue to be sent for microbiological culture. Fresh frozen or glutaraldehyde-fixed tissue may be needed for special investigations (specialised immunohistochemistry, electron microscopy).

Endobronchial /transbronchial biopsies: taken at rigid or flexible bronchoscopy. The rigid bronchoscope ranges from 3 to 9 mm in diameter and may be used for straight-ahead viewing or at 30º or 90º for visualization of the upper lobe bronchi. It is essential for complete examination of the trachea as a flexible bronchoscopy may miss lesions. It may also be used for brush cytology, biopsy, and to trap sputum for cytology and culture.

However, it allows visualization of major lobar orifices only and is usually performed under general anaesthetic. Flexible bronchoscopes have outer diameters ranging from 3 to 6 mm. Light is transmitted through fibre optic bundles. The bronchoscope can be attached to a video camera for large-screen display. The working channel allows the insertion of various diagnostic and therapeutic accessories. Biopsy forceps are inserted to obtain bronchial or transbronchial biopsies. Lesions not accessible to direct biopsy can be approached with a brush to obtain specimens for cytological or microbiologic analysis. Needles may also be used for aspiration and biopsy. Flexible bronchoscopy is the endoscopic procedure of choice as it is simple, quick to use, and is performed under local anaesthetic.

Open lung biopsies: obtained at thoracotomy for the assessment of peripheral lung disease.

Resection Specimens

Video-assisted thoracoscopic surgery (VATS): direct thoracoscopy is being replaced by the video-assisted thoracoscopic surgical (VATS) technique. VATS allows access to peripleural lung nodules, biopsy and sampling of mediastinal nodes especially in the aortapulmonary window, examination of the pleural space for tumour, wedge resection of lung for diagnosis of diffuse lung infiltrates or peripheral nodules and resection of apical pleural blebs for spontaneous pneumothorax.

Wedge/segmental resections: obtained via open lung biopsy or video-assisted closed chest biopsy. They are used to sample focal areas that are suspicious, e.g., pleural-based nodules or to resect tumours if a patient cannot tolerate a more extensive procedure. Recurrence rates of tumour are higher than with more radical surgery.

Bullectomies: used to excise bulla to improve lung function via a median sternotomy approach, posterolateral thoracotomy or VATS.

Bronchoplastic or sleeve resections: used as alternatives to pneumonectomy. They are lung sparing and are typically used to resect proximal endobronchial lesions at, or adjacent to, the carina, in order to preserve distal, uninvolved lung.

Sleeve lobectomy: excision of a lobe with the associated lobar bronchus and subsequent anastomosis of the distal bronchial tree to the proximal airway.

Bronchial sleeve resection: resection of either mainstem bronchus, with anastomosis of the distal airway to the carina or lower trachea.

Sleeve pneumonectomy: resection of the carina with pneumonectomy and anastomosis of the contralateral distal bronchus to the distal trachea.

Lobectomy/bilobectomy: resection of one or two lobes of lung and includes complete resection of hilar (N1) lymph nodes draining the primary tumour.

Pneumonectomy: resection of the whole lung and accounts for 20% of all lung resections. It is indicated when tumour invades hilar structures such as the mainstem bronchus or the main pulmonary artery. It is also indicated when tumour crosses the oblique fissure or when there is lymph node involvement along the mainstem bronchus, proximal to the upper lobe take-off. In the majority of cases it is for the purpose of resecting tumours, an exception being recipient pneumonectomy performed prior to lung transplant.

Extended pulmonary resection: extension of the limits of conventional pulmonary resection with an en-bloc excision of contiguous intrathoracic structures involved by tumour.

Extrapleural pneumonectomy: indications include resection of malignant mesothelioma, or rarely carcinoma of the lung, which is restricted to the lung, pleura and local lymph nodes.

Surgical incisions: the most versatile approach used by the thoracic surgeon is the *posterolateral thoracotomy*. The incision is 8 cm lateral to the sixth thoracic spinous process and curves forward, 2 cm below the tip of the scapula to the mid-axillary line in the line of the ribs. It is used in unilateral lung resection, chest wall tumour resection, unilateral lung volume reduction surgery, bullectomy and tumours of the posterior mediastinum.

Anterolateral thoracotomy and axillary thoracotomy are used with decreasing frequency. *Median sternotomy* is used in mediastinal tumour resection, bilateral lung volume reduction surgery or bullectomy, resection of multiple pulmonary lesions (e.g., metastases) and transpericardial access to the trachea or bronchus, e.g., carinal tumours.

The thoracoabdominal approach is used in procedures where access is needed to both pleural and peritoneal cavities. Bilateral anterior thoracotomies (also known as the clamshell incision) provide maximum exposure of both hemithoraces and mediastinal structures. This approach is used in bilateral lung resections such as lung transplant and lung reduction surgery.

Lung volume reduction surgery (LVRS): a palliative surgical procedure for patients with end-stage emphysema in which 20–30% of each upper lobe is resected.

6. Surgical Pathology Specimens-Laboratory Protocols

Biopsy Specimens

Small biopsies are promptly put into 10% formalin fixative.

Endobronchial/ transbronchial biopsies

- count the number of fragments.
- record the greatest dimension of the largest fragment (mm).
- note the colour and consistency of the fragments.
- place the fragments in cassettes between foam pads or wrapped in filter paper or in molten agar for processing.
- cut through multiple levels, keeping intervening spares for further stains.

Open lung biopsy

- reinflate lung using a formalin injection.
- record the size (cm) and weight (g)/number of fragments.
- describe the colour and consistency.
- serially transverse section at 3 mm intervals and sample representative blocks.

Histopathology Report

- nature of biopsy.
- size of biopsy (mm), number of fragments.
- bronchial wall–epithelium, thickness of wall, goblet cell hyperplasia, malignancy.
- alveoli – count approximate number, type I or II pneumocyte proliferation, inflammation, macrophages in lumen, consolidation, exudate.
- nature of inflammatory cells if present.
- fibrosis if present: type – interstitial, intra-alveolar (BOOP), grade of fibrosis – mild, moderate, severe.
- other pathology – vascular, asbestos bodies, doubly refractile material, granulomas, lymphangitis carcinomatosa.
- if transplant, grade rejection according to the 1995 working formulation.

Resection Specimens

Larger specimens are put into dry containers and brought promptly to the laboratory.

Wedge Resections (or "Cornish Pastie")

- consist of a triangular segment of lung and pleura with two staple lines at the margin (Figure 38.2).
- palpate the specimen to locate the lesion.
- record the dimensions(cm).
- describe the pleura.
- inflate with a syringe of formalin. A disadvantage of inflation fixation is that free cells may be cleared from consolidated alveoli so that diagnoses such as desquamative interstitial pneumonia (DIP) are obscured. Measure the length of the margin. Cut off the staple line as closely as possible. The cut surface of the lung can be taken en face or perpendicularly. The open surface is inked.
- ink the pleural surface over the lesion.
- serially transverse section at 3 mm intervals.
- describe the lesion – size, colour, pleural involvement, distance (mm) from margin.
- describe the remainder of the lung.
- take representative sections of any lesion, of its relationship to the pleura and uninvolved lung, and the closest margin.
- if the lung disease is diffuse submit the vast majority of the specimen for histology.

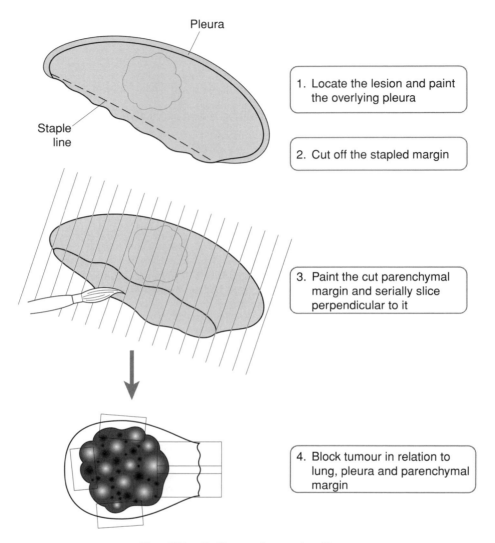

Figure 38.2. Blocking a wedge resection of lung.

Lung Resection for Tumours

Most resections are for tumour: lobectomy, bilobectomy, and pneumonectomy.

Initial procedure

- palpate to locate tumour or areas of abnormality.
- specify which lung or lobe.
- record the weight (g) and dimensions (cm). Ink the pleura overlying the tumour.
- remove the bronchial margin by sectioning transversely, before inflation fixation (Figure 38.3). Sample the hilar nodes.

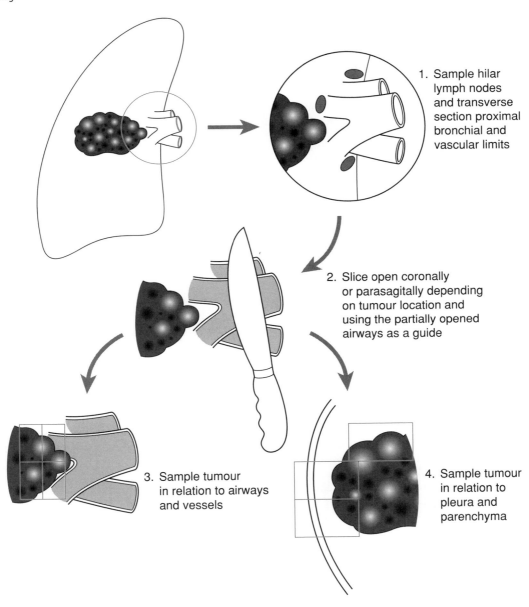

1. Sample hilar lymph nodes and transverse section proximal bronchial and vascular limits

2. Slice open coronally or parasagitally depending on tumour location and using the partially opened airways as a guide

3. Sample tumour in relation to airways and vessels

4. Sample tumour in relation to pleura and parenchyma

Figure 38.3.   Blocking a pneumonectomy specimen.

- inflation: if the specimen is intact instil fixative from a height of about 25 cm via tubing that terminates in a nozzle wedged into the supply bronchus or bronchi. Continue until the pleural surface is smooth. Immerse in a container of fixative overnight with a covering of lint or filter paper to prevent drying. If the specimen is not intact inflate with a syringe. Remember to culture, if appropriate, before fixation.

- allow to fix for 24–36 hours.
- to access airways open from the hilum, pass a probe down to the tumour and then cut along it.
- serially slice the tumour at 3 mm intervals in the plane that best demonstrates its relationship to the anatomical structures. In general, mid-zone and peripheral lesions are sliced parasagitally, hilar lesions coronally.
- with vascular lesions such as pulmonary emboli, approach laterally within fissures cutting towards the hilum until the pulmonary artery is entered.
- photograph.
- ribs – decalcify.

Description

- lesion site – central/peripheral, main/segmental bronchus.
  - endobronchial/bronchial/extrabronchial/extrinsic compression.
  - distances (mm) to the bronchial or parenchymal resection margins/pleura.
- lesion size – length × width × depth or maximum dimension (cm).
- lesion appearance – colour/consistency/necrosis/haemorrhage/cavitation.
- lesion edges – circumscribed/infiltrative.
- lung – emphysema/fibrosis/bullae/bronchiectasis/mucus plugging/post-obstructive pneumonia.
- hilar lymph nodes – number/size/colour/consistency.

Blocks for histology (Figure 38.3)

- transverse section the proximal resection margin, and the pulmonary staple margin, if the specimen is a lobectomy.
- submit all hilar lymph nodes. The surgeon for staging purposes often also submits other separate named lymph node stations, and these are processed separately.
- sample four sections of tumour, showing relationships to uninvolved lung, adjacent bronchi and vessels and the nearest aspect of the pleura.
- sample uninvolved lung (one or two blocks – more if there is suspected asbestosis).
- sample the margins of any attached parietal pleura, chest wall soft tissue or ribs – represent the deepest point of rib invasion.

Histopathology report

- type of procedure – wedge resection, lobectomy, bilobectomy, pneumonectomy.
- tumour type – squamous carcinoma/adenocarcinoma/small cell carcinoma/large cell carcinoma/neuroendocrine tumours/salivary gland type adenocarcinoma/others.
- tumour differentiation – well/moderate/poor.
- tumour edge – pushing/infiltrative.
- extent of local tumour spread. Elastin stain may be helpful in recognising visceral pleural invasion.
  - pTx positive cytology but tumour not visualised by imaging or bronchoscopy.
  - pTis carcinoma in situ.
  - pT1 tumour ≤ 3 cm diameter, surrounded by lung or visceral pleura and not invasive proximal to a lobar bronchus.

- – pT2 tumour > 3 cm diameter or involves main bronchus 2 cm or more distal to the carina or invades visceral pleura. Partial atelectasis extending to the hilum but not involving the entire lung.
- – pT3 tumour of any size that directly invades chest wall, diaphragm, mediastinal pleura or parietal pericardium or tumour of the main bronchus < 2 cm distal to the carina but without involvement of the carina or associated total atelectasis or obstructive pneumonitis of the entire lung.
- – pT4 tumour of any size invading the mediastinum, heart, great vessels, trachea, oesophagus, vertebral body or carina, or tumour with malignant pleural effusion or separate tumour nodule(s) in the same lobe.
- – pM1 distant metastases, including separate tumour nodules in a different lobe (ipsilateral or contralateral).
- lymphovascular invasion – present/not present
- regional nodes – intrathoracic, scalene, supraclavicular.
  - – pN0 no regional lymph node metastases.
  - – pN1 metastases in ipsilateral peribronchial/hilar/intrapulmonary nodes, including involvement by direct extension.
  - – pN2 metastases in ipsilateral mediastinal and/or subcarinal nodes.
  - – pN3 metastases in contralateral mediastinal, contralateral hilar, ipsi-/contralateral scalene or supraclavicular nodes.

At least 6 lymph nodes should be found in the hilar and mediastinal lymphadenectomy specimen. If less than this, and the lymph nodes obtained are negative, classify as pN0.

- excision margins – distances (mm) to the proximal bronchial, vascular and mediastinal limits and pleura.
- other pathology – atelectasis/bronchiectasis/lipid pneumonia/suppurative pneumonia.

39 Pleura

1. Anatomy

The visceral pleura covers the surface of the lungs and the parietal pleura covers the inner surface of the chest wall, mediastinum and diaphragm. Under normal circumstances the cavity contains 5–20 ml of fluid. The lining of the pleura is composed of a continuous layer of flat or low cuboidal cells – the mesothelium.

Lymphovascular supply

Branches of systemic arteries supply the parietal pleura. The bronchial circulation supplies the visceral pleura. Venous blood from the visceral pleura drains into the pulmonary veins and lymph from the visceral pleura passes to a superficial plexus in the lung and then to the hilar nodes. Lymph leaves the pleural cavity mainly via the parietal lymphatic system. The parietal pleura drains to the parasternal, diaphragmatic and posterior mediastinal nodes.

2. Clinical Presentation

Pleural disease may present with pain and breathlessness. Non-specific symptoms such as weakness, anorexia, and fever may be present in 25% of cases of malignant mesothelioma. Paraneoplastic syndromes occasionally arise causing immunosuppression, thrombocytosis, cachexia, amyloidosis or hypoglycaemia.

3. Clinical Investigations

Chest X-ray – to detect pleural effusions and calcified pleural plaques.

CT scan – may identify an effusion undetectable by conventional radiography. It will show pleural thickening and calcification due to asbestos exposure. It is important in detecting invasion of chest wall, ribs and mediastinum by malignant mesothelioma.

Ultrasound – used to localize pleural effusions during thoracentesis.

Thoracentesis – aspiration of pleural fluid using a sterile technique. Fifty to 100 ml are sufficient for diagnosis but more may be removed if the thoracentesis is therapeutic.

Pleural fluid analysis – cytology, biochemistry – total protein, lactate dehydrogenase, amylase, glucose, pH, lipids, complement and antibodies, Gram stain and culture.

Pleural needle biopsy – percutaneous closed needle biopsy with thoracentesis. A diagnosis of malignancy is achieved in 40–70% of cases.

Thoracoscopy and pleural biopsy – thoracoscopy, especially if guided by CT findings, should improve the diagnostic yield to over 95%. Minimally invasive approaches such as video-assisted thoracoscopy (VATS) lead to earlier diagnosis.

Open pleural biopsy (with or without decortication) – occasionally rigid (open tube) pleuroscopy or even minithoracotomy are required to obtain an adequate pleural biopsy.

4. Pathological Conditions

Pleural disease is either primary or secondary, e.g., to an underlying lung lesion or systemic disorder such as SLE.

Pleural effusions: over 90% of effusions are secondary to one of four conditions – congestive heart failure, pneumonia, malignancy or pulmonary emboli. Transudates are effusions containing low concentrations of proteins (< 3 g/dl) and the majority are due to congestive heart failure. Exudates contain higher concentrations of protein (> 3 g/dl) and over 80% are due to pneumonia, neoplasm or pulmonary emboli. Depending on the aetiology effusions can be serous, fibrinous, serofibrinous, purulent or haemorrhagic.

Empyema is the presence of frank pus in the pleural cavity. Non-infective processes such as pulmonary infarction, rheumatoid disease, SLE and uraemia may present with a pleural effusion.

Asbestos-related pleural effusion develops in 3% of asbestos workers. In most it will resolve in one to two years but 20% progress to massive pleural fibrosis and 5% develop malignant mesothelioma. Carcinoma of the lung is the most common malignancy to invade the pleura and produce pleural effusions, followed by carcinoma of the breast.

Pneumothorax: primary spontaneous pneumothorax occurs most commonly in 30 to 40 year old tall, thin males. They are most often due to rupture of blebs or bullae on the apical parts of the upper lobes. Rate of recurrence is 25%. Secondary pneumothorax occurs in chronic obstructive pulmonary disease, cystic fibrosis, asthma, tuberculosis, idiopathic pulmonary fibrosis, lymphangioleiomyomatosis, Langerhans histiocytosis and pneumocystis carinii pneumonia (PCP). Catamenial pneumothorax is associated with menstruation and may be due to focal endometrial deposits on the pleura. Traumatic pneumothorax can be iatrogenic, e.g., secondary to biopsy or otherwise, e.g., penetrating chest trauma.

Pleural plaques: usually but not always associated with asbestos. Histological examination shows hyalinized fibrous tissue with basket-weave collagen fibres. Usually present on the parietal pleura mainly in the intercostal spaces on the anterior and posterolateral aspects of the chest wall and on the dome of the diaphragm.

Diffuse pleural thickening: involves the visceral pleura and is associated with asbestos exposure.

Asbestos-induced mesothelial hyperplasia: consists of a papillary proliferation of the surface mesothelium with cores of connective tissue and a surface lining of regular mesothelial cells. It may be difficult to distinguish from well-differentiated malignant mesothelioma on pleural biopsy.

Neoplastic Conditions

Metastatic tumours, e.g., lung and breast cancer, are the most common tumours of the pleura.

Malignant mesothelioma: most common primary malignant tumour of the pleura. There is a proven relationship with asbestos exposure although 10–20% appear to be unrelated. Rarely they may be associated with therapeutic irradiation or intrapleural thorium dioxide (Thorotrast). In industrialized countries malignant mesothelioma accounts for about 1% of all cancer deaths. There is a latency period of twenty years between exposure to asbestos and development of the tumour.

Malignant mesothelioma occurs usually in the lower half of the hemithorax on the right side more often than the left. It encases the lung and direct extension into the subpleural lung is common. If nodular masses are present within the lung parenchyma a primary lung carcinoma with pleural spread is more likely.

Histological patterns include epithelial, sarcomatoid (or fibrous) and biphasic, a combination of both. The epithelioid pattern appears to be commonest in most series, with tubules, papillae and sometimes psammoma bodies being seen. Spindle cells set in varying amounts of collagenized stroma are seen in the sarcomatoid pattern. Differential diagnosis includes adenocarcinoma, reactive mesothelial hyperplasia and fibrosis. Immunohistochemistry, assessment of radiological findings and disease course are correlated to reach a final diagnosis.

Distant metastases occur late, if at all, the sarcomatous form showing metastatic spread more commonly. Malignant mesotheliomas are rarely operable. Few patients survive longer than two years and the outlook is not significantly affected by current therapy. Occasional patients are suitable for adjuvant chemotherapy with local resection of limited disease. Symptomatic relief is gained by multiple paracentesis of malignant effusions supplemented by intracavitary injection of chemotherapeutic or sclerosant agents.

Solitary fibrous tumour: origin is from the subpleural mesenchyme, from fibroblasts or myofibroblasts and is unrelated to asbestos exposure. It more often arises from the visceral pleura and is often attached by a pedicle. Histological examination shows a low-grade spindle cell neoplasm of variable cellularity with tumour cells dispersed in a collagenous stroma. The most important prognostic factor is the completeness of excision and particularly the presence or absence of a pedicle. Tumour size and cellularity correlate with malignancy. Prognosis is generally good with a minority showing local recurrence.

Calcifying fibrous pseudotumour: occurs in young adults and may be a late stage of inflammatory myofibroblastic tumour.

Pyothorax-associated lymphoma: non-Hodgkin's lymphoma of B cell phenotype. Associated with Epstein Barr virus (EBV).

Body cavity-based lymphoma: presents as a mass lesion. Associated with EBV, human herpes virus 8, and HIV. A high-grade lymphoma of null cell phenotype.

5. Surgical Pathology Specimens – Clinical Aspects

Biopsy Specimens

A number of procedures can be undertaken to obtain pleural biopsies. A special needle, usually an Abrams or Cope needle may be used during thoracentesis, both to drain fluid and obtain a pleural biopsy. A pleural needle biopsy often provides insufficient tissue for diagnosis. When this is the case thoracoscopy and a visually directed pleural biopsy may be required. In some cases an open pleural biopsy is undertaken with or without decortication. *Decortication* is a procedure to remove constricting visceral pleural peel in order to expand the underlying lung. It is of use in very few patients as the morbidity and mortality usually outweigh any benefit. Approximately 10% of cases of malignant mesothelioma that have a biopsy will have seeding of the biopsy tract by tumour with subsequent chest wall recurrence. To prevent this happening radiation therapy is used on the biopsy site.

Resection Specimens

Surgery may be used to treat pneumothorax. The preferred approach is using minimally invasive techniques (VATS) but thoracotomy can be used with an axillary, muscle-sparing approach. Resection of blebs or bullae is achieved using mechanical stapling devices.

Pleurectomy is a procedure used to debulk a malignant mesothelioma or for diagnosis. Multiple fragments or strips of pleural membrane are obtained.

An *extrapleural pneumonectomy (EPP)* is the en-bloc resection of visceral and parietal pleura, lung, ipsilateral hemidiaphragm and pericardium. It has an operative mortality of 5–15%. Combined with postoperative chemotherapy and adjuvant radiotherapy it may improve survival.

6. Surgical Pathology Specimens – Laboratory Protocols

Biopsy Specimens

As for lung biopsies (see page 401).

Resection Specimens

Pleurectomy (Figure 39.1)
- record the number of fragments.
- measure the dimensions (cm) of the fragments unless there are more than three, then note dimensions of the smallest and largest, weigh the fragments (g).

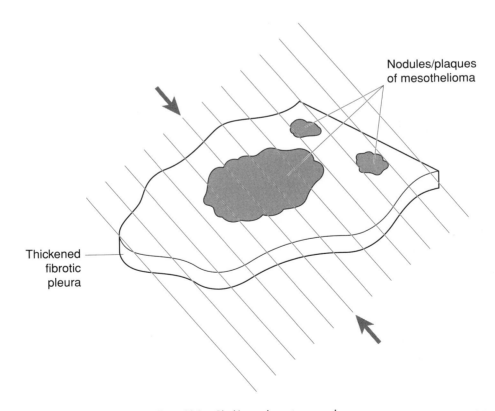

Figure 39.1.   Blocking a pleurectomy specimen.

- describe any lesions – colour, consistency and sizes.
- record the presence of other structures such as muscle, pericardium or fat and any involvement of these by tumour.
- ink margins and note the distances (cm) of any lesion from them.
- submit one section for each cm of tumour to include the margins.

Extrapleural Pneumonectomy

- tissue may be taken for electron microscopy before fixation.
- weigh the specimen (g) and record its dimensions (cm).
- inflate and fix the lung.
- take the bronchial margin and remove hilar lymph nodes (number/size).
- examine the pleura – determine the percentage involvement by tumour.
- examine the pericardium for tumour.
- ink margins close to the tumour.
- serially section the specimen coronally at 1 cm intervals.
- describe involvement of the diaphragm by tumour – distance from the anterior, posterior, medial and lateral margins, depth of invasion into diaphragm, involvement of the peritoneal surface of the diaphragm.
- describe involvement of visceral pleura – extent of fusion of visceral pleura to parietal, size of nodules of tumour.

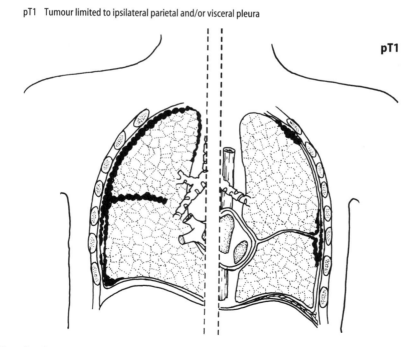

Figure 39.2.   Pleural and interlobar spread of malignant mesothelioma. Reproduced from Hermanek P, Hutter RVP, Sobin LH, Wagner G, Wittekind Ch (eds). TNM Atlas: illustrated guide to the TNM/pTNM classification of malignant tumours, 4th edition. Springer-Verlag: Berlin and Heidelberg, 1997.

- invasion of lung – usually tumour invades along interlobar fissures (Figure 39.2). Describe parenchymal disease such as pneumonia or fibrosis.
- if rib is attached describe the dimensions, and any tumour involvement seen. If lesions are seen in the ribs, X-ray.

Blocks for histology

- take sections perpendicular to the pleura from: the apex of the lung; the anterior, posterior, medial, and lateral pleura at one level; the anterior, lateral, medial, posterior and inferior margins of the diaphragm.
- take sections of rib if involved.
- if chest wall is attached to the specimen take margins.

Histopathology report

- type of specimen – biopsy/pleurectomy/extrapleural pneumonectomy.
- size (cm) and weight (g).
- tumour site – visceral/parietal/parenchymal.
- tumour size – length × width × depth or maximum dimension (cm).
- tumour appearance – localized/diffuse/nodular/plaque/infiltrative/cystic change.
- tumour histological type – malignant mesothelioma–biphasic, epithelioid, sarcomatoid.
- extent of local tumour spread.
  - pT1 tumour limited to ipsilateral parietal and/or visceral pleura.
  - pT2 tumour invades any of: ipsilateral lung, diaphragm, confluent visceral pleura.
  - pT3 tumour invades any of: endothoracic fascia, mediastinal fat, focal chest wall, non-transmural pericardium.
  - pT4 tumour directly extends to any of :contralateral pleura, peritoneum, rib, extensive chest wall, mediastinum, myocardium, brachial plexus, spine, inner pericardium, malignant pericardial effusion.
- lymphovascular invasion – present/not present.
- regional lymph nodes – intrathoracic, internal mammary, scalene, supraclavicular.
  - pN0 no regional lymph node metastases.
  - pN1 metastasis in ipsilateral bronchopulmonary and/or hilar lymph nodes.
  - pN2 metastasis in ipsilateral internal mammary, mediastinal and/or subcarinal lymph nodes.
  - pN3 metastasis in contralateral mediastinal, contralateral internal mammary or hilar, ipsilateral or contralateral scalene or supraclavicular lymph nodes.
- excision margins – distance (mm) to the nearest inked margin of local resection of limited disease.
- other pathology – pleural plaques, asbestosis, bronchogenic carcinoma, fibrosis, emphysema.

40 Mediastinum

1. Anatomy

The mediastinum is that part of the thoracic cavity located centrally between the pleural cavities. It extends anteroposteriorly from the inner aspect of the sternum to the spine and superoinferiorly from the thoracic inlet to the diaphragm. It can be subdivided arbitrarily into anterior, superior, middle and posterior compartments. (Figure 40.1).

The anterosuperior compartment contains the thymus gland, lymph nodes, vessels and fat. The thymus is large at birth but atrophies after puberty and in the adult is variable in size. It can extend down beyond the aortic arch and lie in front of the brachiocephalic veins and left common carotid artery. Parathyroid tissue may be embedded in it. The great vessels, the aorta, the superior vena cava and the azygos vein lie in the anterosuperior compartment.

The middle compartment contains the heart, pericardium, trachea, major bronchi, the pulmonary vessels, phrenic and vagus nerves.

The posterior (paravertebral) compartment contains the sympathetic chain, vagus nerves, oesophagus, thoracic duct, descending aorta, azygous and hemiazygous veins and lymph nodes.

Lymphovascular Drainage

Lymphatic drainage is to tracheobronchial lymph nodes situated at the carina.

2. Clinical Presentation

Almost half of patients with mediastinal cysts or tumours are asymptomatic. Lesions are often discovered incidentally on X-ray.

Local symptoms may result from compression or invasion of mediastinal structures and include cough, dysphagia, recurrent pulmonary infection, dyspnoea, pain and rarely haemoptysis. Most bronchial, gastric and gastroenteric cysts are asymptomatic although the latter can be life threatening because of gastric secretion leading to haemorrhage, peptic ulcer and perforation. Superior vena cava (SVC) syndrome, due to compression or invasion of the superior vena cava usually indicates the presence of malignancy but can be caused by benign fibrosing mediastinitis.

Myasthenia gravis is present in one third of patients with thymomas. Symptoms include fatigability affecting the proximal limb muscles, extraocular muscles, muscles of mastication, speech and facial expression. Respiratory difficulties may occur. Other associated conditions in 5–10% of cases are red cell aplasia with a severe anaemia, hypogammaglobulinaemia resulting in bacterial infections and diarrhoea, and pemphigus foliaceous producing skin blisters.

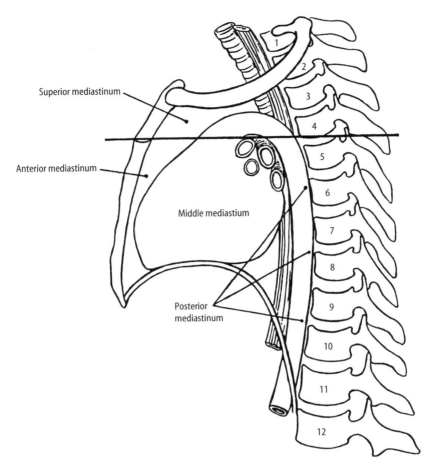

Figure 40.1. Compartments of the mediastinum. Reproduced from Hall-Craggs ECB. Anatomy as a basis for clinical medicine, 3rd edition. Williams and Wilkins: London, 1995.

3. Clinical Investigations

- Chest X-ray – mediastinal masses commonly present on chest X-ray obtained for other purposes or in patients with cancer undergoing CT scan staging of the chest and abdomen.
- CT scan – has limitations when distinguishing between cystic and solid structures.
- MRI scan – particularly useful in determining tumour invasion of vascular or neural structures, when coronal or radial body sections are necessary, or when contrast material cannot be given intravenously due to renal disease or allergy.
- Angiography – used in vascular lesions.
- Barium swallow – used to investigate posterior mediastinal lesions.
- Gallium scan – of value in the diagnosis of lymphoma.

- Blood tests:
  - mediastinal germ cell tumours: AFP (alpha-fetoprotein), β-HCG (beta-human chorionic gonadotrophin).
  - lymphoma/seminoma: LDH (lactate dehydrogenase).
  - parathyroid tumours: serum calcium and alkaline phosphatase.
  - myasthenia gravis: acetylcholine receptor antibody.
- Blood count – normochromic normocytic anaemia – red cell aplasia.
- Single fibre EMG and tensilon test – for suspected myasthenia gravis.
- Percutaneous or thoracoscopic fine needle aspiration – performed under radiological guidance.
- Percutaneous or thoracoscopic core biopsy – using a larger gauge or cutting needle under radiological guidance.
- Oesophagoscopy – for dysphagia or for any mass close to the oesophagus.
- Bronchoscopy – used when there is hilar or peritracheal lymphadenopathy.

4. Pathological Conditions

Infections

Acute mediastinitis: potentially fatal, may affect all three compartments and arise from an adjacent pneumonia or as a complication of oesophageal perforation. *Fibrosing mediastinitis* is characterized by fibrosis causing a variety of symptoms depending on which structures are constricted. Aetiological factors include histoplasma capsulatum and TB.

Mediastinal Masses (Table 40.1)

Anterior Mediastinal Masses

Table 40.1.   Mediastinal masses

Anterior/Superior Compartment	Middle Compartment	Posterior Compartment
Thymomas	Bronchogenic cyst	Neurogenic tumours-neurofibroma, neurilemmoma (schwannoma),ganglioneuroma, ganglioneuroblastoma, malignant schwannoma, neuroblastoma, paraganglioma
Thymolipomas	Enteric cyst	Malignant lymphoma
Carcinoid tumours	Pericardial cyst	Gastroenteric cysts
Thymic cyst	Malignant lymphoma	
Germ cell tumours	Primary cardiac tumours	
Malignant lymphoma	Metastatic carcinoma	
Teratomas		
Metastatic carcinoma		
Thyroid/parathyroid lesions		
Mesenchymal lesions – Lipoma, Haemangioma, Lymphangioma		
Aberrant thyroid		
Thyroid goitre		

Unilocular thymic cysts: of developmental origin and occur more often in the neck than the mediastinum. The lining may be flattened, cuboidal, columnar or (rarely) squamous epithelium with thymic tissue in the wall.

Multilocular thymic cysts: acquired and thought to be secondary to inflammation. Some cases are seen in HIV infection. They can mimic an invasive thymic tumour and occur in about half of thymuses with nodular sclerosing Hodgkin's disease or seminoma. They also occur in other tumours such as thymoma and large cell lymphoma, though less frequently. Exceptionally, true squamous cell carcinoma arises from these cysts.

Thymic hyperplasia: strongly associated with autoimmune disease especially myasthenia gravis. There is extreme variability in size and weight of the thymus with formation of germinal centres, principally in the medulla that expand and cause cortical atrophy.

Thymoma: the most common primary neoplasm of the mediastinum. Seventy-five per cent present in the anterior mediastinum but they can also occur in other compartments (neck, thyroid, pulmonary hilum, lung parenchyma, pleura). It is a mixture of neoplastic thymic epithelial cells and non-neoplastic lymphocytes. Tumours are evaluated on the basis of the morphology of the neoplastic epithelial cells (spindle, plump) and the relative number of these cells, compared with the non-neoplastic lymphocytic component.

Medullary thymomas: composed of epithelial cells that resemble those of the medulla and are elongated or spindle shaped. They are benign.

Mixed thymomas: show a mixture of spindle cells and plumper, rounder, cortical-type epithelial cells. They act in a benign fashion.

Predominantly cortical (organoid) thymomas: have a less prominent epithelial component with lymphocyte-rich organoid corticomedullary areas. Local invasion is common.

Cortical thymomas: have a lesser component of lymphocytes with large round or polygonal epithelial cells. They are frequently locally invasive.

Well-differentiated thymic carcinoma: composed predominantly of epithelial cells with mild nuclear atypia and few lymphocytes. It is locally invasive.

Thymic carcinoma: an epithelial tumour exhibiting cytological features of malignancy. Cytoarchitectural features are no longer specific to the thymus but are analogous to those seen in carcinomas of other organs. No immature lymphocytes are present. Microscopic types of thymic carcinoma include squamous cell carcinoma, non-keratinizing squamous cell carcinoma and lymphoepithelioma-like carcinoma. These account for over 90% of cases.

Lymphoma: accounts for 10–14% of mediastinal masses in adults and is the commonest primary neoplasm of the middle mediastinum. Lymphoma of any type may occur, generally as part of widespread disease.

Mediastinal Hodgkin's disease: the nodular sclerosing variety occurs most frequently with mediastinal involvement in 80% of cases There is a nodular growth pattern, collagen bands and lacunar cells.

Non-Hodgkin's lymphoma: usually high grade. T-lymphoblastic (young patients) or large B-cell and occasionally low grade (MALToma).

Mediastinal large B-cell lymphoma: thought to be of thymic B-cell origin. Histological examination shows a diffuse proliferation of cells, which are compartmentalized into groups by fine bands of sclerosis. There may be thymic remnants. There is an association with nodular sclerosis Hodgkin's lymphoma (composite lymphoma). Biopsy samples are often small and may be obscured by profuse sclerosis with associated cellular crush artefact.

Germ Cell Tumours: make up 20% of mediastinal masses.

Mature cystic teratoma: the most common type of mediastinal germ cell neoplasm comprising a disorganized mixture of derivatives of the three germinal layers – ectoderm, mesoderm and endoderm.

Immature teratoma: a germ cell tumour similar to mature teratoma but also containing immature epithelial, mesenchymal or neural elements.

Seminoma: the most common malignant germ cell tumour to occur in the mediastinum. These arise almost always within the thymus.

Non-seminomatous malignant germ cell tumours: include malignant teratomas, malignant teratocarcinomas, yolk sac tumours, endodermal sinus tumours, choriocarcinomas and embryonal cell carcinomas.

Malignant germ cell tumours are usually treated with chemotherapy and radiotherapy. If a residual mass is left, it is usually a benign teratoma or necrotic tumour mass that can potentially degenerate and redevelop malignancy. Excision may be carried out.

Middle Mediastinal Masses

Pericardial cysts: benign cysts, the inner surface of which are lined by a single layer of mesothelium and contain clear watery fluid.

Bronchial (bronchogenic) cysts: make up 60% of all mediastinal cysts and occur along the tracheobronchial tree, commonly posterior to the carina. They are usually lined by ciliated columnar epithelium but there may be focal or extensive squamous metaplasia. The wall can contain hyaline cartilage, smooth muscle, bronchial glands or nerve trunks.

Oesophageal cysts: usually in the wall of the lower half of the oesophagus. The lining may be squamous, ciliated or columnar epithelium and there is a double layer of smooth muscle in the wall.

Malignant lymphoma and metastatic carcinoma: see above

Posterior Mediastinal Masses

Gastric and *enteric cysts:* located in the posterior mediastinum in a paravertebral location and nearly all are associated with vertebral malformations. The gastric type has the same coats as the stomach, the enteric type similar to the wall of the small intestine. Combined forms of cysts are termed gastroenteric cysts.

Neurogenic tumours: the most common posterior mediastinal masses. Most are asymptomatic. MRI scan may be necessary to rule out intraspinal extension along the nerve roots (dumbbell tumours).

Nerve sheath tumours account for 65% of all mediastinal neurogenic tumours and include *neurilemoma* (schwannoma) and neurofibromas. Of patients with nerve sheath tumours, 25–40% have multiple neurofibromatosis (von Recklinghausen's disease). Malignant tumours such as neurogenic sarcomas and malignant schwannomas may occur and other tumours include neuroblastomas and paragangliomas.

5. Surgical Pathology Specimens – Clinical Aspects

Biopsy Specimens

Percutaneous or thoracoscopic fine needle or *core biopsy:* used to obtain a tissue diagnosis, e.g., malignant lymphoma. The role of needle biopsy for diagnosis of thymoma is controversial. Diagnostic accuracy is 59% but the differentiation between benign and malignant thymoma is difficult. There is also an intra-operative risk of seeding tumour cells in the mediastinum or pleural space.

Open biopsy: in some cases invasive mediastinal incisional biopsy may be required. Surgical approaches include cervical mediastinoscopy, sub-xiphoid mediastinoscopy, anterior mediastinoscopy and videothoracoscopy. *Cervical mediastinoscopy* is performed through a small incision in the suprasternal notch. It is used to sample masses in the superior mediastinum or lymph nodes in the subcarinal and paratracheal area. *Anterior mediastinotomy* (*Chamberlain procedure*) is performed through a small incision over the second or third rib on either side. It is used to sample lymph nodes in the para-aortic position or anterior mediastinal masses. Biopsy of the thymus may cause seeding of tumour into the operative site and violate the tumour capsule. Diagnostic accuracy for thymoma by open biopsy is 81%.

Resection Specimens

Thymectomy: performed for benign or malignant thymic tumours, treatment of myasthenia gravis or may be incidental during thoracic surgery such as open-heart surgery. If the thymus is not very large, thymectomy may be carried out through a transcervical route. The usual surgical approach is through either partial or complete sternotomy. Median sternotomy involves the use of an incision in the midline from the suprasternal notch to just below the xiphoid process with division of the sternum longitudinally. Ideally there should be complete removal of the thymus with surrounding margins of normal tissue. Alternatively, tumour debulking may be undertaken. The clinical ease of excision, and the tumour circumscription or degree of spread into adjacent tissues, are strong indicators of potential for future local recurrence and invasion.

6. Surgical Pathology Specimens – Laboratory Protocols

Biopsy Specimens

- count the number of fragments and measure their length (mm).
- Describe colour, consistency.
- place in cassettes between foam pads or wrapped in filter paper.
- examine histologically through multiple levels and keep intervening sections for stains.

Resection Specimens

Initial procedure and description

- measure and record size – length × width × depth (cm) and weight (g).
- appearance – cystic/haemorrhagic/necrosis.
- capsule/soft tissue invasion.
- adherence to pleura/pericardium.
- photograph.
- fixation by immersion in 10% formalin for 48 hours.
- ink the outer surface.
- serially section the specimen transversely at 3–5 mm intervals.
- describe lesions – size (cm), colour, whether lobulated or smooth, relationship to the capsule and surrounding structures, edges (encapsulated or infiltrating), the presence of calcification, necrosis or haemorrhage.
- describe uninvolved tissue, e.g., thymus – colour, consistency, proportions of fat and parenchyma.
- dissect out and submit lymph nodes in any attached tissue.

Blocks for histology

- sample four or five blocks of the lesion and its relationship to the capsule if present and to the rest of the tissue.
- block the margins.
- sample blocks from uninvolved tissue (at least two).
- sample lymph nodes.
- block pleura and/or pericardium if present.

Histopathology report

- tumour type – metastatic carcinoma, malignant lymphoma, germ cell tumour, neurogenic tumour, thymoma, sarcoma.
- tumour differentiation:
  - metastatic carcinoma: well/moderate/poor.
  - malignant lymphoma: low-grade (MALToma/follicular lymphoma)/high-grade (diffuse large cell lymphoma, lymphoblastic lymphoma).
  - germ cell tumour: seminoma/non-seminomatous: mature, immature, malignant – embryonal carcinoma, yolk sac tumour, choriocarcinoma, MTI.
  - neurogenic tumours: small round blue cell/neuroblastoma component.
  - sarcoma – low-grade/high-grade.
  - thymoma – classify according to morphology (see above)
- tumour edge – pushing/infiltrative.
- extent of local tumour spread

All tumours:

- confined to mediastinal nodes.
- confined to the thymus.
- into mediastinal connective tissues.
- into other organs:pleura, lung, pericardium, main vessels.

Thymoma(WHO):

- *encapsulated* – thymoma completely surrounded by a fibrous capsule of varying thickness which is not infiltrated by tumour; it may infiltrate into but not through.
- *minimally invasive* – thymoma surrounded by a capsule which is focally infiltrated by tumour growth or which invades mediastinal fat.
- *widely invasive* – thymoma spreading by direct extension into adjacent structures such as pericardium, large vessels and lung (may appear invasive to the surgeon – excision may be incomplete).
- *with implants* – thymoma in which tumour nodules separate from the main mass are found on the pericardial or pleural surface.
- *with lymph node metastasis* – a tumour that involves one or more lymph nodes anatomically separate from the main mass (most commonly mediastinal and supraclavicular).
- *with distant metastases* – tumour accompanied by embolic metastases to a distant site (lung, liver, skeletal system).

Encapsulated thymomas with no implants, no lymph node metastases or distant metastases are benign. All other combinations are malignant.

- lymphovascular invasion – present/not present. Note perineural invasion.
- regional lymph nodes – intrathoracic, scalene, supraclavicular nodes.

Thymoma:

- – pT0 no regional lymph nodes involved.
- – pT1 metastasis to anterior mediastinal lymph nodes.
- – pN2 metastasis to intrathoracic lymph nodes other than the anterior mediastinal lymph nodes.
- – pN3 metastasis to extrathoracic lymph nodes.

- excision margins – comment on adequacy of excision.

41   Heart

1. Anatomy

The heart is a muscular pump weighing approximately 300 g. It consists of four chambers: the right and left atria and the right and left ventricles (Figure 41.1). The right side of the heart pumps venous blood through the pulmonary circulation for oxygenation, the left heart oxygenated blood through the systemic circulation for distribution to the tissues.

The superior and inferior vena cavae enter the right atrium. There is a small projection, the right auricle, which overlaps the beginning of the ascending aorta. The atrioventricular valves, the mitral and tricuspid valves each consist of a valve ring or annulus, leaflets, anchoring chordae tendinae and papillary muscles. The semilunar valves, the aortic and pulmonary valves comprise three cusps, each with a sinus. The cusps meet at three commissures. The thickness of the wall of the right ventricle is normally 0.25 to 0.3 cm and the left ventricle 0.9 to 1.5 cm.

The heart is surrounded by the pericardial sac, which is composed of two layers of connective tissue (visceral and parietal pericardia) each covered by a layer of mesothelial cells.

The coronary arteries supply blood to the heart (Figure 41.1). The right coronary artery arises from the anterior coronary sinus and runs over the anterior surface of the heart before crossing the posterior surface, where it finally anastomoses with the left coronary artery. Its major branches are the marginal artery and the posterior interventricular artery. There are also atrial and ventricular branches. The left coronary artery arises from the left posterior aortic sinus.

Major branches include the anterior interventricular artery and the circumflex artery. The anterior interventricular artery descends towards the apex and anastomoses with the posterior interventricular artery. A diagonal branch runs to the left ventricle. The circumflex artery anastomoses with the terminal branch of the right coronary artery. It gives off the marginal artery, which runs along the left border of the heart.

The heart is composed of three layers, the epicardium (serous pericardium), the muscular myocardium and the endocardium.

Lymphovascular drainage

Lymphatic drainage of the heart is to the tracheobronchial lymph nodes.

2. Clinical Presentation

Dyspnoea is an awareness of breathlessness and a symptom of congestive cardiac failure, the end-stage of many cardiac conditions. Orthopnoea and paroxysmal nocturnal dyspnoea are shortness of breath, which arise when the patient has been recumbent due to collection of fluid in the pulmonary circulation (pulmonary oedema).

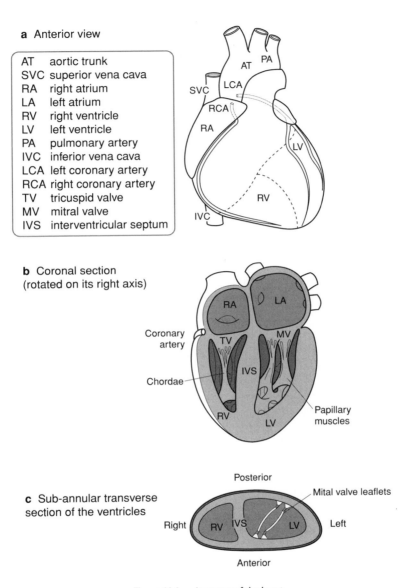

a Anterior view

AT	aortic trunk
SVC	superior vena cava
RA	right atrium
LA	left atrium
RV	right ventricle
LV	left ventricle
PA	pulmonary artery
IVC	inferior vena cava
LCA	left coronary artery
RCA	right coronary artery
TV	tricuspid valve
MV	mitral valve
IVS	interventricular septum

b Coronal section (rotated on its right axis)

c Sub-annular transverse section of the ventricles

Figure 41.1. Anatomy of the heart.

Wheezing (cardiac asthma) is due to swelling of the bronchial lining and ankle swelling is secondary to congestive cardiac failure with systemic venous congestion.

Angina commonly presents as central gripping chest pain radiating to the jaws, neck or arms, provoked by exercise and relieved by rest. It is due to cardiac hypoxia.

Myocardial infarction is similar but is not relieved by rest.

Pericarditis presents with severe, sharp, central chest pain, aggravated by movement, posture, respiration and coughing, and myocarditis with mild pleuritic chest pain and lethargy.

Sudden unexplained death may be the presentation of acute cardiac failure due to ischaemic heart disease, and syncope (fainting episodes) may occur in aortic stenosis, both of which can also be caused by cardiac dysrhythmia.

Infective endocarditis presents with fever, weight loss, malaise, splenomegaly and splinter haemorrhages of the fingernails due to embolic infarcts of the skin. Abdominal pain may be secondary to renal or splenic infarcts. Chest pain due to pulmonary infarcts can occur in tricuspid valve endocarditis.

In hypertrophic obstructive cardiomyopathy the patient may present with atrial fibrillation, ventricular arrthymias or sudden death.

Cardiac myxoma can present with symptoms of mitral stenosis and embolisation of fragments of the tumour or of overlying thrombus. Fever, cachexia and malaise also occur.

Cardiac rhabdomyomas may cause stillbirth or death within the first few days of life.

3. Clinical Investigations

Echocardiocardiography/Doppler flow studies – used to study valvular heart disease, congenital abnormalities, cardiac tumours and pericardial effusions.

Transoesophageal echocardiography (TOE) – used to investigate lesions of the left atrium, the ascending aorta, the aortic valve, and septal defects.

Chest X-ray – used to assess heart size and to identify calcification or fluid in the pericardium.

Electrocardiogram (ECG) – a resting ECG is useful in the diagnosis of myocardial infarction, cardiac hypertrophy or abnormalities of rhythm. An exercise ECG is useful in patients with angina, and an ambulatory ECG made over 24 hours may be used when heart rhythm disturbances occur only intermittently.

Nuclear cardiology – assesses the function of cardiac muscle. Radioactivity from substances injected intravenously into the patient are measured and allow evaluation of cardiac function and assessment of ischaemia and infarction.

Cardiac catherization and angiography – catheters are advanced into the right and left sides of the heart and pressure and oxygen saturation studies performed. During coronary angiography radio-opaque contrast medium is injected through the catheter into the coronary artery ostia.

Magnetic Resonance Imaging (MRI) – synchronised with the ECG gives systolic and diastolic images.

Endomyocardial biopsies – taken via cardiac catheter.

4. Pathological Conditions

Non-neoplastic Conditions

Disorders of the Endocardium

Infective endocarditis: a disorder affecting the endocardial surface of the heart as the result of infection. The characteristic lesion is the vegetation, which consists of thrombus containing microorganisms. In acute bacterial endocarditis large friable vegetations are found on the valves, which can cause erosion or perforation of the underlying tissue. Predisposing factors to endocarditis are valvular anatomical abnormalities (congenital or acquired, e.g., rheumatic heart disease), sepsis, immunosuppression or IV drug abuse.

Non-bacterial thrombotic endocarditis (NBTE): produces small, bland vegetations, attached to the valve surface at the lines of closure. They are seen in cachetic patients, e.g., disseminated tumour. Systemic lupus erythematosus can be associated with *Libman–Sacks endocarditis* with small, bland vegetations located on both surfaces of the valves or cords.

Rheumatic fever: an inflammatory disease, which in the acute phase produces pathognomic Aschoff bodies in the heart. Chronic rheumatic heart disease is characterized by organization of the endocardial inflammation with subsequent fibrosis particularly affecting the valves.

Disorders of the Valves

In valvular disease, assessment of the gross appearance often contributes to the final diagnosis more than microscopic examination.

Mitral valve stenosis: most commonly due to rheumatic fever with commissural fusion, cusp scarring and dystrophic calcification.

Mitral valve regurgitation: due to floppy mitral valve, shows valve cusps which are increased in area, dome shaped and show myxoid change. Other causes include rheumatic fever, rupture of a papillary muscle or chordae tendinae, ventricular enlargement or infective endocarditis.

Aortic valve stenosis: due to calcification of a congenitally bicuspid valve, senile calcific aortic stenosis or post-inflammatory scarring.

Aortic regurgitation: secondary to post-inflammatory scarring, infective endocarditis or abnormalities of the cusps and commissures.

Pulmonary valve abnormalities: consist of stenosis, insufficiency or a combination of the two. Ninety-five per cent of cases are due to congenital heart disease, tetralogy of Fallot being the most common. A bicuspid pulmonary valve is the most common anomaly.

Tricuspid valve abnormalities: most commonly pure insufficiency and caused by post-inflammatory scarring, congenital abnormalities, infective endocarditis or dilatation of the valve ring in cardiac failure.

Disorders of the Myocardium

Myocarditis: viral, bacterial or fungal. In developed countries viral infections predominate. Parasitic aetiologies include toxoplasmosis and the protozoon *Trypanosoma cruzi*. Granulomatous myocarditis can occur due to TB or sarcoidosis. Myocarditis occurs secondary to collagen vascular disease, especially rheumatic fever, and may also be drug or radiation induced.

Idiopathic hypertrophic obstructive cardiomyopathy (HOCM): massive myocardial hypertrophy and classically there is asymmetric ventricular septal hypertrophy. Histological examination shows myofibre disarray with hypertrophy and interstitial fibrosis. A scoring system may be used to quantitatively assess the degree of myocardial abnormality.

Idiopathic dilated cardiomyopathy (congestive cardiomyopathy; DCM): the clinical presentation of DCM is progressive cardiac failure. There is hypertrophy but also marked dilatation of all chambers. Histological examination shows non-specific abnormalities with hypertrophy and degenerative changes in the myocardial fibres. A significant number of cases are thought to be post-viral.

Restrictive cardiomyopathy (RCM): is the least common of the three types of cardiomyopathy in developed countries. The ventricles are of approximately normal size or slightly enlarged and the cavities are not dilated. Histology shows patchy or interstitial fibrosis.

Infiltrative cardiomyopathies: may be due to amyloidosis, haemochromatosis, haemosiderosis, glycogenosis or mitochondrial myopathies.

Right ventricular dysplasia: is a familial idiopathic cardiomyopathy involving mainly the right ventricle. Histological examination shows infiltration of the right ventricular myocardium by adipose and fibrous tissue.

Drug-induced cardiomyopathy: caused by drugs such as adriamycin and cyclophosphamide, which cause characteristic subcellular changes seen on electron microscopy.

Ischaemia: very common due to atheromatous thickening of the coronary arteries. Acute, sub-acute or chronic, and, sub-endocardial or transmural in distribution. Consequences include mural thrombus, papillary muscle or ventricular wall rupture, cardiac tamponade, dysrhythmias, sudden death or chronic ventricular dysfunction (due to diffuse ischaemic fibrosis).

Heart transplant rejection: graded using the International Society for Heart and Lung Transplantation (ISHLT) grading system.

Disorders of the Pericardium

Acute pericarditis: due to infection caused by viruses or bacteria. Viruses include coxsackie B, echoviruses, influenza, mumps and Epstein–Barr virus. Bacterial pericarditis may be due to *Staphylococcus aureus*, Streptococci or *Haemophilus influenza*. Tuberculous pericarditis usually becomes chronic. Acute pericarditis can also be secondary to acute rheumatic fever, myocardial infarction, connective tissue disorders such as systemic lupus erythematosus and rheumatoid disease, uraemia, renal transplantation, irradiation or following cardiac trauma.

Chronic pericarditis: can lead to *constrictive pericarditis* where the heart is encased in a thick layer of fibrous tissue. Surgical removal of pericardium is the only effective means of treatment.

Neoplastic Conditions

Myxoma: accounts for 50% of primary tumours of the heart. Familial or sporadic, they usually occur in the left atrium (86%). Familial cases can be multicentric and have extra-cardiac abnormalities (Carney's syndrome). Histological examination shows round, polygonal or stellate cells in an abundant loose stroma. Mitoses, pleomorphism and necrosis are minimal to absent. Myxomas may show ossification (petrified myxoma), cartilaginous tissue, extramedullary haematopoiesis and thymic or foregut remnants. When myxoma is excised with a partial atrial septectomy, it rarely recurs.

Other Cardiac Neoplasms

Rhabdomyoma: the most common primary tumour of the heart in children, is often congenital and has a close association with tuberous sclerosis. Most rhabdomyomas are multiple, occur in the ventricles and regress spontaneously.

Other benign conditions include mesothelial/monocytic incidental cardiac excrescences (MICE), papillary fibroelastoma, haemangioma, lipomatous hypertrophy (of the atrial septum), mesothelioma of the atrioventricular node, fibroma, paraganglioma, granular cell tumour, lymphangioma and schwannoma.

Primary malignant tumours: very rare and more commonly found in the right side of the heart, benign tumours in the left. Angiosarcoma is probably the commonest, others being leiomyosarcoma, rhabdomyosarcoma and Kaposi's sarcoma. Primary malignant lymphoma of the heart is very rare, most being diffuse large cell especially those occurring in AIDS. Secondary involvement of the heart by systemic lymphoma is more usual.

The pericardium is involved in approximately 8.5% of cases of disseminated malignancy but primary neoplasms are very rare, e.g., mesothelioma of the pericardial sac, germ cell tumour and angiosarcoma.

5. Surgical Pathology Specimens – Clinical Aspects

Endomyocardial biopsies: right heart biopsies (and occasionally left) are taken via cardiac catheter. They are used to evaluate graft status in cardiac transplant patients and to diagnose cardiomyopathies and intracavitary or myocardial tumours. The auricular appendage may also be sampled at the same time as a mitral valve correction. One third of these biopsies, as well as showing myocardial hypertrophy, have necrobiotic Aschoff nodules. Their presence does not correlate with clinical evidence of the activity of the rheumatic process or with the postoperative course.

Cardiac valves: native aortic valves are generally resected because of calcific degeneration and are often bicuspid. Mitral valves are usually replaced because of rheumatic valve disease or because the valve is myxomatous. Valves are also resected due to the sequelae of bacterial endocarditis, e.g., perforation. Prosthetic valves may be removed because of infection, thrombosis, anastomotic or valvular leakage, haemolysis, obstructive fibrous tissue overgrowth or mechanical failure, e.g., fracture.

Open-heart surgical procedures: used in the repair of ventricular aneurysms, septal resection in HOCM and in the removal of atrial myxomas or other tumours. In resection of a myxoma, the tumour and site of origin such as the atrial septum segment or atrial wall segment is removed.

Heart transplant: performed in patients with end-stage cardiac failure due to ischaemic heart disease or idiopathic cardiomyopathy. The resected specimen usually consists of atria and the upper parts of the ventricles.

6. Surgical Pathology Specimens – Laboratory Protocols

Biopsy Specimens

- count the number of fragments.
- measure their size (mm).
- describe colour, consistency.
- place in cassettes between foam pads or wrapped in filter paper.
- examine histologically through multiple levels and keep intervening sections for stains, e.g., Masson trichrome (fibrous tissue), Congo Red (amyloid), Perl's Prussian Blue (iron) or immunoperoxidase (CMV antibody, B/T lymphocytes).
- occasional cases may require fresh frozen tissue or glutaraldehyde fixation for specialist techniques (immunohistochemistry, electron microscopy).

Cardiac Valves

Native valves

Most are received in fragments though some may be submitted intact.

- identify and document the type of valve – aortic, congenital bicuspid aortic, mitral, tricuspid.
- photograph if intact.
- X-ray to document calcification.
- culture.
- measure the dimensions (cm) of the valve and the valve orifice.
- describe the leaflets or cusps
  - number, sizes (mm), consistency,
  - abnormalities, e.g., myxoid changes, fibrosis, calcifications, thrombi, perforations.
- describe vegetations if present – distribution, location, consistency, presence of destruction of the valve leaflet or cusp.
- describe the commissures – relationship to each other – fused or not, completely or partially.
- describe the chordae tendinae – length, status – normal/shortened/thickened/stretched/fused/ruptured.
- describe the papillary muscles – hypertrophy, elongation, scarring – evidence of recent or past myocardial infarction.
- decalcification may be needed.

Blocks for histology:

● representative sections are taken from the free edge of the valve to the annulus.

Prosthetic valves

Mechanical heart valves:

● culture.
● photograph.
● document the type of valve.
● measure the diameter of the external sewing ring.
● check function – ability to open and close fully.
● describe the presence of calcifications, mechanical degeneration, cracks in any of the components.
● describe the presence of tissue overgrowth.
● check for vegetations – colour, site, size, consistency, presence of underlying destruction.

Blocks for histology:
● in most cases it is not possible to submit any tissue for histology unless vegetations are present.

Bioprosthetic heart valve:

● culture.
● photograph.
● X-ray – aids type identification, shows calcification (grade 1 to 4) and ring or stent fracture.
● measure the diameter of the external sewing ring.
● inspect leaflets for thrombi, vegetations, calcifications.
● check for fibrous overgrowth.
● check the valve leaflets for tears or perforations. Document the location and size of any lesions and the effect these appear to have on valve function.

Blocks for histology:

● a portion of the valve cusp is submitted for histological examination. Vegetations are also submitted if present.

Resection Specimens

Specimen

May consist of atrial myxomas and other tumours; portions of heart removed during open-heart surgical procedures such as repair of ventricular aneurysms or septal resection in hypertrophic cardiomyopathy.

● measure the specimen (cm) and weigh (g).
● document the presence of scarring and if transmural.
● document any inflammation and its pattern.
● note the presence of necrosis, calcification, mural thrombus, haemorrhage.
● describe the endocardium – colour, thickness (mm).
● describe the epicardium – colour, thickness (mm).

- section transversely at 3 mm intervals.
- sample representative blocks for histology.

Resection for tumour

- measure the specimen (cm) and weigh (g).
- describe the appearance – myxoid, haemorrhage, necrosis, site of origin – atrial wall/ventricular wall/ atrial septal wall, infiltration into wall.
- photograph.
- fix in 10% formalin for 48 hours.
- ink limits – underlying wall.
- section lesion, noting appearance and attachment to the wall.

Blocks for histology:

- sample representative blocks of tumour, tumour and adjacent myocardium, and specimen limits.

Heart transplants

- weigh (g).
- describe the epicardial surface-fat, petechiae, adhesions.
- fix in 10% formalin for 48 hours.
- use method of cutting appropriate to the specimen:
  - *apical four chamber cut* – cut longitudinally from apex to base bivalving both ventricles and bisecting the tricuspid and mitral valves. This method is useful in cutting specimens showing dilated cardiomyopathy.
  - *serial sectioning* – cut heart transversely beginning at the apex and extending to the level of the mitral valve at approximately 1 to 2 cm intervals. The base of the heart may be cut longitudinally or opened according to the lines of flow. This method is useful in ischaemic heart disease.
- describe each ventricle – hypertrophy, dilatation, fibrosis, infarcts, trabeculation, papillary muscles, mural thrombus.
- measure the thickness of the ventricular walls (mm).
- describe the atria and any endocardial lesions.
- describe the valves (as above).
- dissect atherosclerotic coronary arteries, fix and decalcify them, section transversely at 3–5 mm intervals.
- describe coronary arteries – presence of right or left dominance, thrombi, atheroma, locations.
- describe by-pass grafts if present – type, location, presence of thrombus, atheroma.

Blocks for histology:

- take sections from the left and right ventricular walls, the ventricular septum, native coronary arteries, bypass grafts, other lesions.

42 Vessels

1. Anatomy

Vessels consist of three layers – the lining intima, the musculo-elastic media and the outer connective tissue adventitia.

Coronary arteries: see Chapter 41.

Aorta: the main trunk of the systemic circulation. It arises from the left ventricle and ascends as the ascending aorta, becomes the arch, the descending aorta and then the abdominal aorta. The arch supplies the main vessels of the head and neck, the abdominal aorta the viscera of the abdomen and pelvis and the legs via the femoral arteries.

Temporal artery: the external carotid artery ends behind the neck of the mandible by dividing into the maxillary and superficial temporal arteries. The latter ascends over the posterior end of the zygomatic arch on the lateral aspect of the scalp where it divides into anterior and posterior branches. It supplies the face, the auricle and the scalp.

2. Clinical Presentation

Peripheral vascular disease presents with "intermittent claudication", cramp-like pain in the calf and thigh muscles on exercise, which disappears on resting for a few minutes. It is caused by atherosclerosis which is responsible for multiple symptoms depending on the affected arterial supply – ischaemic heart disease leading to angina or myocardial infarction, stroke, transient ischaemic attacks (TIA) and intestinal ischaemia.

Internal carotid artery atheroma may lead to a transient ischaemic attack or cerebrovascular accident (CVA). A TIA is a transient loss of function in one region of the brain lasting less than 24 hours. The patient can present with aphasia, hemiparesis, hemisensory loss, hemianopic visual loss and amaurosis fugax (transient loss of vision in one eye). A cerebrovascular accident produces similar symptoms lasting longer than 24 hours.

Aortic abdominal aneurysm presents with epigastric or back pain exacerbated by rupture and may be associated with a palpable, pulsatile abdominal mass.

Thoracic aortic aneurysms cause chest pain or evidence of pressure on other organs such as the superior vena cava or oesophagus.

Dissecting aortic aneurysm causes severe central chest pain radiating into the back, arms and neck. There may be neurological signs due to involvement of spinal vessels. Rupture of an aneurysm is a surgical emergency.

Temporal arteritis presents with a headache, which is often localized to, and tender over, the temporal area. Involvement of the ophthalmic artery may lead to blindness and prompt treatment with systemic steroids is necessary.

Vasculitides produce a wide spectrum of symptoms dependent on the location of the affected vessels, including skin rashes, fever, myalgia, arthralgia, malaise, abdominal pain and renal failure.

3. Clinical Investigations

Arteriography – used to localize the site and extent of vessel blockage and presence of collaterals.
  Doppler studies – used to determine the site of blockage and flow rates in vessels.
  Duplex ultrasound – used to measure pressure in small arteries.
  X-ray – plain X-ray of abdomen may show an aortic aneurysm if the wall is calcified.
  Ultrasound – used to diagnose abdominal aortic aneurysm or deep venous thrombosis.
  CT scan – a sensitive imaging method that allows precise measurement of size, e.g., abdominal aortic aneurysm.
  Transoesophageal echocardiography (TOE) – used to diagnose aortic root dissection.
  Ventilation/Perfusion scan (V/Q scan) – detects pulmonary emboli.
  Blood tests:

- Erythrocyte Sedimentation Rate (ESR) – characteristically over 100 mm in the first hour in temporal arteritis.
- c-ANCA – associated with Wegener's granulomatosis and some cases of polyarteritis nodosa.
- p-ANCA – associated with polyarteritis nodosa.

4. Pathological Conditions

Non-neoplastic Conditions

Atherosclerosis: very common and affects the elastic arteries (aorta, carotid, iliac) and large and medium-sized muscular arteries (coronary and popliteal). The vessels show intimal thickening and lipid accumulation producing atheromatous plaques, which may become complicated by calcification, focal rupture or gross ulceration. Debris can be discharged into the bloodstream forming microemboli. Haemorrhage may occur into a plaque or a thrombus may form on the surface, potentially occluding the vessel. With the formation of atheromatous plaques the adjacent media atrophies and aneursymal dilatation may occur.

  Hyaline arteriolosclerosis: occurs in the elderly with an increased incidence in hypertension and diabetes. There is thickening of the walls with deposition of pink homogenous material and narrowing of the lumen. *Hyperplastic arteriolosis* is characteristic of, but not limited to, malignant hypertension.

  Vasculitis: inflammation of the walls of blood vessels due to immune-mediated inflammation or to invasion of the wall by pathogenic organisms.

  Giant cell arteritis (temporal arteritis): a granulomatous arteritis affecting the aorta and major branches especially the extracranial branches of the carotid artery (temporal, vertebral and ophthalmic arteries). Most commonly there is a granulomatous inflammation of the inner half of the media centred on the internal elastic lamina. Up to 40% of patients with good clinical evidence of cranial arteritis have a negative temporal artery biopsy. The diagnostic histological findings are often also only found focally within an involved segment.

  Takayashu arteritis (pulseless disease): a rare granulomatous vasculitis of the aortic arch, its branches and the pulmonary arteries. Morphological changes may be indistinguishable from giant cell arteritis, but the clinical profile differs with the patient usually being female and under the age of forty years but elderly in giant cell arteritis.

Polyarteritis nodosa: a relatively uncommon condition causing necrotising fibrinoid vasculitis of small-to-medium-sized arteries particularly in the kidneys, heart, liver and gastrointestinal tract. Vessel necrosis, thrombosis, rupture and aneurysms occur with fibrous repair resulting in mural nodularity.

Microscopic polyarteritis (leukocytoclastic vasculitis): involves arterioles, capillaries and venules. It affects skin, mucous membranes, lungs, brain, heart, gastrointestinal tract, kidneys and muscle in isolation or various combinations. It is much more common than polyarteritis nodosa and may be precipitated by drugs or infections.

Kawasaki syndrome: a rare arteritis, which affects the large, medium and small arteries (often coronary arteries). Eighty per cent are less than four years old and 20% develop cardiovascular sequelae.

Wegener's granulomatosis: a focal necrotizing or granulomatous vasculitis involving small and medium sized vessels, most prominent in the lungs or upper airways, and associated with a focal or necrotizing (often crescentic) glomerulitis.

Aneurysm: an abnormal widening of a blood vessel wall. In a true aneurysm the walls make up the boundary; in a false aneurysm the boundary is made of haematoma or fibrous tissue.

Abdominal aortic aneurysms: the most common site for atherosclerotic aneurysms, usually below the renal arteries, above the bifurcation of the aorta. Aneurysms less than 5 cm diameter rarely rupture, while about 50% of those more than 5 cm suffer fatal rupture within a ten-year period. Operative mortality after rupture is approximately 50% but 5% prior to it. A small minority are inflammatory in type, with a thick cuff of surrounding fibrous tissue, and associated with obstruction of the ureters.

Dissecting aneurysms: blood enters the wall of the aorta and dissects between layers. It affects two groups of patients – males predominantly between the age of 40 and 60 years with a history of hypertension, and a younger group with an abnormality of the connective tissue, e.g., Marfan's syndrome. Histological examination shows cystic medial degeneration with elastic tissue fragmentation. Surgery involves plication of the aortic wall (65–75% of patients with dissection survive).

Syphilitic aneurysms: obliterative endarteritis affects the vasa vasorum leading to a thoracic aortitis and subsequent aneurysmal dilatation of the thoracic aorta and the aortic annulus. These are now rare in developed countries.

Berry aneurysms occur in the circle of Willis of the brain, due to congenital defects in the vessel wall, and are an important cause of sudden subarachnoid haemorrhage in young adults.

Mycotic aneurysm occurs in the arterial wall secondary to damage caused by sepsis. They are rare in developed countries. *Polyarteritis nodosa* may be associated with multiple microaneurysms. *Kawasaki disease* causes arteritis and aneurysm of the coronary arteries.

Varicose veins: abnormally dilated, tortuous veins due to prolonged intraluminal pressure or loss of support of the vessel wall. They affect a wide range of patients but particularly obese females over 50 years of age. There is also a familial tendency. Varicosities also occur in the oesophagus secondary to portal hypertension in association with liver cirrhosis. Haemorrhoids are varicose dilatations of the haemorrhoidal plexus of veins at the anorectal junction.

Neoplastic Conditions

Benign

- Haemangioma – capillary, cavernous, pyogenic granuloma (lobular capillary haemangioma).
- Lymphangioma.
- Glomus tumour.

- Vascular ectasia.
- Bacillary angiomatosis is a reactive vascular proliferation.

Intermediate Grade Neoplasms

- Kaposi's sarcoma.
- Haemangioendothelioma.

Malignant Neoplasms

- Angiosarcoma.
- Haemangiopericytoma.

These specimens are discussed in the skin and soft tissue chapters.

5. Surgical Pathology Specimens – Clinical Aspects

Dissecting aortic aneurysm: a section of aorta is excised which shows a medial haematoma with an associated intimal flap entrance site and often either an intimal re-entrant or adventitial rupture site.

Abdominal aortic aneurysm: surgical repair involves opening the aneurysm and removing the clot. The graft is sewn inside the aorta and the wall of the aorta is closed. The specimen may consist of clot only, or clot with media.

Internal carotid endarterectomy: considered in symptomatic patients who have carotid artery stenosis that narrows the arterial lumen by more than 70%. The specimen may retain the shape of the bifurcation. It consists of luminal plaque with portions of intima and media attached.

Atherectomy: the removal of atherosclerotic plaque by cardiac catherization. Open thrombectomy or embolectomy of peripheral vessels, e.g., femoral artery, is also undertaken for the acutely ischaemic limb.

Vascular grafts: removed because of thrombosis, fibrous obstruction or infection.

Coronary artery bypass graft (CABG): during a second CABG the saphenous vein or internal artery mammary grafts are occasionally removed.

Temporal artery: a biopsy of approximately 2–10 mm length is taken.

Varicose veins: usually inverted during the procedure and not submitted for histology.

6. Surgical Pathology Specimens – Laboratory Protocols

Vessel specimens:

- measure the length, internal and external diameter (mm) of the vessel.
- examine the lumen for thrombi.
- estimate the percentage of luminal narrowing caused by any lesions.
- examine the media – check for aneurysm formation, fibromuscular hyperplasia, calcification, and rupture.

Blocks for histology:

- sample multiple representative transverse sections of the vessel.

Aortic dissection:
- measure (cm) and weigh (g).
- describe the location of the dissection, intimal flap entrance, intimal re-entrant site or adventitial rupture site.
- take sections from areas of medial separation and from grossly normal tissue. One section should be stained for elastin.
- when embedding, orientate the specimens on edge to ensure the entire thickness can be assessed

Aortic aneurysm:
- measure (cm) and weigh (g).
- describe – thrombus only or aortic wall also present – colour, consistency, organisation (lines of Zahn) and calcification.
- serially section the thrombus to look for tumour or mycotic aneurysm.

Atherectomy specimens:
- count and measure the fragments (mm).
- decalcify plaques.
- submit all fragments.

Endarterectomy:
- if intact, open longitudinally.
- measure (cm).
- describe – shape, colour, calcification, stenosis.
- decalcification may be needed.
- sample representative transverse blocks.

Embolectomy specimens:
- measure (mm).
- examine for tumour fragments.
- serially slice transversely and submit representative blocks.

Temporal artery:
- measure – length and diameter (mm).
- describe – colour, presence of thrombus, wall thickening.
- cut into 2–3 mm cross-sections after processing and before embedding.
- embed each piece on end.
- examine histologically through multiple levels and keep intervening sections for stains, e.g., elastin.

Vascular grafts:
- culture.
- measure – length and diameter (cm).
- describe – type of graft – saphenous vein, Gore-tex grafts, Dacron grafts; colour, tears or holes, thrombus.
- sections of graft may be submitted – saphenous vein and Gore-tex are easy to cut, Dacron is difficult.

Coronary artery bypass grafts:
- measure – length and diameter (mm).
- describe – atherosclerosis, thrombus.
- take multiple cross sections of the graft.

Varicose veins:
- measure – length and diameter (cm).
- describe – thrombus, wall thickening, nodularities.
- take one transverse section.

Osteoarticular and Soft Tissue Specimens

Richard I Davis

43. Joint Space, Bone, Soft Tissues and Special Techniques

43 Joint Space, Bone, Soft Tissues and Special Techniques

1. Joint Space

Anatomy

Most joints are *synovial* joints formed by a thin lining of synovium which secretes fluid into the joint (Figure 43.1). The joint is covered by a capsule. The synovium not only forms the lining of joints but also covers tendon sheaths and bursae.

The synovial membrane consists of an intimal layer and the subintimal supportive layer of fibrofatty tissue. The intima is 1–2 cell layers thick and composed of synoviocytes. About 90% are fibroblast-like but the other 10% have ultrastructural features of macrophages.

The space between the two articulating bone surfaces is occupied by articular hyaline cartilage (Figure 43.1). It is firm, pliable tissue and resists compressive forces. In young people it is bluish-white and translucent but in later life it becomes opaque and yellow. Cartilage is avascular and devoid of nerves and lymphatics, obtaining nutrients by diffusion from the surrounding synovial fluid.

Cartilage is rather poorly cellular tissue composed of chondrocytes laid down within a matrix or ground substance composed of collagen fibres and proteoglycans. The latter are complex biopolymers consisting of a central protein core with attached chains of carbohydrates. These proteoglycans include chondroitin sulphate and keratin sulphate and can absorb large volumes of water to form gels.

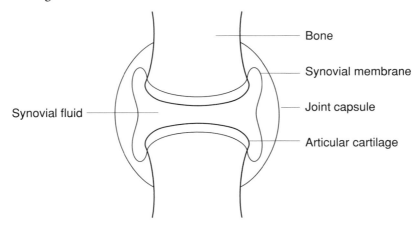

Figure 43.1. Synovial joint.

437

Clinical Presentation

Symptoms of joint disease generally tend to be non-specific and accurate diagnosis depends on detailed clinical history noting the number of joints involved, sites and specific patterns of joint disease. Typical symptoms include pain, stiffness, swelling and reduced range of movement. Severe, acute inflammation such as in septic arthritis results in a red, hot, swollen joint. Effusions due to increased fluid, blood or pus may also be seen.

Clinical Investigations

Routine blood tests such as white cell count, ESR and C-reactive protein to detect active inflammation. Checking the blood for the presence of increased quantities of antibodies (such as rheumatoid factor) is very important in rheumatology. These tests are generally not specific and need to be interpreted carefully in the light of the patient's clinical history and pattern of joint involvement.

Plain X-ray and tomography to detect evidence of arthritis such as loss of joint space (due to destruction of cartilage), osteophytes (bone irregularities), bone sclerosis (thickening) and localised osteoporosis (thinning).

Effusions may be aspirated and investigated for the presence of blood, pus, cell content and crystals. This constitutes *synovial fluid analysis*. In order to detect the presence of crystals the fluid is examined using polarised light with a red filter. The needle-shaped crystals associated with gout exhibit a strong negative birefringence whereas the rhomboid-shaped crystals associated with pseudogout exhibit weak positive birefringence.

In general, biopsy has very little role to play in the investigation and diagnosis of joint disease. Accurate clinical diagnosis seldom depends on histological analysis of the synovium.

Pathological Conditions

Non-neoplastic Conditions

Synovitis: the majority of patients have non-specific synovitis characterised by hyperplasia of the synovium and chronic inflammation. There are really no specific features which can be regarded as pathognomonic of any particular type of synovitis.

Rheumatoid arthritis: a rheumatoid nodule may be seen and is highly suggestive of this condition but only a small number of biopsies (less than 5%) display this feature.

Granulomatous inflammation: the presence of granulomata can indicate infection due to tuberculosis, atypical TB, fungi, sarcoid or reaction to foreign body material such as prosthetic wear products.

Prosthetic reactions: patients who have had knee or hip arthroplasty may suffer from joint loosening years later due to foreign-body reaction and inflammation caused by breakdown of the prosthetic materials. A foreign-body reaction composed of giant cells and macrophages with doubly refractile material can be seen.

Crystal arthropathy: this includes *gout* and *pseudogout*. A giant cell reaction to doubly refractile material may be seen. Synovial fluid analysis can be helpful in this diagnosis. Gout can also be associated with extra-articular soft tissue lesions or tophi, e.g., in the skin overlying the elbows or ears.

Synovial chondromatosis: islands of metaplastic cartilage in the synovium characterised clinically by the presence of loose bodies and reduced joint movement.

Pigmented villonodular synovitis: the presence of haemosiderin pigment with a collection of macrophages and giant cells may indicate a reaction to *haemarthrosis* (haemophilia or trauma) or pigmented villonodular synovitis.

Neoplastic Conditions

Very rarely a benign giant cell tumour of tendon sheath may occur in a joint space. This is seen when the tumour arises within an intra-articular tendon such as the knee. Primary or secondary malignancy is exceedingly rare in the joints.

Surgical Pathology Specimens – Clinical Aspects

Biopsy Specimens

In general, biopsy has very little role to play in the investigation and diagnosis of joint disease. Synovium is difficult to biopsy and sufficient material is only reliably obtained at arthroscopy or at open joint exploration. Most inflammatory arthritides have similar histological features and therefore biopsy will not discriminate one type of arthritis from another. For these reasons synovial biopsy is not routinely performed.

Resection Specimens

Resection of the synovium is seldom undertaken except for a florid synovial chondromatosis or pigmented villonodular synovitis. Partial or total synovectomy is technically difficult and may often lead to damage to the articular cartilage in later life.

Surgical Pathology Specimens – Laboratory Protocols

Biopsy and Resection Specimens

The tissue is submitted in formalin. However, if the clinician strongly suspects the presence of gout, the biopsy should be sent in alcohol and not formalin so as to better preserve the crystals. The size of the biopsy should be recorded and is usually submitted in toto. There are usually no distinctive gross features to note except for the tan colouration associated with a haemarthrosis or pigmented villonodular synovitis or the presence of cartilage as in synovial chondromatosis.

Histopathology report

- presence of hyperplasia.
- inflammation – intensity (mild/moderate/severe), diffuse/focal, acute/chronic/granuloma-tous.
- presence of haemosiderin/crystals/prosthetic wear products/cartilage.

2. Bone

Anatomy

Bones may be classified as long (femur, humerus, radius, ulna), tubular (small bones of hands and feet) or flat (scapula, pelvis, rib, vertebrae). The shell of the bone is called the *cortex* and the interior is known as the *medulla*, which consists of interconnecting bars of bone called *trabec-ulae*. This trabecular bone is also referred to as *cancellous* bone. The thickness of the cortex varies considerably along the length of a given bone and especially between different bones. The proportion of a bone occupied by cortical and cancellous bone also varies between bones and with age. The trabecular bone is set in a fatty marrow containing haemopoietic tissue. The cortex is covered by a thin, tough mesenchymal layer known as *periosteum*. The ends of a bone are known as the *epiphysis*. The *metaphysis* is the region immediately adjacent to the epiphysis and the *diaphysis* is the shaft (area between the two metaphyses) (Figure 43.2).

Clinical Presentation

The symptoms of bone disease are few and rather non-specific. The most common symptom is pain, which may be of variable intensity. Severe unremitting pain continuing at night in bed is insidious and suspicious of malignancy. Pain relieved by non-steroidal inflammatory agents is suggestive of a benign osteoid osteoma. Remember that sometimes pain felt in one bone may be *referred* pain; that is, disease originating elsewhere. A swelling is indicative of a primary bone tumour. Pathological fracture – a fracture occurring due to low-impact trauma – is indicative of a diseased bone and suggests osteoporosis, multiple myeloma or metastatic disease.

Clinical Investigations

Routine blood tests – include white cell count, ESR and C-reactive protein for the presence of inflammation. A *calcium profile* consists of serum calcium, phosphate and alkaline phosphatase. This test is particularly useful in endocrine or metabolic bone disease. *Hypercalcaemia* is seen in primary hyperparathryoidism and metastatic disease. A raised alkaline phosphatase can be indicative of increased osteoblast activity and if very high suggests Paget's disease. The alkaline

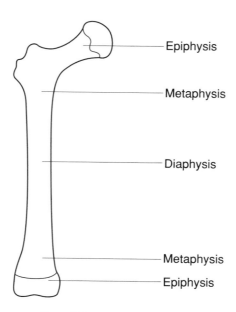

Figure 43.2. A typical long bone.

phosphatase results need to be interpreted in the light of the age of the patient, as a child or adolescent during a growth spurt will have very elevated values. Plasma protein electrophoresis will detect a monoclonal gammopathy indicative of myeloma.

Urinary hydroxyproline – a useful measure of osteoclast activity and is elevated in Paget's disease.

Good-quality plain X-ray – using two views is still the mainstay of skeletal radiology. X-rays should be examined carefully for a periosteal reaction, indicative of osteomyelitis or a tumour.

Isotope bone scan – measures osteoblast activity. A positive bone scan confined to one bone suggests fracture, infection or tumour. A positive result in several long bones indicates metastatic disease, growth spurt or generalised arthritis.

CT scan – extremely valuable in the diagnosis of a primary bone tumour.

Pathological Conditions

Non-neoplastic Conditions

Fracture: not routinely biopsied unless there is non-union, delayed healing or is thought to be pathological. In the former there is little or no new bone formation and only loose fibrous tissue. Sometimes there may be evidence of accompanying infection. Pathological fracture is most often due to metastatic carcinoma or myeloma although occasionally a primary bone tumour such as malignant fibrous histiocytoma, dedifferentiated chondrosarcoma or a benign bone cyst may be the cause.

Osteomyelitis: in the acute stages this disease is not routinely biopsied but when a biopsy is submitted material will be routinely sent to microbiology for culture as well. Infection is most commonly due to Staph. aureus but increasingly, low-virulence organisms are being implicated as in drug addicts or the immuno-suppressed. Chronic osteomyelitis can result in marked bone deformity and usually is characterised by prominent bone formation with quite minimal inflammation. The pathologist should always be aware of tuberculosis, which is increasing in incidence.

Metabolic bone disease: osteoporosis is very effectively diagnosed using DEXA (dual energy X-ray absorptiometry) and is almost never routinely biopsied. Osteomalacia is most uncommon in the UK but may rarely be seen in renal failure or in patients taking long-term phenytoin therapy. Paget's disease is easily diagnosed using plain X-ray, serum alkaline phosphatase and urinary hydroxyproline so it is almost never biopsied.

Avascular necrosis: seen in some fractures (neck of femur, scaphoid, talus), chronic steroid therapy, alcohol abuse, sickle cell anaemia, Caisson disease (dysbarism).

Neoplastic Conditions

Benign tumours: relatively rare and the most common is the *osteochondroma*, a bony polyp with a cap of hyaline cartilage seen usually in long bones. *Enchondromas* are cartilaginous tumours occurring in the medullary cavity of long bones. *Osteoid osteoma* is a painful lesion occurring in the cortex of a long bone, with a central lytic nidus and a margin of sclerotic bone. A *giant cell tumour* of bone is seen in people aged 20 to 40 years of age and characteristically represents a lytic lesion occurring in the epiphysis of long bones. Other benign tumours include osteoblastoma, chondroblastoma and chondromyxoid fibroma but these are very rare.

Tumour-like conditions: includes cysts, reparative granulomas, fibrous dysplasia, benign fibrous histiocytoma and eosinophilic granuloma.

Primary malignant tumour: these are also rare and most commonly seen in young people and children. *Osteosarcoma* is a high-grade sarcoma producing malignant osteoid, typically seen in the metaphysis of long bones and people aged 10 to 25 years old. It is very rare in older people but can be associated with previous radiation exposure and Paget's disease. It is treated by a combination of chemotherapy and surgery. *Ewing's sarcoma* is a poorly differentiated, small, round, blue cell tumour seen in the long bones of children and young adults. It is treated with a combination of chemotherapy, radiotherapy and surgery. *Chondrosarcomas* are usually low-grade sarcomas occurring in long bones and flat bones in middle-aged and older people. They have a tendency for recurrence rather than metastasis. They do not respond to chemotherapy and treatment is surgical removal. The *dedifferentiated* chondrosarcoma is a high-grade tumour, typically large in size occurring in the pelvis and proximal femur of older people. These tumours metastasise early and have an extremely bad prognosis.

Multiple myeloma: this is really a haematological tumour but sometimes classified as a bone tumour. It is a tumour arising from the plasma cells and occurs in multiple skeletal sites. It is treated with chemotherapy.

Metastatic carcinoma: this is by far the most common malignant tumour in bone and presents as bone pain or pathological fracture. The most common primary sites are lung, kidney, breast, prostate and thyroid. Most metastatic tumours produce lytic lesions but prostatic secondaries are often sclerotic. The usual skeletal sites are proximal long bones, rib, pelvis and vertebrae. Metastatic disease is distinctly uncommon in the skeleton distal to the elbow or knee.

Surgical Pathology Specimens – Clinical Aspects

Biopsy Specimens

Fine needle aspiration (FNA) cytology has only a very limited role in the diagnosis of primary bone tumours. Bones are obviously deep-seated and due to the hard nature of the tissue do not avail themselves to aspiration cytology. Although this technique is very well established in breast and head and neck pathology it has almost no role to play in the diagnosis of primary bone tumours. Occasionally, radiologically guided fine needle aspiration can be performed where metastatic disease is suspected.

Needle biopsy (Jamshedi needle or Surecut) under radiological control is the preferred method used to obtain a biopsy. Often the radiologist performs the biopsy. This method has the advantage of saving valuable theatre time, requires minimal anaesthesia and is much less invasive for the patient and for planning future treatment. It is most important that good radiological imaging is available to ensure that the needle is in the right place. Occasionally needle biopsy fails to obtain a good sample to allow definitive diagnosis to be made and then open biopsy is required.

Resection Specimens

Femoral heads removed at hip replacement for arthritis or repair of hip fracture are not routinely submitted for pathology. They are submitted in cases of pathological fracture, avascular necrosis or in rapidly progressive arthropathy occurring in young people.

Malignant tumours need to be removed completely with a tumour-free margin or else they will recur. Characteristically, malignant bone tumours also permeate the soft tissues adjacent to the bone. These soft tissues must also be removed. Detailed preoperative planning and careful examination of MRI scans is required to determine the appropriate dissection. An *intralesional* excision occurs when the surgeon cuts through the tumour. A *marginal* excision is where the tumour is completely removed without any significant margin of normal tissue. A *wide* excision is where the surgeon removes the tumour completely with a cuff of normal tissue. A *radical* excision is where the entire muscle compartment of bone is removed and it usually implies the removal of the joint proximal to the tumour. These are often disarticulations.

Surgical Pathology Specimens – Laboratory Protocols

Biopsy Specimens

Needle biopsy specimens are submitted directly in formalin. If gritty or firm they are put in 4% acetic acid/formalin for 1–4 hours and then in EDTA overnight. Decalcification is clearly important so as to obtain good sections but gentle decalcification is necessary in case immuno-histochemistry is required. Vigorous decalcification using formic acid can destroy the tumour cells and expressed antigens rendering subsequent immunohistochemistry unhelpful.

Small bony fragments, curettings or reamings from a primary bone tumour, infection or metastatic disease are placed into cassettes and decalcified in 10% formic acid after adequate fixation. If the curettings are from a suspect bone cyst or primary tumour it is advisable to use gentler methods of decalcification such as 4% acetic acid/formalin and overnight treatment with EDTA.

Bone biopsy for osteomalacia requires undecalcified sections cut by a sledge microtome, plastic embedding and use of trichrome/toluidine blue stains. Fluorescent tetracycline labelling is also used for the assessment of bone turnover.

The diagnosis of osseous tumours may also be aided by the use of alkaline phosphatase stains. Briefly, air-dried imprints are made from fresh tissue and stained for alkaline phosphatase demonstrated by the naphthol ASBI phosphoric acid method. The alkaline phosphatase appears as bright red intracytoplasmic granules.

Resection Specimens

Femoral heads or large chunks of bone require adequate fixation and are then cut coronally with a junior hacksaw or vibrating table saw. The thin, sawn slices are placed in 10% formic acid for decalcification. The decalcified slices are then serially blocked, labelled and submitted in toto.

Amputation specimens are examined to:

- evaluate the resection margins including vessel involvement.
- determine the extent of bone involvement.
- evaluate the tumour necrosis, a measure of response to prior chemotherapy.

Initial procedure

- ideally, amputation specimens should be properly fixed before attempting dissection but for large specimens, especially above knee amputations, it is not practicable and therefore extreme care must be taken.
- the handedness (left or right) and limb (upper or lower) is recorded.
- palpate for any obvious tumour masses or soft tissue involvement.
- note any previous scars including length and location.
- locate the proximal limit of all major nerves and vessels.
- confirm that the proximal limit is free of tumour.
- cut through the skin and soft tissues to determine if soft tissue spread has occurred; the soft tissue should be incised to the bone.
- locate and trace major nerves and vessels to ensure they are free and not encased by tumour.
- the bone itself is bivalved with a bandsaw or mortuary skull saw. Extreme safety precautions and care must be taken when using the bandsaw and only specifically named personnel, specially trained in its use, should be allowed to use this apparatus.

- measurements:
  - amputated bone: length (cm).
  - tumour: length, width and depth (cm).
  - distance (cm) to proximal resection margin – depth of overlying skin and soft tissues free of tumour.
  - extent of extra-osseous tumour involvement in soft tissues.

Description

- tumour: location (bone surface, cortex, intramedullary canal).
  - site (epiphysis, metaphysis, diaphysis).
  - gross features (osseous, cartilaginous, cystic change, necrosis).

Blocks for histology (Figure 43.3)

- vessel limits.
- marrow and proximal margin of resection.
- any scars related to previous surgery or open biopsy.
- representative blocks of involved soft tissues.
- representative blocks of tumour obviously around or in major vessels.
- blocks to evaluate the tumour characteristics and extent of necrosis for assessing response to chemotherapy.
- the extent of tumour necrosis is roughly estimated by calculating the tumour necrosis present in a whole bone slab 0.4 cm thick. Having bivalved the affected bone this 0.4 cm longitudinal slab is obtained by cutting along the plane of maximum tumour diameter. The slab is drawn out and the whole slab cut into blocks for histology. These blocks are individually labelled and are correspondingly noted and labelled on the written diagram. About 20–40 blocks are required to achieve this properly (Figure 43.3).
- the blocks are properly fixed in formalin prior to decalcification. It is most important that blocks, especially these relatively large bone blocks, are well fixed as the acid used in

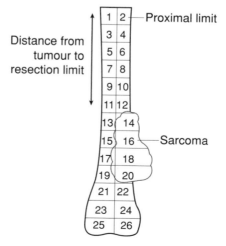

Figure 43.3. Taking blocks from a bone slab containing sarcoma.

- decalcification can destroy the cell morphology. Often about 48 hours fixation is required.
- decalcification is obtained using 10% formic acid. This may take several days.

Histopathology report

- tumour type – osteosarcoma/Ewing's sarcoma/chondrosarcoma.
- tumour subtype – parosteal/small cell osteo/chondroblastic, fibroblastic, dedifferentiated.
- tumour grade – osteosarcoma and Ewing's (nearly all are high grade), chondrosarcoma (grade I-III), dedifferentiated.
- tumour necrosis – response as a percentage for an entire slab (applies only to osteosarcoma).
- extent of local tumour spread – medullary cavity/cortex/extra-osseous soft tissues/proximal marrow involvement.

A TNM system is available to help with staging bone tumours but in practice the more simple Enneking system is much more widely used.

Enneking system:

Stage	Grade	Site
1A	G_1 (low)	T_1
1B	G_1 (low)	T_2
2A	G_2 (high)	T_1
2B	G_2 (high)	T_2
3	G_1 or G_2	Metastases
T_1	intracompartmental	
T_2	extracompartmental	

- lymphovascular invasion including vessel limits.
- excision margins – proximal limit, skin and overlying scars.

3. Soft Tissues

Anatomy

The soft tissues refers to non-epithelial extraskeletal tissue of the body but not including the haemopoietic or brain tissue. It really consists of muscle, fat, fibrous tissue along with blood vessels and peripheral nerves.

Clinical Presentation

Most soft tissue lesions present as a lump or swelling and are usually painless. The lump may reach quite a size before the patient is aware of its existence, particularly if the lump is deep-seated or in the retroperitoneum. From a clinical point the most important aspect is the possibility that the soft tissue lump could be malignant, i.e., a sarcoma. In general, any lump which is more than 5 cm in size, deep-seated, painful or growing rapidly should be considered as a possible sarcoma and investigated accordingly.

Clinical Investigations

Routine blood tests have no useful role to play in diagnosing a soft tissue lump.

Plain X-rays also yield very little information unless there is calcification or ossification within the lump. This may sometimes be seen in synovial sarcomas.

The most useful investigation in assessing soft tissue lumps is magnetic resonance imaging (MRI) but the interpretation of the scans is complicated and depends on a highly trained and experienced radiologist. MRI can define the composition of a lump, identify the location and extent of the mass, provide information on involvement of nearby structures such as nerves and vessels, may help differentiate between benign and malignant tumours and can stage a malignant tumour locally.

Pathological Conditions

Non-neoplastic Conditions

Ganglion: is a fibrous walled cyst typically arising from a tendon in the hands, wrist or feet. They are regarded as herniations of synovium, usually have no recognisable lining, and a focally myxoid fibrotic wall with gelatinous contents.

Bursa: this is a swelling which may be painful, arising from the synovial lining between muscles, tendons or bones. They are especially common near joints. They include Baker's cyst at the back of the knee and housemaid's knee.

Rheumatoid nodule: this is an irregular swelling seen in the soft tissues or in the organs in patients with rheumatoid arthritis. However, not every patient has well-established rheumatoid arthritis. It forms part of the necrobiotic collagen disorders.

Neoplastic Conditions

Benign tumour: there are many different benign soft tissue lesions including lipomas, chondromas, neural tumours, leiomyomas and a range of fibromatoses and fasciitis conditions. *Lipomas* are by far the most common and are usually less than 2–3 cm in size, mobile and superficial. Some lipomas can be quite large, deeper located and may contain small numbers of atypical cells. It may be difficult to determine if these lesions are benign or malignant. *Fibromatoses*, e.g., Dupuytren's contracture, are irregular, poorly defined lesions which can be difficult to remove surgically and have a high rate of recurrence.

Nodular fasciitis is a rapidly growing lump which clinically and microscopically can mimic malignancy.

Sarcomas: these are malignant soft tissue tumours and include such lesions as liposarcomas, fibrosarcomas, synovial sarcoma, malignant fibrous histiocytoma and leiomyosarcomas. They are quite rare and benign soft tissue lumps outnumber sarcomas by a ratio of 50–100:1. The precise classification of sarcomas is very complicated but clinically and prognostically is of limited value. Surgery remains the mainstay of treatment and chemotherapy, except in a few specific tumours such as extra-skeletal Ewing's sarcoma or childhood rhabdomyosarcoma, has little role to play as the toxicity of the therapy outweighs any benefits in increased survival. The most important features are size, grade and stage. Grading in turn depends on differentiation, necrosis and mitotic rates. The five-year survival for most sarcomas is about 40%.

Surgical Pathology Specimens – Clinical Aspects

Biopsy Specimens

Fine needle aspiration cytology has only a limited role to play but in some large national centres, with good clinico-pathological correlation and highly experienced operators, it can be used to reliably distinguish most benign and malignant soft tissue lumps. If FNA is to be relied on it is most important that the cytopathologist is well experienced in dealing with soft tissue lumps. The technique is quick, relatively painless and requires no anaesthesia. It is essential that any soft tissue swelling is properly assessed clinically and radiologically prior to FNA. Many lesions may be too deeply located to rely on FNA. Sometimes only necrotic tissue is obtained. Some benign lesions can contain atypical cells such as nodular fasciitis and some malignant tumours such as synovial sarcoma or well-differentiated liposarcoma have rather bland cytology. Immunohisto-chemistry and, where available, cytogenetic analysis may be performed on fine needle aspiration specimens. FNA is also useful for assessing recurrence or metastases in patients with previously diagnosed sarcoma.

In most UK centres needle core biopsy (Jamshedi or Surecut) performed under radiological control is the preferred method of obtaining a tissue diagnosis. More than 90% of these lesions are diagnosed using this technique. It must be emphasised that FNA and needle biopsy are only used to determine if a swelling is benign or malignant. Biopsy is not a reliable means for precise subdiagnosis. Some soft tissue tumours have a variety of patterns and needle biopsy may result in sampling error.

Open biopsy is used when FNA or closed needle biopsy have failed. It is performed by a surgeon and general anaesthesia is required. Only experienced surgeons specifically trained to deal with soft tissue tumours should perform this procedure, and not by general surgeons. A wedge of tissue is removed, preferably along the long axis of the tumour and directly over the tumour.

Resection Specimens

Intracapsular excision: these are performed inside the tumour, are often piecemeal in nature and local recurrence is almost 100%.

Marginal excision: this refers to removal of the lesion but without any significant margin of normal tissue. Sometimes the excision biopsy is referred to as shelling out. This technique is adequate for superficial tumours or smaller tumours less than 3 cm in diameter.

Wide excision: are excisions through the normal tissue beyond the reactive zone associated with the tumour but still within the muscle compartment of origin. The tumour is never visualised during the procedure.

Radical excision: is the removal of the tumour and entire muscle compartment of origin. A radical amputation usually requires disarticulation of the joint proximal to the involved compartment.

Surgical Pathological Specimens – Laboratory Protocols

Biopsy Specimens

Biopsies are usually in the form of needle-shaped pieces of tissue. They will usually be submitted directly in formalin. The biopsies are examined through levels. Special techniques such as immunohistochemistry, electron microscopy and cytogenetics can be helpful (see later).

Resection Specimens

Specimen types

Most resections for soft tissue tumours will consist of the tumour with a margin of uninvolved soft tissue. It is very unusual to submit any attached bone, and actual amputations are extremely rare.

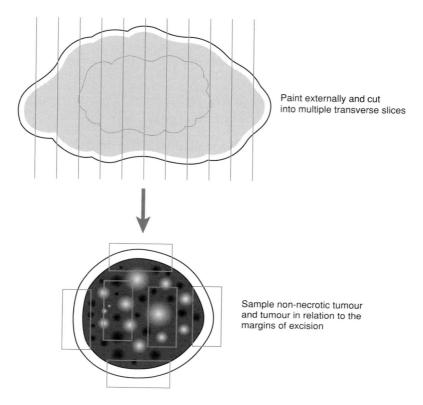

Paint externally and cut
into multiple transverse slices

Sample non-necrotic tumour
and tumour in relation to the
margins of excision

Figure 43.4.   Blocking a wide excision of a soft tissue mass.

Initial procedure

- palpate the soft tissue to locate the tumour.
- paint the outer surface in toto or selectively to assist the assessment of margins.
- note the presence of attached skin ellipse and any scars present.
- serially cut through the specimen making a series of transverse parallel cuts at 0.5 cm intervals (pan-loafing), (Figure 43.4).
- measurements:
    - specimen: length × width × depth (cm), weight (g).
    - tumour: length × width × depth (cm) or maximum dimension (cm).
      distance (cm) from overlying skin.
      distance (cm) from nearest margins.
    - skin: length × width (cm).
      length (cm) of scar.

Description

- tumour: character of cut surface.
    - margins (infiltrating or circumscribed).

- presence of necrosis, haemorrhage, cystic change, mucinous change.
- ulceration of overlying skin.
- relationship to any major vessels or nerves.
- other: note tissues included in the specimen (muscle, fat, major vessels, bone).

Blocks for histology

- limits of any major nerves or vessels included in resection.
- representative blocks of margins.
- sufficient blocks to adequately sample the tumour including different macroscopic appearances such as cystic and necrotic areas (about one block per cm of greatest dimension).
- any bone present.
- overlying skin and scars.

Histopathology report:

- tumour type/subtype (often requires immunohistochemistry, electron microscopy or cytogenetics).
- tumour grade – Trojani grade (I, II, III) based on tumour differentiation, necrosis and mitoses.
- tumour edge – circumscribed or infiltrating.
- extent of local tumour spread:
    - pT1 tumour ≤ 5 cm in greatest dimension.
      a. superficial.
      b. deep.
    - pT2 tumour > 5 cm in greatest dimension.
      a. superficial.
      b. deep.

- note ulceration of overlying skin.
- lymphovascular invasion.
- excision margins – distance (cm) from nearest excision margin.

Special Techniques

Immunohistochemistry

Immunohistochemistry can be useful in diagnosing bone and soft tissue sarcomas. In bone tumours the decalcification process can destroy antigens in the tumour cells and this can limit the usefulness of the technique. As with all tumours the following general points must be emphasised:

- antibodies are not specific to a particular type of tumour, there is often overlap with several other types.
- immunohistochemistry will not directly determine if the tumour is benign or malignant.
- beware of interpretation in the presence of extensive tumour necrosis.
- be careful of edge artefact.
- know whether the antibodies you use should stain on the membrane, within the cytoplasm or nucleus of the cell.
- always use a panel of antibodies.

The use of immunohistochemistry in bone and soft tissue sarcomas is a huge subject and good standard textbooks of soft tissue tumour pathology should be consulted. However, the list below is a very simplified version illustrating some of the uses of the more common antibodies:

LCA (CD45)

- lymphomas, chronic inflammation.

Cytokeratins

- metastatic carcinoma, synovial sarcoma, epithelioid sarcoma.

PRAP/PSA

- metastatic prostate carcinoma.

S100

- neural, lipomatous and cartilaginous tumours.

Smooth muscle actin

- muscle tumours, fibroblastic and myofibroblastic soft tissue lesions.

Desmin

- muscle tumours.

MIC-2 (CD99)

- Ewing's sarcoma but it can be positive in many other tumours.

Electron Microscopy

If sufficient tissue is available, examination of the ultracellular features can give guidance on the tissue of origin. Small (1 mm) cubes of tissue should be transferred to glutaraldehyde and submitted to the electron microscopy laboratory. It is important to ensure that blocks are taken from the tumour but do not include necrotic tissue.

Cytogenetics

Specific chromosomal abnormalities have been identified in some bone and soft tissue sarcomas. The presence of these chromosomal abnormalities can support a particular diagnosis, help to sub-classify a lesion and may provide information associated with a poor prognosis. However, this technology is expensive, available to only a minority of laboratories, depends on successful cell culture of the tumour cells, requires the immediate dispatch of fresh tumour tissue from the operating theatre to the pathology laboratory and in most cases does not provide any additional information that cannot be obtained by histology and immunohistochemistry. Nevertheless, cytogenetics is an interesting technique and major developments are taking place. In time, technological advances will render the technique much more widely available even to smaller laboratories and pathologists should therefore be aware of its applications.

Haemopoietic Specimens

Lakshmi Venkatraman, W Glenn McCluggage, Peter A Hall

44. Lymph Nodes, Spleen and Bone Marrow

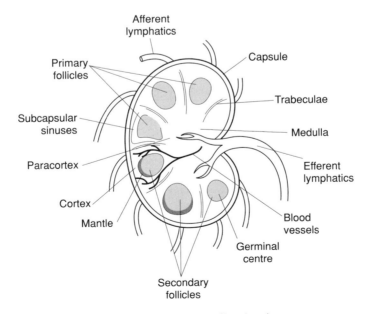

44

Lymph Nodes, Spleen and Bone Marrow

1. Lymph Nodes

Anatomy

Lymph nodes are ovoid encapsulated structures situated at regular intervals along the lymphatic channels. They neutralise, degrade or modify the antigens that are presented to them by the lymphatics before returning them to the blood. The immune response to antigens after birth determines the structure and composition of the node. Each lymph node has a fibrous capsule from which trabeculae extend into the parenchyma. The non-stimulated/minimally stimulated lymph node is composed of a reticulum meshwork supported by fibroblastic dendritic cells. The broad functional and anatomical divisions within a lymph node are the outer cortex and the inner medulla, which are sometimes visible on naked-eye examination (Figure 44.1). The cortex or the B zone contains pale-staining, densely packed aggregates of lymphocytes called primary follicles. These are separated from each other and the sinuses by smaller lymphocytes forming a mantle

Figure 44.1. Architecture of lymph node.

of darkly staining cells, the mantle zone, and yet another zone of paler cells, the marginal zone. Deep to the cortex and between follicles is the paracortex or T zone, composed mostly of T cells mixed with histiocytes, interdigitating reticulum cells and Langerhan's cells. The paracortex also has the characteristic high endothelial venules that are involved in lymphocyte trafficking.

Following antigenic stimulation the cells of the primary B follicles become larger, acquire multiple nucleoli, divide and die. The germinal centres of the secondary follicles thus formed contain immunoblasts, centroblasts, centrocytes and tingible body macrophages. Antigenic stimulation also results in a paracortical T cell response with transformation to blast cells. The medulla contains large numbers of plasma cells, which are the terminally mature B cells.

The afferent lymphatics enter the lymph node through the convex surface on the cortex and drain into the subcapsular venous sinuses. The lymph is conveyed to the efferent lymphatics in the hilum by the intermediate and medullary sinuses.

Three lineages of lymphocytes are recognised in the lymph node, the B, T and NK (natural killer) cells. The B lymphocytes express surface and cytoplasmic immunoglobulins, which mediate humoral immunity. Large quantities of immunoglobulin are produced by the plasma cells. The T cells including the helper and suppressor subsets mediate cellular immunity. The two mechanisms of immunity are interdependent.

Immunophenotyping is essential in characterisation of lymphoid diseases and it is important to be familiar with the normal immunoarchitecture of the lymph node (Figure 44.2).

In general, the follicles stain strongly with B cell markers (CD19, CD20, CD 79a). The interfollicular and paracortical regions express CD3 (T cell marker) predominantly. The developmental stages and immunophenotype of B and T lymphocytes are shown in Figure 44.3.

Lymphovascular supply

The artery enters the lymph node at the hilum where it divides into numerous branches. These follow the trabeculae and reach the cortex to form a capillary network. Some arterioles reach the medulla through the trabeculae. The post-capillary venules draining the cortex and paracortex coalesce to form collecting veins that leave the hilum of the lymph node. The intranodal lymphatic flow is detailed above.

Clinical Presentation

Lymphadenopathy may be a presenting sign or symptom or an incidental finding. Up to two thirds of patients have non-specific causes or upper respiratory illness. Patients may present with sore throat, cough, fever, night sweats and fatigue or weight loss. There are many diseases associated with lymphadenopathy. The major categories are listed in Table 44.1.

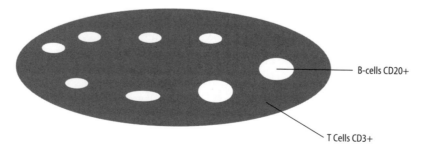

Figure 44.2.   Normal immunoarchitecture of lymph node.

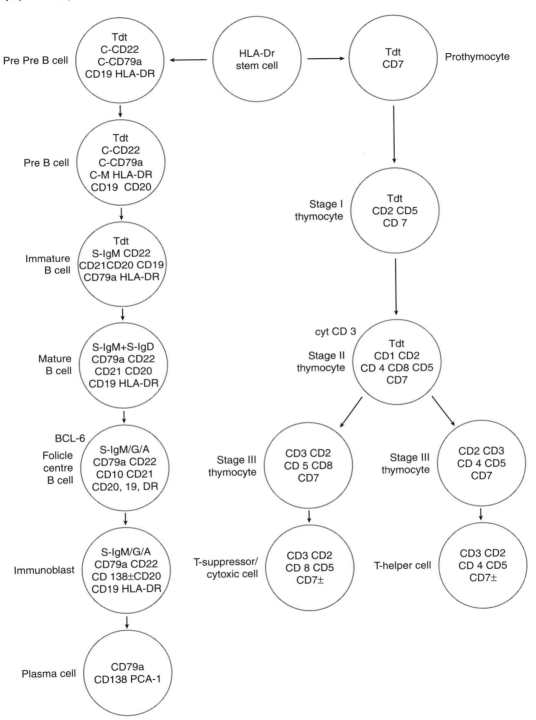

Figure 44.3. Development of B and T lymphocytes.

Table 44.1.   Causes of lymphadenopathy

Infectious Diseases
Viral: Infectious mononucleosis, hepatitis, herpes simplex, HIV, measles, Varicella zoster, rubella. Bacterial: Streptococci, Brucellosis, Tuberculosis, other mycobacterial infection, plague, primary and secondary syphilis. Fungal: Histoplasmosis, cryptococcosis. Chlamydia: Lymphogranuloma venereum. Parasitic: Toxoplasmosis, Leishmaniasis. Rickettsial: Rickettsial pox, scrub typhus.
Immunologic Disorders
Rheumatoid arthritis, lupus erythematosus, dermatomyositis, Sjogren's syndrome, primary biliary cirrhosis Drug hypersensitivity: Diphenylhydantoin, hydralazine, allopurinol, gold, carbamazepine. Graft versus host disease.
Malignancy
Haematological Metastasis: from various sites.
Lipid Storage Disorders
Nieman Pick's, Gaucher's.
Endocrine Diseases
Hyperthyroidism.
Others
Castleman's disease, sarcoidosis, dermatopathic lymphadenitis, Kikuchi's disease, sinus histiocytosis with massive lymphadenopathy, inflammatory pseudotumour.

Pain in a lymph node is usually secondary to inflammation. However, rapid enlargement and pain may be present in lymphomas and leukaemias. Lymphadenopathy can be localised or generalised. The site of enlargement may provide a clue to the cause. Some of the common sites of lymphadenopathy and causes of enlargement are listed in Table 44.2.

Small size (< 1 cm diameter) usually indicates a benign lymph node.

Malignant lymphoma: large, discrete, symetric, mobile, rubbery, non-tender lymph nodes.

Metastatic carcinoma: hard, non-tender lymph nodes fixed to surrounding tissues.

Patients with lymphadenopathy may have splenomegaly as seen in chronic lymphocytic leukaemia, lupus erythematosus, toxoplasmosis and various haematological disorders.

Non-superficial lymphadenopathy: thoracic or abdominal. Thoracic lymph nodes may be secondary to lung diseases and identified on routine chest X-ray. Other symptoms are cough and wheezing from airway compression, hoarseness from recurrent laryngeal nerve involvement, dysphagia from oesophageal compression or swelling of the face due to superior vena cava compression. Abdominal/retroperitoneal lymph nodes if enlarged are usually malignant. However, tuberculosis can also cause mesenteric lymphadenopathy.

Table 44.2. Sites of lymphadenopathy and the related causes

Occipital: scalp infection.
Pre-auricular: conjunctival infection.
Neck: oral, dental and respiratory infections, viral diseases, e.g., infectious mononucleosis.
Malignant neck nodes: drain thyroid, head and neck, breast and lung carcinomas.

Scalene and supraclavicular (Virchow's nodes): always abnormal if enlarged as these drain lung and retroperitoneum.
Causes: infection, lymphomas or other malignancies. Tuberculosis, sarcoidosis and toxoplasmosis are the commonest causes of non-neoplastic enlargement at this site.
Virchow's node: is associated with a gastrointestinal primary. Metastasis from the lung, breast, testes and ovaries may present as lymphadenopathy at this site.

Axillary: Non-neoplastic: trauma, infection of the ipsilateral upper extremity.
Neoplastic: metastasis from malignant melanoma, breast cancer or lymphoma.
Inguinal: Non-neoplastic: trauma, infection of the lower extremities or venereal diseases.
Neoplastic: metastasis from cancers of lower rectum, anal canal, genitalia and melanoma of the lower extremities.

Clinical Investigations

Investigations are done to find the cause suspected from the history and physical findings.

ENT examination: is essential in the work-up of persistent cervical lymphadenopathy.

Full blood picture (FBP): raised WCC count in acute/chronic leukaemias and pyogenic infections.

Serology: raised immunoglobulin titres in EBV, CMV, HIV, toxoplasmosis and brucellosis. ANA (anti-nuclear antibody), anti dsDNA: raised in rheumatoid arthritis and lupus erythematosus.

Chest X-ray: if there is an abnormality suggestive of tuberculosis, sarcoidosis or cancer further investigations are necessary.

USS (ultrasound scan): long axis (L)/short axis (S) ratio < 2 has 95% specificity and sensitivity to detect metastatic disease.

CT (computed tomography) and MRI (magnetic resonance imaging): are 65–90% accurate in the diagnosis of metastatic malignancy.

FNA (fine needle aspiration): has > 90% sensitivity and specificity in diagnosis of metastatic cancer and even lymphoma in some centres. It is extremely useful in selecting patients for lymph node excision biopsy and sometimes can help focus further evaluation. It may also be useful in follow up of patients with known haematological disease.

Indications for lymph node excision biopsy:

1. to make a diagnosis in cases of unexplained, persistent lymphadenopathy, e.g., confirming and typing a suspected lymphoma.
2. to confirm a clinical diagnosis, e.g., metastatic squamous carcinoma in a known case of head and neck cancer.
3. as part of the diagnostic work-up of a systemic disease with lymphadenopathy, e.g., rheumatoid arthritis and lupus erythematosus.
4. staging protocol for cancers.
5. to monitor progress in a previously diagnosed malignant lymphoma.

Pathological Conditions

Non-neoplastic Conditions

These include various patterns of hyperplasia all of which show morphological and immunohistochemical preservation of the nodal architecture. The main patterns are:

Follicular hyperplasia: this is characterised by prominent hyperplastic follicles in the cortex. It is a common non-specific reaction. It is a striking feature of lymph nodes in progressive transformation of germinal centres, HIV-associated lymphadenopathy, rheumatoid arthritis and syphilis.

Mantle zone hyperplasia: the reactive follicles have thick mantles. This is best seen in Castleman's disease and is a common pattern in reactive mesenteric lymph nodes.

Marginal zone hyperplasia: is characterised by monocytoid B lymphocyte proliferation within sinuses. It is seen in toxoplasmosis, HIV-associated lymphadenopathy, granulomatous diseases such as cat scratch disease, lymphogranuloma venereum and CMV lymphadenitis.

Granulomatous inflammation: May be due to infections such as tuberculosis, brucellosis, foreign body reaction, sarcoidosis and in response to malignancy as in lymph nodes draining carcinomas or in patients with Hodgkin's disease.

Caseating granulomas: seen in tuberculosis.

Suppuration and granulomata: seen in non-tuberculous mycobacterial infections and fungal infections due to histoplasmosis, cryptococcosis, aspergillosis, mucormycosis and candidiasis.

Microgranulomata within germinal centres: seen in toxoplasmosis.

Suppurative lymphadenitis with/without granulomata: seen in cat scratch disease, tularaemia and lymphogranuloma venereum.

Necrotising lymphadenitis without neutrophils (Kikuchi's disease): occurs in young women, is of unknown aetiology and shows pale patches of large lymphoid cells with karyorrhectic debris, crescentic histiocytes and plasmacytoid monocytes. It may be confused with a large cell lymphoma.

Paracortical hyperplasia: is commonly a non-specific response but is typical of dermatopathic lymphadenitis which occurs in generalised exfoliative dermatitis.

Immunoblastic proliferation: is characteristic of infectious mononucleosis and prominent in other viral infections, hypersensitivity reactions, post vaccinial and Kikuchi's disease.

Sinus proliferation/sinus histiocytosis: is frequently present in lymph nodes draining carcinomas. Other disorders that show prominent sinus involvement include Rosai–Dorfman disease (sinus histiocytosis with massive lymphadenopathy), Langerhan's histiocytosis, Whipple's disease and virus-associated haemophagocytic syndrome.

Neoplastic Conditions

Malignant lymphomas: Hodgkin's lymphoma and non-Hodgkin's lymphoma (NHL) are the two broad categories of malignant lymphoid neoplasms in the WHO consensus classification. The NHLs are further subclassified as neoplasms of the B, T and NK cells. The disease entities are recognised on the basis of available information using morphology, immunophenotyping, genetics and clinical features.

The WHO classification includes both lymphomas and leukaemias since both solid and circulatory phases are recognised in many lymphoid neoplasms. The practical approach to diagnosis is based on cell size, which correlates with clinical features and response to treatment. Thus, "low-grade lymphomas" present as disseminated disease, respond to treatment and have a median survival in years.

Prognosis may also be related to stage of disease, i.e., the number of regional lymph node groups involved, their anatomical site (viz peripheral versus mediastinal or retroperitoneal) and the presence and extent of extranodal disease.

Up to 90% of the NHLs are B cell neoplasms. The clinical and pathological features of the most frequent *"low-grade" small B cell lymphomas* are listed in Table 44.3.

Marginal zone lymphoma: accounts for 7–8% of lymphoid neoplasms. It is rare in the nodes but nearly always presents at extranodal sites as MALTomas, e.g., stomach, salivary gland and thyroid.

"High-grade" diffuse large B cell lymphomas: are aggressive and present as nodal, extranodal, localised or disseminated disease. Distinctive clinical variants are mediastinal large B cell lymphoma, primary effusion lymphoma and intravascular lymphoma. Morphologic variants are centroblastic, immunoblastic, plasmablastic, T cell rich and anaplastic. The clinical relevance of these is debatable and they are not subdivided in the WHO classification. Early-stage disease is chemoresponsive and potentially curable. Tumour cells are usually CD20 and CD79a positive with a high Ki67 proliferation index.

Burkitt's lymphoma: is a high-grade tumour of medium-sized rapidly proliferating B cells (Ki67~100%). The major clinical subtypes include endemic, sporadic and immunodeficiency related. The type of tumour seen in the West shows greater pleomorphism than the Burkitt's lymphoma described in Africa and has been termed Burkitt-like.

T/NK cell neoplasms: are relatively uncommon and account for approximately 12% of the lymphoid neoplasms in the West. The clinical features are important for subtyping, as the morphology, immunophenotype and genetics are not absolutely specific.

Table 44.3. Low-grade small B cell non-Hodgkin's lymphomas

	Chronic Lymphocytic Leukaemia	Mantle Cell Lymphoma	Follicle Centre Cell Lymphoma	Lymphoplasmacytic Lymphoma
Clinical	≈6% of NHL. Rare under 40 yrs. Disseminated disease at presentation.	≈6% of NHL. M:F ratio 5:1. Disseminated at presentation. Biologically aggressive. Median survival 2–5yrs.	≈22% of NHL. Rare under 20yrs. Disseminated at presentation.	Disseminated at presentation. M protein, Hyperviscosity, cryoglobulinemia
Architecture	Pale staining pseudofollicles. Background diffuse small lymphocytes.	Diffuse, less commonly nodular proliferation.	Closely packed follicles, absent mantles, loss of polarity.	Diffuse, Interfollicular.
Cytology	Paraimmunoblasts, Prolymphocytes. Small lymphoid cells with clotted chromatin minimally larger than mature lymphocytes.	Small-to-medium-sized lymphocytes with slight nuclear irregularity. Scattered histiocytes and hyalinised vessels common. Blasts in blastoid variant.	Centroblasts, centrocytes. Atypia. May have signet ring cells.	Small B lymphocytes. Plasmacytoid lymphocytes
Immunohistochemistry	CD5, CD20, CD23, CD43 positive. CD10, Cyclin D1 negative	CD5, Cyclin D1, CD43 positive. CD10, CD23, bcl6 negative.	CD20, CD10, bcl2, bcl6 positive. CD5/43 negative. CD23+/–	VS38 positive. CD43+/–. CD5, CD10, CD23 negative
Cytogenetics	Trisomy 12 in 20%	t (11:14)	t (14:18)	t (9:14)

The commonest subtypes are peripheral T cell lymphoma, not otherwise specified, and anaplastic large cell lymphoma.

Peripheral T cell lymphoma, NOS: is a heterogeneous group of neoplasms with a broad cytological spectrum. The tumour cells are small-to-medium sized with irregular nuclei and pleomorphic cells that may be Reed–Sternberg-like. CD3 and other T cell antigens are positive and aberrant antigen expression is common. TCR genes are rearranged but there are no markers of monoclonality.

Anaplastic large cell lymphoma: most frequently occurs in the first three decades of life. The tumour cells have pleomorphic horseshoe-shaped nuclei, abundant cytoplasm, and are referred to as "hallmark cells". The tumour grows often within sinuses in a cohesive manner. T cell antigens, EMA, cytotoxic granule proteins, ALK-1 and CD30 are positive. Ninety per cent of cases have clonal rearrangement of TCR genes. ALK-1 expression is due to t (2:5) (q23; 35). Variant translocations involving ALK-1 and other partner genes on chromosomes 1, 2, 3 and 17 also occur. Overall five-year survival rate is 80% in ALK-1-positive patients while ALK-1 negativity is prognostically adverse.

Hodgkin's lymphoma: accounts for 30% of all lymphomas. The new WHO classification divides Hodgkin's lymphoma into two major subtypes.

- Classic Hodgkin's lymphoma (HL).
  - HL, nodular sclerosis, grade I and II.
  - HL, lymphocyte-rich.
  - HL, mixed cellularity.
  - HL, lymphocyte depleted.
- Nodular lymphocyte-predominant HL (NLPHL – a B cell lymphoma).

The clinical and pathological features are detailed in Table 44.4.

Plasma cell neoplasms: include myeloma and its variants, plasmacytoma, immunoglobulin deposition diseases, osteosclerotic myeloma and heavy chain diseases, all of which have a clonal proliferation of immunoglobulin-secreting, terminally differentiated B cells, i.e., plasma cells and plasmacytoid lymphocytes.

Metastatic tumours: lymph nodes are common sites of tumour metastasis, which may be the presenting feature. Nodal spread is common in carcinomas, malignant melanomas and germ cell tumours, and uncommon in sarcomas and mesotheliomas.

Lymphomas mimicking carcinomas: anaplastic large cell lymphoma, diffuse large B cell lymphoma with sclerosis, large cell lymphoma with sinusoidal growth pattern, nodular sclerosing Hodgkin's lymphoma and signet ring lymphoma.

Metastatic carcinoma mimicking lymphoma: nasopharyngeal/lymphoepithelial carcinoma and lobular carcinoma breast.

Cystic metastases in cervical lymph nodes: commonly due to papillary thyroid carcinoma and squamous cell carcinoma.

Surgical Pathology Specimens – Clinical Aspects

Excision Biopsy of Lymph Node

The general principle is to remove a representative lymph node and submit it for histology with minimal tissue distortion – this requires careful surgical expertise.

If only a single enlarged lymph node is identified, it is removed for histological assessment. In cases of widespread lymphadenopathy, excision of a large node is more diagnostically useful than a smaller, easily accessible lymph node, which may be uninvolved or only focally involved by the disease process.

Table 44.4. Subtypes of Hodgkin's lymphoma

	Nodular sclerosis	Lymphocyte rich	Mixed cellularity	Lymphocyte-depleted	NLPHL
Clinical	Most common subtype. Peripheral/mediastinal LN. Usually Stage II.	Stage I/II in peripheral nodes. Rare B symptoms[a]. Mediastinal disease uncommon.	High stage at presentation. B symptoms[a] common. Spleen involved in 30%. Usually peripheral node involvement.	Rarest subtype. Frequently associated with HIV. Involves abdominal organs, retroperitoneal LN and bone marrow. Presents as high-stage disease.	Occurs in young, often single cervical node involved. Stage I common. Frequent relapses, usually chemosensitive.
Architecture	Prominent nodularity. Collagen bands at least around one nodule.	Commonly nodular, rarely diffuse.	Obliterated architecture. No fibrous bands.	May have diffuse fibrosis.	Nodular/nodular and diffuse.
Cytology	Lacunar R-S cells. Grade I: > 75% nodules contain few R-S cells in a lymphocyte-rich, mixed-cellularity or fibrohistiocytic background. Grade II: at least 25% nodules are lymphocyte-depleted and have increased R-S cells.	Scattered R-S cells against a nodular background of small lymphocytes.	Typical R-S cells against a polymorphous background of cells including eosinophils, neutrophils, histiocytes and plasma cells.	Variable numbers of pleomorphic R-S cells and few lymphocytes. Can look anaplastic or fibrohistiocytic.	Nodules contain darkly staining small B-lymphocytes, neoplastic 'popcorn' L&H cells and rare classic R-S cells.
IHC	CD30/15+, BSAP+ in 90% cases. CD20−/+. EMA, ALK neg. EBVLMP1+/−	Same as nodular sclerosis.	Same as nodular sclerosis. EBVLMP1+ in 75% cases.	Same as nodular sclerosis. HIV + patients express EBVLMP1.	CD20/CD79a/EMA/bcl6+, transcription factors Oct2/BoB1 + in L&H cells. CD15/30 usually negative.
Prognosis	Slightly better than mixed cellularity or lymphocyte-depleted. Bulky mediastinal disease is an adverse risk factor.	As good as NLPHL	Intermediate between nodular sclerosis and lymphocyte-depleted but differences not observed with modern chemotherapy.	Aggressive in HIV + patients but with modern chemotherapy prognosis similar to other subtypes in immunocompetent patients.	Excellent prognosis in Stage I. High-stage disease is rare but death occurs in 1–2 yrs.

[a] Symptoms, e.g., weight loss, night sweats, pain.

Some lymph node groups are virtually always pathological, i.e., Virchow's/supraclavicular. Inguinal lymph nodes usually show non-specific lymphadenitis or scarring and are unlikely to be informative except when markedly enlarged or the patient has a previous history of malignancy.

Obtaining biopsies from deep lymph nodes is difficult and it may not be possible to distinguish lymphadenopathy from visceral or soft tissue malignancies. In such situations, FNAs and needle core biopsies may be taken under radiological guidance. Note that interpretation may be hindered by handling artefact and cell size/lymphoma grade underestimated, diagnosis being limited to lymphoma without further typing possible.

Surgical Pathology Specimens – Laboratory Protocols

Lymph Node Biopsy

- preferably received intact and fresh soon after excision.
- after assigning a lab number, dissect the lymph node free from surrounding fat/connective tissue.
- count the number of nodes and measure their size (length × width × depth (mm)).
- make parallel cuts along the transverse axis at 2–3 mm intervals with a sharp blade.
- a small portion is submitted for microbiological investigations if infectious disease is suspected clinically. If not submitted immediately, store at 4 °C. Make smears for Gram's/ Ziehl–Nielsen stain.
- make imprints of the cut surface on coated, alcohol-cleaned slides. Touch the glass slide gently to the cut surface of the node after ensuring it is not too wet or bloody. Avoid using force. Dry the slides in air. Heating or blow-drying is unnecessary and creates artefacts. For wet fixation, the smears are dipped in alcohol-based fixative immediately after taking imprints.
- submit the slices for histology. Fix in 10% formalin for 24–48 hours prior to paraffin processing. Prolonged fixation can bind antigenic sites and hamper immunohistochemistry. Good quality, thin (3–4 µm) sections are required for H & E morphology. Correlate imprint findings with histology of the slice from which it was obtained.

Frozen section for immunohistochemistry: usually no longer necessary as the vast majority of diagnostic antibodies are readily applicable to good-quality paraffin sections, particularly with the advent of newer, robust antibodies and antigen-retrieval techniques (e.g., pressure cooking/ microwave).

Cytogenetics/flow cytometry: place a 0.5–1-cm^3 piece of tissue in a bottle containing a culture medium such as RPMI/DMEM and send to the appropriate laboratory. Snap freeze tissue at −70 °C if tissue is not immediately processed.

Immunoglobulin heavy chain and T cell receptor gene rearrangement studies can be carried out using both fresh and paraffin-processed material as determined by local protocols.

Needle Biopsy

- count number of fragments, search the container well for all tissue.
- handle tissue gently, take care not to squeeze or transect the biopsy.
- record the length and diameter of all cores of tissue.
- note the colour and any other distinctive feature.
- submit all tissue for histology. Cores may be painted with alcian blue prior to processing so that they are readily apparent when facing the block and vital tissue is not lost. Cut through three levels and keep the intervening ribbons pending morphological assessment and any need for immunohistochemistry.

Description

- size of the node – not very helpful in determining if the lymph node is benign or malignant.
- capsule present/intact.
- appearance of the cut surface and colour – pink or grey in normal nodes, variegated with distinct nodules in metastatic carcinomas, uniformly whitish with fish-flesh appearance in lymphomas. Can be black in metastatic melanomas.
- nodularity – prominent in Hodgkin's lymphoma, sometimes follicles are prominent in follicular lymphoma.
- haemorrhage.
- necrosis – caseous /cheesy in tuberculosis, pale friable areas in high-grade lymphomas, also seen sometimes in Kikuchi's disease.

Blocks for histology

- cross section of the node including capsule.
- 1–3 slices submitted depending on size and whether the abnormality is focal or diffuse on gross examination.

Histopathology report

- indication for investigation – primary diagnosis, staging, relapse/progression, re-staging.
- type of biopsy – excision, needle biopsy, endoscopic biopsy, bone marrow biopsy, extra-nodal resection, splenectomy or other biopsy.
- site and size of – lymph node, skin, bone marrow trephine and other extra-nodal biopsies.
- size and weight of spleen.
- tumour type – lymphoma or others. If lymphoma specify type using a combination of clinical features, morphology, immunohistochemistry and cytogenetics as necessary to characterise entities included in the WHO classification. In general, Hodgkin's or non-Hodgkin's lymphoma, and characterise the latter as nodular or diffuse, small cell or large cell, low/intermediate or high-grade, and B, T, NK or ALCL.
- bone marrow – involved or not involved.

2. Spleen

Anatomy

The spleen is an encapsulated reticuloendothelial organ located in the left upper quadrant of the abdominal cavity. Anatomically, it has two compartments – the red pulp and the white pulp with an intervening poorly defined marginal zone. The white pulp comprises T lymphocytes in the periarteriolar lymphoid sheath and B lymphocytes that form primary follicles eccentrically around this sheath. The red pulp consists of cords and a complex network of venous sinuses that contain splenic macrophages. Specialised endothelial cells known as littoral cells line the sinuses. The lining is discontinuous in order to facilitate cell traffic between cords and sinuses. The important physiological roles of the spleen are removal of abnormal and senescent red blood cells mounting an antibody response to immunogens, removal of antibody-coated bacteria and other antibody-coated particles from the blood. Haemopoiesis occurs in the foetal spleen, stops within two weeks after birth and may begin again when haemopoiesis in the bone marrow is insufficient to meet the body's needs. Increased normal function of the spleen can cause splenomegaly.

Clinical Presentation

Patients may be symptomatic either as a result of splenic enlargement or the underlying disease causing it.

- pain in the left upper quadrant of abdomen. Rupture of the spleen may be painless and yet cause intra-abdominal haemorrhage, shock and death. Severe pain due to infarction is common in children with sickle cell disease or adults with CML.
- early satiety or a feeling of fullness.

A palpable spleen is a major physical sign and may be due to hyperfunction, passive congestion or infiltration by infectious disease, benign and malignant haematological disorders, metastatic carcinoma (rare) and storage diseases (Table 44.5). Rarely, the cause is unknown.

Clinical Investigations

Clinical methods – palpation and percussion to detect splenomegaly.

CT scan, MRI or USS to confirm a palpable swelling as spleen, detect non-palpable splenomegaly and exclude other causes. These methods may also show alteration in splenic texture.

Cytopenias: may result from hypersplenism or hyposplenism.

Hypersplenism – splenomegaly, cytopenia(s), normal/hyperplastic marrow, responds to splenectomy.

Hyposplenism: can be caused by surgical removal, sickle cell disease, and splenic irradiation for neoplastic/autoimmune disease.

Full blood picture: red blood cell counts and indices, i.e., MCV, MCH, MCHC, reticulocyte index.

WBC and platelet counts – may be normal, increased/decreased depending on underlying disorders.

Table 44.5.   Causes of splenomegaly

Hyperfunction: removal of RBCs, e.g., spherocytosis, sickle cell disease, haemoglobinopathies, paroxysmal nocturnal haematuria, nutritional anaemias.

Immune hyperplasia: Viral – infectious mononucleosis, hepatitis, CMV.
Bacterial – infective endocarditis, septicaemia, abscess, tuberculosis.
Fungal – histoplasmosis.
Parasitic – Malaria, Leishmaniasis.

Disordered immune regulation: Rheumatoid arthritis, lupus erythematosus, immune haemolytic anaemias, immune thrombocytopenia, drug hypersensitivity, sarcoidosis.
Extramedullary haemopoiesis: Chronic myeloid leukaemia, myelofibrosis, marrow failure due to any cause.
Increased splenic blood flow: Portal hypertension of any cause – cirrhosis, splenic vein obstruction, portal vein obstruction including due to schistosomiasis, congestive heart failure.
Infiltration: Amyloid, Gaucher's, Nieman–Pick's, hyperlipidemias.
Benign and malignant infiltrations: Leukaemia, lymphoma, myeloproliferative disorders, metastatic carcinoma, angiosarcoma, histiocytosis X.
Unknown.

Pathological Conditions

Non-neoplastic Conditions

Traumatic rupture of spleen and iatrogenic removal: are the most frequent reasons for splenectomy, e.g., road traffic accident, and splenic damage or creating access at abdominal surgery. Spontaneous rupture can occur in diseases such as infectious mononucleosis, infective endocarditis, malaria, lymphoma/leukaemia and primary non-lymphoid splenic neoplasms.

Congestive splenomegaly: is due to portal venous hypertension, commonly secondary to liver cirrhosis but may also result from portal venous thrombosis, inflammation, sclerosis or stenosis.

Amyloidosis: secondary involvement of the spleen results in a characteristic gross appearance, i.e., the sago or lardaceous spleen.

Hypersplenism: refers to a condition in which the blood cells are culled excessively within the spleen. It usually occurs when the haemopoietic cells are intrinsically abnormal – as in idiopathic thrombocytopenic purpura (ITP), congenital spherocytosis and acquired haemolytic anaemias (due to various leukaemias, Hodgkin's lymphoma, sarcoidosis, lupus erythematosus, etc.).

Neoplastic Conditions

Benign Tumours

Haemangioma: is the commonest primary splenic tumour. It may be an incidental finding and is often less than 2 cm in size. It is usually of cavernous type and may be associated with haemangiomas elsewhere. Rupture and bleeding are common complications.

Littoral cell angioma: is a multinodular tumour that resembles splenic venous sinuses histologically.

Other benign tumours include: hamartoma, epidermoid cysts, inflammatory mycobacterial pseudotumour, lymphangioma and lipoma.

Malignant Tumours

Malignant lymphoma: is the commonest malignant tumour involving the spleen and represents secondary spread in most cases, although primary splenic lymphomas do occur. The gross pattern of involvement often corresponds to the microscopic type of lymphoma: homogeneous in small lymphocytic lymphoma, miliary in follicular lymphoma, solitary nodules or multiple masses in large cell lymphoma and Hodgkin's lymphoma.

Primary splenic marginal zone lymphoma: is the splenic equivalent of MALT lymphoma in other sites. It involves the splenic hilar lymph nodes and bone marrow frequently and lymphoma cells often circulate in peripheral blood as villous lymphocytes. It infiltrates the red and white pulp. It is composed of small lymphocytes, which overrun the germinal centres in the white pulp and merge with the transformed larger cells in the peripheral marginal zone. The prognosis is similar to other low-grade lymphomas in that patients often have long-term survival after splenectomy but do not respond well to chemotherapy.

Leukaemia: any leukaemia can involve the spleen. However, marked splenomegaly is typical of chronic myeloid leukaemia, hairy cell leukaemia and myelofibrosis. In the latter there is bone marrow fibrosis and extramedullary haemopoiesis occurs in the spleen.

Systemic mastocytosis: almost always involves the spleen. The mast cell nodules are seen as fibrotic masses on gross examination.

Other haematolymphoid conditions involving the spleen include: Hodgkin's lymphoma particularly the nodular sclerosis subtype, Langerhan's histiocytosis and follicular dendritic reticulum cell tumour, which is usually EBV associated at this site.

Non-haematological malignancies: angiosarcoma is the commonest non-lymphoid primary splenic malignancy. It may present with spontaneous splenic rupture or mimic a haemopoietic disease. Other malignancies are rare.

Metastatic carcinoma: is uncommon. Malignant melanoma, lung (small cell) and breast cancers are the commonest primaries to involve the spleen and can be mistaken for a haemopoietic disease. Gastric and pancreatic cancers may also show direct spread to the spleen.

Surgical Pathology Specimens – Clinical Aspects

Splenectomy may be a diagnostic procedure. The common indications for splenectomy are: traumatic rupture, suspected primary lymphoma, symptom control in massive splenomegaly, e.g., CML and correction of cytopenias in hypersplenism.

Contraindication: marrow failure where haemopoiesis in the spleen is a source of circulating blood cells.

Immediately after splenectomy an increase in WCC and platelet counts occur but this normalises in 2 or 3 weeks. In the long term there are erythrocyte abnormalities including anisocytosis, poikilocytosis, Howell–Jolly bodies and Heinz bodies. A major consequence of splenectomy is increased susceptibility to bacterial infections due to S. pneumoniae, H. influenzae and sepsis. This requires pneumococcal vaccination and lifelong antibiotic prophylaxis.

Surgical Pathology Specimens – Laboratory Protocols

Splenectomy Specimens

Usually of three types:

- incidental.
- traumatically ruptured.
- diseased spleen.

The specimen is received fresh in the laboratory and fixed according to established protocols.

- measurements:
    - length × width × depth (cm).
    - number/maximum dimensions (cm) of any capsular deficits, infarcts, cysts or tumour nodules.

- weight (g) must be taken before slicing, as blood loss from the cut surface reduces the splenic weight considerably.
- photograph if required.
- look for splenic lymph nodes and dissect them off the hilum.
- fixation: make parallel, thin slices 5 mm thick with a sharp knife. Examine each slice for focal lesions. Do not wash in tap water. Submit a 1 × 1 cm section for culture if infectious disease is suspected. Make imprints for immediate assessment.
- fix each slice flat in a container of 10% buffered formalin. For suspected sickle cell disease fix in formalin immediately after slicing.

Description

- hilum: nature of blood vessels, presence of lymph nodes and accessory spleen.
- capsule: colour, thickened with perisplenitis (sugar icing). If defect/laceration is present, record location, length, depth. Record any other focal changes.

- examine the cut surface for:
  - colour: infarcts are pale.
  - consistency: soft/diffluent in sepsis, firm in portal hypertension, wax-like in amyloidosis.
  - white pulp: size of individual nodules if prominent.
  - fibrous bands: present/ absent.
  - nodules/masses: record number, size, colour, presence of haemorrhage or necrosis.
  - diffuse involvement.

Blocks for histology

- a general recommendation is to sample any nodule larger than the adjacent white pulp.
- no abnormality in an incidental splenectomy: 4 blocks including samples of the superior, inferior borders, the hilum and the lateral convex border.
- focal gross abnormality: 2 or 3 blocks of the abnormal area depending on size and 2 blocks from uninvolved parenchyma.
- diffuse abnormality: 4 blocks.

Histopathology report

Specify: type of splenectomy, i.e., laparoscopic, partial, total. Mention reason for splenectomy, i.e., incidental, traumatic or therapeutic removal of diseased spleen. For incidental and traumatic splenectomies mention the presence or absence of tears/lacerations and any other pathology related to the cause of surgery. For therapeutic splenectomies, confirm the primary diagnosis and exclude additional pathology. Classify lymphoma/leukaemia in the spleen according to the WHO classification incorporating immunohistochemical findings.

3. Bone Marrow

Anatomy

The bone marrow is a specialised tissue of haemopoietic elements, and comprises bony and stromal tissue with definite spatial organisation. The supporting stromal tissue consists of a fine reticulin meshwork, fat and blood vessels. The amount of fat varies with age and quantity of haemopoiesis. From 50 to 80% fat is seen in marrows of adults and elderly patients. Little or no fat is seen in marrows of children and neonates as haemopoiesis occurs throughout the marrow in all bones. In adults, haemopoiesis is limited to certain areas within bone marrow of skull, vertebrae, sternum, ribs, pelvic bones and proximal long bones. The row of fat cells separating haemopoietic cells from bone trabeculae is called the first fat space. This is lost in leukaemic infiltration. The lamellar bone trabeculae contain osteoblasts and multinuclear osteoclasts on the endosteal surface and osteocytes within lacunae. In elderly patients with osteoporosis the trabeculae are thinned. Thin-walled venous sinuses are seen throughout the marrow and mature haemopoietic cells have a perisinusoidal location. Small muscular arteries and capillaries are also present.

Haemopoietic elements include the myeloid, erythroid, megakaryocytic and lymphoid cells; all of these have a common precursor stem cell. The committed stem cells give rise to the distinct cell lines. The various stages of maturation are shown in Figure 44.4. The morphology of haemopoietic cells in general is better appreciated in Giemsa-stained thin/semi-thin sections. The different types of cells and some of their features are presented in Table 44.6.

Artefacts including non-haemopoietic cells such as epidermis, skin appendages, muscle and bone tissue may be introduced into the trephine biopsy inadvertently during the biopsy procedure. The presence of epithelial elements can result in confusion with metastatic malignancy.

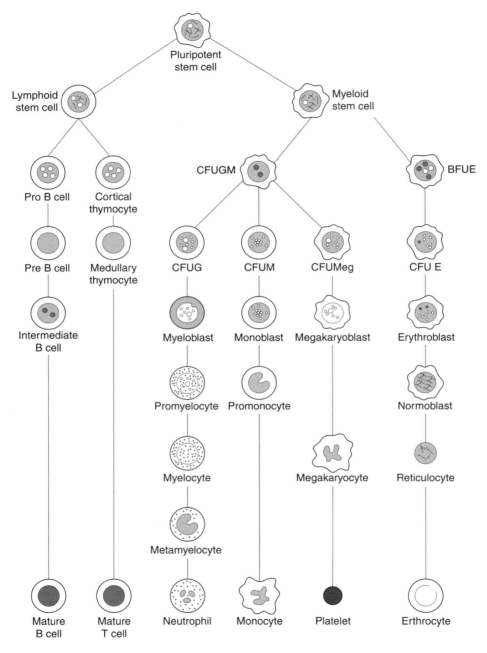

Figure 44.4. Development and maturation of haemopoietic cells.

Table 44.6. Haemopoietic cells

	Precursors	Usual location within marrow	Numbers	Cytology	Clues to pathological proliferation
Granulocytes including neutrophils & eosinophils	Myeloblasts	Immature-paratrabecular. Mature-central.	2 to 4 times the number of erythroid cells	Immature cells – high N/C ratio and granular cytoplasm. Mature – lobated nuclei and specialised granules in cytoplasm.	Excess of blasts, present in both paratrabecular and central areas.
Erythroid	Erythroblasts	Colonies in central intertrabecular areas.	1/3 to1/4 of the myeloid cells.	Immature cells – dark blue cytoplasm, round nuclei, coarse chromatin, and nucleoli attached to nuclear membrane. Mature – dark, densely staining, perfectly round nuclei.	Paratrabecular proliferation.
Megakaryocytes	Megakaryoblast	Perisinusoidal	Variable, usually at least 1 per field	Largest cells. Occur singly. Multilobated nuclei with abundant cytoplasm.	Clustering, paratrabecular location and nuclear hypolobation.
Lymphoid	Lymphoblast	Interstitial infiltrates or < 3 nodular aggregates	Up to 50% in children, 5–10% in adult marrows	Mixed population of small mature and larger lymphoid cells ± germinal centres.	> 3 aggregates/ diffuse heavy interstitial proliferation particularly if monoclonal.
Plasma cells	Lymphoblast	Perivascular	Up to 2% in adult marrows.	Mature plasma cells – eccentric nuclei with clock face chromatin, no nucleoli. Immature plasma cells – nucleolated.	Large clusters and nucleolated plasma cells.
Mast cells	Myeloblast	Perivascular or paratrabecular	Few	Basophilic coarse granules in cytoplasm, round/oval nucleus.	Increased numbers, spindle cells, fibrosis.

Clinical Presentation

Anaemia: most often detected on routine blood examination. Acute anaemia due to blood loss or haemolysis presents with signs of haemodynamic instability. Severe back pain, renal failure and haemoglobinuria may occur in acute haemolysis. Chronic anaemia irrespective of cause is associated with tiredness, shortness of breath and tachycardia. Often the symptoms are due to the underlying cause of the anaemia such as rheumatoid arthritis causing joint pains.

Polycythaemia: is defined as an increase in circulating red blood cells. The patients may be asymptomatic, have thrombotic symptoms or neurological symptoms such as vertigo, tinnitus, headache and visual disturbances.

Bleeding disorders: usually there is a history of prolonged blood loss during menstruation or following tooth extraction, childbirth or minor surgery. Bleeding into body cavities, particularly joints, causes deformity and limited mobility.

Thrombotic disorders: ischaemia of critical organs, such as gastrointestinal tract, brain and myocardium, caused by unregulated clotting within blood vessels.

Fever, malaise, weight loss, night sweats, bleeding, fatigue and increased susceptibility to infections are common features of white blood cell disorders.

Clinical Investigations

Evaluation of anaemia is directed toward its classification as a hypoproliferative disorder (e.g., aplasia or hypoplasia), maturation disorder (e.g., megaloblastic anaemia), due to blood loss or due to haemolysis (e.g., haemoglobinopathies).

Full blood picture, red blood cell indices, reticulocyte count and red cell morphology aid classification.

Reticulocyte index < 2.5 suggests a maturation disorder or a hypoproliferative disorder. High reticulocyte index is usual in haemolytic anaemias.

Iron levels and iron storage indices: low in iron deficiency anaemia.

Serum erythropoietin levels and red cell mass: increased in polycythemia.

Bleeding time: is a sensitive measure of platelet function.

Platelet count: normal ranges 150,000–450,000/μL. Decreased platelet count increases risk of bleeding from severe trauma or spontaneously – petechiae in skin or intracranial haemorrhage.

Prothrombin time, partial thromboplastin time, thrombin time, clot lysis, clot solubility: are tests for detecting coagulation defects.

White blood cell count and differential leukocyte counts: valuable in diagnosing acute and chronic leukaemias, infections and inflammatory disorders such as lupus erythematosus.

Marrow aspirate: for definitive diagnosis of haematological disorders and haematological malignances.

Role of the trephine biopsy: complementary to the aspirate. Main uses are – evaluation of cellularity particularly if there has been a dry tap due to a packed, fibrotic or empty marrow, spatial relationships between constituent cell types, enumeration and distribution of cells, staging of lymphomas, assessing lymphoid aggregates, staging other malignant disease, assessing fibrosis and post-chemotherapy changes (residual disease/remission/relapse).

Other investigations are directed by clinical suspicion.

Pathological Conditions

Many haematological diseases can be diagnosed on microscopy of the bone marrow aspirate and ancillary investigations including flow cytometry and molecular biological techniques. The following paragraphs emphasise those conditions in which the trephine biopsy has a definite diagnostic role. Aspirate, trephine and peripheral blood findings must be closely correlated.

Non-neoplastic Conditions

Reactive hyperplasia: occurs commonly in a wide range of infections, autoimmune disorders including immune thrombocytopenias, haemolytic anaemia, and megaloblastic anaemia and as a non-specific response to systemic malignancy. A variation is the occurrence of reactive/benign lymphoid aggregates. These are non-paratrabecular and polyclonal.

Granulomatous inflammation: the causes and histological features are similar to granulomas that occur elsewhere in the body, e.g., tuberculosis, sarcoidosis, reaction to malignancy.

HIV and AIDS: The marrow can show specific features such as neoplastic infiltration, opportunistic infections, absent iron stores and Parvovirus-induced red cell aplasia.

Aplastic anaemia: is diagnosed when marrow cellularity is < 25% of normality for the age. It may be congenital or acquired from exposure to toxins, viral infections or drugs. There is marked reduction in erythroid, myeloid and megakaryocytic series and increase in fat, perivascular plasma cells and lymphocytes.

The trephine biopsy is useful in diagnosis of megaloblastic anaemia but the features can be mistaken for acute leukaemia, hence, correlation with aspirate findings is mandatory.

Neoplastic Conditions

Acute leukaemias: the FAB and the EGIL systems of classification are widely used and most acute leukaemias can be diagnosed as prognostically distinct entities on peripheral blood and bone marrow aspirate examination with immunophenotyping. The trephine is useful when marrow aspiration fails due to a dry tap. The presence of undifferentiated/poorly differentiated blast cells is diagnostic of leukaemia even in hypocellular marrows where the differential diagnosis includes aplastic anaemia and myelofibrosis. The morphological classification and recognition of well-defined FAB entities is difficult on biopsies but can be done using a broad panel of immuno-histochemical stains. Post-chemotherapy, if the disease is sensitive, the tumour cells die and the marrow becomes hypocellular. Regeneration of stromal/fat cells occurs followed by restoration of haemopoiesis. Growth factors and chemotherapeutic regimens used can cause alarming changes in the quantity and quality of haemopoiesis. After bone marrow transplantation, the changes are similar.

Myelodysplastic syndromes (MDS): a group of heterogeneous disorders classified according to the FAB system into five types based on bone marrow smears. These are: refractory anaemia (RA), refractory anaemia with ring sideroblasts (RARS), chronic myelomonocytic leukaemia (CMML), refractory anaemia with excess blasts (RAEB) and refractory anaemia with excess blasts in transformation (RAEB-t). The diagnostically helpful features in the trephine biopsy are: ALIPs (abnormally located immature precursors), hypercellularity, trilineage dysplasia – particularly striking in megakaryocytes – and increased reticulin fibrosis. Patients present with persistently decreased blood counts. The MDS are preleukaemic disorders and have a variable potential to transform to acute leukaemia.

Myeloproliferative disorders: include chronic myeloid leukaemia, essential thrombocythemia and polycythemia rubra vera. These are characterised by increased leukocyte count and Philadelphia chromosome, marked thrombocythaemia and an increased red cell mass respectively. The marrow findings overlap in all three diseases; usually there is panmyeloid hyperplasia with abnormal clustering of megakaryocytes.

Primary/chronic idiopathic myelofibrosis: a disease of unknown aetiology, with a prolonged clinical course and presents in adults at a mean age of 60 years. Secondary myelofibrosis evolves from pre-existing myeloproliferative disorders, some lymphoproliferative disorders and acute leukaemia. Dense reticulin fibrosis and pan myeloid hyperplasia are features seen in the trephine biopsy.

Lymphoproliferative malignancies: include acute and chronic lymphoid leukaemias, special types such as hairy cell leukaemia and lymphomas secondarily involving the bone marrow.

Hairy cell leukaemia is a chronic B-cell lymphoproliferative disorder involving the blood, bone marrow and the spleen simultaneously. It presents with pancytopenia and splenomegaly. The hairy cytoplasmic projections are seen in peripheral blood but the cells have characteristic haloes and there is increased reticulin fibrosis in the trephine biopsy.

Lymphomatous involvement of the marrow is common in low-grade lymphomas, i.e., follicular lymphoma and lymphocytic lymphoma (diagnosed arbitrarily as chronic lymphocytic leukaemia when absolute lymphocyte count in the peripheral blood exceeds 5,000/µl), mantle cell lymphoma and some high-grade lymphomas such as peripheral T-cell lymphoma and Burkitt's lymphoma. The pattern of involvement may be obvious or subtle, diffuse, focal, non-trabecular, focal paratrabecular or interstitial. Sometimes appropriate immunostains are required to demonstrate involvement, e.g., CD30 in anaplastic large cell lymphoma, CD 20/CD3 in T-cell-rich B-cell lymphoma. The cytology and architecture may be similar to the lymph node involved or discordant. Classic Hodgkin's lymphoma involves the marrow in approximately 5% of cases. This is more common in the lymphocyte-depleted subtype and requires the same diagnostic criteria as in a lymph node for a definite diagnosis.

Metastases: are most common from breast, prostate, lung, stomach, colon and renal cancers in adults. In children the most common metastatic tumours in the marrow are neuroblastoma, Ewing's sarcoma, rhabdomyosarcoma, retinoblastoma and clear cell sarcoma of the kidney.

Myeloma: is a monoclonal proliferation of plasma cells that form nodules, large aggregates and sheets in the trephine biopsy. The diagnosis is based on a combination of clinical, morphologic features, laboratory data and radiological findings. It is usually incurable with a median survival of 3 years and 10% survival at 10 years.

Miscellaneous: some bony abnormalities such as osteoporosis and Paget's disease can be diagnosed in a trephine biopsy.

Surgical Pathology Specimens – Clinical Aspects

Trephine Biopsy

There are several reusable and disposable commercially available instruments for performing a bone marrow trephine biopsy procedure in adult and paediatric patients. The choice is based on safety, convenience and quality of the specimen obtained.

Smaller-gauge needles are used in children and patients with severe osteoporosis.

The procedure should be done under sterile conditions. The patients are given suitable local anaesthesia/analgesia and positioned properly for the procedure. The posterior superior iliac spines are the most favoured sites for aspiration. Anterior iliac crest or sternal puncture are also used. The aim is to obtain a biopsy specimen of adequate length (usually 1–1.5 cm in length) avoiding crushing and excess haemorrhage.

Surgical Pathology Specimens – Laboratory Protocols

All material should be submitted for histology. If the biopsies are obtained from multiple sites, these are submitted separately.

Make imprints prior to fixation.

Description

- number and length (mm) of each fragment.
- colour, consistency and whether homogeneous.

Procedure

- fixation: routinely fixed immediately in 10% buffered formalin or B5 fixative. Other fixatives in use include Zenker's fixative and 2% formol acetic acid.
- fixation time: 48–72 hrs. Further fixation results in loss of antigenicity and lesser fixation yields poor morphology.

- decalcification: should be carefully controlled and limited to softening the bone enough to permit even sectioning.
- embedding: the choice between plastic resin and paraffin wax largely depends on individual laboratory preference. The morphology is better preserved in plastic-embedded semi-thin sections but many pathologists are unfamiliar with this preparation. The advantage of paraffin embedding lies in familiarity, cost effectiveness and antigen preservation that allows for better immunohistochemistry.
- sectioning: 2–4 μm sections are ideal for good morphological detail.
- staining: both Giemsa and H&E are essential for routine interpretation. Additional stains for iron and reticulin are commonly used.

Histopathology report

Should contain all clinical details including aspirate findings as stated on the request form, comment on technical preparation and whether the sample is representative. A proforma helps in maintaining uniformity and serves as a checklist for all items that need to be mentioned in the report. These include: length of the trephine; number of intertrabecular spaces; cellularity; normality or otherwise of erythroid, myeloid and megakaryocytic series; presence and distribution of lymphocytes, plasma cells, and other lymphoid cells; other cells including extramedullary cells if present; granulomata; reticulin; iron stores; sinusoids and results of immunohistochemistry if used. The report should present a unifying conclusion and suggest further investigation for appropriate management of the patient.

Miscellaneous Specimens

Damian T McManus

45

Miscellaneous Specimens and Ancillary Techniques

- Needle Core Biopsies.
- Fine Needle Aspirates.
- Cytospins, Liquid-based Cytology and Cell Blocks.
- Specimen Photography.
- Specimen Radiography.
- Frozen Section.
- Ancillary Techniques: Immunohistochemistry and immunofluorescence.
  - Flow Cytometry.
  - In-situ hybridisation including FISH.
  - Electron Microscopy.
  - Cytogenetics.
  - Molecular Genetics and Proteomics.
- Tissue Banking and the use of surplus tissue for research.

1. Needle Core Biopsies

Minimally invasive techniques for diagnosis and treatment are increasingly important in many fields of medicine and this has implications for the types of specimens received by pathologists.

Biopsy needles range in calibre from 22 gauge (skinny core needle) through 18 gauge to the standard 14 gauge Tru-Cut needle. The introduction of automated, spring-loaded 18 gauge core biopsy guns has been accompanied by a dramatic increase in the use of core needle biopsy of the breast, prostate and bone or soft tissue masses. Such biopsies are increasingly performed by a radiologist or specialist clinician using ultrasound guidance. Stereotactic core biopsy is frequently used by radiologists in the investigation of breast lesions such as microcalcification detected by screening mammography.

CT-guided percutaneous biopsy is an invaluable tool in the assessment of deep-seated, inaccessible tumours. It may be used to evaluate peripherally located lung lesions, anterior mediastinal masses or retroperitoneal/mediastinal lymph node masses. Percutaneous liver or kidney biopsy are well established techniques both in the investigation of tumours and medical conditions.

Core biopsy may establish a specific histological diagnosis of malignancy prior to radical surgical excision/resection or enable radical or palliative radiotherapy and/or chemotherapy to be administered by oncologists. It may also confirm metastatic disease, although fine needle aspiration cytology can often represent a less invasive alternative. The increasing use of sophisticated radiological imaging modalities such as PET scanning may reduce the need for needle core biopsy to confirm metastatic disease. Core biopsy may also be used to stage lymphoma or to detect recurrent disease. Although excision biopsy of an easily accessible superficial lymph node is still recommended to make a primary diagnosis of lymphoma and for subtyping, it is increasingly acknowledged that core biopsy may be more appropriate for deeply situated lesions or in the elderly and infirm.

Transrectal ultrasound-directed biopsy is commonly used in the evaluation of the prostate in patients with a raised serum PSA. Smaller-calibre 18G biopsy needles can reduce the complications associated with this procedure including infection and clot retention without compromising sensitivity and specificity. However, it can be difficult to embed multiple fine tissue cores in a single wax block and a variety of techniques have been proposed to check that they are fully faced on sectioning including marking the biopsies with ink so that they are more easily seen.

The trend towards small-gauge needle core biopsies has been accompanied by the increasing use of immunohistochemistry and other ancillary investigations in the diagnosis and classification of cancer. The conservation of tissue for these techniques must be balanced by the need to examine an adequate number of levels to detect focal areas of involvement by cancer. These two somewhat conflicting requirements may be resolved by carefully levelling into the tissue and storing intervening sections as ribbons. These can be used subsequently for immunohistochemistry if needed and it is also possible to select the most representative level for the appropriate stains. Such an approach is particularly relevant to prostate needle core biopsies and endoscopic biopsies from the upper gastrointestinal tract.

Concerns have been raised about tumour diagnosis using small biopsies. Clearly, tumour heterogeneity is not uncommon and small biopsies may not be representative of a large lesion. Correlation with radiological and other clinical findings is important. It can be difficult to assess cell size and to accurately subtype malignant lymphomas in needle core biopsies; they are also particularly susceptible to compression artefact.

2. Fine Needle Aspirates

Fine needle aspiration cytology (FNAC) may also be used as an alternative to core biopsy. Air-dried slides may be stained immediately with a modified May Grünwald Giemsa stain and examined in a small side room in an outpatient setting. Slides may also be fixed in alcohol-based fixatives. This should be done immediately to avoid drying artefact. Papanicolaou and H&E stains are routinely used.

FNAC is particularly useful in the assessment of superficial, palpable breast lumps and lesions around the head and neck such as thyroid nodules, salivary gland lesions or enlarged lymph nodes. FNA may also be performed under radiological guidance and is generally less traumatic than core biopsy. However, the technique has its limitations. Diagnostic accuracy depends on adequate sampling of the lesion under investigation, good preparation and staining of the slides and careful interpretation by an experienced cytopathologist with due consideration given to the clinical and radiological findings. It is not possible to provide a detailed review here but in general, best results are obtained when a large volume of aspirates is examined by a limited number of pathologists. If pathologists are not actively involved in aspiration then ideally rapid review will provide immediate feedback to the aspirator on the quantity of aspirated material and on the preparation.

It can be difficult to obtain sufficient material for extended panels of immunohistochemical markers. It is generally not possible to reliably distinguish between in situ and invasive malignancy in the breast, and often material from areas of microcalcification detected at screening is scant. Precise categorisation of borderline lesions discovered in breast screening programmes can also be problematic. FNA and core biopsy may be performed simultaneously for impalpable, screen-detected breast lesions and provide complementary information.

3. Cytospins, Liquid-based Cytology and Cell Blocks

The interpretation of non-gynecological cytology specimens, (FNA, cell effusions and respiratory specimens) may be greatly facilitated by the use of immunocytochemical staining techniques, described in more detail below.

A variety of techniques have been used to prepare such specimens. A cytospin can be used to make slides from cell suspensions obtained from effusions, needle washings from FNAs or other specimens. The cells may be partially obscured by blood or proteinaceous debris and the preparation can be improved by lysis of red cells and/or the addition of agents such as polyethylene glycol to the cell suspension. Alternative methods of processing are also available such as liquid-based cytology, exemplified by the proprietary Thin Prep system in which vortexing of the cell suspension is followed by transfer to a slide by a membrane using gentle vacuum suction. This is claimed to reduce obscuring debris and to produce a representative cell sample on the slide. Cell blocks may be prepared from effusions or FNAs if a clot forms. This is transferred to formalin for fixation and processed through paraffin wax as a small biopsy, providing complementary morphological information to that of the direct smear preparations and also suitable for conventional immunohistochemistry.

4. Specimen Photography

An accurate macroscopic description of a gross specimen is often vital in making the correct diagnosis (e.g., the pattern of involvement in inflammatory bowel disease) and in accurately staging a malignant tumour. With the decline of the autopsy and the controversy surrounding organ retention, macroscopic specimen photographs also play an important role in undergraduate teaching, and may be correlated with radiological images in today's integrated courses. Macroscopic specimen photography has also been used to audit the quality of mesorectal excision in rectal cancers and it is an important communication medium in multidisciplinarian team meetings. Another factor that may contribute to its increasing use includes participation of BMSs in specimen dissection and in the selection of tissue for histology; specimen dissection is inherently destructive and sequential pictures can be used to record key features of the specimen.

The principles of specimen photography are described in many standard textbooks of surgical pathology and some reviews. It is important that there is a clean, textureless background that is suitably illuminated. Reflective glare and wet highlights should be avoided by switching off the room lights, correctly positioning the illumination system and blotting the cut surface of the specimen. The specimen should be properly centred and orientated. In general, the cut surface usually provides more information than the external aspect of a specimen. It is important to trim away fat and other extraneous tissue and to slice the tissue cleanly. It may be advantageous to open ducts, etc. to highlight these structures but the inclusion of probes and forceps or other objects can be distracting.

The use of a stand is recommended. A 35 mm camera may be used. A smaller lens aperture (higher f-stop) will maximise the depth of field for specimens of a substantial height and many photographers will use a number of slightly different exposures. Polaroid cameras offer a convenient method to produce specimen pictures rapidly that can then be marked as to the origin of blocks for histology. However, such pictures are often of poor quality and it is not easy to produce 35 mm slides from the prints. Digital photography can be used to produce high-quality images relatively cheaply and hard copy rapidly. Digital images may be archived easily on CD ROM and software systems exist that allow the incorporation of digital images into biopsy files. Non-specialised equipment can give good results and the use of a simple scanner has recently been advocated.

5. Specimen Radiography

Specimen radiography may be used in a variety of different specimens for a range of purposes:

- breast: to identify and confirm excision of small impalpable lesions detected by screening mammography or to localise areas of microcalcification in excision and core biopsies.
- bone and joint: to delineate the extent of a tumour involving bone.
- bioprosthetic heart valves: to document the degree of calcification.

6. Frozen Section

The number of frozen sections appears to be declining in the United Kingdom, due in part to improved preoperative diagnosis of breast lumps and many other tumours by FNA, needle core or endoscopic biopsy. This is in contrast to the situation in North America where frozen sections and intra-operative consultations are very common.

The use of frozen section should be restricted to those cases where the result will change the intra-operative management of the patient.

Frozen sections are used in a wide variety of clinical situations

- confirmation of excised tissue, e.g., parathyroidectomy versus lymph node or a thyroid nodule.
- evaluation of a suspicious lymph node, liver or lung nodule as part of an operative staging procedure, or prequel to consideration of radical surgery.
- determination of a lung, pancreatic or ampullary mass prior to proceeding to lobectomy or a Whipple's procedure.
- clearance of resection margins, e.g., gastrectomy, pulmonary lobectomy or resections for squamous cell carcinoma of the upper aerodigestive tract.
- diagnosis of suspicious abdominopelvic masses at laparotomy, e.g., ovarian tumours.

Specimens for frozen section are best examined using a safety cabinet. As the tissue is not fixed, full precautions must be taken against blood-borne Category Three infections. Thin fragments of tissue (no more than 2–3 mm thick and no wider than the diameter of the chuck) should be removed by a scalpel and placed on the surface of a metal chuck in a blob of embedding medium such as OCT compound (Tissue Tek) so that the tissue is covered. The chuck is rapidly cooled by standing it in a small volume of liquid nitrogen or using a proprietary aerosol spray such as CryoSpray Freezer Spray (Cell Path PLC). The sections are then cut using a microtome and cryostat and stained routinely by haematoxylin and eosin.

Touch imprints can be made by gently smearing the fresh tissue against a glass slide. This is allowed to air dry and then stained by Giemsa or proprietary stains such as Diff Quick. This can be very useful in the evaluation of lymph nodes and many tumours providing complementary cytological detail that cannot be appreciated on frozen section. Immunocytochemistry and FISH may be performed on touch imprints of tumours made onto suitable adhesive coated slides (e.g., APES).

Relative contra-indications to frozen section include certain infections such as suspected tuberculosis or where the frozen section is unlikely to yield a clinically useful result and may compromise the final diagnosis (e.g., an impalpable breast lesion containing microcalcification picked up at screening). Some diagnoses cannot be readily made on frozen section; classical examples being the distinctions between follicular carcinoma and adenoma of the thyroid and lymph node hyperplasia and follicular lymphoma.

7. Ancillary Techniques

Immunohistochemistry and Immunofluorescence

The development of antigen-retrieval techniques and the increasing range of monoclonal and polyclonal antibodies have been accompanied by widespread application of immunohistochemistry to routinely fixed paraffin wax-embedded material. Adequate, controlled fixation is still crucial in obtaining the best results from immunohistochemistry, but there is little indication for the use of fixatives other than formalin outside a research setting.

Heat-mediated antigen-retrieval techniques (HMAR) are particularly important for the detection of nuclear antigens such as ER (oestrogen receptor) and Ki67, low-density surface antigens, e.g., CD5 and other surface antigens such as CD20. Both microwaving and pressure cooking have been used for HMAR, with citrate or EDTA buffer. HMAR avoids the risk of over digestion and loss of morphology that may accompany pretreatments with proteolytic enzymes but can lead to loss of adherence of the section to the slide in a significant fraction of cases. This technical problem may be circumvented by the use of slides pretreated with an adhesive material such as APES.

Other technical advances in immunohistochemistry include the development of highly sensitive detection systems and the increasing use of automated immunostainers. New, polymer-based detection systems (e.g., Envision, Dako) may give superior sensitivity to existing methods but many laboratories will continue to use more established ABC techniques (e.g., Duet, Dako) which appear adequate for routine use. The use of immunohistochemistry has been reported to have risen 600% over the last few years in some laboratories and automation is helpful in managing this rising workload. It may also offer more reproducible staining with less batch-to-batch variation, particularly important with stains for predictive markers such as ER or HER2, which are assessed in a semi-quantitative fashion.

The use of immunohistochemistry continues to increase rapidly. It plays a crucial role in tumour diagnosis in particular and especially in the differential diagnosis of tumour types with similar morphological appearances. For example, in the diagnosis of small round blue cell tumours and soft-tissue lesions and in the differentiation of malignant mesothelioma and metastatic adenocarcinoma. The accurate classification of lymphoma subtypes is crucially dependent on the use of appropriate antibody panels and interpretation of the results; indeed, the latest classifications of lymphoma fully incorporate both immunophenotyping and genotyping results. Panels of immunohistochemical stains may also be used to help determine the likely origin of metastatic carcinoma where the primary remains occult (Table 45.1).

The increasing use of diagnostic immunohistochemistry can cause problems. Anomalous or unexpected patterns of staining may be potentially confusing or indeed misleading and result in an erroneous diagnosis, unless the pathologist is aware of such a possibility. It is generally better to use panels of markers rather than to rely on one or two isolated stains. The use of very extended antibody panels with little consideration given to a differential morphological diagnosis is likely to confuse and be very expensive. Standardised panels are easier to order and to organise on automated immunostainers and may assist in the calculation of costs. Technical pitfalls may also trap the unwary and the results of immunohistochemistry should always be considered critically. Judicious use of positive and negative controls, and correlation with morphological, clinical and radiological findings are essential.

Immunohistochemistry has also been used to detect prognostic and predictive biomarkers in malignant tumours and in pre-malignant conditions. The use of prognostic factors is mainly a research activity with the exception of ER/PR receptors in breast cancer and proliferation indices (Ki67) in lesions such as non-Hodgkin's lymphoma, gastrointestinal stromal tumours and haemangiopericytoma. In multivariate analysis, many new "prognostic biomarkers" do not show effects on prognosis independent of histological grade or tumour stage.

Table 45.1. Immunoprofile of cancer types

System	Tumour/Condition	Marker Panel
Head and Neck	Salivary Gland Tumours	Calponin, S100, SmActin, AE1/AE3
	Thyroid Tumours	Thyroglobulin, Calcitonin, CEA, TTF1
Gastrointestinal	Oesophageal Tumours	AE1/AE3, CAM5.2, CK7, CK20
	Barrett's Oesophagus	Villin, Ki67, cyclinD1, p53
	Gastric and Small bowel	CK7, CK20, CEA
	Colorectal Tumours	CK7, CK20, CEA
	Hepatocellular Carcinoma	αFetoprotein, HEPAR1, CEA polyclonal
	Pancreatico-biliary Carcinoma	CK7, CK20, CEA, CA19.9, CA125
	Gastrointestinal Stromal Tumours	CD117, CD34, Sm Actin, Desmin, S100, Ki67, vimentin
	Neuroendocrine Carcinoids	Chromogranin, CD56, gastrin, insulin, glucagon
Respiratory	Small Cell Carcinoma	CD45, CAM5.2, CD56, chromogranin
	Non-small Cell Carcinoma	TTF1, PE10, EP4
	Malignant Mesothelioma	Calretinin, Thrombomodulin, HBME1, CK5/6, WT1, EMA, EP4, CEA
	Salivary Gland-type Tumours	Calponin, S100, SmActin, AE1/AE3
Gynaecological	Ovarian Carcinoma	CK7, CK20, CEA, CA125, WT1
	Sex Cord Stromal	Calretinin, Vimentin, AE1/AE3, Inhibin, EMA
	Uterus, Mesenchymal	CD10, Desmin, Sm actin
	Endometrial Carcinoma	CK7, CK20, CD10, ER, p53
	Cervix-GGIN	BCL-2, P16, Ki67
	Cervical Adenocarcinoma	CEA, vimentin and ER (both –)
Genitourinary	Renal Carcinoma	CK7,CK20, EMA, vimentin
	Prostate	PSA, PSAP, 34βE12
	Transitional Carcinoma	CK7, CK20, p53
	Testicular Tumours	PLAP, αFetoprotein, CAM5.2, EMA, CD30
Breast	Breast Carcinoma	ER, PR, HER2/neu, SmActin, CK5/6, CK14, CK8/18, E-cadherin
Soft Tissue	Spindle Cell Sarcomas	Vimentin, CD34, SmActin, desmin, CAM5.2, AE1/AE3, S100
	Small round blue cell tumours	CD 45, S100, CD99, desmin, WT1, NB84, vimentin, SmActin, CD56
Skin	Melanoma	S100, MelanA, HMB45
Haematopoetic	Lymphomas	CD45, CD43, CD5, CD10, CD20, CD21, CD23, CD3, CD15, CD30, CD56, CD57, ALK, cyclinD1, MIB1, κ&λ, BCL-2, BCL-6, BCL-10, LMP-1, EBER, granzyme B, myeloperoxidase

These panels can be adapted and modified to suit individual cases and preferences. It is not really possible to summarise this rapidly expanding and complex area with a simple table. Queries about immunohistochemical staining may be answered by logging onto www.immunoquery.com. Alternatively, a vade mecum, in the form of a help file, may be downloaded from http://ourworld.compuserve.com/homepages/paul.bish/

A tissue microarray consists of an array of small-calibre core biopsies of tumours (or other tissues) prepared either prospectively from resected tumour specimens or retrospectively from paraffin-embedded tumour tissue. High-density arrays can have hundreds of cores on a single glass slide. This innovation represents an "industrial revolution" for such biomarker investigations and should greatly facilitate large-scale immunohistochemical investigations.

Predictive biomarkers are used to predict the response of a malignancy to either conventional treatments such as chemotherapy and radiotherapy or novel targeted therapies. Examples include CD 20 and Rituximab in certain B cell lymphomas, CD 117 (c-kit) and STI 571 in gastrointestinal stromal tumours and HER2/neu and Trastuzumab in breast cancer. ER/PR and HER2/neu are good examples of biomarkers that are both prognostic and predictive and that have clinical utility in the choice of treatments for patients with breast cancer. The expression levels of such markers in tumours vary both within and between tumours and both technical issues and inter-observer variation may affect the validity and reproducibility of the results.

The increasingly important role of immunohistochemistry and the need for standardisation of assays for predictive markers such as ER has prompted the development of external quality-assurance schemes to ensure acceptable technical standards. Methods have also been developed to improve the reproducibility of scoring, the best examples being the "Histo" and "Quick Score" methods used to score ER expression in breast cancer.

Immunofluorescence continues to be used in many laboratories for the evaluation of renal biopsies and skin biopsies in conditions characterised by the deposition of immune complexes or auto-antibody binding, fluorescence providing high resolution and precise localisation. Immunofluorescence ideally requires frozen sections and specialised fluorescence microscopy equipment. As fluorescent preparations fade, photomicroscopy is needed to provide a permanent record and some laboratories have abandoned this technique for conventional immunoperoxidase.

Flow Cytometry

Flow cytometry is a technique that allows the measurement of fluorescence intensity of large numbers of cells in suspension. Cells may be labelled using antibodies conjugated to fluorescent reporter molecules and it is possible to accurately detect the fraction of cells in a population expressing an antigen. Two or more antigens can also be examined simultaneously. This technique has found an important diagnostic role in leukaemia and lymphoma subtyping. Propidium iodide is a fluorescent dye that binds stoichiometrically to DNA. Tumour cell suspensions can be prepared from paraffin blocks and it is possible to produce DNA histograms based on the analysis of thousands of tumour cells. This can be used to measure S phase fraction or to detect aneuploid DNA content although they generally do not emerge as prognostic markers independent of stage and grade and therefore this technique is not routinely used. Detection of a triploid DNA content is of value in the differentiation between complete and partial hydatidiform mole but this distinction can often be made on histology and is not vital clinically.

In-situ Hybridisation including FISH

This technique has been regarded as a research tool but improved technologies (proprietary kits and integrated instruments for automated immunohistochemistry and in-situ hybridisation) are leading to clinical applications. In-situ hybridisation may be used to detect viral nucleic acid, examples being the detection of EBV in post-transplant lymphoproliferative disorders or HPV subtyping in cervical biopsies. In-situ hybridisation for κ and λ light chain mRNA may have advantages over conventional immunohistochemistry. Fluorescence in-situ hybridisation (FISH) may be used to detect karyotypic abnormalities in the intact interphase nucleus such as HER2/neu amplification in breast cancer, particularly in patients with equivocal immunohistochemistry, and n-myc amplification in neuroblastoma. It can also be used to detect translocations but this is technically very difficult and has not been adopted widely. The development of antibodies detecting fusion gene proteins (e.g., NPM-ALK) and the availability of PCR and rt PCR (reverse transcriptase polymerase chain reaction) based methods for translocation detection may prevent the further development of such assays. FISH requires access to a good fluorescence microscope with appropriate filter sets and a low-light CCDTV camera to capture and digitise images. It is a specialised technique only available in a small number of large centres. Routinely fixed and processed paraffin sections may be used but the technique is equally applicable to touch imprints or similar cytological preparations.

Electron Microscopy

The increasing application of immunohistochemistry and pressures to contain costs have led to a decline in the use of electron microscopy, which is usually only available in large institutions.

Nonetheless, EM can still be very useful in the evaluation of renal biopsies and in the differential diagnosis of paediatric small round blue cell tumours and high-grade pleomorphic sarcomas. It can also help in the differentiation of malignant mesothelioma from adenocarcinoma and can be used on cytology specimens. Although paraffin-embedded material can be processed for EM, the best results are obtained when small cubes (~1 mm^3) of fresh tissue are fixed without delay in a solution such as 3% glutaraldehyde in cacodylate buffer.

Cytogenetics

Metaphase cytogenetics has become an established technique in the evaluation of leukaemias and other haematological conditions. Although it is not used routinely in solid tumours, the detection of specific translocations or other cytogenetic abnormalities may be useful in paediatric and soft tissue tumours. Metaphase cytogenetics requires fresh tissue which should be taken under sterile conditions. Small cubes of minced tissue are placed in tissue culture medium and sent to the cytogenetics laboratory. More detailed karyotypes can now be gleaned from metaphase spreads due to improved chromosome banding techniques and technical innovations such as chromosome painting and spectral karyotyping. These techniques have an established role in the classification of leukaemias, lymphomas and myeloproliferative disorders in large centres and may be used in solid tumours such as kidney tumours, small round blue cell tumours of childhood and soft tissue lesions.

Molecular Genetics and Proteomics

Nucleic acid and protein may be extracted from fresh tissue and used as substrate for a wide range of investigative techniques usually performed as part of a research study. However, certain tumour types such as lymphomas, paediatric small round cell tumours and soft tissue sarcomas harbour tumour-specific genetic abnormalities, usually translocations that may be of diagnostic and prognostic relevance.

RNA extracted from tumours and tissues can be hybridised to cDNA or oligonucleotide arrays, techniques variously described as transcriptional profiling or molecular fingerprinting. These high-throughput techniques generate enormous quantities of data and have necessitated new bioinformatics approaches. The pattern of gene transcription – "the transcriptome" – may be used to predict prognostic or behavioural differences within morphologically homogeneous or indistinguishable groups.

It is also possible to test for clonality and cell lineage in lymphomas by detecting immunoglobulin heavy chain or T-cell receptor gene rearrangements. Many of these assays now routinely use PCR or rt-PCR technology and can be adapted so that the impure, partially degraded DNA and mRNA that is extracted from paraffin-embedded material can serve as a template. However, there will be a significant failure rate of such assays from paraffin and some techniques will only work on unfixed material. It is therefore preferable to prospectively collect snap-frozen tissue from lesions where the use of such techniques is anticipated. Even relatively small biopsies can be used for a wide range of investigative techniques, if handled carefully. Small biopsies can be bisected. One half can be used to make touch imprints for FISH or immunocytochemistry and further bisected for EM and snap freezing. The other half can be processed through to paraffin wax.

Protein may also be extracted from tissues and analysed by 2D PAGE, western blotting and variants of mass spectroscopy such as SELDI. These are specialised research techniques and require fresh tissue as formalin fixation irreversibly denatures proteins.

8. Tissue Banking and the Use of Surplus Tissue for Research

The increasing use of minimally invasive techniques and the advent of screening programmes for breast and cervical carcinoma have been accompanied by a reduction in the size and amount of tumour tissue submitted and an increased range of investigative techniques. Radiotherapy and/or neoadjuvant chemotherapy has been used in the treatment of oesophageal, rectal, breast and cervical carcinoma and when successful there may be very little evidence of residual tumour. Pathologists have an important role in the triage of tissue and in the selection of the most appropriate ancillary techniques to assist diagnosis. Moreover, pathologists must ensure that the removal of tissue for research projects (which may be led by basic scientists and usually involve exciting, cutting-edge technologies as described above) does not compromise the diagnosis, staging or assessment of resection margins, which remain fundamental to optimal patient care.

The controversy in the United Kingdom related to the use of retained organs and tissues removed at autopsy for research and teaching has led to a reconsideration of the ethical and legal framework surrounding the use of surplus biopsy tissue for research. Detailed guidelines are available from the MRC and the Royal College of Pathologists. Generally, prospective investigations involving the procurement of fresh tissue should have been considered and approved by an official ethics committee. Informed consent from the patient is usually needed. It is not always feasible to obtain consent retrospectively for archived tissue and suitably anonymised studies may be permitted. Some Trusts have convened tissue committees specifically to deal with the ethical and practical issues outlined above.

Clinical Request Form Abbreviations

General

adeno	adenocarcinoma
AIDS	acquired immune deficiency syndrome
B9	benign
Bx	biopsy
Ca	carcinoma
CIS	carcinoma in situ
C/O	complaining of
coronal	at right angles to the sagittal plane dividing into anterior and posterior halves
CT scan	computerised tomography scan
CXR	chest X-ray
CXT	chemotherapy
Δ	(differential) diagnosis
DXT	radiotherapy
FNAB	fine needle aspiration biopsy
FNA(C)	fine needle aspiration (cytology)
FUP	follow up
HIV	human immunodeficiency virus
H/O	history of
HPE	histopathology examination
Ix	investigation
L (t)	left
MAI	mycobacterium avium intracellulare
MRI	magnetic resonance imaging
NAD	nothing abnormal detected
NCB	needle core biopsy
NG	neoplasm, new growth
O/E	on examination
P/C	presenting complaint
PET	positron emission tomography
P(M)H	past (medical) history
1°	primary neoplasm
PUO	pyrexia (fever) of unknown origin
?	query
R (t)	right
R/O	rule out

Rx	resection
sagittal	anteroposterior plane
SCF	supraclavicular fossa
2°	secondary neoplasm
∴	therefore
Tx	treatment
U and E	urea and electrolytes
USS	ultrasound scan
x/7	x days
x/52	x weeks
x/12	x months
yr	year

Gastrointestinal Specimens

AFP	alpha fetoprotein: serum/tissue marker of hepatocellular carcinoma or germ cell tumour
AIN	anal intraepithelial neoplasia
ALT	alanine aminotransferase
APC	adenomatous polyposis coli (see FAP)
AP(R)	abdominoperineal (resection)
AR	anterior resection
AST	aspartate aminotransferase
AXR	abdominal X-ray
Ba enema	barium enema
Ba meal	barium meal
CA19–9	serum/tissue marker of pancreatic or upper GI malignancy
CD	Crohn's disease or coeliac disease
CEA	carcinoembryonic antigen – serum/tissue marker of intestinal malignancy
(C)IBD	(chronic) inflammatory bowel disease
CLO	columnar lined oesophagus (Barrett's)
CMV	cytomegalovirus
CRM	circumferential radial margin
D1–4	parts of the duodenum
DALM	dysplasia associated lesion or mass
DU	duodenal ulcer
EATCL	enteropathy associated (or type) T cell lymphoma
ECL	enterochromaffin-like cell
EGC	early gastric cancer
ELUS	endoluminal ultrasound
EMR	endoscopic mucosal resection
ERCP	endoscopic retrograde cholangiopancreatography
FAP	familial adenomatous polyposis coli (also APC)
GANT	gastrointestinal autonomic nerve tumour
GFD	gluten-free diet
GIST	gastrointestinal stromal tumour
GOR	gastroesophageal reflux
GU	gastric ulcer
haematemesis	blood in vomitus

HBV, HCV	hepatitis B, C infection
HH	hiatus hernia
HP	helicobacter pylorii
IBS	irritable bowel syndrome
IRA	ileo-rectal anastomosis
KS	Kaposi's sarcoma
lap. chole	laparoscopic cholecystectomy
LFTs	liver function tests
MALToma	lymphoma of Mucosa Associated Lymphoid Tissue
melaena	altered blood passed per rectum
NSAIDs	non-steroidal anti-inflammatory drugs
OGD	oesophago-gastro-duodenoscopy
OGJ	oesophago-gastric junction
PD	pancreaticoduodenectomy
PP	pseudomyxoma peritonei
PR	per rectum
PTC	percutaneous transhepatic cholangiogram
PUD	peptic ulcer disease
Σ or siggy	sigmoidoscopy
SRUS	solitary rectal ulcer syndrome
TART	transanal resection of tumour
UC	ulcerative colitis
ZE syndrome	Zollinger–Ellison syndrome

Breast Specimens

ANC	axillary node clearance
ANS	axillary node sampling
BCS	breast conserving surgery
DCIS	ductal carcinoma in situ
ER	oestrogen receptor
FNAC	fine needle aspiration cytology
LCIS	lobular carcinoma in situ
LVI	lymphovascular invasion
NAC	nipple areolar complex
NCB	needle core biopsy
NPI	Nottingham prognostic index
PM	partial mastectomy
PR	progesterone receptor
TCB	trucut biopsy
TM	total mastectomy
WLE	wide local excision

Head and Neck Specimens

AG	apical granuloma
apic.	apicectomy or apical
B (tooth)	buccal surface

C/-	upper complete denture
-/C	lower complete denture
C/C	upper and lower complete denture
D (tooth)	distal surface
DIGO	drug-induced gingival overgrowth
DIH	denture-induced hyperplasia
FE	fibrous epulis
FEP	fibroepithelial polyp
EC	ethyl chloride
EPT	electric pulp tester
FOM	floor of mouth
GP	gutta percha
K-cyst	keratocyst
L (tooth)	lingual surface
LA	lymphadenopathy
LL (+ numeral)	lower left (tooth designated by numeral)
LN	lymph node
LP	lichen planus
LR	lichenoid reaction
LR (+ numeral)	lower right (tooth designated by numeral)
M (tooth)	mesial surface
MNG	multinodular goitre
MRND	modified radical neck dissection
NG	tumour
O (tooth)	occlusal surface
OKC	keratocyst
P/-	upper partial denture
-/P	lower partial denture
P/P	upper and lower partial dentures
PE (tooth)	partially erupted
PJC	porcelain jacket crown
P(S)A	pleomorphic (salivary) adenoma
Q	quadrant of jaw
RAS/RAU	recurrent aphthous ulceration
RND	radical neck dissection
RRF	retrograde root filling
RCT	root canal treatment
SCC/SCCa	squamous cell carcinoma
SS	Sjögren's syndrome
TTP	tenderness to percussion
UE (tooth)	unerupted
UL (+ numeral)	upper left (tooth designated by numeral)
UR (+ numeral)	upper right (tooth designated by numeral)
WSN	white sponge naevus

Tooth nomenclature:

A	deciduous central incisor
B	deciduous lateral incisor
C	deciduous canine
D	deciduous first molar

E	deciduous second molar
1	permanent central incisor
2	permanent lateral incisor
3	permanent canine
4	permanent first premolar
5	permanent second premolar
6	permanent first molar
7	permanent second molar
8	permanent third molar

Gynaecological Specimens

A = x/52	amenorrhoea = x weeks
AIS	adenocarcinoma in situ
AWE	acetowhite epthelium
(α) AFP	alpha fetoprotein – serum marker of yolk sac tumour
BTB	breakthrough bleeding
CA125	serum/tissue marker of ovarian malignancy
CIN	cervical intraepithelial neoplasia
CGIN	cervical glandular intraepithelial neoplasia
D & C	dilatation and curettage
DUB	dysfunctional uterine bleeding
EDC	expected date of confinement
EIN	endometrial intraepithelial neoplasia
ET	endometrial thickness
EUA	examination under anaesthesia
HCG	human chorionic gonadotrophin – serum/tissue marker of pregnancy or trophoblastic tumour
HPV	human papilloma virus
HRT	hormone replacement therapy
HSV	herpes simplex virus
IMB	intermenstrual bleeding
LMP	last menstrual period
NDMCS	no dyskaryotic or malignant cells seen
PCB	post coital bleeding
PLND	pelvic lymph node dissection
PMB	post menopausal bleeding
POC	products of conception
PV	per vagina
SIL	squamous intraepithelial lesion
TAHBSO	total abdominal hysterectomy with bilateral salpingo-oophorectomy
TBA	therapeutic balloon ablation of the endometrium
TCRE	transcervical resection of endometrium
TVS	transvaginal ultrasound scan
UBT	uterine balloon dilatation therapy
VAIN	vaginal intraepithelial neoplasia
VIN	vulval intraepithelial neoplasia

Urological Specimens

ADPKD	adult polycystic kidney disease
AFP	alpha fetoprotein – tissue/serum marker of germ cell tumour
ALL	acute lymphoblastic leukaemia
AML	angiomyolipoma
ARF	acute renal failure
BCG	intravesical attenuated tubercle Bacille–Calmette–Guerin
BNH	benign nodular hyperplasia
BOO	bladder outlet obstruction
BTTP	British testicular tumour panel
BXO	balanitis xerotica obliterans
CAPD	continuous ambulatory peritoneal dialysis
CIS	carcinoma in situ
CRF	chronic renal failure
CRM	circumferential resection margin
DMSA	dimercaptosuccinic acid – radionucleotide renal function test
DPTA	diaminopropanoltetraacetic acid – radionucleotide renal test
DRE	digital rectal examination
ELUS	endoluminal ultrasound
EM	electron microscopy
FNAC	fine needle aspiration cytology
G1, G2, G3	WHO cytological grade I, II, III (transitional cell carcinoma)
haematuria	blood in the urine
Hb	haemoglobin
HCG	human chorionic gonadotrophin – serum/tissue marker for germ cell tumour
HIFU	high-intensity focussed ultrasound
HPV	human papilloma virus
IF	immunofluorescence
ITGCN	intratubular germ cell neoplasia
IVC	inferior vena cava
IVP	intravenous pyelogram
IVU	intravenous urogram
LDH	lactate dehydrogenase
LM	light microscopy
LUTS	lower urinary tract symptoms
MSSU	mid-stream specimen of urine
MTD	malignant teratoma differentiated
MTI	malignant teratoma intermediate
MTU	malignant teratoma undifferentiated
NSGCT	non-seminomatous germ cell tumour
NSS	nephron-sparing surgery
PA(N)	polyarteritis (nodosa)
PIN	prostatic intraepithelial neoplasia
PLAP	placental alkaline phosphatase – tissue marker of seminoma and carcinoma in situ
pneumaturia	gas in the urine usually from a gut fistula
post BCG	following therapy with intravesical attenuated tubercle (Bacille–Calmette–Guerin).

PSA	prostate specific antigen – tissue/serum marker of prostatic tumour
PU	pass urine
PUJ	pelviureteric junction
RBC	red blood cells
RCC	renal cell carcinoma
RPLND	retroperitoneal lymph node dissection
TCC	transitional cell carcinoma
TRUS	transrectal ultrasound of the prostate
TURB(T)	transurethral resection bladder (tumour)
TURP	transurethral resection prostate
UTI	urinary tract infection
VUR	vesicoureteric reflux
WHO	World Health Organisation
XGP	xanthogranulomatous pyelonephritis

Pelvic and Retroperitoneal Specimens

ACTH	adrenocorticotrophic hormone
MEN	multiple endocrine neoplasia syndrome
RPLND	retroperitoneal lymph node dissection

Skin Specimens

AFX	atypical fibroxanthoma
AK	actinic (solar) keratosis
BCC	basal cell carcinoma
BCE	basal cell epithelioma
BCP	basal cell papilloma (seborrhoeic keratosis)
CMN	congenital melanocytic naevus
C & C	curettage and cautery
CBCL	cutaneous B-cell lymphoma
CTCL	cutaneous T-cell lymphoma
DFSP	dermatofibrosarcoma protuberans
DH	dermatitis herpetiformis
DLE	discoid lupus erythematosus
DMN	dysplastic (atypical) melanocytic naevus
EED	erythema elevatum diutinum
EM	erythema multiforme
EPD	extramammary Paget's disease
GA	granuloma annulare
GVHD	graft-versus-host disease
KA	keratoacanthoma
KP	keratosis pilaris
LE	lupus erythematosus
LM	lentigo maligna
LMM	lentigo maligna melanoma
Ly P	lymphomatoid papulosis
LP	lichen planus

LSC	lichen simplex chronicus
LS et A	lichen sclerosus et atrophicus
MFH	malignant fibrous histiocytoma
MF	mycosis fungoides
MM	malignant melanoma
MPD	mammary Paget's disease
MZL	marginal zone B cell lymphoma
NLD	necrobiosis lipoidica diabeticorum
PLC	pityriasis lichenoides chronica
PLE	polymorphous light eruption
PLEVA	pityriasis lichenoides et varioliformis acuta
PLC	pityriasis lichenoides chronica
PRP	pityriasis rubra pilaris
PRPPP	pruritic urticarial papules and plaques of pregnancy
SALE	subacute lupus erythematosus
SCC	squamous cell carcinoma
Seb K	seborrhoeic keratosis
SSM	superficial spreading melanoma
SLE	systemic lupus erythematosus
TEM	toxic epidermal necrolysis

Cardiothoracic Specimens

ARDS	adult respiratory distress syndrome
BAC	bronchioloalveolar carcinoma
BAL	bronchoalveolar lavage
COPD	chronic obstructive pulmonary disease
CS	Churg–Strauss syndrome
CVA	cerebrovascular accident
FEV_1	forced expiratory volume in one second
FVC	forced vital capacity
haemoptysis	blood in sputum
LVRS	lung volume reduction surgery
MI	myocardial infarction
NSCLC	non-small cell lung cancer
PE	pulmonary embolus
SCLC	small cell lung cancer
SVCO	superior vena cava obstruction
TB	tuberculosis
TOE	transoesophageal echocardiography
TTNA	transthoracic needle aspiration
TTNB	transthoracic needle biopsy
VATS	video-assisted thorascopic surgery
V/Q Scan	ventilation/perfusion scan
WG	Wegener's granulomatosis

Osteoarticular and Soft Tissue Specimens

ABC	Aneurysmal bone cyst
AKA	Above-knee amputation
AS	Ankylosing spondylitis
FD	Fibrous dysplasia
GCT	Giant cell tumour
LCH	Langerhan's cell histiocytosis
MFH	Malignant fibrous histiocytoma
NOF	Neck of femur
OA	Osteoarthritis
PSC	Primary synovial chondromatosis
PVNS	Pigmented villonodular synovitis
RA	Rheumatoid arthritis
THR	Total hip replacement
TKR	Total knee replacement
#	Fracture

Haemopoietic Specimens

AL	acute leukaemia
ALL	acute lymphoblastic leukaemia
AML	acute myeloid leukaemia
ALCL	anaplastic large cell lymphoma
BM(T)	bone marrow trephine
BMTx	bone marrow transplant
BT	bleeding time
CLL	chronic lymphocytic leukaemia
CML	chronic myeloid leukaemia
CT	clotting time
DC	differential count
DLBCL	diffuse large B cell lymphoma
(D)WCC	(differential) white cell count
ESR	erythrocyte sedimentation rate
ET	essential thrombocythemia
FBP/FBC	full blood picture/count
HCL	hairy cell leukaemia
HD	Hodgkin's disease
ITP	idiopathic thrombocytopenic purpura
IVL	intravascular lymphoma
LD(HD)	lymphocyte depleted (Hodgkin's disease)
MC(HD)	mixed cellularity (Hodgkin's disease)
MCTD	mixed connective tissue disorder
MDS	myelodysplastic syndrome
MF	mycosis fungoides
MM	multiple myeloma
NHL	non-Hodgkin's lymphoma
NLPHL	nodular lymphocyte predominant Hodgkin's lymphoma

NS(HD)	nodular sclerosis (Hodgkin's disease)
PRV	polycythaemia rubra vera
PT	prothrombin time
RA	rheumatoid arthritis
SLE	systemic lupus erythematosus
TCRBCL	T-cell-rich B-cell lymphoma
TT	thrombin time
WCC	white cell count

Bibliography

General

Allen DC. Histopathology reporting. Guidelines for surgical cancer. London: Springer-Verlag, 2000

Domizio P, Lowe D. Reporting histopathology sections. London: Chapman and Hall, 1997

Fletcher CDM (ed). Diagnostic histopathology of tumours. 2nd edn. London: Churchill Livingstone, 2000

Hermanek P, Hutter RVP, Sobin LH, Wagner G, Wittekind C (eds). TNM atlas: illustrated guide to the TNM/pTNM classification of malignant tumours. UICC. 4th edn. Berlin, Heidelberg, New York: Springer, 1997

Hruban RH, Westra WH, Phelps TH, Isacson C. Surgical pathology dissection. An illustrated guide. New York: Springer, 1996

Lester SC. Manual of surgical pathology. New York: Churchill Livingstone, 2001

McKee PH, Chinyama CN, Whimster WF, Bogomoletz WV, Delides GS, de Wolf CJM (eds). Comprehensive Tumour Technology Handbook. UICC. New York: Wiley-Liss, 2001

Rosai J. Ackerman's Surgical Pathology. 8th edn. St Louis: Mosby, 1996

Silverberg SG (ed). Principles and practice of surgical pathology. 2nd edn. New York: Churchill Livingstone, 1990

Sobin LH, Wittekind Ch (eds). TNM classification of malignant tumours. 6th edn. New York: Wiley-Liss, 2002

Spence RAJ, Johnston PG (eds). Oncology. Oxford: Oxford University Press, 2001

The Royal College of Pathologists Working Party Report: Draft guidelines for the involvement of biomedical scientists in the dissection of specimens and selection of tissues. London: Royal College of Pathologists, 2001

Vollmer RT. Pathologists' assistants in surgical pathology. The truth is out. Am J Clin Pathol 1999; 112:597–598

Gastrointestinal Specimens

Albores-Saavedra J, Henson DE, Klimstra DS. Tumors of the gall bladder, extrahepatic bile ducts and ampulla of vater. Atlas of tumor pathology. 3rd series. Fascicle 27. Washington: AFIP, 2000

Bateman AC. How to handle and report pancreatic specimens. CPD Cellular Pathology 2001; 3:94–98

Beckingham IJ (ed). ABC of liver, pancreas and gall bladder diseases. London: BMJ Books, 2001

Biddlestone LR, Bailey TA, Whittles CE, Shepherd NA. The clinical and molecular pathology of Barrett's oesophagus. In: Kirkham N, Lemoine NR (eds). Progress in pathology 5. London: Medical Media Limited. 2001;57–80

Birbeck KF, Quirke P. Reporting protocols in colorectal cancer. CPD Bulletin Cellular Pathology 1999;1:58–64

Burnand KG, Young AE (eds). The new Aird's companion in surgical studies. London: Churchill Livingstone, 1992

Burroughs SH, Williams GT. Examination of large intestine resection specimens. J Clin Pathol 2000;50:344–349

Carter D, Russell RCG, Pitt HA, Bismuth H (eds). Rob and Smith's operative surgery: hepatobiliary and pancreatic surgery. 5th edition. London: Chapman and Hall, 1996

Cotton P, Williams C. Practical gastrointestinal endoscopy. 4th edition. London: Blackwell Science, 1996

Day DW, Dixon MF. Biopsy pathology of the oesophagus, stomach and duodenum 2nd edn. London: Chapman and Hall Medical, 1995

Dudley H, Pories W, Carter D (eds). Rob and Smith's operative surgery: alimentary tract and abdominal wall. 4th edition. London: Butterworths, 1993

Fenoglio-Preiser CM, Noffsinger AE, Stemmermann GN, Lantz PE, Listrom MB, Rilke FO. Gastrointestinal pathology. An atlas and text. 2nd edn. Philadelphia: Lippincott, Williams and Wilkins, 1999

Fielding LP, Goldberg SM (eds). Rob and Smith's operative surgery: surgery of the colon, rectum and anus. 5th edition. London: Butterworth-Heinemann, 1993

Goldman H. Gastrointestinal mucosal biopsy. New York: Churchill Livingstone, 1996

Haggitt RC, Glotzbach RE, Soffer EE, Wruble LD. Prognostic factors in colorectal carcinomas arising in adenomas: implications for lesions removed by endoscopic polypectomy. Gastroenterology 1985;89:328–336

Ibrahim NBN. Guidelines for handling oesophageal biopsies and resection specimens and their reporting. J Clin Pathol 2000;53:89–94

Ishak KG, Goodman ZD, Stocker JT. Tumors of the liver and intrahepatic bile ducts. Atlas of tumor pathology. 3rd series. Fascicle 31. Washington: AFIP, 2001

Jones DJ (ed). ABC of colorectal diseases. 2nd edition. London: BMJ Books, 1999

Lewin KJ, Appelman HD. Tumors of the esophagus and stomach. Atlas of tumor pathology. 3rd series. Fascicle 18. Washington: AFIP, 1996

Logan RPH, Harris A, Misciewicz JJ, Baron JH (eds). ABC of the upper gastrointestinal tract. London: BMJ Books, 2002

MacSween RNM, Burt AD, Portmann BC, Ishak KG, Scheuer PJ, Anthony PP (eds). Pathology of the liver. 4th edn. London: Churchill Livingstone, 2002

Mann CV, Russell RCG, Williams NS (eds). Bailey & Love's short practice of surgery. 22nd edition. London: Chapman and Hall Medical, 1995

Quirke P. The pathologist, the surgeon and colorectal cancer: get it right because it matters. In: Kirkham N, Lemoine NR (eds). Progress in pathology 4. Edinburgh: Churchill Livingstone, 1998:201–213

Scheuer PJ, Lefkowitch JH. Liver biopsy interpretation. 6th edn. London: WB Saunders, 2000

Schlemper RJ, Riddell RH, Kato Y et al. The Vienna classification of gastrointestinal epithelial neoplasia. Gut 2000;47:251–255

Shepherd NA. Pathological mimics of chronic inflammatory bowel disease. J Clin Pathol 1991;44:726–733

Snell RS. Clinical anatomy for medical students. 3rd edition. Boston: Little, Brown and Company, 1986

Solcia E, Capella C, Klöppel G. Tumors of the pancreas. Atlas of tumor pathology. 3rd series. Fascicle 20. Washington: AFIP, 1997

Standards and minimum datasets for reporting common cancers. Minimum dataset for colorectal cancer histopathology reports. London: The Royal College of Pathologists, 1998

Standards and minimum datasets for reporting common cancers. Minimum dataset for oesophageal carcinoma histopathology reports. London: The Royal College of Pathologists, 1998

Standards and minimum datasets for reporting common cancers. Minimum dataset for gastric cancer histopathology reports. London: The Royal College of Pathologists, 2000

Standards and minimum datasets for reporting common cancers. Minimum dataset for the histopathological reporting of pancreatic, ampulla of vater and bile duct carcinoma. London: The Royal College of Pathologists, 2002

Breast Specimens

Dixon M. ABC of breast diseases. 2nd edn. London: BMJ books, 2000

Elston CW, Ellis IO (eds). The breast. Systemic pathology. 3rd edn. Vol 13. Edinburgh: Churchill Livingstone, 1998

Fitzgibbons PL, Page DL, Weaver D et al. Prognostic factors in breast cancer. College of American Pathologists consensus statement 1999. Arch Pathol Lab Med 2000;124:966–978

Guidelines for non-operative diagnostic procedures and reporting in breast cancer screening. Non-operative diagnosis subgroup of the National Coordinating Group for breast screening pathology. NHSBSP publication no. 50. June 2001

Rosen's Breast Pathology. 2nd edn. Philadelphia. Lippincott, Williams and Wilkins, 2001

Sainsbury JRC, Anderson TJ, Morgan DAL. ABC of breast diseases. Breast cancer. BMJ 2000; 321:745–750

Shousha S. Reporting breast biopsies. Current Diagnostic Pathology 2000;6:140–145

Standards and minimum datasets for reporting common cancers. Minimum dataset for breast cancer histopathology reports. London: The Royal College of Pathologists. 1998

Van Diest PJ. Histopathological workup of sentinel lymph nodes: how much is enough? J Clin Pathol 1999;52:871–873

Head and Neck Specimens

British Association of Otorhinolaryngologists – Head and Neck Surgeons. Effective head and neck cancer management. Second Consensus Document. London: Royal College of Surgeons, 2000

Gnepp DR (ed). Diagnostic surgical pathology of the head and neck. Philadelphia: WB Saunders, 2001

Gnepp DR, Barnes L, Crissman J, Zarbo R. Recommendations for the reporting of larynx specimens containing laryngeal neoplasms. Am J Clin Pathol 1998;110:137–139

Helliwell TR, Woolgar JA. Minimum dataset for head and neck carcinoma histopathology reports. London: Royal College of Pathologists, 1998

Shah JP. Head and neck surgery. 2nd edn. London: Mosby-Wolfe, 1996

Sneed DC. Protocol for the examination of specimens from patients with malignant tumors of the thyroid gland, exclusive of lymphomas. Arch Pathol Lab Med 1999;123:45–49

Eye, Muscle and Nerve Specimens

Eye

Barcroft JD. Histochemical Technique. London: Butterworths, 1967

Lee WR. Ophthalmic Histopathology. London: Springer-Verlag, 1993

Lucus DR. Greer's Ocular Pathology. Oxford: Blackwell Scientific, 1989

Muscle

Croker BP, Bossen EH, Brinn NT, Hammon FA. A fixative for use in muscle histochemistry. J Histochem Cytochem 1983;31:110

Dubowitz V, Brooke MH. Muscle Biopsy. London: WB Saunders, 1973

Nerve

Jennekins FGI, Tonkinson BE, Walton JN. Histochemical aspects of five limb muscles in old age; an autopsy study. J Neurol Sci 1971;14:259

Lascelles RG, Thomas PK. Changes due to age in internodal length in the sural nerve in man. J Neurol Neurosurg Psychiat 1966;29:40

Ochoa J, Mair WGP. The normal sural nerve in man. Part 2 (Changes in axons and Schwann cells due to ageing). Acta Neuropath 1969;13:217

Gynaecological Specimens

Histopathology reporting in cervical screening. NHSCSP Publication, No 10; April 1999

Kurman RJ, Norris HJ, Wilkinson E. Tumors of the cervix, vagina and vulva. In: Atlas of tumor pathology. 3rd series. Fascicle 4. Washington DC: AFIP, 1992

Kurman RJ, Amin MB. Protocol for the examination of specimens from patients with carcinoma of the cervix. Arch Pathol Lab Med 1999;123:55–66

Lage JM. Protocol for the examination of specimens from patients with gestational trophoblastic malignancies. Arch Pathol Lab Med 1999;123:50–54

Robboy SJ, Anderson MC, Russell PR. Pathology of the female reproductive tract. London: Churchill Livingstone, 2002

Scully RE. Protocol for the examination of specimens from patients with carcinoma of the vagina. Arch Pathol Lab Med 1999;123:62–67

Scully RE, Bonfiglio TA, Kurman RJ, Silverberg SG, Wilkinson EJ. International histological classification and typing of female genital tract tumors. New York: Springer-Verlag, 1994

Scully RE, Young RH, Clement PB. Tumors of the ovary, maldeveloped gonads, fallopian tube and broad ligament. In: Atlas of tumour pathology. 3rd series. Fascicle 23, Washington DC: AFIP, 1998

Scurry J, Patel K, Wells M. Gross examination of uterine specimens. J Clin Pathol 1993;46:388–393

Silverberg SG, Kurman RJ. Tumors of the uterine corpus and gestational trophoblastic disease. In: Atlas of tumor pathology. 3rd series. Fascicle 3. Washington DC: AFIP, 1992

Silverberg SG. Protocol for the examination of specimens from patients with carcinomas of the endometrium. Arch Pathol Lab Med 1999;123:28–32

Staging Announcement: FIGO staging of gynecological cancers; cervical and vulval. International Journal of Gynecological Cancer 1995;5:319 (see erratum – International Journal of Gynecological Cancer 1995;5:465)

The Royal College of Pathologists. Minimum dataset for the histopathological reporting of atypical hyperplasia and adenocarcinoma in endometrial biopsy and curettage specimens and for endometrial cancer in hysterectomy specimens. March 2001

The Royal College of Pathologists. Minimum dataset for the histopathological reporting of cervical neoplasia. March 2001

The Royal College of Pathologists. Minimum dataset for the histopathological reporting of vulval biopsy specimens and vulvectomy specimens for vulval cancer. March 2001

Urological Specimens

Bostwick DG, Dundore PA. Biopsy Pathology of the Prostate. London: Chapman and Hall Medical, 1997

Bostwick DG, Eble JN. Urologic Surgical Pathology. St Louis: Mosby, 1997

Campbell MF, Walsh PC, Retik AB. Campbell's Urology. 8th edn. Philadelphia: W B Saunders, 2002

Fleming ID, Cooper JS, Henson DE, et al (eds). AJCC Manual for Staging of Cancer. 5th edn. Philadelphia: Lippincott-Raven, 1997

Fuhrman SA, Lasky LC, Limas C. Prognostic significance of morphologic parameters in renal cell carcinoma. Am J Surg Pathol 1982;6:655–663

Kovacs G, Akhtar M et al. The Heidelberg Classification of Renal Cell Tumours. J Pathol 1997;183:131–133

Lawrence WD, Young RH, Scully RE. Sex cord – stromal tumors. In: Talerman A, Roth LM (eds). Pathology of the Testis and its Adnexa. New York: Churchill Livingstone, 1986, pp 67–92

Mostofi FK, Sesterhenn IA, Sobin LH. Histological typing of testis tumours. 2nd edn. Berlin: Springer-Verlag, 1998

Murphy WM, Beckwith JB, Farrow GM. Tumors of the adult kidney. In: Tumors of the Kidney, Bladder and Related Structures. Atlas of Tumor Pathology. 3rd series. Fascicle 11. Washington, D C: Armed Forces Institute of Pathology, 1994, pp 98–124

Sternberg SS. Histology for Pathologists. 2nd edn. Philadelphia: Lippincott-Raven, 1997

Tanagho EA, McAninch JW. Smith's General Urology. 15th edn. New York: McGraw-Hill, 2000

Ulbright TM, Roth LM. Testicular and paratesticular neoplasms. In: Sternberg SS (ed). Diagnostic Surgical Pathology. 2nd edn. New York: Raven Press, 1994, pp 1885–1947

Young RH, Talerman A. Testicular tumours other than germ cell tumours. Semin Diagn Pathol 1987;4:342–360

Pelvis and Retroperitoneum Specimens

Cullen MH, Stenning SP, Parkinson MC, Fossa SD, Kaye SB, Horwich AH et al. Short-course adjuvant chemotherapy in high-risk stage I nonseminomatous germ cell tumors of the testis: a Medical Research Council report. J Clin Oncol 1996;14:1106–1113

Hruban RH, Westra WH, Phelps TH, Isacson C: Surgical Pathology Dissection: an illustrated guide. New York: Springer Verlag, 1996

Lester SC. Chapter 10: Adrenal Glands. In: Manual of Surgical Pathology. Philadelphia: Churchill Livingstone, 2001, pp 103–107

Parkinson MC, Harland SJ, Harnden P, Sandison A. The role of the histopathologist in the management of testicular germ cell tumour in adults. Histopathology 2001;38:183–194

Rodrigues-Bigas MA, Petrelli NJ. Pelvic exenteration and its modifications. Am J Surg 1996; 171:293–298

Rosai J. Chapter 26: Peritoneum, Retroperitoneum and Related Structures. In: Rosai J. Ackerman's Surgical Pathology, 8th ed. St Louis: Mosby, 1996

Stenning SP, Parkinson MC, Fisher C, Mead GM, Cook PA, Fossa SD et al. Post-chemotherapy residual masses in germ cell tumor patients: content, clinical features, and prognosis. Medical Research Council Testicular Tumour Working Party. Cancer 1998;83:1409–1419

Temple WJ, Saettler EB. Locally recurrent rectal cancer: role of composite resection of extensive pelvic tumors with strategies for minimizing risk of recurrence. J Surg Oncol 2000;73:47–58

Skin Specimens

Balch CM, Buzaid AC, Soong SJ, Atkins MB, Cascinelli N, Coit DG, Fleming ID, Gershenwald JE, Houghton A Jr, Kirkwood JM, McMasters KM, Mihn MF, Morton DL, Reintgen DS, Ross MI, Sober A, Thompson JA, Thompson JF. Final version of the American Joint Committee on cancer staging system for cutaneous melanoma. J Clin Oncol 2001;19(16):3635–3648

McKee PH. Pathology of the skin with clinical correlations. 2nd edition. London: Mosby-Wolfe, 1996

Motley R, Kersey P, Lawrence C. Multiprofessional guidelines for the management of the patient with primary cutaneous squamous cell carcinoma. Br J Dermatol 2002;146(1):18–25

Roberts DL, Anstey AV, Barlow RJ, Cox NH, Newton Bishop JA, Corrie PG, Evans J, Gore ME, Hall PN, Kirkham N. UK guidelines for the management of cutaneous melanoma. Br J Dermatol 2002;146(1):7–17

Shriner DL, McCoy DK, Goldberg DJ, Wagner RF Jr. Mohs' micrographic surgery. J Am Acad Dermatol 1998;39(1):79–97

Sober AJ, Chuang Tsu-Yi, Duvic M, Farmer ER, Grichnick JM, Halpern AC, Ho V, Holloway V, Hood AF, Johnson TM, Lowery BJ. Guidelines of care for primary cutaneous melanoma. J Am Acad Dermatol 2001;45(4):579–586

Telfer NR, Colver GB, Bowers PW. Guidelines for the management of basal cell carcinoma. Br J Dermatol 1999;14(3):415–423

The Royal College of Pathologists. Minimum dataset for the histopathological reporting of common skin cancers. Standards and minimum datasets for the histopathological reporting of common skin cancers. February 2002

Weedon D. Skin pathology. 2nd edition. London: Churchill Livingstone, 2002

Cardiothoracic Specimens and Vessels

Association of Directors of Anatomic and Surgical Pathology. Recommendations for the reporting of resected primary lung carcinoma. Hum Pathol 1995;26:937–939

Baumgartner WA, Reitz B, Kasper E, Theodore J. Heart and lung transplantation. 2nd edn. Saunders: London, 2001

Billingham M, Carey N, Stewart S, Goddard M. Atlas of biopsy histopathology for heart and lung transplantation. 1st edn. Arnold: London, 2000

Billingham ME, Cary NRB, Hammond ME et al. A working formulation for the standardisation of nomen-
    clature in the diagnosis of cardiac and lung rejection: heart rejection study group.
    J Heart Transplant 1990;9:587–593
Casson AG, Johnston MR. Key topics in thoracic surgery. 1st edn. Oxford, Washington DC: Bios Scientific
    Publishers, 1999
Corrin B. Pathology of the lungs. 1st edn. London: Churchill Livingstone, 2000
Fishman AP, Elias JA, Fishman JA, Grippi MA, Kaiser LR, Senior RM. Fishman's manual of pulmonary
    diseases and disorders. 3rd edn. New York: McGraw-Hill, 2002
Forbes CD, Jackson WF. Atlas and text of clinical medicine. 2nd edn. London: Mosby-Wolfe, 1997
Hall-Craggs ECB. Anatomy as a basis for clinical medicine. 3rd edn. London: Williams and Wilkins,
    1995
Muller-Hermelink HK, Marx A, Kircher Th. Advances in the diagnosis and classification of thymic epithe-
    lial tumours. In: Anthony PP, MacSween RNM (eds). Recent advances in histopathology 16. Edinburgh:
    Churchill Livingstone, 1994, pp 49–72
Nash G, Otis CN. Protocol for the examination of specimens from patients with malignant pleural mesothe-
    lioma. Arch Pathol Lab Med 1999;123:39–44
Standards and minimum datasets for reporting common cancers. Minimum dataset for lung cancer
    histopathology reports. The Royal College of Pathologists: London, 1998
Travis WD, Colby TV, Corrin B, Shimosata Y, Brambilla E. Histological typing of lung and pleural tumours.
    3rd edn. WHO: International histological classification of tumours. Berlin: Springer, 1999
West JB. Pulmonary pathophysiology – the essentials. 5th edn. Baltimore: Williams & Wilkins, 1995
Yousen SA, Berry GJ, Cagle PT et al. A revision of the 1990 working formulations for the classification of
    lung allograft rejection. J Heart Lung Transplant 1996;15:1–15

Osteoarticular and Soft Tissue Specimens

Akerman M, Domanski HA. Fine needle aspiration (FNA) of bone tumours: with special emphasis on defi-
    nite treatment of primary malignant bone tumours based on FNA. Current Diagnostic Pathology
    1998;5:82–92
Athanasou NA. Colour Atlas of Bone, Joint and Soft Tissue Pathology. Oxford: Oxford University Press, 1999
Bullough PG. Orthopaedic Pathology. 4th edn. St Louis: Mosby Wolfe, 1998
DAKO. Immunohistochemistry in the Diagnosis of Soft Tissue Sarcomas. Glostrup: DAKO, 1999
Dorfman HD, Czerniak B. Bone Tumours. St Louis: Mosby-Wolfe, 1998
Enzinger FM, Weiss SW. Soft Tissue Tumors. 4th edn. St Louis: Mosby-Wolfe, 2000
Fechner RE, Mills SE. Tumors of the Bones and Joints. 3rd series: Fascicle 8. Washington DC: Armed Forces
    Institute of Pathology, 1993
Kempson RL, Fletcher CDM, Evans HL, Hendrickson MR, Sibley RK. Tumors of the Soft Tissues. 3rd series:
    Fascicle 30. Washington DC: Armed Forces Institute of Pathology, 2001
McCarthy EF, Frassica FJ. Pathology of Bone and Joint Disorders. Philadelphia: Saunders, 1998
Pringle JAS. Osteosarcoma: the experiences of a specialist unit. Current Diagnostic Pathology 1996;3:127–136
Rydholm A. Chromosomal aberrations in musculoskeletal tumours: clinical importance. J Bone Joint Surg
    1996;78B:501–504
Soderlund V, Tani E, Domanski HA, Kreicbergs A. Representativeness of radiologically guided fine needle
    aspiration biopsy of bone lesions. Sarcoma 2002;6:61–68
Unni KK. Dahlin's Bone Tumours. 5th edn. Philadelphia: Lippincott-Raven, 1996
Wold LE. Practical approach to processing osteosarcomas in the surgical pathology laboratory. Paediatric
    and Devolopmental Pathology 1998;1:449–454

Haematopoietic Specimens

Braunwald E, Fauci AS, Kasper DL, Hauser SL, Longo DL, Jameson JL (eds). Harrison's Principles of Internal
    Medicine. 15th edn. Volume 1. USA: McGraw-Hill, 2001, pp 348–74

Adamson JW, Longo DL. Anaemia and polycythemia. In: Harrison's Principles of Internal Medicine. 15th edn. Volume 1. USA: McGraw-Hill, 2001

Handin RI. Bleeding and thrombosis. In: Harrison's Principles of Internal Medicine. 15th edn. Volume 1. USA: McGraw-Hill, 2001

Henry PH, Longo DL. Enlargement of the lymph nodes and spleen. In: Harrison's Principles of Internal Medicine. 15th edn. Volume 1. USA: McGraw-Hill, 2001

Holland SM, Gallin JI. Disorders of granulocytes and monocytes. In: Harrison's Principles of Internal Medicine. 15th edn. Volume 1. USA: McGraw-Hill, 2001

Brunning RD. Bone marrow. In Rosai J (ed). Ackerman's surgical pathology. 8th edn. Volume 2. New York: Mosby, 1996, pp 1797–1915

Chan JKC. Tumours of the lymphoreticular system, including spleen and thymus. In Fletcher CDM (ed) Diagnostic Histopathology of Tumours 2nd edn. Volume 2. London: Harcourt. 2000, pp 1099–1245

Gatter K. Brown D. An illustrated guide to bone marrow diagnosis. Oxford: Blackwell Science, 1997, pp 153–157

Hall JG. The functional anatomy of lymph nodes. In Stansfield AG, d' Ardenne AJ (eds). Lymph node biopsy interpretation, 2nd edn. Edinburgh: Churchill Livingstone, 1992, pp 3–28

Jaffe ES, Harris NL, Stein H, Vardiman JW. (eds). World Health Organization Classification of Tumours. Pathology and Genetics. Tumours of Haematopoietic and Lymphoid tissues. Lyon: IARC Press, 2001, pp 119–253

Rosai J. Lymph nodes, spleen. In Rosai J (ed). Ackerman's surgical pathology. Volume 2. 8th edn. New York: Mosby, 1996, pp 1661–1796

Wilkins BS, Wright DH. Illustrated pathology of the spleen. Cambridge: Cambridge University Press, 2000, pp 1–31.

Miscellaneous

Barnes DM, Millis RR. Oestrogen receptors: the history, the relevance and the methods of evaluation. In: Kirkham N, Lemoine NR (eds). Progress in Pathology, Vol. 2. Edinburgh: Churchill Livingstone, 1995, pp 89–114

Bostwick DG, Dundore PA. Biopsy Pathology of the Prostate. London: Chapman & Hall, 1997

De Kerviler E, Guermazi A, Zagdanski AM et al. Image-guided core-needle biopsy in patients with suspected or recurrent lymphoma. Cancer 2000;89:647–652

Dodson A. Modern methods for diagnostic immunocytochemistry. Current Diagnostic Pathology 2002;8:113–122

Domizio P, Lowe D. Frozen Sections. In: Domizio P, Lowe D (eds). Reporting Histological Sections. London: Chapman and Hall, 1997, pp 396–404

Ellis IO, Dowsett M, Bartlett J, Walker R, Cooke T, Gullick W, Gusterson B, Mallon E, Barrett Lee P. Recommendations for HER2 testing in the UK. J Clin Path 2000;53:890–892

Heim S, Mitelman F. Cytogenetics of Solid Tumours. In: Anthony PP, Mac Sween RNM (eds). Recent Advances in Histopathology 15. Edinburgh: Churchill Livingstone, 1992, pp 37–66

Herrington CS. Demystified . . . In situ-hybridisation. Mol Pathol 1998;51:8–13

Human tissue and biological samples for use in research: operational and ethical guidelines. Medical Research Council. London, 2001. http://www.mrc.ac.uk/pdf-tissue_guide_fin.pdf

Jaffe ES, Harris NL, Stein H, Vardiman JW. WHO Classification of Tumours Pathology and Genetics. Tumours of Haematopoietic and Lymphoid Tissues. Lyon: IARC Press, 2001

Jasani B, Rhodes A. The role and mechanism of high-temperature antigen retrieval in diagnostic pathology. Current Diagnostic Pathology 2001;7:153–160

Lester SC. Chapter 6: Operating Room Consultations, In: Manual of Surgical Pathology. Philadelphia: Churchill Livingstone, 2001, pp 35–52

Matthews TJ, Denney PA. Digital Imaging of Specimens using a wet scanning technique. J Clin Pathol 2001;54:326–327

McKay B. Electron microscopy in tumour diagnosis. In: Fletcher CDM (ed) Diagnostic Histopathology of Tumours. Volume 2, 2nd edn. London: Churchill Livingstone, 2000, pp 1785–1823

McManus DT, Anderson NH. Fine Needle Aspiration Cytology of the breast. Current Diagnostic Pathology 2001;7:262–271

Micklem K, Sanderson J. Digital Imaging in Pathology. Current Diagnostic Pathology 2001; 7:131–140

Mount SL, Cooper K. Beware of biotin: a source of false positive immunohistochemistry. Current Diagnostic Pathology 2001;7:161–167

Nocito A, Kononen J, Kallioniemi OP, Sauter G. Tissue microarrays for high-throughput molecular pathology research. Int J Cancer 2001;94:1–5

Pecciarini L, Giulia Cangi M, Doglioni C. Identifying the primary sites of metastatic carcinoma: the increasing role of immunohistochemistry. Current Diagnostic Pathology 2001;7:168–175

Perou CM, Sorlie T, Eisen MB et al. Molecular portraits of human breast tumours. Nature 2000;406:747–752

Shipp MA, Ross KN, Tamayo P et al. Diffuse large B-cell lymphoma outcome prediction by gene-expression profiling and supervised machine learning. Nature Medicine 2002;8:68–74

Rosai J. Chapter 2: Gross techniques in surgical pathology. In: Rosai J (ed) Ackerman's Surgical Pathology, 8th ed. St Louis: Mosby, 1996, pp 21–22

Russell GA. Specimen Photography. *ACP News* 1994; Autumn Issue:19–22

Symposium " Minimally Invasive Techniques and Pathology". Royal College of Pathologists. Spring, 2002

Transitional guidelines to facilitate changes in procedures for handling "surplus" and archival material from human biological samples. Royal College of Pathologists. June, 2001

Van Dam P, Tjalma WAA. Clinical Applications of Flow Cytometry. In: Lowe DG, Underwood JCE (eds). Recent Advances in Histopathology 18. London: Churchill Livingstone, 1999, pp 131–146

Index

Punch excision, 378, 380
Pupil of eye, 221
Pyelonephritis, 288
Pyogenic abscess, 115
Pyogenic epididymo-orchitis, 333
Pyonephrosis, 289
Pyosalpinx, 245

R

Radiation therapy, 72
Radical maxillectomy, 170
Radiography, 480
Rectal mucosa in prolapse, 80
Rectal stump, 80
Redcurrant jelly stool, 52
Reflux oesophagitis, 6, 15–16
Reidel's thyroiditis, 200
Reinke's oedema, 178
Reinke's space, 175
Renal cysts, 289
Renal stones, 288
Respiratory bronchiolitis-associated interstitial
    lung disease, 397
Restorative proctocolectomy, 79
Restrictive cardiomyopathy, 423
Rete testis, 331, 337
    see also Testis
Retina, 221
Retinoblastoma, 228, 229
Retroperitoneum, 359–64
    anatomy, 359, 360
    biopsy, 361, 362
    clinical investigations, 360
    clinical presentation, 359
    pathological conditions, 360–1
    resection specimens, 361–4
Rhabdomyoma, 424
Rheumatic fever, 423
Rheumatoid arthritis, 438
Rheumatoid nodules, 446
Rhinorrhoea, 145
Right hemicolectomy, 90
Right ventricular dysplasia, 423
Rim resection, 170, 171
Rivinus ducts, 188

S

S100, 450
Salivary duct obstruction, 190
Salivary gland-type adenocarcinoma, 147
Salivary glands, 188–97
    anatomy, 188–9
    biopsy, 192–3, 193–4
    clinical investigations, 190

clinical presentation, 189
lymphovascular drainage, 189
neoplasia, 191–2, 398
pathological conditions, 190–2
resection specimens, 193, 194–6
Sarcoidosis, 397
Sarcomatoid carcinoma, 291
Scanning electron microscopy, 386
Schistosomiasis, 71
Schlemm's canal, 221, 224
Sclera, 221
Sclerosing haemangioma, 397
Seminoma, 334
Sentinel node biopsy, 134, 390
Sertoli cell tumour, 336
Serum tumour markers, 332–3
Sex cord-stromal tumours, 335
Sexually transmitted diseases, 344
Shave biopsy, 378, 379
Sigmoid notch, 164
Sigmoidoscopy, 74
Siliconoma, 130–1
Silicosis, 396
Singer's node, 178
Sinonasal adenocarcinoma, 147
Sinonasal cancer, 146
Sinusitis, 145–6
Sinusoids, 107
Sister Mary Joseph's nodule, 120
Sjögren's syndrome, 191, 193
Skin, 375–90
    anatomy, 375
    appendages, 95, 97, 375, 378
    biopsy, 378–82
    clinical investigations, 376
    clinical presentation, 375–6
    dermis, 375
    electron microscopy, 386
    epidermis, 375
    lymphovascular drainage, 375
    pathological conditions, 376–8
    special techniques, 382–9
Skin grafts, 385
Skin rashes, 375–6
Skin scrapings, 386
Small intestine, 51–64
    anatomy, 51–2
    biopsy, 56, 58
    clinical investigations, 52–3
    clinical presentation, 52
    intussusception, 57, 63
    ischaemia, 59, 61
    lymphovascular supply, 52
    neoplasia, 55–6
    obstructive enteropathy, 59